Hormonal Carcinogenesis III

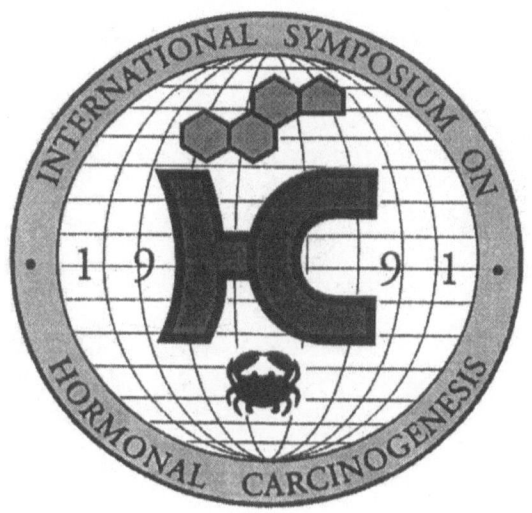

Springer

New York
Berlin
Heidelberg
Barcelona
Hong Kong
London
Milan
Paris
Singapore
Tokyo

Jonathan J. Li, Ph.D.

Professor of Pharmacology, Toxicology, and Therapeutics
Director, Division of Etiology and Prevention of Hormonal Cancers
Hormonal Carcinogenesis Laboratory, University of Kansas Cancer Center

Sara Antonia Li, Ph.D.

Associate Professor of Pharmacology, Toxicology, and Therapeutics
Division of Etiology and Prevention of Hormonal Cancers
Hormonal Carcinogenesis Laboratory, University of Kansas Cancer Center

Janet R. Daling, Ph.D.

Division of Public Health Sciences
Fred Hutchinson Cancer Research Center
University of Washington
Editors

Hormonal Carcinogenesis III

Proceedings of the
Third International Symposium

With 147 Illustrations

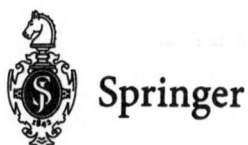 Springer

Jonathan J. Li, Ph.D.
Professor of Pharmacology,
  Toxicology, and Therapeutics
Director, Division of Etiology &
  Prevention of Hormonal Cancers
Kansas Cancer Institute
University of Kansas Medical Center
Kansas City, Kansas 66160
USA

Sara Antonia Li, Ph.D.
Associate Professor of Pharmacology,
  Toxicology, and Therapeutics
Division of Etiology &
  Prevention of Hormonal Cancers
Kansas Cancer Institute
University of Kansas Medical Center
Kansas City, Kansas 66160
USA

Janet R. Daling, Ph.D
Division of Public Health Sciences
Fred Hutchinson Cancer Research Center
University of Washington
Seattle, Washington 98101
USA

Library of Congress Cataloging-in-Publication Data
Hormonal carcinogenesis III : proceedings of the third international symposium / editors,
Jonathan J. Li, Sara Antonia Li, Janet R. Daling.
      p. ; cm.
    Includes bibliographical references and index.
    ISBN-13:978-1-4612-7411-7   e-ISBN-13:978-1-4612-2092-3
    DOI: 10.1007/978-1-4612-2092-3

     1. Generative organs—Cancer—Congresses.   2. Breast—Cancer—Etiology—Congresses.
  3. Hormones, Sex—Carcinogenicity—Congresses.   4. Cancer—Endocrine
  aspects—Congresses.   I. Title: Hormonal carcinogenesis 3.   II. Title: Hormonal
  carcinogenesis three.   III. Li, Jonathan J.   IV. Li, Sara Antonia.   V. Daling, Janet R.   VI.
  International Symposium on Hormonal Carcinogenesis (3rd : 1998 : Seattle, Wash.)
      [DNLM: 1. Neoplasms, Hormone-Dependent—Congresses.   2. Breast
  Neoplasms—etiology—Congresses.   3. Neoplastic Processes—Congresses.   4. Prostate
  Neoplasms—etiology—Congresses.   5. Receptors, Cell Surface—physiology—Congresses.
  6. Sex Hormones—adverse effects—Congresses. QZ 200 H8113 2001]
  RC280.G4 H67 2001
  616.99'4071—dc21   00-058849

Printed on acid-free paper.

© 2001 Springer-Verlag New York, Inc.
Softcover reprint of the hardcover 1st edition 2001

Production managed by Allan Abrams; manufacturing supervised by Jerome Basma.
Camera-ready copy supplied by the editors.

9 8 7 6 5 4 3 2 1

ISBN-13:978-1-4612-7411-7   SPIN 10778265

Springer-Verlag   New York Berlin Heidelberg
A member of BertelsmannSpringer Science+Business Media GmbH

The real voyage of discovery consists not in seeking new landscapes but in having new eyes.

−Marcel Proust

Christopher and Stephanie
− Jonathan J. Li
− Sara Antonia Li

Lane
− Janet R. Daling

Acknowledgments

Patrons

Fred Hutchinson Cancer Research Center
National Cancer Institute
Division of Cancer Biology
Division of Cancer Control & Population Sciences
Wyeth-Ayerst Research
National Institute of Environmental Health Sciences
National Institute of Environmental Health Sciences -
International Programs

Sponsors

National Institute of Child Health & Human Development
Office of Research on Women's Health
Hoechst Marion Roussel
Seattle Breast Cancer Research Program

Contributors

Alza Corporation
National Institute of Diabetes & Digestive & Kidney Diseases
Nitta Gelatin Inc.
The Council for Tobacco Research
Amgen
DAKO

Participants of the Third International Hormonal Carcinogenesis Symposium

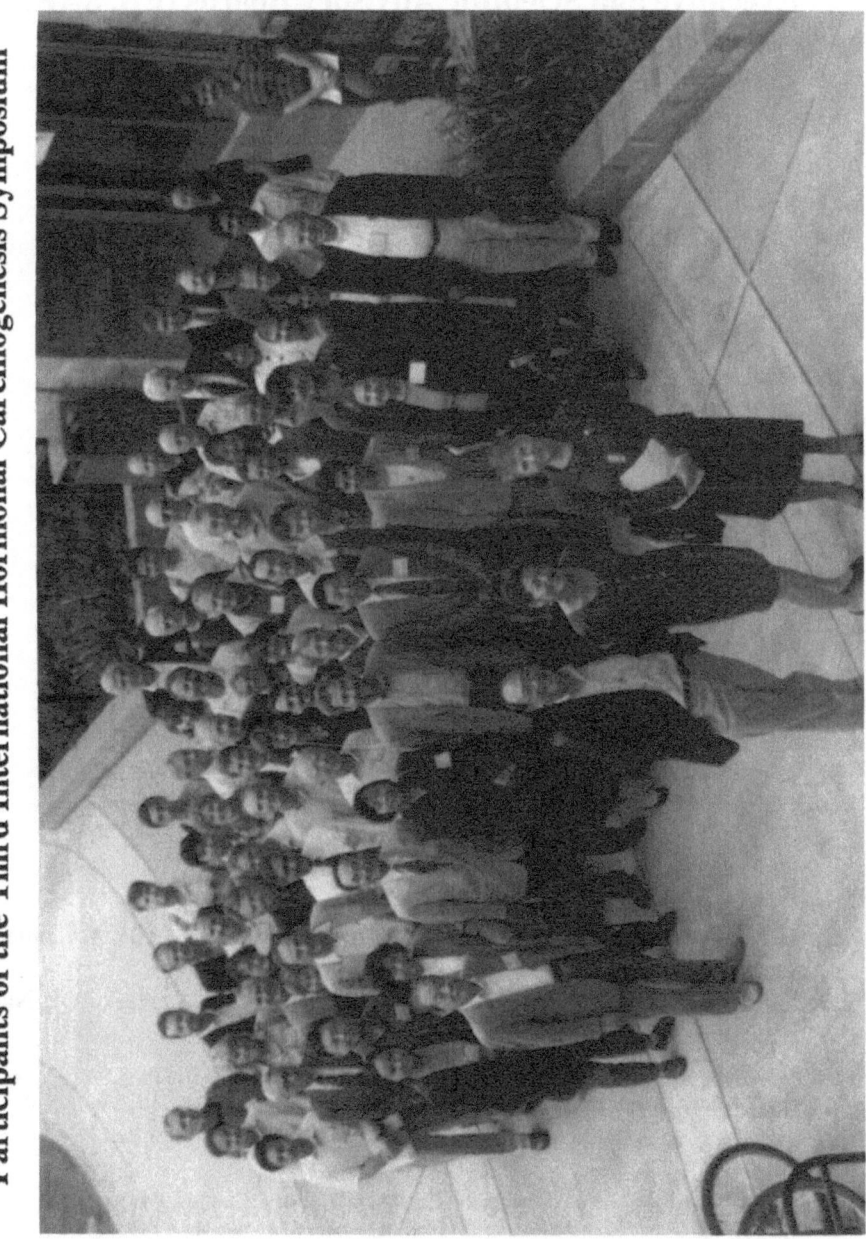

Executive and Scientific Advisory Boards (EB, SAB) and Consultants (C)

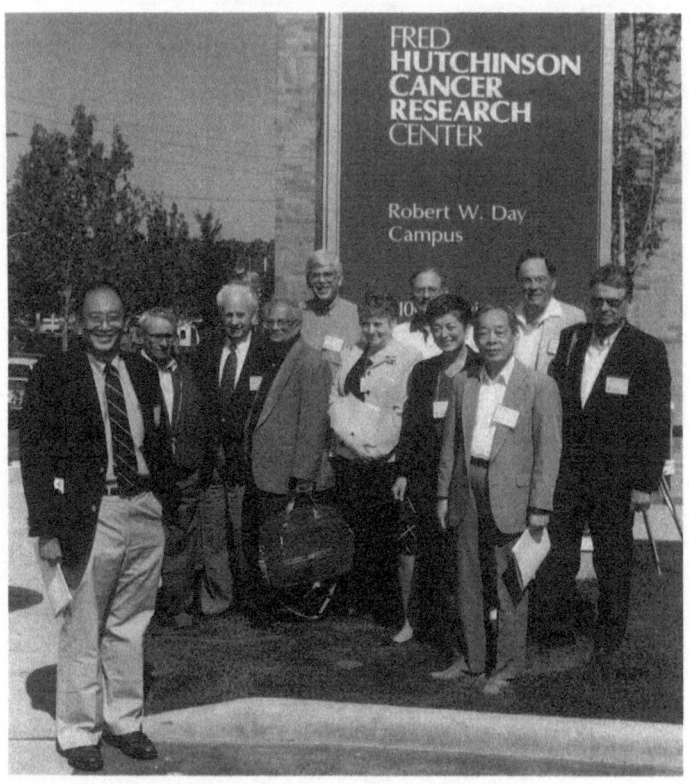

Top Row, L to R: J. Rosen (SAB), J. Pickar (SAB), E. Jensen (SAB), A. Llombart-Bosch (SAB)

Bottom Row, L to R: J.J. Li (EB), H. Rochefort (SAB), G. Mueller (C), S. Nandi (C), J. Daling (EB), S.A. Li (EB), S. Liao (SAB)

SAB members not present: P. Chambon, G. Colditz, S. J. Collins, M. Gallo, J.Å. Gustafsson, L. Hartwell, H.C. Pitot, R. Sutherland, F. Waldman

Preface

Since our previous symposium in 1995, the pace of research in hormones and cancer has accelerated. Progress in our understanding of hormonal carcinogenic processes has been a direct result of the advances made in cell biology, endocrinology, and carcinogenesis at the molecular level. The newer fields of molecular genetics and cytogenetics already have and are expected to continue to play a major role in furthering our understanding of the cellular and molecular events in hormonal carcinogenesis.

It has become increasingly clear that the risk of naturally occurring sex hormones in carcinogenic processes, both in human and in animal models, requires only minute quantities of hormones, at both the serum and tissue levels. Moreover, hormone target tissues for neoplastic transformation, perhaps with the exception of the liver, generally have relatively modest ability to metabolize sex hormones, such as the breast and prostate.

Table 1 summarizes the serum, and in most cases, the tissue levels of sex hormones, both endogenously and exogenously ingested, which are associated with increased risk for endocrine-associated cancers such as breast, endometrium, and prostate, as well as the hormone levels of four experimental models that have been shown to elicit high tumor incidences. In contrast to the human, in which the hormone levels are cyclic, however, the latter require continuous hormone exposure at these relatively low levels.

Although likely multi-factorial, it is increasingly evident that estrogens and perhaps to a lesser extent progestins are critical etiologic agents in breast cancer development. While the association of estrogens has been well established for endometrial cancer, it was not until after 1990 that endogenous estrogen levels have been associated with increased breast cancer risk. These studies, drawn from larger case-control studies, many of them nested within prospective cohorts, have now firmly established this association. Moreover, European and American studies such as the Nurse's Health Study, have also shown that both ERT and HRT ingestion also increases breast cancer risk. In regard to prostate cancer, there is substantial evidence, both from human and animal studies, that androgens are essential during the initiation and promotion stages of this neoplasm. In all of these endocrine-associated cancers, much needs to be known concerning the precise role of these hormones in neoplastic processes. This remains the primary subject of these symposia.

Table 1. Normal serum, breast and endometrial tissue levels and those required for experimental hormonal carcinogenesis

Hormone	Species	Serum (ng/ml)	Organ	Tissue (pg/mg P)
17β-E$_2$	Human, ♀			
	Cycling	0.02 - 0.36	Breast &	114 (8)
E$_1$-SO$_4$	ERT	(1)	Endometrium	
	Post-Meno	2.5 (2)		95 (8)
Testosterone	Human, ♂	30 - 110 (1)	Prostate	ND^2
17β-E$_2$	Hamster, ♀			
	Cycling	0.06-0.36 (4)	Kidney	5.7-12.3
	H. impl.^{5} ♂	2.5 (4)	Kidney	3.9-5.5
17β-E$_2$	Rat, ACI, ♀			
	Cycling	0.04-0.12 (5)	Mam Gland	ND^2
	H. impl.^{5}	0.18-0.21 (5)		
17β-E$_2$	Rat, Noble, ♂	$\leq$ 0.04 (6)	Prostate	0.10^3
	H. impl.^{5}			
+Testosterone		2.3 (6)		0.90^4
17β-E$_2$	Mouse, ♂			
	transgenic	0.006 (7)	Testes	ND^2

^{2} ND, not determined ^{3} pg/g tissue ^{4} mg/g tissue ^{5} Hormone(s) implanted

1. Schiff I, Walsh B (1995) Menopause. In: Becker KL (ed) Principles and Practice of Endocrinology and Metabolism, 2nd Edition. J.B. Lippinicott Co, New York, pp. 916.
2. Mistry JS, Ranadive G, Saujahl G et al (1997) Estrone sulfate as a marker of estrogenicity in women. Proc. Endocrine Soc 79:P3-418.
3. Hankinson SE, Manson JE, Spiegelman D et al (1995) Reproducibility of plasia hormone levels in postmenopausal women over a 2-3-year period. Cancer Epidemiol Biomarkers Prevent 4:649-654.
4. Li SA, Xue Y, Xie Q et al (1994) Serum and tissue levels of estradiol during estrogen-induced renal tumorigenesis in the Syrian hamster. J Steroid Biochem Molec Biol 48:283-286.

5.   Shull JD, Spady TJ, Snyder MC et al (1997) Ovary-intact, but not ovariectomized female ACI rats treated with 17β-estradiol rapidly develop mammary carcinoma. Carcinogenesis 18:1595-1601.

6.   Leav I, Ho SM, Ofren P et al (1988) Biochemical alternatives in sex hormone-induced hyperplasia and dysplasia of the dorsolateral prostate of Noble rats. J Nat Cancer Inst 80:1045-1053.

7.   Fowler KA, Gill K, Kirma N et al (1999) Overexpression of aromatase leads to development of testicular Leydig cell tumors: An in-vivo model for hormone-mediated testicular cancer. Am J Path (in press).

8.   Thussen JHH, Van Landeghem, Poortman J (1996) In: Ann NY Acad Sci. Angeli A, Bradlow HL, Dogiotti L (eds) Volume 464. New York, pp. 106-116.

Once again, we would like to express our deep gratitude to the members of the Scientific and Advisory Boards for their time and effort in assisting us in selecting speakers which provided a truly outstanding, cohesive program. The editors are grateful to Drs. M. Aldaz, J. Daling, S. Liao, G. Mueller, S. Nandi, J.S. Norris, C. Walker, and F. Waldman for their assistance in critically reviewing the manuscripts presented herein. We again are deeply indebted to Dr. J.H. Pickar, Wyeth Ayerst, and G.A. Lucier, NIEHS, for their continuous generous support of these symposia. We thank Dr. L. Hartwell and the Weiss/Daling staff at the Fred Hutchinson Cancer Center for providing the fine facilities, technical support, and both time and effort on behalf of this symposium. Special thanks to Ms. Carolyn Burns for unstinting help in keeping this symposium on course. We are indebted to Ms. Stephanie Parks for her dedication and gracious equanimity during all stages of this symposium. We are grateful to Ms. Tandria Price for her excellent assistance in bringing this volume to the accustom high standard expected. We are also very grateful to the organizations listed separately for their contributions to this symposium, without their help this meeting could not have taken place.

Kansas City, Kansas

Jonathan J. Li, Ph.D.
Sara Antonia Li, Ph.D.

Seattle, Washington

Janet Daling, Ph.D.

Contents

PART 1. EPIDEMIOLOGY:
BREAST AND PROSTATE CANCER 59

PART 2. MOLECULAR GENETICS OF
HORMONAL CANCERS 97

PART 3. ESTROGEN RECEPTOR INTERACTIONS

COMMUNICATIONS

Participants

C. MARCELO ALDAZ Department of Carcinogenesis, MD Anderson, Science Park, University of Texas, Smithville, TX, USA

BENJAMIN D. ANDERSON University of Washington, Seattle, WA, USA

GARNET ANDERSON Fred Hutchinson Cancer Research Center, Seattle, WA, USA

J. CARL BARRETT Laboratory of Molecular Carcinogenesis, National Institute of Environmental Health Sciences, NIH, Research Triangle Park, NC, USA

HELEN BRADY Bone Metabolism and Functional Genomics, Signal Pharmaceuticals, San Diego, CA, USA

ROBERT W. BRUEGGEMEIER College of Pharmacy, The Ohio State University, Columbus, OH, USA

TRUDY BUSH Department of Epidemiology, University of Maryland, Baltimore, MD, USA

CHU CHEN Fred Hutchinson Cancer Research Center, Seattle, WA, USA

SHIUAN CHEN Beckman Research Institute, City of Hope National Medical Center, Duarte, CA, USA

BARBARA COCHRANE Fred Hutchinson Cancer Research Center, Seattle, WA, USA

JOHN E. COE Laboratory of Persistent Viral Diseases, NIAID, Hamilton, MT, USA

GRAHAM A. COLDITZ Channing Laboratory, Brigham and Women's Hospital, Boston, MA, USA

STEVEN J. COLLINS Fred Hutchinson Cancer Research Center, Seattle, WA, USA

EVA COREY Department of Urology, University of Washington, Seattle, WA, USA

GERALD R. CUNHA Department of Anatomy, University of California, San Francisco, CA, USA

JANET R. DALING Division of Public Health Sciences, Fred Hutchinson Cancer Research Center, Seattle, WA, USA

RICHARD P. DIAUGUSTINE Laboratory of Biochemical Risk Assessment, National Institute of Environmental Health Sciences, NIH, Research Triangle Park, NC, USA

YVONNE DRAGAN School of Public Health, Ohio State University, Columbus, OH, USA

JACK FISHMAN Department of Biochemistry, Rockefeller University, New York, NY, USA

ANNETTE FITZPATRICK Department of Biostatistics, University of Washington, Seattle, WA, USA

PATRICK FRIEL Department of Genetics and Cell Biology, Washington State University, Pullman, WA, USA

ROBIN FUCHS-YOUNG University of Texas, MD Anderson Cancer Center, Smithville, TX, USA

HIROMI FUJITA Nakano Eye Clinic, Kyoto, Japan

JACK GORSKI Department of Biochemistry, University of Wisconsin, Madison, WI, USA

BAIBI GRUBE Division of Immunology, Beckman Research Institute, City of Hope National Medical Center, Duarte, CA, USA

JAN-ÅKE GUSTAFSSON Department of Medical Nutrition, Huddinge University Hospital, NOVUM, Huddinge, Sweden

STEPHEN E. HARRIS Division of Endocrinology, University of Texas, San Antonio, TX, USA

LEE HARTWELL Fred Hutchinson Cancer Research Center, Seattle, WA, USA

NEILANN HENDERSON Fred Hutchinson Cancer Research Center, Seattle, WA, USA

ROBERT N. HOOVER Environmental Epidemiology Branch, National Cancer Institute, NIH, Bethesda, MD, USA

CHAD E. HUDSON Department of Microbiology, Medical University of South Carolina, Charleston, SC, USA

FRIEDRICH HUSMANN Division of Endocrinology, Klinik am Malerwinkel, Bad Sassendorf, Germany

KAZUHIRO IKEDA Department of Biochemistry, Saitama Medical School, Saitama, Japan

HERBERT JACOBSON Reproductive Studies Laboratory, Albany Medical College, Albany, NY, USA

ELWOOD V. JENSEN IHF Institute for Hormone and Fertility Research, Hamburg, Germany

HELENA JERNSTRÖM Department of Oncology, University of Lund, Lund, Sweden

OLLI-P. KALLIONIEMI Laboratory of Cancer Genetics, National Human Genome Research Institute, National Institutes of Health, Bethesda, MD, USA

MARION KAVANAUGH-LYNCH University of California, Oakland, CA, USA

SEEMA A. KHAN Department of Surgery, Northwestern Memorial Hospital, Chicago, IL, USA

MICHAEL KLEEREKOPER Division of Endocrinology, Wayne State University, Detroit, MI, USA

ALAN R. KRISTAL Fred Hutchinson Cancer Research Center, Seattle, WA, USA

SABINE E. KULLING Institute of Food Chemistry, University of Karlsruhe, Karlsruhe, Germany

SUE-MIN LAI Department of Preventative Medicine, Kansas Cancer Institute, University of Kansas Medical Center, Kansas City, KS, USA

JOHANNA LAMPE Fred Hutchinson Cancer Research Center, Seattle, WA, USA

JONATHAN J. LI Division of Etiology and Prevention of Hormonal Cancers, University of Kansas Medical Center, Kansas City, KS, USA

SARA ANTONIA LI Division of Etiology and Prevention of Hormonal Cancers, University of Kansas Medical Center, Kansas City, KS, USA

SHUTSUNG LIAO The Ben May Institute for Cancer Research, University of Chicago, Chicago, IL, USA

ANTONIO LLOMBART-BOSCH Department of Pathology, Instituto Valenciano de Oncologia, University of Valencia, Valencia, Spain

MARGARET MADELEINE Fred Hutchinson Cancer Research Center, Seattle, WA, USA

KATHY E. MALONE Division of Public Health Sciences, Fred Hutchinson Cancer Research Center, Seattle, WA, USA

MARGARET T. MANDELSON Center for Health Studies, University of Washington, Seattle, WA, USA

POLLY A. MARCHBANKS Centers for Disease Control, Atlanta, GA, USA

CHARLES P. MARTUCCI Strang Cancer Research Laboratory, Rockefeller University, New York, NY, USA

DORIS MAYER Division of Cell Pathology, Deutsches Krebsforschungszentrum, Heidelberg, Germany

ANNE MCTIERNAN Fred Hutchinson Cancer Research Center, Seattle, WA, USA

MANFRED METZLER Laboratory of Environmental Toxicology, Department of Chemistry, University of Kaiserslautern, Germany

ANDREI MIKHEEV Fred Hutchinson Cancer Research Center, Seattle, WA, USA

SURESH MOHLA National Institutes of Health, National Cancer Institute, Rockville, MD, USA

GERALD C. MUELLER McArdle Laboratory for Cancer Research, University of Wisconsin, Madison, WI, USA

SATYABRATA NANDI Cancer Research Laboratory, University of California, Berkeley, CA, USA

POLLY A. NEWCOMB Fred Hutchinson Cancer Research Center, Seattle, WA, USA

JAMES S. NORRIS Department of Microbiology and Immunology, Medical University of South Carolina, Charleston, SC, USA

ELAINE OSTRANDER Fred Hutchinson Cancer Research Center, Seattle, WA, USA

ARTHUR B. PARDEE Dana-Farber Cancer Institute, Harvard University, Boston, MA, USA

INGEMAR R. PERSSON Department of Medical Epidemiology, Stockholm, Sweden

ERIKA PFEIFFER Institute of Food Chemistry, University of Karlsruhe, Kalrsruhe, Germany

JAMES H. PICKAR Clinical Research and Development, Wyeth-Ayerst Research, Philadelphia, PA, USA

HENRY C. PITOT McArdle Laboratory for Cancer Research, University of Wisconsin, Madison, WI, USA

PEGGY PORTER Fred Hutchinson Cancer Research Center, Seattle, WA, USA

OWEN W.J. PRALL Cancer Research Program, Garvan Institute of Medical Research, St. Vincent's Hospital, Sydney, Australia

GREGORY A. REED Department of Pharmacology, Toxicology and Therapeutics, University of Kansas Medical Center, Kansas City, KS, USA

M. J. REED Unit of Metabolic Medicine, Imperial College, London, United Kingdom

JUERGEN K.V. REICHARDT Department of Biochemistry and Molecular Biology, University of Southern California, Los Angeles, CA, USA

HARVEY A. RISCH Department of Epidemiology and Public Health, Yale University School of Medicine, New Haven, CT, USA

HENRI ROCHEFORT INSERM U 148, Montpellier, France

MARIANNA RODOVA Division of Etiology and Prevention of Hormonal Cancers, University of Kansas Medical Center, Kansas City, KS, USA

JEFFREY M. ROSEN Department of Cell Biology, Baylor College of Medicine, Houston, TX, USA

MARY ANNE ROSSING Fred Hutchinson Cancer Research Center, Seattle, WA, USA

JACQUES E. ROSSOUW Office of Prevention, Bethesda, MD, USA

CAROLYN RUTTER Center for Health Studies, Seattle, WA, USA

DIPAK K. SARKAR Department of Veterinary and Comparative Anatomy, Pharmacology and Physiology, Washington State University, Pullman, WA, USA

DAVID A. SCHWARTZ Department of Microbiology, Medical University of South Carolina, Charleston, SC, USA

STEPHEN SCHWARTZ Fred Hutchinson Cancer Research Center, Seattle, WA, USA

LEA I. SEKELY National Cancer Institute, National Institutes of Health, Bethesda, MD, USA

ROBERT P. C. SHIU Protein and Polypeptide Hormone Laboratory, University of Manitoba, Winnipeg, Canada

JAMES D. SHULL Cancer Institute, University of Nebraska Medical Center, Omaha, NE, USA

PENTTI SIITERI Somona, CA, USA

GARY J. SMITH Department of Pathology, University of North Carolina, Chapel Hill, NC, USA

THOMAS C. SPELSBERG Department of Biochemistry and Molecular Biology, Mayo Graduate School of Medicine, Rochester, MN, USA

GEORGE M. STANCEL Department of Integrative Biology, Pharmacology, and Physiology, University of Texas Medical School, Houston, TX, USA

JANET L. STANFORD Division of Public Helath Sciences, Fred Hutchinson Cancer Research Center, Seattle, WA, USA

BERND STEIN Bone Metabolism and Functional Genomics, Signal Pharmaceuticals, Inc., San Diego, CA, USA

JOHN C. STEVENSON Cecil Rosen Research Laboratories, Imperial College School of Medicine, London, United Kingdom

JAY M. SULLIVAN Cardiovascular Diseases, University of Tennessee, Memphis, TN, USA

KALYAN SUNDARAM Central Biomedical Research, Population Council, New York, NY, USA

ROBERT L. SUTHERLAND Cancer Research Program, Garvan Institute of Medical Research, St. Vincent's Hospital, Sydney, Australia

RAJESHWAR RAO TEKMAL Department of Gynecology and Obstetrics, Emory University School of Medicine, Atlanta, GA, USA

DAVID B. THOMAS Fred Hutchinson Cancer Research Center, Seattle, WA, USA

WAYNE D. TILLEY Flinders Cancer Centre, Division of Surgery, Flinders Medical Centre, Bedford Park, Australia

MARTIN TOCHACEK Cancer Institute, University of Nebraska Medical Center, Omaha, NE, USA

TAKEKI TSUTSUI The Nippon Dental University, Department of Pharmacology, Tokyo, Japan

PRISCILLA VELENTGAS Cardiovascular Health Study, University of Washington, Seattle, WA, USA

FREDERIC M. WALDMAN Department of Laboratory Medicine, University of California - San Francisco, San Francisco, CA, USA

CHERYL LYN WALKER Department of Carcinogenesis, MD Anderson Cancer Center, Smithville, TX, USA

MIAN-YING WANG Department of Biomedical Sciences, UIC College of Medicine, Rockford, IL, USA

NOEL S. WEISS Fred Hutchinson Cancer Research Center, Seattle, WA, USA

ALESSANDRO WEISZ Instituto di Patologia Generale e Oncologia, Seconda Universitá degli Studi di Napoli, Napoli, Italy

HEATHER-MARIE P. WILSON Department of Pathology, University of Washington, Seattle, WA, USA

Y.C. WONG Department of Anatomy, University of Hong Kong, Hong Kong, Peoples Republic of China

B. XIE Department of Anatomy, University of Hong Kong, Hong Kong, Peoples Republic of China

CHUN YANG Division of Immunology, Beckman Research Institute, City of Hope National Medical Center, Duarte, CA, USA

YUTAKA YASUI Fred Hutchinson Cancer Research Center, Seattle, WA, USA

FU-LI YU Department of Biomedical Sciences, UIC College of Medicine, Rockford, IL, USA

DUJIN ZHOU Division of Immunology, Beckman Research Institute, City of Hope National Medical Center, Duarte, CA, USA

Contributors

RAFFAELE ADDEO Instituto di Patologia Generale e Oncologia, Seconda Universitá degli Studi di Napoli, Napoli, Italy

C. MARCELO ALDAZ Department of Carcinogenesis, MD Anderson, Science Park, University of Texas, Smithville, TX, USA

LUCIA ALTUCCI Instituto di Patologia Generale e Oncologia, Seconda Universitá degli Studi di Napoli, Napoli, Italy

MASSIMO ANCORA Instituto di Patologia Generale e Oncologia, Seconda Universitá degli Studi di Napoli, Napoli, Italy

BENJAMIN D. ANDERSON University of Washington, Seattle, WA, USA

GARNET ANDERSON Fred Hutchinson Cancer Research Center, Seattle, WA, USA

PETER BANNASCH Division of Cell Pathology, Deutsches Krebsforschungszentrum, Heidelberg, Germany

J. CARL BARRETT Laboratory of Molecular Carcinogenesis, NIEHS, Research Triangle Park, NC, USA

ANDRZEJ BEDNAREK Department of Carcinogenesis, MD Anderson, Science Park, University of Texas, Smithville, TX, USA

WANDA BENDER Department of Biomedical Sciences, UIC College of Medicine, Rockford, IL, USA

DIANE F. BIRT Center for Designing Foods, Ames, IA, USA

DEBAJIT K. BISWAS Dana-Farber Cancer Institute, Harvard Medical School, Boston, MA, USA

HOLLY L. BOETTGER-TONG Department of Integrative Biology, Pharmacology, and Physiology, University of Texas Medical School, Houston, TX, USA

ÅKE BORG Department of Oncology, University of Lund, Lund, Sweden

RAPHAELLE BORGO Instituto di Patologia Generale e Oncologia, Seconda Universitá degli Studi di Napoli, Napoli, Italy

HELEN BRADY Bone Metabolism and Functional Genomics, Signal Pharmaceuticals, Inc., San Diego, CA, USA

FRANCESCO BRESCIANI Instituto di Patologia Generale e Oncologia, Seconda Universitá degli Studi di Napoli, Napoli, Italy

ROBERT W. BRUEGGEMEIER College of Pharmacy, Ohio State University, Columbus, OH, USA

LUKAS BUBENDORF Laboratory of Cancer Genetics, National Human Genome Research Institute, National Institute of Health, Bethesda, MD, USA

GRANT BUCHANAN Flinders Cancer Centre, Division of Surgery, Flinders Medical Centre, Bedford Park, Australia

TRUDY BUSH Department of Epidemiology, University of Maryland, Baltimore, MD, USA

MASSIMO CANCEMI Instituto di Patologia Generale e Oncologia, Seconda Universitá degli Studi di Napoli, Napoli, Italy

MARILYN CANSLER Department of Pathology, University of Kansas Medical Center, Kansas City, KS, USA

CARMEN CARDA Department of Pathology, Instituto Valenciano de Oncologia, University of Valencia, Valencia, Spain

APRIL CHARPENTIER Department of Carcinogenesis, MD Anderson, Science Park, University of Texas, Smithville, TX, USA

CHU CHEN Fred Hutchinson Cancer Research Center, Seattle, WA, USA

SHIUAN CHEN Beckman Research Institute, City of Hope National Medical Center, Duarte, CA, USA

TAE-YON CHUN Department of Biochemistry, University of Wisconsin, Madison, WI, USA

LUIGI CICATIELLO Instituto di Patologia Generale e Oncologia, Seconda Universitá degli Studi di Napoli, Napoli, Italy

BARBARA COCHRANE Fred Hutchinson Cancer Research Center, Seattle, WA, USA

JOHN E. COE Laboratory of Persistent Viral Diseases, NIAID, Hamilton, MT, USA

GRAHAM A. COLDITZ Channing Laboratory, Brigham and Women's Hospital, Boston, MA, USA

WILLIAM B. COLEMAN Department of Pathology, University of North Carolina, Chapel Hill, NC, USA

STEVEN J. COLLINS Fred Hutchinson Cancer Research Center, Seattle, WA, USA

EVA COREY Department of Urology, University of Washington, Seattle, WA, USA

N. CORREIA Department of Medical Epidemiology, Stockholm, Sweden

GERALD R. CUNHA Department of Anatomy, University of California, San Francisco, CA, USA

KARA CUSHING Fred Hutchinson Cancer Research Center, Seattle, WA, USA

JANET R. DALING Division of Public Health Sciences, Fred Hutchinson Cancer Research Center, Seattle, WA, USA

RICHARD P. DIAUGUSTINE Laboratory of Biochemical Risk Assessment, National Institute of Environmental Health Sciences, NIH, Research Triangle Park, NC, USA

YVONNE P. DRAGAN School of Public Health, Ohio State University, Columbus, OH, USA

D. DUBIK Protein and Polypeptide Hormone Laboratory, University of Manitoba, Winnipeg, Canada

JACK FISHMAN Department of Biochemistry, Rockefeller University, New York, NY, USA

ANNETTE FITZPATRICK Department of Biostatistics, University of Washington, Seattle, WA, USA

HEIDE L. FORD Dana-Farber Cancer Institute, Harvard Medical School, Boston, MA, USA

PATRICK FRIEL Department of Genetics and Cell Biology, Washington State University, Pullman, WA, USA

ROBIN FUCHS-YOUNG University of Texas, MD Anderson Cancer Center, Smithville, TX, USA

HIROMI FUJITA Nakano Eye Clinic, Kyoto, Japan

M.W. GHILCHIK Unit of Metabolic Medicine, Imperial College, London, United Kingdom

KIRAN GILL Department of Gynecology and Obstetrics, Emory University School of Medicine, Atlanta, GA, USA

ITSUO GORAI Department of Biochemistry, Saitama Medical School, Saitama, Japan

JACK GORSKI Department of Biochemistry, University of Wisconsin, Madison, WI, USA

JOE W. GRISHAM Department of Pathology, University of North Carolina, Chapel Hill, NC, USA

GARY D. GROSSFELD Department of Anatomy, University of California, San Francisco, CA, USA

BAIBA GRUBE Beckman Research Institute, City of Hope National Medical Center, Duarte, CA, USA

JAN-ÅKE GUSTAFSSON Department of Medical Nutrition, Huddinge University Hospital, NOVUM, Huddinge, Sweden

RAPHAEL GUZMAN Department of Molecular and Cell Biology, University of California, Cancer Research Lab, Berkeley, CA, USA

RANDALL E. HARRIS College of Pharmacy, Ohio State University, Columbus, OH, USA

STEPHEN E. HARRIS Division of Endocrinology, University of Texas, San Antonio, TX, USA

LEE HARTWELL Fred Hutchinson Cancer Research Center, Seattle, WA, USA

DJUANA M.E. HARVELL Cancer Institute, University of Nebraska Medical Center, Omaha, NE, USA

KATHLEEN HAWKINS Department of Carcinogenesis, MD Anderson, Science Park, University of Texas, Smithville, TX, USA

SIMON W. HAYWARD Department of Anatomy, University of California, San Francisco, CA, USA

THERESA E. HEFFERAN Department of Biochemistry and Molecular Biology, Mayo Graduate School of Medicine, Rochester, MN, USA

NEILANN HENDERSON Fred Hutchinson Cancer Research Center, Seattle, WA, USA

SHANE T. HENTGES Department of Veterinary and Comparative Anatomy, Pharmacology and Physiology, Washington State University, Pullman, WA, USA

YASUHIRO HIGASHI Department of Biochemistry, Saitama Medical School, Saitama, Japan

RICHARD A. HIIPAKKA The Ben May Institute, Chicago, IL, USA

HISAHIKO HIROI Department of Biochemistry, Saitama Medical School, Saitama, Japan

ROBERT N. HOOVER Environmental Epidemiology Branch, National Cancer Institute, NIH, Bethesda, MD, USA

CHAD E. HUDSON Department of Microbiology, Medical University of South Carolina, Charleston, SC, USA

FRIEDRICH HUSMANN Division of Endocrinology, Klinik am Malerwinkel, Bad Sassendorf, Germany

SALMAN M. HYDER Department of Integrative Biology, Pharmacology, and Physiology, University of Texas Medical School, Houston, TX, USA

KAZUHIRO IKEDA Department of Biochemistry, Saitama Medical School, Saitama, Japan

SATOSHI INOUE Department of Biochemistry, Saitama Medical School, Saitama, Japan

KAMAL G. ISHAK Laboratory of Persistent Viral Diseases, NIAID, Hamilton, MT, USA

B. IWASIOW   Protein and Polypeptide Hormone Laboratory, University of Manitoba, Winnipeg, Canada

ERIC JACOBS Institute of Food Chemistry, University of Karlsruhe, Karlsruhe, Germany

HERBERT JACOBSON Reproductive Studies Laboratory, Albany Medical College, Albany, NY, USA

ELWOOD V. JENSEN IHF Institute for Hormone and Fertility Research, Hamburg, Germany

HELENA JERNSTRÖM Department of Oncology, University of Lund, Lund, Sweden

FARAHNAZ S. JOARDER College of Pharmacy, Ohio State University, Columbus, OH, USA

O. JOHANNSSON Department of Oncology, University of Lund, Lund, Sweden

THORA JONNASDOTTIR Fred Hutchinson Cancer Research Center, Seattle, WA, USA

V. CRAIG JORDAN Robert H. Lurie Cancer Center, Northwestern University Medical School, Chicago, IL, USA

OLLI-P KALLIONIEMI Laboratory of Cancer Genetics, National Human Genome Research Institute, National Institute of Health, Bethesda, MD, USA

YEH-CHIH KAO Beckman Research Institute, City of Hope National Medical Center, Duarte, CA, USA

MARION KAVANAUGH-LYNCH University of California, Oakland, CA, USA

SEEMA A. KHAN Department of Surgery, Northwestern Memorial Hospital, Chicago, IL, USA

NAMEER KIRMA Department of Gynecology and Obstetrics, Emory University School of Medicine, Atlanta, GA, USA

MICHAEL KLEEREKOPER Division of Endocrinology, Wayne State University, Detroit, MI, USA

DIANE M. KLOTZ Laboratory of Biochemical Risk Assessment, National Institute of Environmental Health Sciences, NIH, Research Triangle Park, NC, USA

JOHN M. KOKONTIS The Ben May Institute, Chicago, IL, USA

ALAN R. KRISTAL Fred Hutchinson Cancer Research Center, Seattle, WA, USA

SABINE E. KULLING Institute of Food Chemistry, University of Karlsruhe, Karlsruhe, Germany

KENDRA LAFLIN Department of Carcinogenesis, MD Anderson, Science Park, University of Texas, Smithville, TX, USA

SUE-MIN LAI Department of Preventative Medicine, Kansas Cancer Institute, University of Kansas Medical Center, Kansas City, KS, USA

JOHANNA LAMPE Fred Hutchinson Cancer Research Center, Seattle, WA, USA

ATHENA M. LEMUS-WILSON Cancer Institute, University of Nebraska Medical Center, NE, USA

JOSEPH LEWCOCK Bone Metabolism and Functional Genomics, Signal Pharmaceuticals, Inc., San Diego, CA, USA

JUAN LEYVA Instituto di Patologia Generale e Oncologia, Seconda Universitá degli Studi di Napoli, Napoli, Italy

DONG-HUI LI McArdle Laboratory for Cancer Research, University of Wisconsin, Madison, WI, USA

JONATHAN J. LI Division of Etiology and Prevention of Hormonal Cancers, University of Kansas Medical Center, Kansas City, KS, USA

SARA ANTONIA LI Division of Etiology and Prevention of Hormonal Cancers, University of Kansas Medical Center, Kansas City, KS, USA

DEZHONG JOSHUA LIAO Lombardi Cancer Center, Georgetown University Medical Center, Washington, D.C., USA

SHUTSUNG LIAO The Ben May Institute for Cancer Research, University of Chicago, Chicago, IL, USA

YOUNG C. LIN College of Pharmacology, Ohio State University, Columbus, OH, USA

STEPHANIE LIPPS   Bone Metabolism and Functional Genomics, Signal Pharmaceuticals, Inc., San Diego, CA, USA

ANTONIO LLOMBART-BOSCH   Department of Pathology, Instituto Valenciano de Oncologia, University of Valencia, Valencia, Spain

MICHAEL MACLEOD   Department of Carcinogenesis, MD Anderson, Science Park, University of Texas, Smithville, TX, USA

MARGARET MADELEINE   Fred Hutchinson Cancer Research Center, Seattle, WA, USA

C. MAGNUSSON   Department of Medical Epidemiology, Stockholm, Sweden

SARI MÄKELÄ   Department of Integrative Biology, Pharmacology, and Physiology, University of Texas Medical School, Houston, TX, USA

KATHLEEN E. MALONE   Fred Hutchinson Cancer Research Center, Seattle, WA, USA

MARGARET T. MANDELSON   Center for Health Studies, University of Washington, Seattle, WA, USA

POLLY A. MARCHBANKS   Centers for Disease Control, Atlanta, GA, USA

KATHERINE J. MARTIN   Dana-Farber Cancer Institute, Harvard Medical School, Boston, MA, USA

CHARLES P. MARTUCCI   Strang Cancer Research Laboratory, Rockefeller University, New York, NY, USA

DORIS MAYER   Division of Cell Pathology, Deutsches Krebsforschungszentrum, Heidelberg, Germany

RODNEY D. MCCOMB   Cancer Institute, University of Nebraska Medical Center, NE, USA

ANNE MCTIERNAN   Fred Hutchinson Cancer Research Center, Seattle, WA, USA

CHRISTEL METZGER   Division of Cell Pathology, Deutsches Krebsforschungszentrum, Heidelberg, Germany

MANFRED METZLER   Institute of Food Chemistry, University of Karlsruhe, Karlsruhe, Germany

ANDREI MIKHEEV Fred Hutchinson Cancer Research Center, Seattle, WA, USA

SURESH MOHLA National Institutes of Health, National Cancer Institute, Rockville, MD, USA

GERALD C. MUELLER McArdle Laboratory for Cancer Research, University of Wisconsin, Madison, WI, USA

MASAMI MURAMATSU Department of Biochemistry, Saitama Medical School, Saitama, Japan

KRISTEN L. MURPHEY Department of Cell Biology, Baylor College of Medicine, Houston, TX, USA

ELIZABETH A. MUSGROVE Cancer Research Program, Garvan Institute of Medical Research, St. Vincent's Hospital, Sydney, Australia

SATYABRATA NANDI Cancer Research Laboratory, University of California, Berkeley, CA, USA

DIRK NEHRBASS Division of Cell Pathology, Deutsches Krebsforschungszentrum, Heidelberg, Germany

POLLY A. NEWCOMB Fred Hutchinson Cancer Research Center, Seattle, WA, USA

JAMES S. NORRIS Department of Microbiology and Immunology, Medical University of South Carolina, Charleston, SC, USA

EMILE NUWAYSIR McArdle Laboratory for Cancer Research, University of Wisconsin, Madison, WI, USA

H. OLSSON Department of Oncology, University of Lund, Lund, Sweden

AKIRA ORIMO Department of Biochemistry, Saitama Medical School, Saitama, Japan

ELAINE OSTRANDER Fred Hutchinson Cancer Research Center, Seattle, WA, USA

JANETTE K. PADGITT Department of Pharmacology, Toxicology, and Therapeutics, University of Kansas Medical Center, Kansas City, KS, USA

ARTHUR B. PARDEE Dana-Farber Cancer Institute, Harvard Medical School, Boston, MA, USA

MICHELLE L. PARRETT College of Pharmacy, Ohio State University, Columbus, OH, USA

KAREN L. PENNINGTON Cancer Institute, University of Nebraska Medical Center, Omaha, NE, USA

INGEMAR R. PERSSON Department of Medical Epidemiology, Stockholm, Sweden

VALERIA BELSITO PETRIZZI Instituto di Patologia Generale e Oncologia, Seconda Universitá degli Studi di Napoli, Napoli, Italy

AMANDO PEYDRO-OLAYA Department of Pathology, Instituto Valenciano de Oncologia, University of Valencia, Valencia, Spain

ERIKA PFEIFFER Institute of Food Chemistry, University of Karlsruhe, Karlsruhe, Germany

JAMES H. PICKAR Clinical Research and Development, Wyeth-Ayerst Research, Philadelphia, PA, USA

HENRY C. PITOT McArdle Laboratory for Cancer Research, University of Wisconsin, Madison, WI, USA

PEGGY L. PORTER Fred Hutchinson Cancer Research Center, Seattle, WA, USA

OWEN W.J. PRALL Cancer Research Program, Garvan Institute of Medical Research, St. Vincent's Hospital, Sydney, Australia

SHARON C. PRESNELL Department of Pathology, University of North Carolina, Chapel Hill, NC, USA

A. PUROHIT Unit of Metabolic Medicine, Imperial College, London, United Kingdom

ANNE L. QUINN College of Pharmacy, Ohio State University, Columbus, OH, USA

LAKSHMANASWAMY RAJKUMAR Cancer Research Laboratory, University of California , Berkeley, CA, USA

LYNN RANSONE Bone Metabolism and Functional Genomics, Signal Pharmaceuticals, Inc., San Diego, CA, USA

GREGORY A. REED Department of Pharmacology, Toxicology, and Therapeutics, University of Kansas Medical Center, Kansas City, KS, USA

M.J. REED Unit of Metabolic Medicine, Imperial College, London, United Kingdom

JUERGEN K.V. REICHARDT Department of Biochemistry and Molecular Biology, University of Southern California, Los Angeles, CA, USA

TANYA M. REINDL Cancer Institute, University of Nebraska Medical Center, Omaha, NE, USA

GREGORY G. REINHOLZ Department of Biochemistry and Molecular Biology, Mayo Graduate School of Medicine, Rochester, MN, USA

R. GREGG RICHARDS Laboratory of Biochemical Risk Assessment, National Institute of Environmental Health Sciences, NIH, Research Triangle Park, NC, USA

DAVID J. RICKARD Department of Biochemistry and Molecular Biology, Mayo Graduate School of Medicine, Rochester, MN, USA

HARVEY A. RISCH Department of Epidemiology and Public Health, Yale University School of Medicine, New Haven, CT, USA

FREDIKA M. ROBERTSON College of Pharmacology, The Ohio State University, Columbus, OH, USA

HENRI ROCHEFORT INSERM U 148, Montpellier, France

MARIANNA RODOVA Division of Etiology and Prevention of Hormonal Cancers, University of Kansas Medical Center, Kansas City, KS, USA

EILEEN M. ROGAN Cancer Research Program, Garvan Institute of Medical Research, St. Vincent's Hospital, Sydney, Australia

JEFFREY M. ROSEN Department of Cell Biology, Baylor College of Medicine, Houston, TX, USA

M.J. ROSS Laboratory of Persistent Viral Diseases, NIAID, Hamilton, MT, USA

MARY ANNE ROSSING Fred Hutchinson Cancer Research Center, Seattle, WA, USA

JACQUES E. ROSSOUW Office of Prevention, Bethesda, MD, USA

CAROLYN RUTTER Center for Health Studies, Seattle, WA, USA

RUTH SAGER Dana-Farber Cancer Institute, Harvard Medical School, Boston, MA, USA

LINDA SARGENT McArdle Laboratory for Cancer Research, University of Wisconsin, Madison, WI, USA

DIPAK K. SARKAR   Department of Veterinary and Comparative Anatomy, Pharmacology and Physiology, Washington State University, Pullman, WA, USA

DAVID A. SCHWARTZ Department of Microbiology, Medical University of South Carolina, Charleston, SC, USA

STEPHEN SCHWARTZ Fred Hutchinson Cancer Research Center, Seattle, WA, USA

LEA I. SEKELY National Cancer Institute, National Institutes of Health, Bethesda, MD, USA

FANGCHEN SHEN Cancer Institute, University of Nebraska Medical Center, NE, USA

ROBERT P.C. SHIU Protein and Polypeptide Hormone Laboratory, University of Manitoba, Winnipeg, Canada

JAMES D. SHULL Cancer Institute, University of Nebraska Medical Center, Omaha, NE, USA

PENTTI SIITERI Somona, CA, USA

A. SINGH Unit of Metabolic Medicine, Imperial College, London, United Kingdom

GARY J. SMITH Department of Pathology, University of North Carolina, Chapel Hill, NC, USA

MARY C. SNYDER   Cancer Institute, University of Nebraska Medical Center, Omaha, NE, USA

THOMAS J. SPADY   Cancer Institute, University of Nebraska Medical Center, Omaha, NE, USA

J. SPARLING Protein and Polypeptide Hormone Laboratory, University of Manitoba, Winnipeg, Canada

THOMAS C. SPELSBERG Department of Biochemistry and Molecular Biology, Mayo Graduate School of Medicine, Rochester, MN, USA

GEORGE M. STANCEL Department of Integrative Biology, Pharmacology, and Physiology, University of Texas Medical School, Houston, TX, USA

JANET L. STANFORD Division of Public Health Sciences, Fred Hutchinson Cancer Research Center, Seattle, WA, USA

BERND STEIN Bone Metabolism and Functional Genomics, Signal Pharmaceuticals, Inc., San Diego, CA, USA

JOHN C. STEVENSON Cecil Rosen Research Laboratories, Imperial College School of Medicine, London, United Kingdom

SCOTT STICKLES University Surgical Associates, SUNY Health Science Center, Syracuse, NY, USA

TRACY E. STRECKER Cancer Institute, University of Nebraska Medical Center, NE, USA

MALAYANNAN SUBRAMANIAM Department of Biochemistry and Molecular Biology, Mayo Graduate School of Medicine, Rochester, MN, USA

YASURO SUGIMOTO College of Pharmacology, The Ohio State University, Columbus, OH, USA

JAY M. SULLIVAN Cardiovascular Diseases, University of Tennessee, Memphis, TN, USA

KALYAN SUNDARAM Central Biomedical Research, Population Council, New York, NY, USA

NICOLA M. SUTER Fred Hutchinson Cancer Research Center, Seattle, WA, USA

MAY SUTHERLAND Bone Metabolism and Functional Genomics, Signal Pharmaceuticals, Inc., San Diego, CA, USA

ROBERT L. SUTHERLAND Cancer Research Program, Garvan Institute of Medical Research, St. Vincent's Hospital, Sydney, Australia

YUKIKO TAMURA The Nippon Dental School, Department of Pharmacology, Tokyo, Japan

RAJESHWAR RAO TEKMAL Department of Gynecology and Obstetrics, Emory University School of Medicine, Atlanta, GA, USA

DAVID B. THOMAS Fred Hutchinson Cancer Research Center, Seattle, WA, USA

GUDMUNDUR THORDARSON Cancer Research Laboratory, University of California, Berkeley, CA, USA

WAYNE D. TILLEY Flinders Cancer Centre, Division of Surgery, Flinders Medical Centre, Bedford Park, Australia

THEA TLSTY Department of Anatomy, University of California, San Francisco, CA, USA

MARTIN TOCHACEK Cancer Institute, University of Nebraska Medical Center, Omaha, NE, USA

S.W. TSAO Department of Anatomy, University of Hong Kong, Hong Kong, Peoples Republic of China

FUJIKO TSUCHIYA Department of Biochemistry, Saitama Medical School, Saitama, Japan

TAKEKI TSUTSUI The Nippon Dental School, Department of Pharmacology, Tokyo, Japan

ERIC A. VANDERWOUDE Cancer Institute, University of Nebraska Medical Center, Omaha, NE, USA

PRISCILLA VELENTGAS Cardiovascular Health Study, University of Washington, Seattle, WA, USA

M. VENDITTI Protein and Polypeptide Hormone Laboratory, University of Manitoba, Winnipeg, Canada

FREDERIC M. WALDMAN Department of Laboratory Medicine, University of California - San Francisco, San Francisco, CA, USA

CHERYL LYN WALKER Department of Carcinogenesis, MD Anderson Cancer Center, Smithville, TX, USA

MIAN-YING WANG Department of Biomedical Sciences, UIC College of Medicine, Rockford, IL, USA

KATRINA M. WATERS Department of Biochemistry and Molecular Biology, Mayo Graduate School of Medicine, Rochester, MN, USA

PETER H. WATSON Protein and Polypeptide Hormone Laboratory, University of Manitoba, Winnipeg, Canada

COLIN K.W. WATTS Cancer Research Program, Garvan Institute of Medical Research, St. Vincent's Hospital, Sydney, Australia

E. WEIDERPASS Department of Medical Epidemiology, Stockholm, Sweden

NOEL S. WEISS Fred Hutchinson Cancer Research Center, Seattle, WA, USA

ALESSANDRO WEISZ Instituto di Patologia Generale e Oncologia, Seconda Universitá degli Studi di Napoli, Napoli, Italy

DOUGLAS WENDELL Department of Biochemistry, University of Wisconsin, Madison, WI, USA

S. JOHN WEROHA Division of Etiology and Prevention of Hormonal Cancers, University of Kansas Medical Center, Kansas City, KS, USA

ANGELA M. WILSON Department of Pharmacology, Toxicology, and Therapeutics, University of Kansas Medical Center, Kansas City, KS, USA

HEATHER-MARIE P. WILSON Department of Pathology, University of Washington, Seattle, WA, USA

Y.C. WONG Department of Anatomy, University of Hong Kong, Hong Kong, Peoples Republic of China

B. XIE Department of Anatomy, University of Hong Kong, Hong Kong, Peoples Republic of China

CHUN YANG Beckman Research Institute, City of Hope National Medical Center, Duarte, CA, USA

JASON YANG Cancer Research Laboratory, University of California, Berkeley, CA, USA

YUTAKA YASUI Fred Hutchinson Cancer Research Center, Seattle, WA, USA

FU-LI YU Department of Biomedical Sciences, UIC College of Medicine, Rockford, IL, USA

DUJIN ZHOU Beckman Research Institute, City of Hope National Medical Center, Duarte, CA, USA

Symposium Address

Hormonal Carcinogenesis:
Perceptions, Challenges, and Anticipations

Gerald C. Mueller

Cancer, whether it develops following an exposure to chemical carcinogens, ionizing irradiation, oncogenic viruses, nutritional insults, or to a prolonged hormonal imbalance, reflects a shift in the balance between cell replication and cell death processes. If a cell is going to exhibit any aspect of malignant behavior, the rate of cell replication has to exceed any proneness to go down the path to cell death.

A second property of malignancies, the most important, is their propensity to undergo progressive changes in their genomic state, i.e., the cells are genetically unstable. This progression process usually selects for combinations of gene expressions that provide the malignant cell with a growth advantage, and in many cases, facilitates the invasion and destruction of their normal neighbors. Such changes may involve many genes, some that reflect their roles in embryonic development.

In this Symposium, we shall focus on the role of hormones in these processes. We shall attempt to identify ways in which hormones contribute to or control the development of malignancies, and hopefully, to elucidate new routes for the prevention and treatment of hormonally responsive malignancies. In this presentation, I shall also attempt to provide a road-map for understanding many aspects of how cancer and normal development are inter-related. **A theory of interactive growth regulators is offered which poses cancer as product of their descriptions.**

To engage in this analysis, let us first review some of the fundamental aspects of carcinogenesis, as already revealed through studies of cancer induction using a spectrum of carcinogenic systems. Perhaps, the best defined principles have come out of studies of skin cancer induction by aryl-hydrocarbons in mice. From the studies of many investigators, we now know that a single application of a low dose of an aryl-hydrocarbon such as 7, 12-dimethylbenz[a]anthracene (DMBA), benzopyrene (BP), or 3-methylcholanthrene (MCA) can produce an irreversible change in the skin cells (i.e., the initiation event). With a low dose of the carcinogen, tumors may fail to develop, but even so, a certain number of cells will have suffered a mutation in their *Harvey ras* genes. Chemically, this has come about through the metabolic activation of the chemical carcinogen via a cytochrome P-450 enzyme mediated formation of a diol epoxide of the procarcinogen, which metabolite in turn attacks the DNA through adduct formation. A mutation at codon 61 in the *Harvey ras* gene appears to be the mutation of importance, although a range of other, as yet undefined, mutations may also have occurred.

In the initiation event, the affected cells are switched to a state of growth dependency on a tumor promoting agent such as 12-O-tetradecanoylphorbol-13-acetate (TPA). This agent by itself does not induce tumors in un-initiated skin cells, but its repeated application to hydrocarbon-treated epithelial cells produces many tumors on the backs of the mice. Since the phorbol ester effects seem to be relatively transient, this tumor promoter, and similar agents, must be applied repeatedly for maximal effectiveness (1).

In addition, this combination of treatments give rise to two classes of proliferative growth, non-invasive papillomas and full-fledged invasive carcinomas. The papillomas, like many of the early malignancies observed in hormonal carcinogenesis, are agent dependent in that they require the continued application of the tumor promoter for their continued growth. With the cessation of the TPA applications, the papillomas regress. Such cells appear to undergo a terminal differentiation with cell death by apoptosis being the usual fate. This situation is quite analogous to a number of early estrogen- and androgen-dependant malignancies, both in experimental animals and in humans. Again, in such situations, the withdrawal of the growth promoting stimulus is attended by retreat down the path to cell differentiation, to a state in which the rate of cell death surpasses the rate of cell replication.

In the case of aryl-hydrocarbon carcinogenesis, we know, from studies of phorbol ester receptors in skin cells, that the tumor promoting agent, TPA, acts in all probability through the formation of a complex with and the activation of the protein kinase C class of enzymes (2). In particular, genetic transfection studies have revealed that the most implicated member of this family is protein kinase C-epsilon. The experimental elevation of this enzyme genetically appears to favor tumor development. In estrogen- or androgen-dependant malignancies, however, hormone specific receptors are involved in the responses We shall hear much about them in the course of this Symposium. As yet, however, we have not really identified the next steps of these agents by which they exert their growth promoting actions or, more important, their roles in the tumor progression responses.

Additionally, in aryl-hydrocarbon carcinogenesis, we know that phosphorylation of some target protein by the activation of protein kinase C is likely to be important. This view is also supported by the observation that okadaic acid, a representative of a different class of tumor promoters appears to act by inhibiting dephosphorylation of some essential protein in the growth response.

A prize winning question in these studies is: *Which is the target protein and its role in the growth promotion of the early agent-dependant malignancies.?* It is important to note, however, that as long as the malignancies exhibit the agent-dependant states, whether it be in mice or humans, life with cancer is a relatively simple situation since controlling the state of such a protein could limit the growth of the tumor.

The real problem with cancer, however, lies with the propensity of altered cells to progress to states in which they can no longer be controlled by the elimination of the tumor promoting agent or the growth supporting hormones (1). Most catastrophic in this phenomena of progression is the associated expression of genes which facilitate the metastasis of the tumor cells to new locations, and the enhancement of their ability to destroy the structure and function of the tissues that they invade. Such progressive changes are often attended by permeable proteins such as tumor necrosis factor, proteolytic enzymes, high levels of certain growth factors or aberrant hormones, factors that program disaster for the host organism. Such changes constitute the real problem of cancer, and thus, our most important challenge is to elucidate the underlying mechanisms that operate in tumor progression, and to design therapies that either prevent or correct these important parameters of the cancerous growth dyscrasia.

Before proceeding to an analyses of the tumor progression events, it is important for investigators of hormonal carcinogenesis to be fully aware of the contribution of our early forebears in this quest. In 1953, Jacob Furth summarized his biological findings on *"Conditioned and autonomous neoplasms: A review"* (3). He clearly demonstrated, in the induction of pituitary tumors by estrogens, that the initial tumor growth was estrogen-dependent, requiring available hormone for continued proliferation. He also showed that with continued diethylstilbesterol (DES) treatment, autonomous pituitary tumors developed which grew out of control (i.e., a product of tumor progression), causing the death of the host. These tumors were often heterogeneous and were found to produce pituitary hormones according to the phenotypes of their cells of origin. These products produced remarkable remote effects on target tissues (4). These early hormonal carcinogenesis studies are reviewed by Kirschbaum (5) and Clifton (6). Such surveys announced to the carcinogenesis field that practically every hormone could play a role in carcinogenesis, amid a vast array of responsive cell types. Not only estrogens and androgens were implicated, but also peptide hormones or those belonging to the secondary agonist class. In practically all cases, a long repeated exposure to the hormonal agent was required, and the hormonal agents often synergized with ionizing radiation. Importantly, the usual responses entailed the development of an initial hormone-dependent state that progressed, after prolonged treatments, to flagrant malignancies that, ultimately, killed the hosts.

Thus, the hallmark of tumor progression is the recruitment of changes reflecting an underlying genomic instability. Whether the tumor progression took place in highly controlled studies of carcinogenesis on the backs of mice, irradiation-induced tumors, diet-provoked malignancies, or cancer arising from unidentified provocators in humans, the life defying malignant states reflect the selection and accumulation of cells, which through the sequential recruitment of mutations, came to have a growth and a direct competition advantage over their normal neighbors. In the case of human colon cancer, the progression towards greater malignant character has been correlated with the recruitment of five or more genetic mistakes (Figure 1) (7). It is of interest that the order of recruitment for the mutations is not as important as the total number. Also, a very significant feature is that the type of mutations ranges widely (i.e., point mutations, deletions, transpositions, loss or gain of whole chromosomes, and reduplication of chromosomal segments). Perhaps most amazing is that the recruited errors arise with a very high frequency in a relatively small number of progenitor cells. These observations, that genetic instability correlates with the development of increasingly malignant tumors, has prompted Loeb (8) to hypothesize that tumor progression is the reflection of a mutator phenotype.

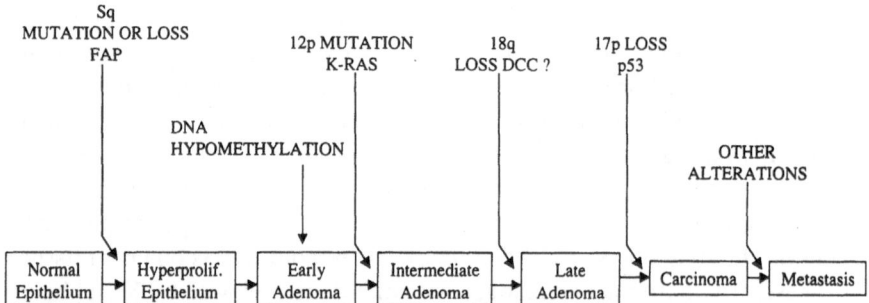

Figure 1. A genetic model for colorectal tumorigenesis from Fearon and Vogelstein (7). Tumorigenesis progresses towards an increasingly malignant character by the recruitment of more and more mutations. While mutations in an oncogene (*ras*) or a suppressor gene may lead the progression, a wide variety of chromosomal defects may contribute to the most malignant states. The order of recruitment is clearly less important than the number of errors recruited.

In other words, true and devastating malignancies arise from some event(s) that lead to genetic instability on a broad scale, and to the recruitment of more and more errors in the genome. It is then the nature of biology to select for the fittest (i.e., most malignant) competitors.

As cited in the introduction, a basic change involves a shift in the balance between cell replication versus cell death. In any case, the result is accumulative growth through either increased cell replication rates or decreased cell death events, changes in either parameter may be casual. An additional point is that, the mechanics of the basic metabolic processes, which continue to operate in either direction, are for the most part fairly normal, except for the shifts in rates or changes in the frequency of triggered events.   In other words, DNA replication, RNA and protein synthesis, other metabolic processes, or cell death events are executed rather normally, but at altered rates of competitive triggering.

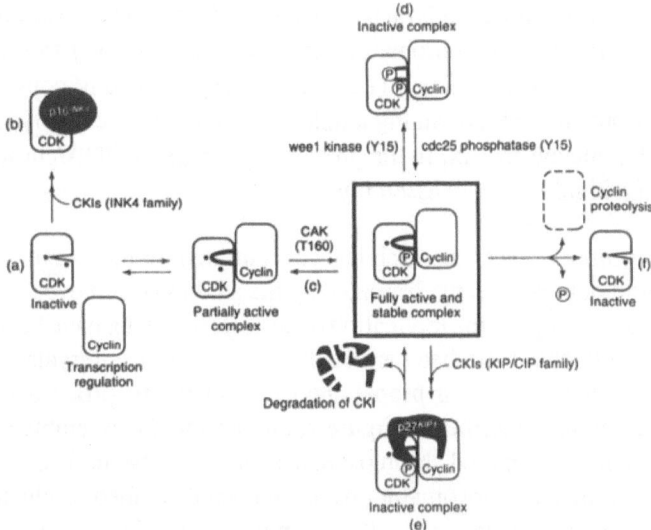

Figure 2. Control mechanisms regulating the cdk-cyclin complex activity (9). Cells triggered by a mitogenic signal proceed into DNA and chromosome replication, and on through the mitotic process by the sequential activation, inactivation, or degradation of specific kinases and their inhibitors belonging to the cyclin/cyclin kinase families. While initiated in nature by a wide number of mitogenic stimuli, the replication response reflects a remarkable convergence of the final steps of nuclear replication.

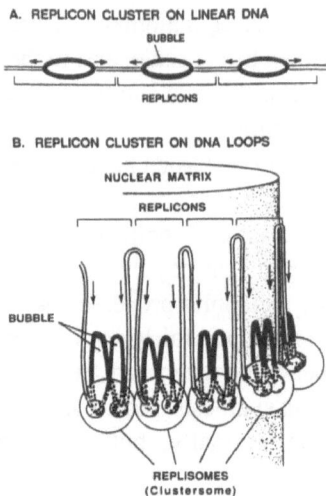

Figure 3. Clustersome model of DNA replication (19). DNA replication in the S-phase of the cell cycle depends on the assembly of DNA replicase components at the site where the DNA/chromatin complexes are attached to the nuclear matrix. The replication machinery (i.e., replisomes) proceed to copy the DNA in a bi-directional manner, retaining a tight association of the newly replicated DNA with the nuclear matrix. In the process, the loops of DNA/chromatin are reeled out in a highly ordered assembly.

In recent times, cancer research has concentrated on the events leading to cell replication or to cell death. Prompted by the studies of cell cycle mutants in yeast, many of the steps in the replication of eukaryotic nuclei have been defined (9). In brief, cells that have been arrested in the G_1 or G_0 intervals of the cell cycle can be stimulated by a proper inductive factor to proceed through a cascade of reactions, described in Figure 2, that lead to the assembly of a DNA replicase machine at prepared chromosomal sites. Such assemblies, localized to specific sites in the chromosomal loops, have been described as clustersomes, and lie in unique associations with the nuclear matrix (Figure 3). DNA replication from such sites proceeds bi-directionally, with a long advancing strand, and the operation of a repair back type synthesis mechanism on the opposing template strand (10). The whole process involves the timely synthesis, phosphorylation, and execution of a cascade of molecular interactions of the proteins that not only carry out DNA replication, but also handle the dissembling and re-assembling of the protein associations that go into the formation and distribution of a new set of chromosomes. In 1978, a scheme (Figure 4) proposing a coupling of chromatin replication, hormone action, and the control of cell phenotype was proposed by Mueller (11).

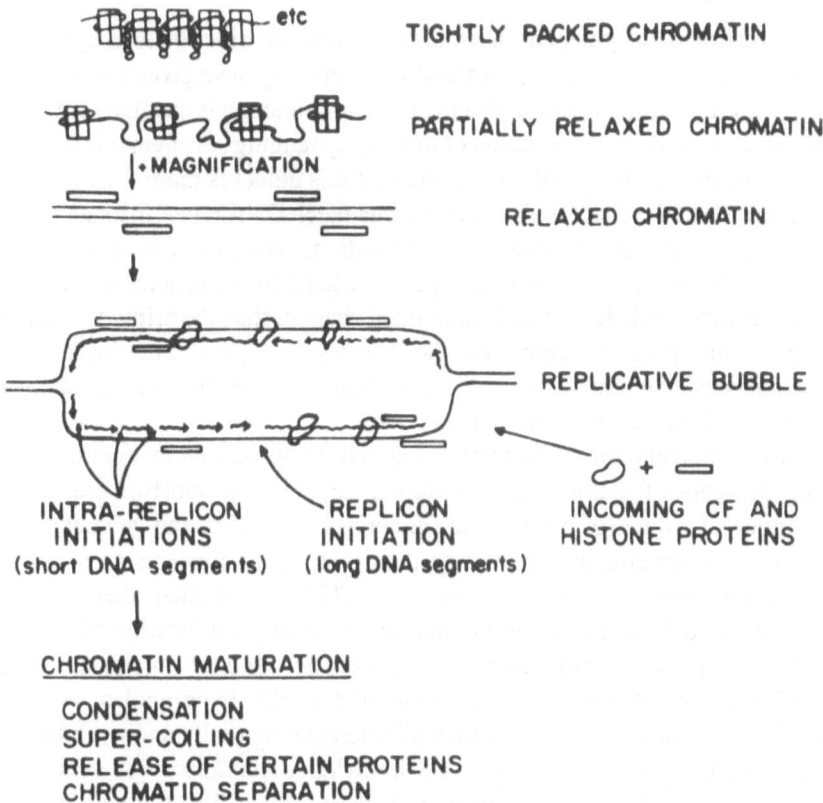

Figure 4. 1978 Model of chromatin replication (11). In the proposed scheme, the DNA, amid its chromosomal protein setting, has to be initially relaxed (i.e., freed up from certain protein associations), whereupon bi-directional DNA replication starts with the help of DNA replicase complexes. This replication process depends critically on the availability of phase specific non-histone proteins. The latter assemble on newly replicated DNA to yield an immature chromatin that has 30% more protein than mature chromatin. Maturation of the chromatin is correlated with the entry of new histones and the partial displacement of non-histones of temporary association.

The karyotypic observations that correlate wide ranging chromosomal abnormalities with malignancy, point to the likelihood that phenomena of tumor promotion and progression are more closely related to errors in the mechanics of chromosome and chromatin handling, than to errors in the actual copying of the DNA code into daughter strands. This author favors the view that cancer, particularly the progression phenomenon, reflects the malfunction of the processes which should guarantee the assembly and distribution of chromatin in the formation of daughter chromosomes, and their distribution to daughter cells. This is not to exclude that, primary coding errors may have given rise to the later aberrancy, but suggest instead that the latter malfunction is one that provides for the recruitment and accumulation of the widely ranging set of genetic errors that characterizes the malignant tumor, and that this defect is more fundamental to the outcome of the disease. Errors of the mismatch DNA repair mechanism (12), chromatin assembly, chromosome segregation, reconstitution of sub-nuclear associations, or errors of a grosser type in the handling of genetic materials may be more responsible for the truly malignant changes than the primary mutations, such as the point mutation of the Harvey *ras* gene that initiates skin carcinogenesis in the mouse model system, or provided an initial growth advantage for a factor-dependant cell.

Unfortunately, the analysis of this area is compromised by the fact, that, in spite of years of study of chromosomal and nuclear substructure, and the multitude of studies of genetic and functional replication and gene expression systems, we are still in our infancy relative to clear concepts as to how the nuclear/chromosomal system really works (13). In particular, there is a great need for solid information on the identity, function, and location of each sub-nuclear component that operates in the carrying out of normal nuclear replication and distribution of genetic material to daughter cells. In particular, we need to develop new concepts as to how they all interact temporally and work together. The new concepts emerging from such knowledge should provide a framework for understanding how genes interact in the on-going life of a cell, cancer or normal, and even more importantly, they should provide the basis for understanding the biology of organismal development. What is needed for the future of biology is a code for development as played out in embryogenesis, and the directional aspects of cell differentiation. With respect to the problem of cancer, the code should provide insights to the biological changes that accompany the accidents and errors that play a causal role in the development of malignancies and their growth. In brief, we need a four-dimensional code for development that would help us understand how genes, important to cell life and death, are coordinated to function in time and space in a manner that sustains the existence of organized cells and tissue growth. The code needs to be four-dimensional in order to provide for the three-dimensional growth of the cells plus a fourth-dimension related to time, in that it deals with the coordinated and timely expression of genes that contribute to specialization among cells with a common genome, the appearance of cells with unique phenotypes. Finally, with respect to the topic of this Symposium, the code should provide some insights as to how hormonal agents can play such powerful roles in the development of tumors, as well as the regulation of normal growth processes in both normal and tumor tissues.

To engage in this, perhaps an impossible quest, I have been called upon to review some aspects of our present knowledge of nuclear structure and function as have been established through the beautiful studies of such investigators and their associates as Sheldon Penman (14), Gordon Hager (15), Alan Wolfe (16), Jan-Ake Gustafasson (17), William Brinkley (13), Donald Coffey (18), Ronald Berenzey (19), and others. In fact, there are many more contributors to our present knowledge of sub-nuclear state and physiology than I can give proper credit here, but let me start by a consideration of the studies cited in the above references, which can lead us further.

In the first place, the best structural studies of eukaryotic nuclei point to the conclusion that the animal cell nucleus is a highly compartmentalized structure that maintains a constant communication with the cytoplasm via diffusing and/or transporting molecules. In its interphase state, the DNA of the genome is partitioned in a functionally important manner among the different chromosomes. Each chromosome, however, resides in a three-dimensionally defined region of the nucleus (20). The orientation of one chromosome with respect to each of the other chromosomes, and to other nuclear sub-structures, retains these relationships significantly through a restricted anchoring to the nuclear matrix. We know from the studies of Boulikas (21) and Bode, *et al.* (22) that such chromosomal anchoring takes place through high affinity associations of matrix/scaffold attachment regions (MARS/SARS, unique DNA sequences) with specific proteins of the nuclear matrix (19).

Each chromosome, while a linear (i.e., two-dimensional) and sequentially ordered array of genes, contains regions in which the potential for expression is structurally regulated. Thus, segments in which the chromatin is highly compacted, the heterochromatin regions, the access of polymerases and proteins that are required for transcription is severely limited, resulting in the lack of expression of the contained genes. Other sections of each chromosome possess bases that have been differentially methylated, a state which again regulates the ease of gene expression given the proper availability of other transcriptional components.

Perhaps most important to our interest in hormones is the fact that, genes of interest can exist in expressible or non-expressible states depending upon the manner that such chromosomal regions are cloaked with nucleosomes or punctuated with high mobility group (HMG) proteins (23). In this setting, the molecular processes such as phosphorylation versus dephosphorylation, acetylation versus deacetylation, can play dominant roles in the modulation of gene expression through a structural remodeling of the chromatin. Thus, we find that the acetylation of histones amid a nucleosomal array contributes to revision of such structures by a mechanism which may be implemented by such elements as steroids, other hormones, and their receptors (16, 24). Rather importantly, whether a particular protein can fit or not into a functional assembly can often depend on a strategic phosphorylation or dephosphorylation of particular amino acids amid its polypeptide structure. In fact, there is probably no more powerful regulator of the conformational state of proteins than the presence or absence of the negatively charged phosphate groups at strategic locations. Hormones, particularly the peptides, frequently exercise their effects through the activation of specific kinases. Since the functional parameters of growth are so dependant on the combined interaction of polymerases, transcription enhancing proteins, and product processing proteins, cells are almost continually the pawns of their selective states of protein phosphorylation. Thus, the control of selective or faulty phosphorylation versus dephosphorylation of the keystone proteins underlies many cellular aberrations in the expression of critical genes.

In addition to the structural localization and functional compartmentalization of the chromosomes and their component genes (20), it is important to note that the initial transcriptional products are practically always processed further by structural changes that render them transportable and ultimately, translatable as meaningful messages for the synthesis of specific proteins. Here again the sub-structure of the nucleus is nothing less than amazing. As revealed in the elegant studies of Penman, *et al.* (25), and others, we know that the RNA processing factories are distributed throughout the nucleus, and appear to be anchored at specific sites amid the nuclear matrix (Figure 5). In fact, it appears that much of the nuclear matrix, as we presently know it, is composed of RNA-protein associations that are imminently associated with the RNA processing foci which also contain proteins that are essential for message splicing and polyA tailing (14).

Combining these observations from the elegant electron microscopic studies of Penman (25) with those of Coffee (18), Berenzey (19), Brinkley (13) and many others, one can begin to see the cell nucleus is a sort of micro-universe in itself. A universe in which the chromosomes and RNA processing factories exist as constellations throughout the nuclear matrix, in situations in which the interactions between such loci are controlled, in a large part, by their relative proximity to each other and the concentrations of communicating molecules. Within these constellations, the potential for all interactions depends a great deal on the proximity of the components, the ranges of the concentrations of potential interacting macromolecules, and their conformational readiness to match a partner in the formation of a significantly functional machine. In any case, the actual affinity is a summation of all the attractive forces over the sum of repulsive forces.

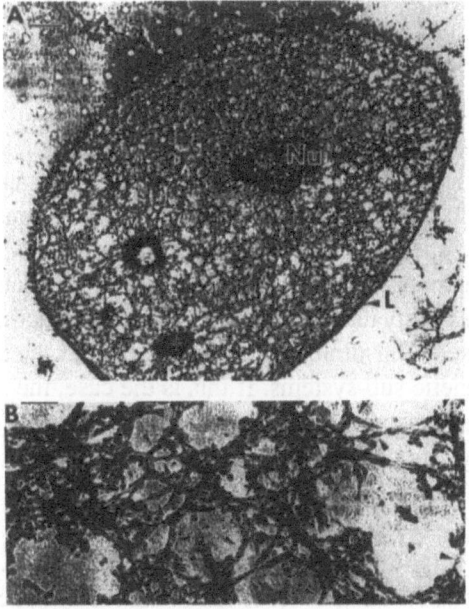

Figure 5. Ultra-structure of the nuclear matrix as revealed by resinless section electron microscopy (25). The nucleus of a Ca5Ki cell was prepared by formaldehyde cross linking and sectioning in the absence of an embedding agent. A. Low magnification reveals the nucleolite (NU), the nuclear lamina (L) and a complex net-work of ribonucleoprotein containing filaments. B. High magnification shows the filament structures to be branched and associated with subnuclear granules. Ribonucleoproteins and RNA processing machines are distributed throughout the nuclear matrix.

In addition, the force of molecular interaction when making contact, like any other mass interaction, transmits a directional impact which relates to the relative masses of the interacting molecules. Similarly, when an affinity complex breaks up by any forces facilitating diffusion, the escaping particles leave tangentially into an ion-charged aqueous environment. The latter is important in that any localized concentration of small ions can be expected to influence the breathing conformational states of the macromolecules of interest. Perhaps the best example of this influence is seen in the regulation of gene expression in the puffs of the giant chromosomes of insect salivary glands by inorganic salts.

Also, within such a substructured nucleus must lie a similar four-dimensional code of other animal cells that operates in their programmed living, developmental changes, and dying of cells on schedule. *But, how might one imagine such a code to present itself when the prime carrier of genetic informa-*

tion, with respect to sequentially dictated assembling of the ribonuclotides and amino acids in the synthesis of RNA and proteins, is contained in a linear array of DNA nucleotides? An important aspect of bridging from the linear state and synthesis of these polymers is the introduction of a time dimension into the three-dimensional structural organization of the primary genetic materials, DNA, RNA and associating proteins that are imbedded in the nuclear matrix.

The observation that the animal cell nucleus is cris-crossed by mesh of highly structured fibers with connections to the nuclear lamina (14), that provide attachment sites to specific DNA sequences in the formation of the loops of chromatin in the regionally confined compartments of each chromosome, makes one ponder the possibility that the whole system of interacting structures might be in itself the elusive four-dimensional map that codes the timed development of the different genetic sub-systems. If this is the case, the relative position of any unit (i.e., a chromosome, a chromatin loop, a gene sequence, and an RNA processing factory) should be important and be definable by distinct sets of coordinates amid the global structure of the nucleus. In brief, each gene informing the synthesis of unique cellular components would have a sub-nuclear address based on proximity or accessibility to each other. Furthermore, the success of moving an adequate level of one product from one site to another for functional interaction (i.e., such as an activator or suppressor of a specific gene transcription) could easily be expected to depend on the concentration of the macromolecule of interest, intermediate barriers, and the functional efficiency of any intranuclear or nuclear/cytoplasmic transport system that might be involved.

Thus, any abnormal translocation of a set of genes from one chromosome to another, the intranuclear migration or exchange of one chromosome or subsection with another at such sites, the acquisition or loss of a chromosome, as occurs in many malignant transformations, could be anticipated to cause imbalances in such subnuclear communication processes, and result in a significant shift in the pattern of a cell's gene expressions. If the shift favors the cascade of gene expressions leading to cell replication, a higher potential for an increased growth rate might result. A shift towards increasing the potential for apoptotic phenomena would have the opposite result.

Thus, mutations, as we know them in carcinogenesis, would impact on these relationships because they would upset the order that evolution and development had selected for. Also, any deficit in DNA repair systems (i.e., miss-match repair, excisional repair, or helicase malfunctions) as appear to be correlated with the proneness to develop cancer (7, 8), might lead to a structural revision of the nuclear intergenic controls that would give rise to a malignant cell behavior. Again, alterations which shift the balance of processes towards a higher frequency of cell replication versus those processes that lead to a higher frequency of apoptosis or cell death, would lead to tumor growth, true malignant character, however, would still lie in the cancer cell's ability to grow autonomously and to destructively attack its normal neighbors. Both aberrations of growth would likely to arise out of the same faulty nuclear processes for handling chromatin.

With respect to the role of hormones, particularly the steroid hormones, in the control of such expression mechanisms, we are particularly fortunate to have the creative efforts of Gordon Hager, *et al.* (15), and the fundamental studies of Alan Wolffe, *et al.* (16), to draw upon. Using the mouse mammary tumor virus system (MMTV) Hager, *et al.* (15) have has demonstrated that newly transfected MMTV constructs have nucleosomal structures that are not subject to regulation by glucocorticoid and progesterone receptor-mediated interactions in the same manner as are characteristic of the constructs that have undergone replication *in vivo* and have taken on the more complex chromatin structure of endogenously replicated chromatin (26, 27). Their experiments clearly demonstrate that the glucocorticoid receptors are also involved in causing changes of the nucleosomal organization that are reflected in the ability of the steroid receptors to induce the expression of these two states of transfected templates.

In a brilliant set of experiments using endogenously produced glucocorticoid receptors (GR) that have been tagged genetically as fusion proteins with the green fluorescent protein (GFP), Hager *et al.* (15), have also described changes in distribution patterns that attend the titration of GR with a ligand steroid, while they function both as modulators of gene expression and chromatin structure. In the case of the unoccupied GR, exclusively localized in the cytoplasm, however, on titration of the GR with dexamethasone, the GR translocates rapidly to the nucleus. Initially, it appears widely distributed throughout the nucleus, apparently reacting with many target sites, but ends up to be localized asymmetrically to the bottom half of the cell, near the supported surface. This finding correlates nicely with the localization of the MMTV target constructs of the transfected 3134 cells. In contrast to dexamethasone, the GR antagonist, RU486, causes the translocation of the GR to the nucleus, but fails to establish the asymmetric subnuclear distribution characteristic of the agonist. In this case, it is concluded that the GR-green fluorescent protein (GFP) appears to be distributed more broadly, by entering into nonfunctional complexes with yet unidentified macromolecular targets (15).

Using the same approaches to the study of progesterone controlled distribution of the progesterone receptor (PR), Hager *et al.* (27) have observed four separate states for this receptor: 1. Nuclear localization without association with chromatin; 2. Association with chromatin that has not undergone an activation transition; 3. Nonliganded receptors that are associated with unknown targets amid chromatin; and 4. Association of the liganded receptors with fully activated and expressible chromatin. The major partner molecules in such localizations of the PR remain to be identified. Clearly, the isolation and identification of these partners is a high priority in elucidating the events whereby PR, as well as other known receptors, effect the changes in chromatin structure that lead to an optimum expression of the contained genetic information. The clever use of the GFPs in such studies promises to make such identification possible, and thus, provide an opening wedge for prying loose some of nature's most conserved secrets. Through such studies, the molecular mechanisms by which hormones modulate the structure of chromatin to activate or inactivate the expression of specific genes will be unveiled. At hand, to assist in such transitions are the fundamental processes of phosphorylation versus dephosphorylation, acetylation versus deacetylation, and methylation versus demethylation, whose actions lead to the conformational changes in structure that guide the association or dissociation of the macromolecules that are critical components in the end states.

In a series of beautiful experiments, Wolffe *et al.* (16) have provided evidence for the mechanisms by which the thyroid hormone receptor system mediates a revision of chromatin surrounding a target gene. Their studies show clearly the dependence of the nucleosomal structure of a target gene on the timely action of acetylation and deacetylation of histones.

The involvement of hormones in the carcinogenesis process would seem to follow two action paths: 1. The stimulation of cell replication or inhibition of cell death pathways; or 2. An indirect involvement in which a hormone receptor mediates changes in chromatin structure that labilize critical regions of specific chromosomes, facilitating the occurrence of the gross genetic accidents that are associated most frequently with the progression of an initiated cell towards a more malignant phenotype (i.e., a hormone mediated genomic destabilization). As stated earlier, the events of significance for the development of cancer are those that either enhance the replication rate or decrease the probability of cell death, and with respect to host effects, changes that lead to the pathology of tissue invasion by the malignant cell.

Future Challenges

Considering the multiplicity of different genetic changes (i.e., the oncogenes) (28) that have been correlated as playing a contributory role to the cancer state, a situation that is almost matched by the identification of the alterations in the function of an increasing number of suppressor genes, one is hard pressed to visualize a single route to malignancy. Overall, however, the basic requirements for malignant growth seem to center on two classes of genetic results, mutations that tend towards accumulative growth (i.e., cell replication exceeds cell death), and mutations that favor the acquisition of invasive growth characteristics (i.e., metastatic properties). In addition, it is of considerable interest that the malignant transformation, depending on the cell phenotype of origin, often appear to reactivate genes of an earlier embryonic state (i.e., a re-ordering of the developmental relationships). This unusual array of observations prompts the view that if there is a common denominator in the array of mutations leading to cancer, it may be a malfunction that impinges functionally on the most basic requirements of organized growth, the balanced expression of genes, many genes. While recent advances in molecular genetics have shown how competitions can arise with certain limited expression systems, the more complex situations seen in the multi genic changes of cancer have defied understanding. Accordingly, it seems appropriate, at this point, to speculate as to how cells might balance their genetic expressions in a manner that sustains normal growth and development, or on disruption, leads to the growth dyscrasia called cancer.

With respect to understanding how cells balance their gene expressions, perhaps one of the greatest challenges is to elucidate mechanisms by which organismal development takes place. Starting from the catalog of genetic information contained in the fertilized zygote, development uses mechanisms that can mediate the sequential and timely activation of the genes, and thus, provide for the development of the different cell phenotypes. Such mechanisms would appear to proceed, guided by an elusive four-dimensional code that also has to be contained primarily in the linear DNA of the original primordial cell. Also, this performance must be highly exact in that it can program the development of even cloned adult organisms reproducibly. Thus, the temporal ordering of such changes requires some method of time keeping for the orderly turn on and turn off of the genes which define the specific cell phenotypes, over a full range of organized growth events.

This code clearly has to reside and retain activity in each individual cell. It has to account for the timely activation and distribution of cell functions that relate to a cell's phenotype, irrespective of when the demand occurs relative to embryonic development. While some of the elements involved in the code initially may well be changed as the cell phenotype specification takes place (i.e., loss of specific chromosomes in insect development or formation of mini or giant chromosomes), the structural remnants of the code have to persist and operate throughout the life of each cell. This situation erects a very fundamental requirement, the need for of a master grid in the temporal activation or repression of potentially expressible genes in accord with cell phenotypes specification. To this end, one can postulate that all animal cells operate with at least two classes of genes: 1. The first class of genes are those that provide the basic mechanisms of life (i.e., chemical energy derivation from food products, the synthesis of DNA, RNA, proteins, carbohydrates, and the lipids common to all cells, and basic mechanisms of transport related to the maintenance of a cell in its environmental setting). This first class of genes also includes genes that inform for the common processes of post-synthetic modification of some macromolecular components, such processes as methylation, acetylation, phosphorylation, and protein degradation. 2. The second class of genes are those that provide the unique properties of a cell, and account for any specialized functions. In this class of genes we have genes that are, in most instances, not necessarily essential for the life of the cell itself, but whose expression provides some product or function that is essential for the life and normal function of neighboring cells such as exist in structure of any organ. Whereas the first class of genes (i.e., the housekeeping genes) are essential in all cells, just to stay alive in hostile environments, the second class of genes provide for the variations in cellular life forms that arise as nature has partitioned the specialized functions among the different cell types of a multi-cellular organism. These are the genes that are involved in setting the nature of the mitogenic stimulus required for cell replication, and the ground rules for apoptosis onset.

In development, it is the second class of genes for which nature especially has the need for a four-dimensional code, required to achieve the degree of orderly growth and function characteristic of multicellular, multi organ life forms. While the four-dimensional code is most important for development, also, it clearly provides the mechanisms for balancing the expression of both classes of genes throughout a cell's life.

As intimated above, this scientist feels that each zygote cell, and each surviving progeny cell in a developing organism contains the fundamental mechanism for programming the meaningful chain of developmental changes that evolution has selected over time. While other subcellular components may play important roles in the periodic operation of the whole system, it appears that the source of order resides structurally within the eukaryotic nucleus. The nuclear matrix is by far the best candidate for providing the required spatial and temporal partitioning of different genetic potentials. This sponge-like mesh appears to have a structural stability, while still likely subject to many perturbations of the physical components (i.e., ribonucleoproteins, chromosomal scaffolding proteins, and the existence of specific and site localized RNA processing machines), nonetheless, this maze appears sufficiently stable to harbor and provide the Rosetta stone for development.

To hypothesize a strategy in which nature might use the nuclear matrix to program development, one needs to first postulate that the distribution of the genes belonging to the second class are localized in the nuclear matrix in a manner that bears a structural relationship to the temporal patterns of their expression. A pattern in which diffusible macromolecules, essential to the expression of these genes, have to overcome concentration limitations imposed by intranuclear diffusion distances or competing opportunities for sequestration in order to activate the genes of interest. In this postulation the localization of particular gene sets relative to each other becomes important for the ordering process.

In addition, it appears likely that nature must have evolved a class of macromolecules that possess sufficient virtuosity in presenting a proper interactive surface topology for targeting. Accordingly, the relative concentrations and proximity of such a group of macromolecules might guide the assembly of structurally distinct macromolecular complexes for the temporal regulation of specific gene expressions. Considering the range of macromolecules, the most likely candidate molecule for such a role is single stranded RNA. Not only is this macromolecule able to enter into a tremendous range of base-pairing combinations with DNA and RNA molecules, but because of its flexibility, it can fold and internally base pair in a manner that provides a fantastic potential for the generation of complementary structures that like antibodies, can complex proteins. In this connection, it should be noted that the 10-13 nm filaments that make up the nuclear matrix consist of RNA/protein complexes, as yet undefined (14).

RNA's have an added qualification, the capacity for self-modification, as evidenced in ribozymes. Finally, single-stranded RNA is easily cleaved into fragments that could still contain potential recognition sequences, which would be capable of physically moving more easily from one site to another, for the formation of molecular complexes with other targets. Accordingly, it is proposed that RNA's and selected fragments, produced in distinct and localized compartments within the nuclear matrix, are the functional components that mediate the fourth-dimension of the genetic code for development. This material would appear to be the only substance, which produced in regulated amounts at restricted nuclear matrix sites, would have the marvelous functional virtuosity and adaptability for recognizing other genetic polymers via base pairing or by folding internally into three-dimensional polymers capable of the topological recognition of proteins involved in sequential gene activation and expression. This virtuosity places RNA in position to play the dominant role as an intranuclear communicator in the ordering of timed gene expressions.

Figure 6 attempts to summarize the major aspects of the hypothesis being set forth as an explanation of how the development and maintenance of organized growth patterns among the cells of multicellular systems operate. First, it is proposed that each chromosome (and thus each chromatin loop or cluster of genes) resides at a specific location within the globular nuclear matrix. In this situation, each subunit of genetic material is anchored in a nuclear space in a fixed relationship to each other. Their relative positions could be defined by subnuclear coordinates. As a result, the potential for interaction of products from one gene site with a targetable component at another site would be determined in part by the proximity of the sites to each other. Diffusion and intranuclear transport should figure prominently in the system. In addition, the concentration of an interacting molecule would be important in such events.

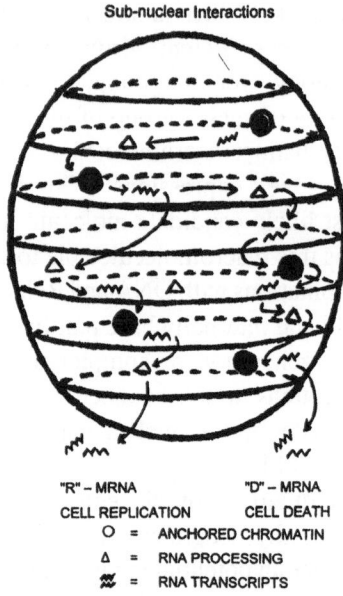

Figure 6. Hypothetical description of sub-nuclear interaction. An animal cell nucleus is depicted as containing chromatin which is anchored to specific sites in the nuclear matrix. The products of transcription move to RNA processing sites from which the modified RNA species can translocate to distant loci where they may target another gene expression complex. For example, such interactions can be competitively directed to emphasize the expression of genes leading to cell replication or events in the cell death pathway.

In Figure 6, single-stranded RNA is postulated as being the primary regulator or communicator. A subfragment of RNA containing the necessary recognition sequences for base pairing with DNA or another RNA, or a tertiary structure capable of forming a complex with a specific protein could also be so involved. Whatever the target, the important point is that the target must play a role in the timely expression of a gene of interest in cell phenotype maintenance.

It is also postulated that nature, through time, has selected constellations in which the hierarchy of interactions has given rise to patterns of balanced gene expressions that give rise to the specialized cell phenotypes that make up organized and functional tissues. Each case is a reproducibly balanced system, arising from and perpetuated by the spatial structure of the genetic sources within the nuclear matrix, and the unique properties of single-stranded RNA molecules as gene products and as communicators between gene sites.

In this hypothetical portrayal, it is visualized that any genetic mistake that disrupts or alters the nuclear matrix relationships, among genes involved in timed events, would also alter the successful balance of other important gene expressions that nature has selected for in each cell or species over time.

When the altered balances lead to an increased probability of triggering cell replication, or when the new state is one of decreased apoptosis, one has the essentials of a malignant state. How malignant the state really is depends on what additional genes have been activated or inactivated that lead to the expression of tissue-invasive pathology. While a single mutation can give a cell a growth advantage and set it on a course towards a malignant state, it is the deranged stability of the whole genetic system that contributes to the progression of the cell to a more malignant state, a state that ends in the recruitment and selection of the multiple mutations that characterize the particular resulting phenotype of the malignant cells. Thus, one can have many routes to cancer, all initiated and promoted through mutations that disrupt the order in gene balances set by evolution in the establishment of each cell phenotype.

Future Research Strategies to Deal with Hormonal Carcinogenesis and Associated Malignancies

1. A much greater understanding of the structural components and functional interactions of the nuclear matrix is required. Just as in the case of the massive celestial universe, we must define the locations and concentrations of the components making up the subnuclear universe. There is a need to establish meaningful coordinates for understanding the probabilities of their interactions. The work of Hager et al.(15), using green-fluorescent-labeled hormone receptors to provide an on-line record of localized and targeted interactions, provides a model of the kind of studies that are needed. The use of this labeling strategy must be expanded and applied to many of the other proteins that make up the cell nucleus, particularly the ones playing a role in cell phenotype specification. The strategic labeling of the proteins such as the chromosomal scaffold and the RNA processing enzymes are examples of entities whose location and variations thereof need to be understood.

With respect to the genes belonging to the second class and accounting for the specification of cell phenotype, we need to apply such strategies for identifying their activating associates. The invention of new technology for extending such studies should be among our highest priorities.

2. Since aberrations in chromosome mechanics and the processes that lead to abnormal fragments or their errant distributions are so closely tied to tumor progression, we are in desperate need to identify the mechanism and targets

involved in such changes. The usual range of genetic engineering techniques should be aimed at exposing the roles of each such component.

3. The prevention of malignancy is clearly of importance and it can be approached by the elimination of environmental hazards (i.e., carcinogenic chemicals, genotoxic drugs, ionizing radiation, food toxins, and exogenous hormonal mimics). However, it is doubtful whether such measures will have much impact on the endogenous hazards associated with aging.

4. In the direction of dealing with human malignancies as they present themselves from any background, a much greater effort should be made to use such agents as hormones or their antagonists to selectively shift or stage the genetic expression products of the malignancies, in a manner that would be useful for a secondary directing of ablative therapies to the tumor tissue. It should be possible to re-direct many gene expression patterns of many genes through the synthesis and delivery of molecules that recognize and mimic the topology of critical interaction sites. Even without a total elimination of tumors, it should be possible to reduce the pathology and contribute to the useful life state of the cancer patient. Some exciting ideas are surfacing in this area for application, even without understanding the full dimensions of the malignant state.

Finally

We Must Learn to Think Like Astro-physicists in the Micro-universe of the Cell Nucleus.

Acknowledgments

The author wishes to thank Ms. Kristen Adler and Ms. Mary Jo Markham for their wonderful help in the preparation of this manuscript. The author is also especially grateful to Dr. Gerald Sattler whose expertise in photography made the preparations of slides and figures a reality. Finally, thanks to the McArdle Laboratory for tolerating an emeritus professor.

References

1. Fusenig NE, Petrusevska RT, Pohlman N (1988) Spontaneous and phorbol ester induced chromosomal alterations in normal and transformed mouse keratinocytes in culture. In: Langenbach R (ed) Tumor promoters: Biological approaches for mechanistic studies and assay systems. Raven Press, New York, pp. 259-273.

2. Mischak H, Goodnight J, Kolch W et al (1993) Overexpression of protein kinase C (delta and epsilon) in NIH 3T3 cells induces opposite effects on growth, morphology, anchorage dependence and tumorigenicity. J Biol Chem 268:6090-6096.

3. Furth J (1953) Conditional and autonomous neoplasms: a review. Cancer Res 13:477-492.

4. Furth J, Clifton KH, Gadsden El et al (1956) Dependent and mammotropic pituitary tumors in rats; their somatropic features. Cancer Res 16:608-616.

5. Kirschbaum A (1957) The role of hormones in cancer: laboratory animals. Cancer Res 17:432-453.

6. Clifton KH (1959) Problems in experimental tumorigenesis of pituitary gland, gonads, adrenal cortices and mammary glands: A review. Cancer Res 19:2-22.

7. Fearon ER, Vogelstein BA (1990) Genetic model for colorectal tumorigenesis. Cell 61:759-767.

8. Loeb LA (1994) Microsatellite instability: Marker of a mutator phenotype in cancer. Cancer Res 54:5059-5063.

9. Martin-Castellanos C, Moreno S (1997) Recent advances on cyclins, cdks and cdk inhibitors. Trends Cell Biol 7:95-98.

10. Dijkwel PA, Hamlin JL (1995) Origins of replication and the nuclear matrix: the DHFR domain as a paradigm. In: Berenzney R, Jeon KW (eds) Nuclear matrix. Academic Press, New York, pp. 455-484.

11. Mueller GC, Kajiwara K, Kim NH et al (1978) Proposed coupling of chromatin replications, hormone action and cell differentiation. Cancer Res 38:4041-4045.

12. Prolla TA (1998) DNA mismatch repair in cancer. Curr Opin Cell Biol 10:311-322.

13. He D, Zeng C, Brinkley BR (1995) Nuclear matrix proteins as structural and functional components of the mitotic apparatus. In: Berezney R, Jeon KW (eds) Nuclear matrix, Part B. Academic Press, New York, pp. 1-74.

14. Penman S (1995) Rethinking cell structure. Proc Natl Acad Sci USA 92:5251-5257.

15. Hager GL, Smith CL, Fragoso G et al (1998) Intranuclear trafficking and gene targeting by members of the steroid/nuclear receptor superfamily. J Steroid Biochem Molec Biol 65:125-132.

16. Wong J, Patterton D, Imhof A et al (1998) Distinct requirements for chromatin assembly in transcriptional repression by thyroid hormone receptor and histone deacetylase. EMBO J 17:520-534.

17. McEwan LJ, Wright APH, Gustafsson JA (1997) Mechanism of gene expression by the glucocorticoid receptor: Role of protein-protein interactions. BioEssays 19:153-160.

18. Berezney R, Coffee DS (1976) The nuclear protein matrix: isolation, structure and functions. In: Weber G (ed) Advances in enzyme regulation. Pergammon Press, New York, vol.14, pp. 63-100.

19. Berezney R, Mortillaro MJ, Ma H et al (1995) The nuclear matrix: a structural milieu for genomic function. In: Berezney R, Jeon KW (eds) Nuclear matrix, Part A. Academic Press, New York, pp. 1-65.

20. Belmont AS, Straight AF (1998) In vivo visualization of chromosomes using lac operator-repressor binding. Trends Cell Biol 8:121-24.

21. Boulikas T (1995) Chromatin domains and predictions of MAR sequences. In: Berezney R, Jeon KW (eds) Nuclear matrix. Academic Press, New York, pp. 279-388.

22. Bode J, Schlake T, Rios-Ramirez M et al (1995) Scaffold/Matrix-attached regions: structural properties creating transcriptionally active loci. In: Berezney R, Jeon KW (eds) Nuclear matrix. Academic Press, New York, pp. 389-454.

23. Ghidelli S, Claus P, Thies G et al (1997) High mobility group proteins cHMB1a, cHMG1b and cHMG1 are distinctly distributed in chromosomes and differentially expressed during ecdysone dependent cell differentiation. Chromosome 105:369-379.

24. Varga-Weisz PD, Becker PB (1998) Chromatin-remodeling factors: Machines that regulate? Curr Opin Cell Biol 10:346-353.

25. Nickerson JA, Krockmalnic G, Wan KM et al (1997) Nuclear matrix revealed by eluting chromatin from a cross-linked nucleus. Proc Natl Acad Sci USA 94:4446-4450.

26. Smith CL, Hager GL (1997) Transcriptional regulation of mammalian genes in vivo: a tale of two templates. J Biol Chem 272:27493-27496.

27. Smith CL, Htun H, Wolford RG (1997) Differential activity of progesterone and glucocorticoid receptors on mouse mammary tumor virus templates differing in chromatin structure. J Biol Chem 272: 14227-14135.

28. Schwab M (1998) Amplification of oncogenes in human cancer cells. BioEssays 20:473-479.

STATE OF THE ART LECTURES

1

The Numbers Game with Estrogen Receptors and Growth Regulation

Jack Gorski, Tae-Yon Chun, and Douglas Wendell

Introduction

It is apparent that estrogens (Es) differentially regulate cell growth compared to other physiological end points such as the induction of specific gene expression. The hypersensitivity of growth to Es is especially critical in human breast cancer where it has long been known that post menopausal patients, whose normal reproductive function has ceased, still respond to endocrine ablation or antiestrogen therapies. This differential sensitivity of growth implies that most of the current studies of E action that examine the regulation of specific gene inductions may not be pertinent to understanding growth regulation. We would like to discuss some work with a system that illustrates these differential effects of E, and in turn raises some interesting questions about numbers in relation to the estrogen receptor (ER).

The numbers game has been played with the ER since the 1960s when the first biochemical characterization of the ER was made. We determined the number of receptors per cell and the affinity of the estrogenic ligands for the ER and were pleased to find that the results fit our theoretical models based on the physiological concentrations of Es found in most mammalian vascular systems (1). These values of ~20,000 ER/cell in the rat uterus and the equilibrium dissociation constants of ~10^{-9} to 10^{-10} M for ~17β-estradiol (E$_2$) or diethylstilbestrol (DES) have remained relatively unchanged with some variations among various cell types and methods of measurement.

Quantitative measurements of the response to E were less satisfactory because much of the earlier literature dealt with *in-vivo* experiments. In these studies, the amount of E reaching the cells was difficult to ascertain. With the development of organ and cell culture systems in the 1970s and 1980s, studies of specific E-induced responses provided results that were quantitatively appropriate for the ER as it had been previously characterized. Thus, induction of the progesterone receptor (PR) by 1 to 10 nM E_2 was within the range of E_2 equilibrium affinity for the ER (2).

In the 1980s, we first saw data concerning the E regulation of growth of target cells, and the results were both startling and intriguing. It should be noted that before the landmark observations of the Katzenellenbogen's (3) on the estrogenicity of the phenol red dye, a pH indicator, in cell culture media, the E induction of the growth of cultured cells was not detectable. It appeared that the small amount of E activity contributed by the phenol red dye maximally stimulated growth and hence additional E had no effect. It is important to note, however, that other responses such as inductions of specific gene expression had been observed in the presence of phenol red. Welshons in V.C. Jordan's lab reported an E dose response curve of MCF-7 cell growth in phenol red free medium (4). The one-half maximal growth occurred at 10^{-12} M or lower E_2. Similarly, Soto and Sonnenschein (5) reported that half maximal growth of their MCF-7 cells occurred at 10^{-14} M E_2. It was not clear in these studies whether the cells were just generally more responsive or whether growth differed in some way from other E responses. Recently, we examined a new cell line, PR1 cells which are derived from a pituitary tumor found in Fischer 344 rats (F344). Growth regulation in this cell line is clearly differentiated from E induction of prolactin gene expression and subsequent prolactin secretion, which is the principal physiological function of these cells.

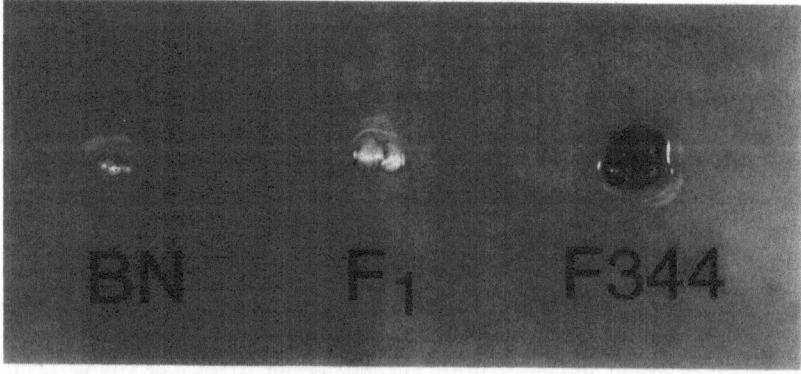

Figure 1. Strain-dependent effects of DES treatment on rat pituitaries. Representative pituitaries of DES-treated BN, F344, and their F1 hybrid. Reprinted by permission of PNAS and the authors (17).

Figure 1 displays the pituitary glands from two inbred strains of rat treated with E for 10 weeks; F344 which develop tumors, with E treatment, Brown Norway (BN) which do not develop tumors and the F1 cross of the two strains which develop intermediate size tumors. Other laboratory rat strains, such as Holtzman, which we used in earlier studies, do not develop tumors either. DeNicola (6) showed that this tumor induction was due specifically to the proliferation of prolactin producing lactotrope cells. Investigations by Wiklund (7) showed that these tumors were directly regulated by E when the pituitary was transplanted to the kidney capsule of either F344 or crossbred females (F344/Holtzman). As illustrated in Figure 2, further studies indicated that the tumors were due to a failure of some normal control mechanism that turns off DNA synthesis even in the presence of E while still controlling prolactin gene expression (8). The similarity that this pituitary tumor system has to human breast tumors is exemplified by the fact that removal of E from the F344 rats results in a dramatic decrease in size and DNA content of the pituitary tumor within one week (8).

Because tumor development is strain specific, we have used genetic approaches to gather additional information about the E induction of this tumor. Wiklund. *et al.* (9) showed, through the use of breeding experiments, that a limited number of genes, but more than one were probably involved in the differential response of the 344 rats to E. Recently, Wendell and Gorski (10) used newer genetic marker approaches to show that there are five genetic loci on four chromosomes that accounted for approximately 5% of the genetic variation between the F344 and BN strains in their pituitary growth response to E (Figure 3). A single loci accounted for over 20% of the genetic variation in growth. These genetic sites still represent large segments of DNA, and at present it is still not possible to identify the specific genes involved. It is possible to state that the two ER genes, α and β, are not involved because their chromosomal location eliminates this possibility. These observations do show that the unregulated growth response to E is surprisingly complex and not the result of a single mutated gene.

The F344 rat pituitaries have been the source of several E responsive cell lines. Best known are the GH cell lines established some time ago from a radiation induced pituitary tumor. GH3 and GH4C1 cells appear to be derived from a somatotrope/lactotrope stem cell, and thus produce both growth hormone and prolactin (11, 12). Prolactin production is stimulated by E in these cells as its growth, but the responses are variable, depending on the strain of cells studied.

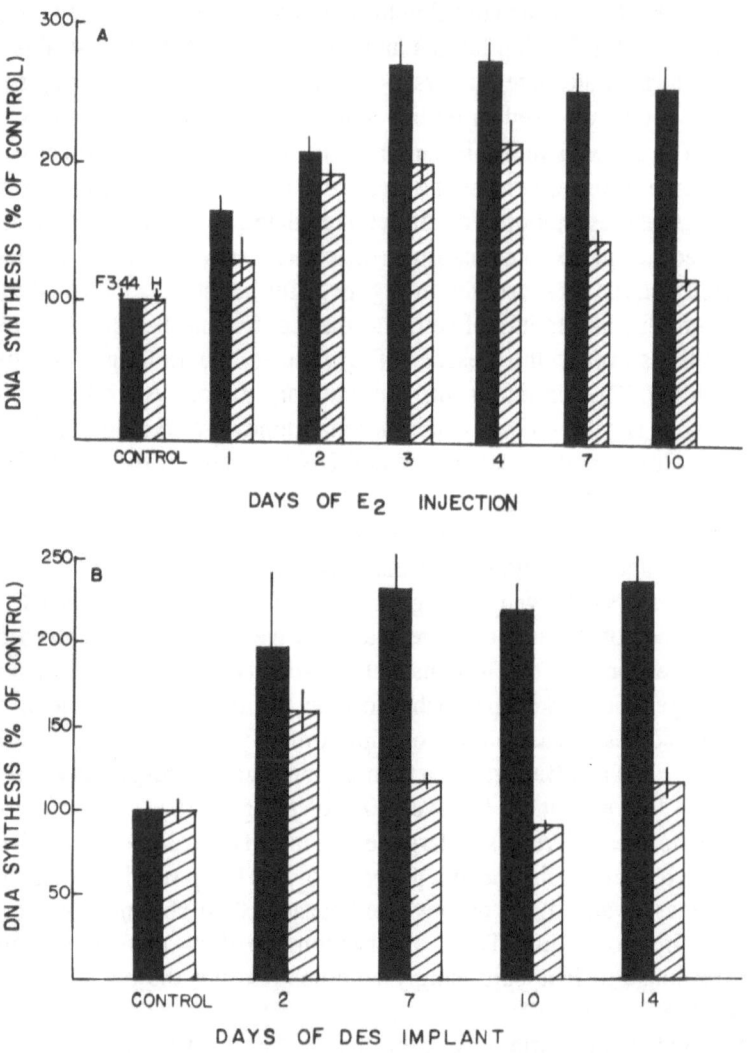

Figure 2. Comparison of pituitary weight gain (A) and DNA synthesis (B) in F1 hybrids and F344 and Holtzman parental strains after daily E treatment. Male rats (42-49 days of age) were given daily sc injections of 10 mg E_2 in sesame oil. Male F1 animals from three separate litters were distributed equally to the different treatment groups. DNA synthesis determinations represent the mean ± SEM of two groups of animals (three animals/group). Pituitary weights represent the mean ± SEM of six pituitaries. Reprinted by permission from The Endocrine Society and the authors (8).

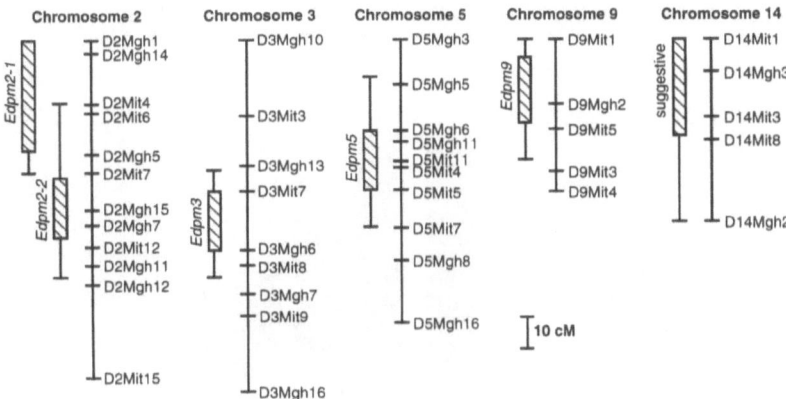

Figure 3. Quantitative trait loci (QTL) for E-dependent pituitary tumor growth. The trait of tumor mass, in log10 (mg), of female rats treated with DES for 10 weeks was mapped in a F2 intercross of F344 and BN. 1-LOD support intervals of Edpm (E-dependent pituitary mass) loci are indicated by rectangles with extended lines indicating the 2-LOD support interval. All Edpm QTL have LOD scores with genome-wide significance by the criteria of Lander and Kruglyk (16). Reprinted by permission from Mamm Genome and the authors (10).

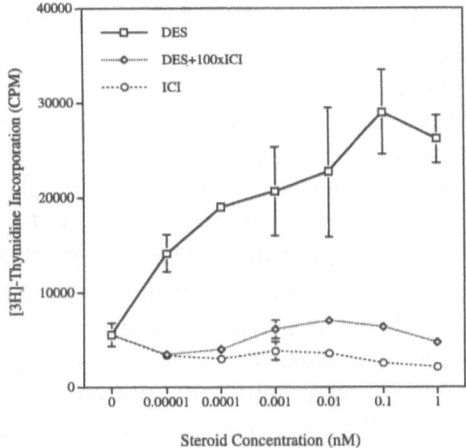

Figure 4. DES, ICI, and DES + 100-fold ICI dose responses of PR1 cell growth. Each point is the mean ± SD of quadruplicate samples. Reprinted by permission from PNAS and the authors (4).

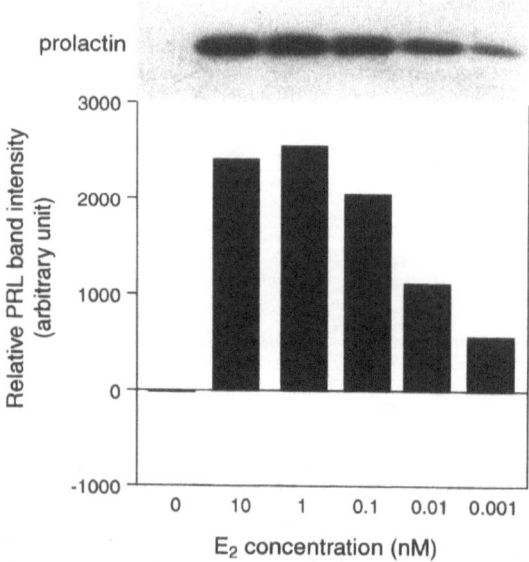

Figure 5. E_2 dose response of intracellular PRL expression using Western blot analysis. Reprinted by permission from PNAS and the authors (16).

More recently, Sarkar (13) developed what appears to be a pure lactotrope cell line, designated PR1, from E-induced F344 tumors. Using these cells, Chun, *et al.* (14), showed that their growth response to Es was hypersensitive (Figure 4). Both E_2 and DES showed one-half maximal growth response at approximately 10 fM (10^{-14} M); whereas prolactin synthesis required 1000 times more E for half maximal induction (Figure 5). Additional studies using the pure antiestrogen ICI 182,780 indicated that inhibition of growth required considerably more antiestrogen than was necessary to inhibit prolactin production (Figure 6). This suggests that only a small number of ER sites need to be occupied by an active E to control growth whereas a greater number of sites need to be occupied to induce prolactin gene expression. E binding in these cells is shown in Figure 7 and indicates that their E binding characteristics are similar to those seen in other cells with one-half maximal binding at approximately 10^{-10} or 10^{-11} M E_2. This is similar to the concentration of E required to induce prolactin production. Immunoblotting studies indicate that the ER form present in these cells is ER-α, not ER-β.

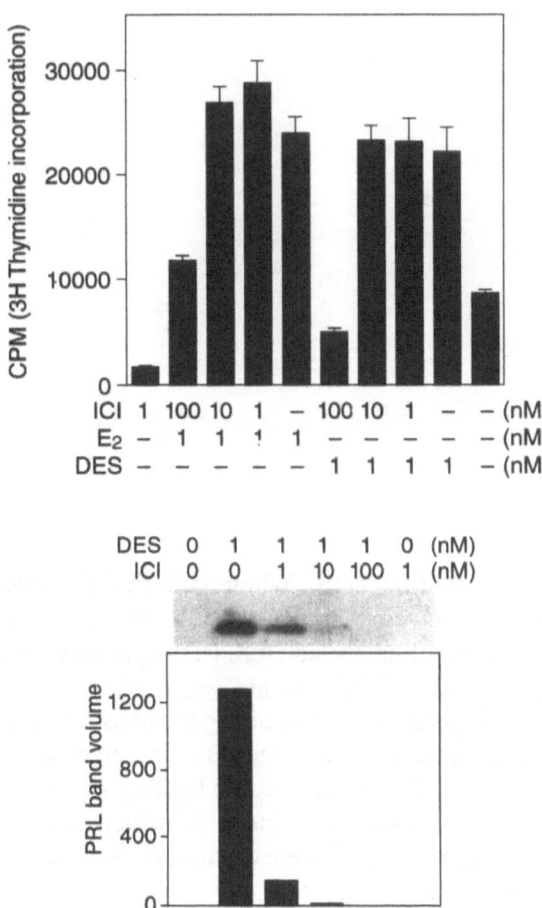

Figure 6. Differential effects of E on PRL expression and cell proliferation. PR1 cells were incubated with either 1 nM of E_2 or DES alone, or with 1-, 10-, or 100-fold more ICI. (A) [^{3}H]-Thymidine incorporation (mean ± SD of quadruplicate samples) and (B) secreted PRL were analyzed. Solid line, no addition. One repesentative data of three. Reprinted by permission from PNAS and the authors (14).

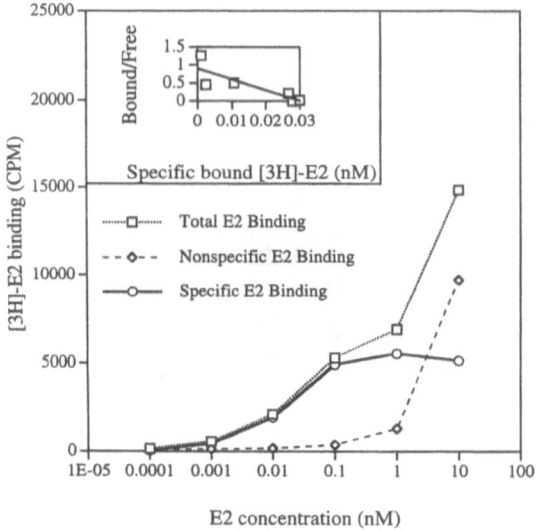

Figure 7. E_2 binding in PR1 cells. Whole cell [^{3}H]-E_2 uptake assay was performed. Cells were allowed to bind increasing concentrations of [^{3}H]-E_2 or [^{3}H]-E_2 + 100-fold excess of unlabeled DES. [^{3}H]-E_2 counts were used as total binding and [^{3}H]-E_2 + 100-fold DES counts were used as nonspecific binding. Specific binding was calculated by subtracting the nonspecific count from the total count. The binding data were run in the EBDA program to calculate Kd and Bmax. The binding curve shows that specific binding was saturable, whereas total and nonspecific binding were not. (Inset) Scatchard plot. By using Bmax, the total number of ER in PR1 cells were calculated. Reprinted by permission from PNAS and the authors (14).

What do these numbers mean? Table 1 presents estimated ER occupancy with the different concentrations of E in the culture media required to either stimulate cell growth or prolactin synthesis. Estimates of receptor occupancy are based on the E binding characteristics observed in this study. Clearly, growth regulation requires fewer occupied receptors than does the induction of prolactin gene expression. It was surprising that such an extremely low number of occupied receptors were sufficient to induce growth of these cells. It should be noted that human breast cancer cells (MCF-7) respond to similar doses of E (4, 15). This small number of binding sites raises a number of questions about E action. *Could there be still another ER with a much higher affinity for E?* While this is possible because a small pool of ER could easily be lost in studies of E binding as currently carried out, it seems unlikely because of the pharmacological characteristics of the growth response. E and antiestrogen specificity suggest that the characteristics of the response are most similar to that of ER-α.

Table 1. E response numbers*. Reprinted by permission from PNAS and the authors (14).

E$_2$ (M)	10^{-9}	10^{-11}	10^{-12}	10^{-14}
E$_2$-occupied ER/Cell	30000	15000	3000	30
PRL synthesis (%)	100	50	10	0
Growth (%)	100	100	90	50

* The total number of ER/PR1 cells is approximately 30,000.

A more likely possibility is that some other cell component with a very high affinity (approximately 10^{-12} M) for occupied ER exists and that this component when complexed with ER in some way regulates growth. At the present time no candidate for this other component has been identified. A specific DNA segment or estrogen response element (ERE) with an extremely high affinity for the ER is only a remote possibility because the vittelogenin response element which has an affinity for the ER of about 10^{-10} M is the highest affinity ERE identified to date. There are many components of cell replication and cell cycle systems which could be involved, but to date most reports of E effects on such systems occur only at much higher E concentrations than we have found to be involved in growth regulation. Also, there have been a number of reports of so-called coactivators and corepressors that are associated with the ER that might be involved with the ER in growth regulation. However, there is little or no quantitative information about the characteristics of these interactions with the ER to suggest that they have high enough affinity to explain the hypersensitivity of growth.

A question that relates to the other side of this numbers problem is, *Why does prolactin gene induction require 15,000 occupied receptors for one-half maximal stimulation?* If there is only one prolactin promoter in the genome containing one to three EREs, then there is little room for more than a small number of receptors to be associated with this DNA segment. This may just represent an equilibrium issue with a requirement for a certain concentration of ER to obtain the one-half saturation of the ERE. If this is true, it leaves open the question of the function of the other 14,900+ occupied receptors. We do know that they are all tightly bound to the nucleus and in a different physical state than the unoccupied receptors.

Another question concerns the state of the ER. Most work has indicated that ER are found as dimers in solution. It is not clear as to the state of the ER in intact cells. If ER-α is the receptor involved in growth, at 1% occupancy of E binding sites, one would predict that only 0.01% of dimeric receptors would have both receptor sites occupied. This is based on the assumption that each site would have an equal chance to bind the ligand. If there was cooperativity of binding in which the binding of one site caused a change in a second site to increase its affinity then a higher number of occupied dimers might occur. However, although cooperativity of E binding has been observed in cell free systems, no such cooperativity has been observed in intact cells (2). One can devise models in which only one member of a dimer pair can be occupied to give full biological activity. These models shift the response curve to the left or make it more sensitive but not more than 10-fold at the lower dose range. We have not observed such curves nor the steeper slope associated with them. We believe that the data are most compatible with a model in which the ER is functionally a monomer.

Most recent work on steroid hormone action has concerned specific gene expression. In most of these cases the doses of steroid used are at the higher end of the dose response curves. We question whether such studies will help elucidate how Es regulate growth at the extremely small doses have been observed. Perhaps thinking about regulation of growth as a separate phenomenon is the best way to approach this problem at the present time.

This means more work needs to be carried out in growth systems that reflect these low dose responses. More consideration should be given to different models such as tthe one proposed by Sonneschein and Soto (5) in which E is proposed to stimulate growth by removing the growth inhibitory effects of serum albumin. It is also of interest whether some of the developmental effects of Es, which are in many cases irreversible, are regulated in a similar way to growth or to specific gene expression. Since it is not even clear that known ERs are implicated in the hypersensitive growth response or whether other molecules must be involved, it is clear that considerably more work is required to reveal the underlying truths as to how Es regulate cell growth.

References

1. Gorski J, Toft D, Shyamala G et al (1968) Hormone receptors: Studies on the interaction of estrogen with the uterus. Recent Prog Hormone Res 24:45-80.
2. Kassis JA, Walent JH, Gorski J (1986) Estrogen receptors in cultured rat uterine cells: Induction of progesterone receptors in the absence of estrogen receptor processing. Endocrinology 118:603-608.

3.   Berthois Y, Katzenellenbogen JA, Katzenellenbogen BS (1986) Phenol red in tissue culture media is a weak estrogen: implications concerning the study of estrogen-responsive cells in culture. Proc Natl Acad Sci 82: 2496-2500.
4.   Welshons W, Jordan C (1987) Adaptation of estrogen -dependent MCF-7 cells to low estrogen (phenol red-free) culture. Eur J Cancer Clin Oncol 23:1935-1939.
5.   Soto AM, Sonnenschein C (1985) The role of estrogens on the proliferation of human breast tumor cells (MCF-7). J Steroid Biochem 23: 87-94.
6.   DeNicola AF, von Lawzewitsch I, Kaplan SE et al (1978) Biochemical and ultrastructural studies on estrogen-induced pituitary tumors in F344 rats. J Natl Cancer Inst 61:753-763.
7.   Wiklund J,Wertz N, Gorski J (1981) A comparison of estrogen effects on uterine growth and pituitary growth and prolactin synthesis in F344 and Holtzman rats. Endocrinology 109:1700-1707.
8.   Wiklund, J, Gorski J (1982) Genetic differences in estrogen induced DNA synthesis in the rat pituitary: Correlations with pituitary tumor susceptibility. Endocrinology 111:1140-1149.
9.   Wiklund J, Rutledge J, Gorski J (1981) A genetic model for the inheritance of pituitary tumor susceptibility in F344 rats. Endocrinology 109:1708-1714.
10.   Wendell DL, Gorski J (1997) Quantitative trait loci for estrogen-dependent pituitary tumor growth in the rat. Mamm Genome 8:823-829.
11.   Tashjian AH, Hinkle PM, Dannies PS (1979) Endocrinology 1979 ed. Scow, R.O. (Excerpta Medica, Amsterdam) pp.648-665.
12.   Scammell JG, Burrage TG, Dannies PS (1986) Hormonal induction of secretory granules in a pituitary tumor cell line. Endocrinology 119:1543-1548.
13.   Sarkar DK, Kim KH, Minami S (1992) Transforming growth factor-beta 1 messenger RNA and protein expression in the pituitary gland: its action on prolactin secretion and lactotropic growth. Mol Endocrinol 6:1825-1833.
14.   Chun T, Gregg D, Sarkar D et al (1998) Differential regulation by estrogens of growth and prolactin synthesis in pituitary cells suggest that only a small pool of estrogen receptors is required for growth. Proc Natl Acad Sci 95:2325-2330.
15.   Sonnenschein C, Szelei J, Nye T et al (1994) Control of cell proliferation of human breast MCF-7 cells; Serum and estrogen Resistant Variants. Oncol Research 6:373-381.

16. Lander ES, Kruglyk L (1995) Genetic dissection of complex traits: guidelines for interpreting and reporting linkage results. Nature Genet 11:241-247.

17. Wendell DL, Herman A, Gorski J (1996) Genetic separation of tumor growth and hemmorragic phenotypes in an estrogen-induced tumor. Proc Natl Acad Sci USA 93:8112-8116.

2

Expression Genetics of Hormone Dependent Human Tumors

Arthur B. Pardee, Heide L. Ford, Debajit K. Biswas, Katherine J. Martin, and Ruth Sager

> *"Expression genetics is a conceptually different approach to the identification of cancer-related genes than the search for mutations at the genomic level. ...Cancer geneticists have... ignored the productive potential of examining downstream events based on screening for differential gene expression."* R. Sager, 1997

Proliferation of some cells in organs such as prostate, breast, and ovary is stimulated by hormones. The hormones function by binding to their receptors, thereby activating them to form complexes with other proteins. These complexes bind to response elements in DNA promoter regions and activate transcriptions of target downstream genes. For example androgen binds to the androgen receptor (AR) which then binds to the androgen response element (ARE) and activates transcription of a set of genes including prostate specific antigen (PSA). Growth of some tumors is hormone dependent, like the hormone dependent normal cells from which they were derived. But other tumors are hormone-unresponsive. For example, prostate tumors initially often are hormone dependent and respond to treatments based on drugs that block androgen production and function. But these tumors progress to develop hormone independence. About half of breast tumors are stimulated by estrogen (E) and the others are not. This property can be correlated in general with presence or absence, respectively, of the estrogen receptor (ER) (1, 2). But about 40% of ER-positive breast tumors are not affected by E or antiestrogens such as Tamoxifen, thereby posing a serious clinical problem.

Why should we discuss hormone dependent tumors as distinct from hormone independent ones? One reason is that hormone dependent tumors can be treated therapeutically with antihormones, to which tumors from most tissues don't respond. These studies also provide a novel approach to understanding the molecular basis of cancer.

Gene Expression

Approximately 20% of the estimated 80,000 genes encoded by the human genome are expressed as mRNAs in a given cell. This subset is a major determinant of a cell's properties. Alterations in gene transcription (induction or repression) underlie the etiology of diverse pathological processes, as well as normal physiological processes of an organism including differentiation and modifications of cellular phenotype. Therefore, general techniques for ready detection of the mRNAs produced under various conditions of health or disease are valuable (3). In the present context we discuss one of these techniques, differential display (DD) of mRNAs, to ask which genes are transcribed in normal and tumor cells under the influence of hormones.

Technical advances over the past two decades have led to the development of several powerful methods capable of identifying novel molecules relevant to both biological and pathological processes. Such molecules can provide new information regarding these processes, and identify targets potentially suitable for biological markers, and for pharmacological manipulation. Methods include assays of enzyme activities, immunochemical methods, and molecular biological techniques such as nucleic acid hybridization and the polymerase chain reaction.

DD is a reverse transcription-polymerase chain reaction with the products displayed on a sequencing gel. It is a "fingerprinting" technology that facilitates the identification of mRNAs present in a cell or tissue (4, 5). In contrast to conventional techniques, DD can be used to study simultaneously mRNA expressions in many samples created under multiple experimental conditions. The method requires relatively small amounts of starting material. In 1000 publications to date, DD has identified genes that encode numerous mRNAs that are involved in the molecular control of differentiation, proliferation, senescence and apoptosis, by coding for putative chemokines, growth factors, adhesion molecules proteases, etc (6). It constitutes a valuable tool for scientists who are interested in the identification of novel molecular mechanisms suitable for therapeutic modulation. The characterization of these molecules may lead to the development of selective antagonists and inhibitors with clinical utility in the treatment of a wide variety of disorders including cancer, cardiovascular disease, CNS disorders and inflammation and tissue repair.

Detailed accounts of protocols used in the DD procedure have been described (7). Essentially the DD protocol consists of a series of conventional molecular biological procedures modified to facilitate the identification of differentially expressed mRNA species. These procedures include, in order of application, the generation of DNA-free total RNA, cDNA generation by mRNA reverse transcription, amplification by the polymerase chain reaction (PCR), separation and visual display of amplified cDNAs by denaturing polyacrylamide gel electrophoresis, extraction and recovery of differentially expressed PCR products, generation of probes for confirmation by Northern analysis, subcloning, and sequencing of differentially expressed cDNAs.Utilization of this technique has encountered the problem of frequent isolation of "false-positive" transcripts, PCR products that appear to be differentially expressed on a polyacrylamide gel but which cannot be verified when subsequent Northern analysis is performed using the same RNA source. PCR is highly sensitive to minor variations in experimental procedures. Reproducibility, to obtain truly positive bands, depends, to a large degree, on great care in achieving consistency, in pipetting, the use of core reagent preparations, duplicate assays, etc. Many modifications of the original protocol have been described such as primer design, PCR parameters, electrophoretic separation, alternatives to Northerns, etc., the implementation of which have resulted in enhanced fidelity and overall utility of this evolving technique (8).

Identifications of Molecular Targets from Hormone Related Cancers

As examples, DD has been applied to study gene expressions in the androgen dependent prostate cancer cell line LNCaP. The gels revealed a cDNA band, initially absent, that appeared within one hour after androgen addition; the great majority of bands did not change. This result was confirmed by Northern blotting. Sequencing and comparison with a data base determined that this gene codes for a known calcium binding protein S100P (9). The mRNA for PSA appeared with very similar kinetics. A novel similarly identified gene was shown to reveal prostate cancer cells in a tissue section, as contrasted to normal cells (Zhang, unpublished). The protease M gene was expressed differently in breast and ovarian tumor cells depending on their stage (10).

Genes, some of which are novel, that are over- and under-expressed, also have been identified in breast cancers by application of DD. We illustrate with a study of function and properties of HSIX1, a recently discovered member of a new homeobox gene subfamily (11). We identified it as increasing in late S-phase of human mammary carcinoma cells. Transfection and constitutive overexpression of HSIX1 in MCF7 cells led to an abrogation of the G2/M cell cycle checkpoint in response to DNA damage, suggesting that this gene may affect chromosomal stability in cancer cells. HSIX1 has utility as a marker of metastasis in tumor biopsies and blood samples. Examination of 35 breast tumor biopsy samples and several normal controls determined that HSIX1 expression was absent or very low in normal mammary tissue, but was overexpressed in 44% of primary (metastatic or non-metastatic) breast cancers, and in 90% of metastatic lesions. Expression of HSIX1 in several different types of cancers suggests that it is involved in numerous tumors. These data together with several recent homeobox gene studies support the argument that genes involved in developmental processes also play roles in cell cycle and tumor progression.

Expression Genetic Changes in Cancer

An extensive search is being conducted to find genes that are differentially expressed in breast cancer. By comparing with DD normal and highly tumorigenic cell lines grown in culture at similar rates in the same medium, about 150 genes have currently been found (12). These include ones, found in several laboratories, with significant homologies to known chemokines (interferon-g), growth and cell cycle-associated factors (heparin-binding, EGF, IGF-binding factors, helicases, Tyr and Ser/Thr kinases, thymidine kinase), and especially proteins involved in cellular adhesion, extracellular matrix production and protease function (integrins, fibronectin, collagen, laminin, osteonectin, TIMPs, tissue factor, tPA and PAI).

About 4% of the observed gene products were expressed differently in a normal vs a cancer breast cell. .Extrapolating from an estimated 15,000 different mRNAs expressed in a cell, this number suggests that 500 gene expressions may be affected in a cancer cell. The underexpressed (tumor suppressor) genes outnumbered the overexpressed ones (oncogenes) by 1.5x (Martin, unpublished). Two criteria for selecting genes of further interest from the set of 500 genes with altered expression are: (1) at least 5x overexpression; for detection in mixed cell tissues there is less interest in underexpressed genes than in overexpressed ones if one plans to identify mRNAs useful as markers. (2) The majority of tumor specimens should show the change. A calculation by the DFCI Statistics Deptartment is that 20 randomly picked samples are needed to distinguish with a probability of 80% between a marker being found in 60% vs. 30% of all tumors.

These studies are now focused on examining tumor biopsy specimens for their expressions of a set of 100+ genes. For this purpose, dot blots on membrane "chips" are being utilized to score the presence or absence of the corresponding mRNAs. One conclusion from these results is that most breast cancers do not display the same expression genetic patterns, and therefore they could differ in their fundamental genetic defects. A second conclusion is that some genes are highly over expressed in many breast cancers. Their mRNAs might provide markers for detecting the disease. These two subjects will be now be further discussed.

A Function-based Reclassification of Breast Cancers

Are there different classes of breast cancers? Some cancers have the ER protein (ER+) and other do not (ER-) (13). The former are often treated with antiestrogens such as Tamoxifen, but the latter are not because they are not able to respond to hormone or antihormone. *Are there two completely different molecular origins of these breast cancers?* We propose that these two are basically different. In the ER+ tumors, a defect in the signaling by E produces a fundamental progression of their growth. In ER- tumors the defect is proposed to be like that in tumors of hormone-independent tissues, and has nothing to do with the E system. After all, *why should the breast be insensitive to a carcinogenic process that takes place in tumors from other tissues?* Most normal breast cells are ER-, and a tumor of the second type would retain this ER-characteristic. This does not rule out that ER- tumor cells will arise from ER+ cells, because of their additional mutations during tumor progression. And other mutations could eliminate the requirement of growth stimulation by E. Such a progression is seen with prostate tumors, which are initially androgen dependent and become insensitive to anti-androgens with time.

Two subclasses of ER+ tumors are recognized. One is responsive to antiestrogens (60%) and the other is not (40%). Differences in expression genetics of ER+ tumor cells were noted. The former subclass requires E for transcription of hormone responsive genes, and the latter subclass does not and transcribes constitutively. For example, the reticulocalbin gene which is overexpressed in more invasive breast cancer cells (14) was inducible by E in the first type and constitutive in the second (15). The hormone independent cells' growth was not inhibited by Tamoxifen. The difference is based on hormone dependent vs. independent binding of ER to ERE and the subsequent activation of gene transcription (15). These findings have evident implications for the decision of whether or not to apply anti-estrogen therapy.

Early Detection

The finding mentioned above, that expressions of some genes are increased in many breast tumors, suggests the possibility of identifying expression markers for earlier detection of cancers. This is important because generally the earlier the stage of a tumor the more successfully it can be treated. Markers that detect, distinguish prognostically (i.e., whether the tumor is likely to metastasize) or therapeutically (to which drugs it will best respond), are good objectives for gene expression studies with tumor biopsies, lymph nodes, fine needle aspirates, blood, etc. Currently used detection methods for cancers are mainly performed on tumor tissues. But sampling a tumor requires that one knows that the tumor exists and believes that it can be located; the results obtained then may be too late to be very useful. Current methods are similar to trying to put out a fire after the house is in flames. We need to invent "smoke detector" techniques that detect tumors at stages earlier than by the current methods, so then the far fewer cancer cells could be treated prior to their invasion of surrounding tissues, development of distant metastases, and of drug resistance. The presently applied therapeutic techniques of surgery, radiation, chemotherapy and perhaps immunology, antisense, and differentiation should be successful more often if applied to earlier detected tumors.

We are devising several early detection systems. Each is potentially capable of finding a very few tumor cells in the presence of vast numbers of normal blood cells, about 1 per million. With these tests we are looking for and finding a few circulating tumor cells in a few cc blood sample. Tumor cells are proposed to appear in blood before metastases are apparent, or even are formed, because most shed cells die before they can seed metastatic tumors. Thus, cancer cells may appear in blood early in disease progression of solid tumors.

Our goal, to identify early-warning markers and develop sensitive detection-diagnostic methods, is based first upon the use of differential display to find tumor- and metastasis- related genes with frequently increased expression levels. Then, with these identified markers, circulating tumor cells in small blood samples are being sought using PCR and hybridization based approaches. The same techniques could be applied to other body fluids. Solid tumors might also be found, by applying these methods to small tissue biopsies, using radiology to tell one where to obtain the sample.

References

1. Jensen EV(1996) Steroid hormone receptors and antagonists. Ann NY Acad Sci 761:109-120.
2. Brown M (1994) Estrogen receptor molecular biology. Hematol Oncol North Am 8:101-111.
3. Sager R (1997) Expression genetics: shifting the focus from DNA to RNA. Proc Natl Acad Sci USA 94:952-955.
4. Liang P, Pardee AB (1992) Differential display of eukaryotic messenger RNA by means of the polymerase chain reaction. Science 257: 967-971.
5. Welsh JK, Chada K, Dalal S et al (1992) Arbitrarily primed PCR fingerprinting of RNA. Nucleic Acids Research 20:4965-4970.
6. Liang P, Pardee AB eds (1997) Differential Display Methods and Protocols, Totowa, N J: Humana Press.
7. Zhao S, Ooi SL, Pardee AB (1995) New primer strategy improves precision of differential display. BioTechniques 18:840-850.
8. Martin K, Kwan C-P, O'Hare M et al (1998) Identification and verification of differential display cDNAs using gene-specific primers and hybridization arrays. BioTechniques 24:1018-1026.
9. Averboukh L, Liang P, Kantoff P et al (1996) Regulation of S100P expression by androgen. Prostate 29:350-355.

10. Anisowicz A, Sotiropoulou G, Stenman G et al (1996) A novel protease homolog differentially expressed in breast and ovarian cancer. Molecular Med 2:624-636.

11. Ford HL, Kabingu EN, Bump EA et al (1998) Abrogation of the G2 cell cycle checkpoint associated with overexpression of HSIX 1: A possible mechanism of breast carcinogenesis. Proc Natl Acad Sci USA 95:12608-12613.

12. Zhang M, Martin KJ, Sheng S et al (1998) Expression genetics: a different approach to cancer diagnosis and prognosis. Trends Biotechnol 66-71.

13. Tsai M-J, O'Malley BW (1994) Molecular mechanisms of action of steroid/thyroid receptor superfamily members. Ann Rev Biochem 63:451-486.

14. Liu Y, Brattain MG, Appert H (1997) Differential display of reticulocalbin in the highly invasive cell line MDA-MB-435s, versus the poorly invasive cell line, MCF-7. Biochem Biophys Res Comm 231:283-289.

15. Biswas DK, Averboukh L, Sheng S et al (1998) Classification of breast cancer cells on the basis of a functional assay for estrogen receptor. Mol Medicine 4:454-467.

3

New Directions in Epidemiologic Studies of Hormonally-related Cancers

Janet R. Daling, Kathleen E. Malone, Elaine A. Ostrander, Peggy L. Porter

Introduction

During the past ten years, advances in science and technology have changed the types of studies epidemiologists are conducting. New directions for epidemiology include genetic studies, studies of tumor markers, and studies of cancer survival. Although the field of epidemiology is rapidly turning toward these new directions, there are still relatively few published reports in some of these areas. Therefore, this overview will by necessity rely heavily on examples from two population-based, case-control studies of women in Seattle who developed breast cancer (BC) under age 45 (i.e., the Seattle BC studies). Examples from the literature or work in progress from other investigators focusing on breast and ovarian cancer will also be included.

Genetics

Traditional epidemiologic studies on breast and ovarian cancer have consisted primarily of interview studies that focus on hormone-related factors such as number of live births, lactation, age at first and last birth, use of oral contraceptives (OCs) and hormone replacement therapy (HRT), diet, and more recently, exercise and use of alcohol and tobacco (1). These interview studies established that nulliparous women and women with a late age at first pregnancy are at increased risk of breast and ovarian cancer. The risk of these cancers decreases as the number of live births increases. Lactation also decreases a woman's risk of these diseases. OC use may increase the risk of BC in young women but provides protection against ovarian cancer.

One of the strongest and most consistent risk factors observed for BC has been having a mother or sister with a history of BC. Table 1 illustrates in the Seattle data how the association between first-degree family history of BC and BC risk varies by age. The relative risk is very high among women diagnosed with BC at age 30 and under. Twenty-one percent had a mother or sister who also had a history of the disease. The relative risk decreases with age primarily due to the increasing proportion of controls who have a family history of BC. Among women diagnosed with their cancer after age 29 approximately 16% report a mother or sister who had the disease. This proportion stays fairly constant with increasing age. Relative risks of about the same magnitude associated with first-degree family history of ovarian cancer have been reported for ovarian cancer (RR = 3.6, 95% CI = 1.8 – 7.1). However, in contrast to the 16% of BC cases with family history, only 3% of ovarian cancer cases have a mother or sister with a history of ovarian cancer (2).

Table 1. BC risk in relation to family history of BC by proband age[1].

Age of Proband	Family Hx. of BC	Cases % (n = 1,451)	Controls % (n = 1,535)	OR[2]	95% C.I.
20-30	None	66.0	83.9	1.0	Ref.
	1st Degree	21.0	2.5	11.4	4.1 - 31.9
31-35	None	63.9	79.2	1.0	Ref.
	1st Degree	14.1	5.3	3.3	1.8 – 5.9
36-40	None	61.1	79.0	1.0	Ref.
	1st Degree	15.9	5.8	3.5	2.3 – 5.3
41-45	None	62.7	74.5	1.0	Ref.
	1st Degree	16.6	7.3	2.7	1.7 – 4.3

[1] Excludes adopted women.
[2] Adjusted for reference age of study subjects.

These strong patterns of familial aggregation led researchers to search for genes that may predispose women to these diseases. The identification of the locus of the first BC gene in 1990 (3) and the cloning of the first two BC genes, *BRCA1* and *BRCA2* in 1994 and 1995 (4,5), opened up new areas of relevant questions that could be answered using population-based studies of breast and ovarian cancer.

Prior to 1990, few studies of breast and ovarian cancer included the collection of blood in their protocol. Today, most study protocols include a blood collection effort with specific aims directed at this resource. One goal of these studies is to determine the frequency of germline mutations (*BRCA1*, *BRCA2*, ATM, and other genes) in a population-based group of women diagnosed with BC and women in the general population.

Geneticists used very unusual high-risk families with multiple affected members to search for these genes (6,7). Such rare families were gleaned from a variety of sources, including large studies that had identified a few very high-risk families from among hundreds of BC cases, as well as from clinics that encountered the families for counseling purposes. With at least two inherited susceptibility genes identified, researchers are now interested in finding out what proportion of BC cases have a mutated gene and what is the frequency of mutations in the general population. Estimates derived from these very high-risk families, however, may not be predictive of what is going on in the general population.   Two population-based studies in the USA have published information relating to this goal. In the Seattle studies of women diagnosed with BC under age 45, we found that between 6-7% of women with either a mother or sister with BC or who were diagnosed with their disease under age 35 had a mutation in the *BRCA1* gene (8). In North Carolina, 3.3% of white women and 0% of black women diagnosed with BC at ages 20-74 had a *BRCA1* mutation (9). The proportion of women in the North Carolina Study with a family history of BC who had a *BRCA1* mutation was similar to that found in Seattle (6.6%). Most of the women in the Seattle study, who had a family history of BC, did not have a mutation in the *BRCA1* or *BRCA2* genes. In neither study has a control been identified with a mutation; however, the numbers tested are limited. In 1995, Ford *et al.* (10) estimated the *BRCA1* gene frequency in the general population to be less than one per thousand, and the contribution of mutations in *BRCA1* to breast and ovarian cancer to be between 5 and 6% of cases diagnosed prior to age 40 and decreasing with age. Similar information on *BRCA2* is only now becoming available. In the Seattle studies of young women with BC, slightly less than 4% of our high-risk women with BC have a *BRCA2* mutation (11). It is thought that the population frequency of *BRCA2* is also less than 1/1000. In contrast, however, it is estimated that approximately 2-3% of the Ashkenazi Jewish population has a mutation in *BRCA1* or *BRCA2* (12, 13).

Epidemiologists are also looking at the role that the more common but less penetrant gene polymorphisms play in the etiology of BC. Although these types of genes may confer a more modest lifetime risk of developing cancer in carriers, they potentially account for a larger proportion of BCs because of their overall frequency. Although not an exhaustive list, Table 2 shows that the frequency of the high-risk genotypes varies from 40% to over 60%. Two examples of early work assessing BC risk associated with gene polymorphisms are studies of the vitamin D receptor (VDR) and the Nat 2 genes.

Table 2. Susceptibility genes that are currently being explored for possible contributions to BC risk.

Gene	High Risk Genotype Frequency
NAT2	55%
GSTM1	50%
CYP17	66%
CYP1a1	40%
Estrogen receptor	50%
Vitamin D receptor	40%
Androgen receptor	30-50%

The VDR gene is a member of the steroid hormone receptor family. It is a transcription factor involved in the regulation of a variety of genes. It is also a regulator of cellular differentiation and replication. Vitamin D is best known for the role it plays in bone metabolism. Although controversial, it has been hypothesized that polymorphisms in the VDR gene may account for a large part of the variation in bone density (14-16). Two recent prospective cohort studies have reported an association between greater bone mass and BC risk, so it was logical to look at the role that the VDR plays in the etiology of BC (17, 18). A recent epidemiologic study typed two polymorphic sites of the VDR gene, bsmI and the 3'UTR poly-A microsatellite, among 47 African-American BC cases and 100 controls (19). Although there was no association with the bsmI allele, there was an over two-fold risk of BC associated with the poly-A alleles. These investigators have extended this work to include 257 African-Americans and 215 Hispanics and have found that the absence of one or more long poly-A allele was associated with an increased risk of BC (OR = 2.22) in both racial groups (20). Mutations in various VDR alleles have also been associated with colon and prostate cancer risk (21, 22).

Past observations that smokers have an earlier menopause, lower body mass index, and different endogenous hormone profiles have long raised interest in the relationship of smoking to BC risk. However, only a few epidemiologic studies have observed an association between cigarette smoking and BC risk, and any relationship remains controversial. Ambrosone *et al.* (23) have addressed this issue among women who have differences in their inherited ability to activate and detoxify tobacco-specific carcinogens. In a case-control study examining the risk of BC associated with NAT2, an enzyme involved in the detoxification of aromatic amines, the authors found no overall association between BC risk and cigarette smoking or between NAT2 status and BC. However, among postmenopausal women with the slow acetylator genotype, there was a significant dose-dependent increase in risk associated lifetime pack years of smoking (Table 3). This example demonstrates the importance of taking into account differences in genetic susceptibility when evaluating environmental exposures and cancer risk. However, subsequent studies by Hunter *et al,* (24) and Millikan *et al.* (25) have not confirmed these results. It is not surprising to see discrepant results between studies that seek to assess a relationship between smoking and disease, as study participants are frequently exposed to environmental smoke, which is difficult to quantify. In addition, many of the studies that have attempted to evaluate even the more common gene polymorphisms have not included adequate sample sizes to reach definitive conclusions.

Table 3. BC risk and pack years smoked in post-menopausal women by NAT2 genotype[1].

	Rapid Acetylators			Slow Acetylators		
	Case/ control	OR	95% CI	Case/ control	OR	95% CI
Lifetime pack years						
None	43/50	1.0	---	41/59	1.0	---
≤183	4/12	0.4	0.1 – 1.6	5/9	0.9	0.3 – 3.0
184-365	10/10	1.5	0.5 – 4.2	10/14	1.1	0.4 – 2.7
>365	14/23	0.9	0.4 – 2.1	36/23	2.8	1.4 – 5.5
p for trend		0.98			<0.01	

[1] Adjusted for age, education, menarche, age of first pregnancy, age of menopause, BMI, and family history of BC (23).

Gene Environment Interactions

One area of great promise in elucidating the etiology of BC is the identification of gene-environment interactions. It is important to identify factors that influence the penetrance of genes or that modify the age at onset of disease. The low population frequency of *BRCA1* and *BRCA2* carriers makes this difficult and dictates that epidemiologists will have to form collaborations and pool data across studies in order to have sufficient numbers to succeed.

We have begun to address these issues in the Seattle studies, although the work is preliminary and limited by small numbers. We currently have identified 23 women who have a mutation in the *BRCA1* gene. Women who had this mutation were twice as likely to be nulliparous, as compared to the women without a *BRCA1* or *BRCA2* mutation or control women (Table 4). Among the women who had a pregnancy, *BRCA1* mutation-positive women were more likely to have had their first birth after age 30. Over half of the parous women with a *BRCA1* mutation had a live birth within two years of diagnosis, as compared to 12% of the BC cases without a mutation and 27% of controls. Johannsson *et al.* (26) also investigated pregnancy-associated BC in pedigrees of 29 *BRCA1* families and 10 *BRCA2* families, comparing 175 women of similar age whose BC was not related to *BRCA1* or *BRCA2* mutations. The odds of having pregnancy-related BC was 3.9 (95% CI = 1.4 - 10.0) and 1.9 (95% CI = 0.5 – 7.0) for *BRCA1* and *BRCA2* cancers, respectively. Presently, we can only speculate that the hormones associated with pregnancy may enhance growth of an existing tumor or that the lack of an intact *BRCA1* protein during the growth and differentiation of breast tissue during pregnancy may promote tumor development due to a lack of DNA repair function.

Table 4. Pregnancy history among women with BC and controls, by *BRCA1* status.

Characteristic	BRCA1+ n=23 (%)		BRCA1-, 2- n=290 (%)		Controls n=522 (%)	OR[1] 95% CI		OR[2] 95% CI	
Parity									
1+	11	---	183	---	323 ---				
Nulliparous	12	(52.2)	107	(36.9)	199 (38.1)	2.0	(0.8-4.9)	2.7	(1.1-6.7)
Age at 1st birth									
<30 years	8	---	152	---	291 ---				
30+ years	3	(27.3)	31	(16.9)	34 (10.5)	2.1	(0.5-9.0)	2.6	(0.6-10.5)

[1] Risk relative to *BRCA1*- and 2-BC cases adjusted for age and family history of BC.

[2] Risk relative to controls adjusted for age and family history of BC.

In contrast, women in the Seattle cohort who had a *BRCA2* mutation were more likely than cases without a mutation or control women to have had at least one live birth (85% compared to 60%). Among the women who had live births, the relationships with age at first birth and recency of birth were similar to that of women with *BRCA1* mutations; however, the magnitude of risks was lower (Table 5).

Also of great interest is whether women who are carriers of a mutated gene can safely use OCs. Ursin *et al.* (27, 28) recently reported that the BC cases who were *BRCA1* or *BRCA2* mutation positive in their study were seven times more likely to have used OCs for long durations than the BC cases who did not have a *BRCA1* or *BRCA2* mutation. There was approximately a two-fold increase in risk of *BRCA1* or 2 related BC associated with OC use when compared to population controls in the Seattle data.

Table 5. Pregnancy history among women with BC and controls, by *BRCA2* status.

	BRCA2+ n=14 (%)	BRCA1-, 2- n=290 (%)	Controls n=522 (%)	OR[1] 95% CI	OR[2] 95% CI
Characteristic					
Parity					
1+	12 ---	183 ---	323 ---		
Nulliparous	2 (14.3)	107 (36.9)	199 (38.1)	0.3 (0.1-1.3)	0.4 (0.1-1.9)
Age at 1st birth					
<30 years	9 ---	152 ---	291 ---		
30+ years	3 (25.0)	31 (16.9)	34 (10.5)	1.8 (0.4-7.3)	2.3 (0.6-9.2)

[1] Risk relative to *BRCA1*, 2-BC cases adjusted for age and family history of BC.
[2] Risk relative to controls adjusted for age and family history of BC.

It is well known that OC use protects against ovarian cancer in general. Narod and the Hereditary Ovarian Cancer Group (29) recently reported that OC use may substantially reduce the risk of ovarian cancer in women with mutations in the *BRCA1* or *BRCA2* gene. *BRCA1* or *BRCA2* carriers who had used OCs for six or more years had one-third the risk of ovarian cancer as compared to women who had never used OCs. Although this result is intriguing, there are several major concerns with this analysis. Most of the women with ovarian cancer were prevalent cases, therefore survivors. If OC use is related to poor prognosis, this could bias the results, as the prevalent cases would have fewer OC users. In addition, 72 of the 161 controls had undergone oophorectomy and were at very little risk of developing ovarian cancer. This topic will be an important area for epidemiologic research in the future.

A final exposure that has been looked at for its modifying effect on cancer risk in *BRCA1* and *BRCA2* carriers is cigarette smoking. Burnet, *et al.* (30), using a registry of prevalent mutant *BRCA1* and *BRCA2* BC cases and unaffected gene carriers, found that *BRCA1* and *BRCA2* carriers who smoked were half as likely to develop BC. Again, if smoking was related to prognosis of BC, this could account, in part, for this finding. Since nicotine has been found to inhibit apoptosis (31), smoking after diagnosis could interfere with treatment and affect survival.

In the Seattle studies, there was not a protective effect of smoking on BC risk among *BRCA1* and *BRCA2* carriers. If anything, the risk was higher when the comparison group was women with BC unrelated to *BRCA1* and *BRCA2* genes (OR = 1.8, 95% CI 0.8 to 3.9).

Gene Discovery

A final goal of epidemiologists in conducting genetic studies is collaborating with molecular geneticists to identify new genes using our population-based studies. It is clear that other putative BC genes exist. Most of the women in our studies who had a family history of BC did not have a mutation in the *BRCA1* or *BRCA2* genes. The great resources of DNA collected in past and current epidemiologic studies will be crucial for the identification of additional genes.

Tumor Markers: Relation to Risk Factors and Survival

Another new data collection effort in current epidemiologic studies of hormonal-related cancers is the collection of tumor blocks for BC cases who have been interviewed. One major goal of these studies is to determine if patient exposures are related to tumor characteristics. While tumor markers have mainly been used to subdivide cases for prognostic purposes, researchers are increasingly using markers for etiologic investigation. Tumor markers may show differences in their relationship to epidemiologic risk factors, thus helping us understand the mechanisms involved in the etiology of the tumors. Also, if factors can be identified that correlate with prognosis, this information could be used by patients and their physicians in planning treatment. In the late 1980s and early 1990s, Hakan Olsson (32, 33) of Sweden hypothesized that reproductive risk factors for BC would correlate with the tumor biology of cancers that occurred decades later. Olsson, *et al.* (34) collected the breast tumors of 72 women and evaluated them for amplification of the Her-2/neu and INT2 genes, proto-oncogenes implicated in mammary tumorigenesis. He then correlated the tumor markers with use of OCs before a woman's first-term pregnancy. The findings of this relatively small study suggested that there was a higher rate of Her-2/neu gene amplification among the tumors of early OC users. The tumors of the women who used OCs at age 20 or less were almost seven times as likely to have amplification of the Her-2/new gene. INT2 was amplified in the tumors of women who had an abortion before their first-term pregnancy.

One tumor characteristic that is frequently related to patient characteristics is estrogen (ER) and progesterone receptor (PR) status. These tumor markers are related to patient survival and are frequently evaluated by pathologists and available in the patient's medical record. Using the BC cases that occurred in the Iowa Women's Health Cohort, John Potter and colleagues related PR and ER status of the tumors to risk factors for the disease (35). They found that receptor status defined fundamental types of breast tumors, each with different risk factors and, therefore, potentially different etiologies. Potter, *et al.* (35) found that women with late age at first birth were more likely to be ER$^+$PR$^+$, the tumors

of OC users were ER⁺PR⁻, and the tumors of women who used alcohol were ER⁻
PR⁻.

It has been suggested that a woman's number of ovulatory cycles is related to
her risk of ovarian cancer. Repair of the ovarian surface after ovulation requires
cellular proliferation that may lead to mutations in the DNA. Shildkraut, *et al.*
(36) evaluated the relationship of the number of lifetime ovulatory cycles in 197
patients with invasive ovarian cancer to p53 status of the tumors. They found
a direct relation between the number of ovulatory cycles and cancer risk among
the women with p53 positive tumors (Table 6), whereas there was no such
relationship in the p53 negative tumors. This analysis suggests etiologic
differences according to the p53 status of the tumors. Stratifying epidemiologic
analyses by tumor markers may aid us in understanding the various pathways to
disease.

Table 6. Case-control comparisons of number of lifetime ovulatory cycles in
197 patients with invasive ovarian cancer and 3,363 control subjects by p53
status[1].

Exposure No. of Ovulatory Cycles	p53+	Controls	OR[2]	95% CI
≤234	4	840	1.0	
235 – 375	29	1222	4.3	(1.4 – 13.0)
376 – 533	67	1159	9.1	(2.7 – 30.9)

[1] Schildkraut J, et al. (36).

[2] Adjusted for age, menopausal status, and nulliparity.

Another goal of the tumor marker studies is to determine the relationship of
tumor characteristics to survival. Clinicians have been doing this for the last
decade, but epidemiologists would like to integrate into this effort patient
characteristics and exposures into the analysis of prognostic markers.

Malone *et al.* (37) contrasted the survival of women with BC who have a
mother or sister with BC to that of women with BC who do not have a family
history of BC. Women diagnosed with BC under age 45 who had a mother or
sister with the disease were at half the risk of dying of their disease as compared
to women without this history (OR = 0.5, 95% CI = 0.3 to 0.9). This favorable
outcome was independent of age at diagnosis, disease stage, mammographic
history, treatment, relative type, or number of affected relatives. The tumor
markers for these women were also consistent with a better prognosis (Table 7).
None of the tumor markers studied was significantly elevated in the women with
family history of BC. Twenty-three of the 305 high-risk women (those

diagnosed under age 35 or with a family history of BC) in this cohort, who have been tested for *BRCA1*, had a germline mutation in this gene. The survival was even more favorable for these women. Interestingly, the tumors from the women with *BRCA1* mut related disease were more likely than the tumors unrelated to *BRCA1* to be ER and PR negative, to have other adverse prognostic markers, and to be of high histologic grade. This adverse tumor marker profile, as well as the better prognosis, has been noted by others (38-40).

Table 7. Family history in relation to tumor characteristics (n = 811).

	No Family	1st Degree Family History	
		OR	95% CI
ER⁻	1.0	0.8	0.5 – 1.2
PR⁻	1.0	0.9	0.6 - 1.3
p53⁺	1.0	0.7	0.5 – 1.1
Ki-67	1.0	1.0	0.7 – 1.5
↓BLC-2	1.0	0.7	0.4 – 1.0
c-erb-B2⁺	1.0	0.7	0.3 – 1.3

In the Seattle cohort, the histology of the *BRCA1*-positive cases also differed from that of the whole cohort. Five, (22%) of the *BRCA1*-related cases were of medullary histology, as compared to 4.2% of the entire cohort. This histologic type of BC is known for its bad prognostic markers yet good survival. The relationship of *BRCA1*-related tumors to medullary histology has been noted by others (40-42).

Women who have *BRCA1*-related ovarian tumors may also have better survival. Rubin *et al.*, (43) followed 53 women with *BRCA1*-associated ovarian tumors and found the median survival time to be more than twice that of age and stage-matched control ovarian tumors. The survival advantage for women who have *BRCA1* and *BRCA2*-associated tumors, as well as women in general who have familial cancer, should be explored further by clinical and basic scientists, as it may give clues to effective therapeutic regimens.

Other exposures have also been evaluated in relation to survival. In contrast with studies of postmenopausal BC, premenopausal women in the highest quartile of body mass index have a lower risk of BC, compared to women in the lowest quartile (44, 45). However, consistent with postmenopausal BC, the heaviest women have a worst prognosis (46, 47). In the Seattle cohort of women diagnosed with BC prior to age 45, the women in the highest quartile of BMI had almost twice the risk of dying of their disease within five years. After adjusting for age, year of diagnosis and stage of disease at diagnosis, the five-year hazard ratio was 1.9, 95% CI 1.2 to 2.9. The tumors of these women were more likely to be ER negative and p53 positive. In this study, nulliparous women were at higher risk than parous women of being diagnosed with BC, OR = 1.4, but they survive better than parous women, five-year hazard ratio for parous women compared to nulliparous women = 1.5, 95% CI 1.0 to 2.1 (Table 7). Women who had a late age at first birth also were at higher risk of dying of their disease, five-year adjusted hazard ratio = 1.9, 95% CI 1.2 to 3.1. Over 40% of the 47 women who had a live birth within one year of diagnosis have died of their disease, compared to 20% of the nulliparous women in our study, adjusted five-year hazard ratio = 2.7, 95% CI 1.5 to 5.0. The tumors of parous women were more likely to be p53 positive, OR = 1.5, 95% CI 1.0 to 2.1, as were those of women whose last birth occurred over age 40, OR = 4.3, 95% CI 1.1 to 18.8. Kroman, et al. (48) also reported an increased risk of dying of BC among parous women who had given birth within two years of diagnosis, RR = 1.6, 95% CI 1.2 to 2.0, adjusted for age, year of treatment, tumor size, number of positive nodes, and histologic grade. Similar results have been reported by Olson, et al. (49), who found a 3.1-fold increase in risk (95% CI 1.8 to 5.4) of dying of BC if the woman had given birth within two years of diagnosis. In this study, parous women were also at increased risk of death from their disease compared to nulliparous women, RR = 1.8 (95% CI 1.2 to 2.9).

In the Seattle study, OC use had no effect on the survival of women diagnosed with BC at age 35 or older; however, women diagnosed under age 35 had poorer survival if they had used OCs. Long-term users had over three times the risk of dying of their disease, compared to women who never used OCs or used them for less than one year. The tumors of OC users were more likely to be estrogen and progesterone receptor negative and p53 positive. In contrast to what Olsson reported (50), use at a young age did not affect survival.

It has been established that factors related to a woman's hormone status and inherited genes are associated with her risk of breast and ovarian cancer. Despite this knowledge, most of the variation in the incidence of breast and ovarian cancer remains unknown. The relationship of tumor markers, patient characteristics and exposures, and genetic factors to prognosis are just beginning to be explored. The studies that have been described in this brief, and not exhaustive, overview illustrate the types of interdisciplinary studies conducted by epidemiologists in conjunction with laboratory-based scientists and with clinicians. The use of these molecular epidemiologic methods should help subdivide BC cases into strata based on markers of genetic susceptibility or tumor characteristics that will help elucidate the various pathways to disease as well as provide prognostic indicators useful in the clinical setting. These studies require large sample sizes, the collection of blood and tissue, and laboratory analyses. More efficient laboratory testing techniques are currently under development. It is the hope of the scientists working in this field that these interdisciplinary studies will advance our knowledge of the etiology, prevention, and treatment of hormonally-related cancers.

References

1. Kelsey JL ed (1993) Breast cancer. In: Epidemiologic Reviews, Vol 1. The Johns Hopkins University School of Hygiene and Public Health, Baltimore, MD .
2. Shildkraut JM, Thompson WD (1988) Familial ovarian cancer: A population-based case-control study. Am J Epidemiol 128:456-466.
3. Hall JM, Lee MK, Newman B et al (1990) Linkage of early-onset familial breast cancer to chromosome 17q21. Science 250:1684-1689.
4. Miki Y, Swensen J, Shattuck-Eidens D et al (1994) A strong candidate for the 17q-linked breast and ovarian cancer susceptibility gene *BRCA1*. Science 266:66-71.
5. Wooster R, Bignell G, Lancaster J et al (1995) Identification of the breast cancer susceptibility gene *BRCA2*. Nature 378:789-791.
6. Narod SA, Feunteun J, Lynch HT (1991) Familial breast-ovarian cancer locus on chromosome 17q12-23. Lancet 338:82-83.
7. Wooster R, Neuhausen SL, Mangion J (1994) Localization of a breast cancer susceptibility gene, *BRCA2*, to chromosome 13q12-13. Science 265:2008-2090.
8. Malone KE, Daling JR, Thompson JD (1998) *BRCA1* mutations and breast cancer in the general population: Analyses in women before age 35 years and in women before age 45 years with first-degree family history. J Am Med Ass 279:922-929.
9. Newman B, Mu H, Butler LM et al (1998) Frequency of breast cancer attributable to *BRCA1* in a population-based series of American women. J Am Med Ass 270:915-921.
10. Ford D, Easton DF, Peto J (1989) Estimates of the gene frequency of *BRCA1* and its contribution to breast and ovarian cancer incidence. Am J Hum Genet 62:676-689.
11. Malone KE, Daling JR, Neal, C et al (2000) Frequency of *BRCA1/BRCA2* mutations in a population-based sample of young breast carcinoma cases. Cancer 88:1393-1402.
12. Struewing JP, Abeliovich D, Peretz T et al (1995) The carrier frequency of the *BRCA1* 185delAG mutation is approximately 1 percent in Ashkenazi Jewish individuals. Nature Genetics 11:198-200.

13. Struewing JP, Hartge P, Wacholder S et al (1997) The risk of cancer associated with specific mutations of *BRCA1* and *BRCA2* among Ashkenazi Jews. N Engl J Med 336:1401-1408.
14. Spector TD, Keen RW, Arden NK et al (1995) Influence of vitamin D receptor genotype on bond mineral density in postmenopausal women: a twin study in Britain. Br Med J 310:1357-1360.
15. Viitanen A-M, Karkkainen M, Laitinen K et al (1996) Common polymorphism of the vitamin D receptor gene is associated with variation of peak bone mass in young Finns. Calcif Tissue Int 59:231-234.
16. Morrison NA, Qi JC, Tokita A et al (1994) Prediction of bone density from vitamin D receptor alleles. Nature 367:284-286.
17. Cauley JA, Lucas FL, Kuller LH et al (1996) Bone mineral density and risk of breast cancer in older women the study of osteoporotic fractures. J Am Med Ass 276:1404-1408.
18. Zhang Y, Kiel DP, Kreger BE et al (1997) Bone mass and the risk of breast cancer among postmenopausal women. N Engl J Med 336:611-617.
19. Ingles SA, Nakaichi GK, Yu MC et al (1996) Polymorphism in the 3' UTR region of the vitamin D receptor is associated with breast cancer risk in African-American women. Abstract presented at 21st meeting of the International Assoc. for Breast Cancer Research. Paris, France, July, 1996.
20. Ingles SA, Haile RW, Henderson B et al (1997) Association of vitamin D receptor polymorphisms with breast cancer risk in African-American and Hispanic women. In: Vitamin D: Chemistry, Biology, and Clinical Applications. Proc. of the 10th workshop on vitamin D, 1997.
21. Taylor JA, Hirvonen A, Watson M et al (1996) Association of prostate cancer with vitamin D receptor gene polymorphism. Cancer Res 56:4108-4110.
22. Ingles SA, Ross RK, Yu MC et al (1997) Association of prostate cancer risk with genetic polymorphisms in vitamin D receptor and androgen receptor. J Natl Cancer Inst 89:166-170.
23. Ambrosone CB, Freudenheim JL, Graham S et al (1996) Cigarette smoking, *N*-Acetyltransferase 2 genetic polymorphisms, and breast cancer risk. J Am Med Ass 276:1494-1501.
24. Hunter DJ, Hankinson SE, Hough H et al (1997) A prospective study of NAT2 acetylation genotype, cigarette smoking, and risk of breast cancer. Carcinogenesis 18:2127-2132.
25. Millikan RC, Pittman GS, Newman B et al (1998) Cigarette smoking *N*-Acetyltransferases 1 and 2, and breast cancer risk. Cancer Epidemiol Biomarkers & Prevention 7:371-378.

26. Johannsson O, Loman N, Borg A et al (1998) Pregnancy-associated breast cancer in *BRCA1* and *BRCA2* germline mutation carriers. The Lancet 352:1359-1360.
27. Ursin G, Henderson BE, Haile RW et al (1997) Does oral contraceptive use increase the risk of breast cancer in women with *BRCA1/BRCA2* mutations more than in other women? Cancer Res 57:3678-3681.
28. Ursin G, Henderson BE, Haile RW et al (1998) Correction. Cancer Research 58:375.
29. Narod SA, Risch H, Moslehi R et al (1998) Oral contraceptives and the risk of hereditary ovarian cancer. N Engl J Med 339:424-428.
30. Brunet J-S, Ghadirian P, Rebbeck TR et al (1998) Effect of smoking on breast cancer in carriers of mutant *BRCA1* or *BRCA2* genes. J Natl Cancer Inst 90:761-766.
31. Wright SC, Zhong J, Zheng H et al (1993) Nicotine inhibition of apoptosis suggests a role in tumor promotion. FASEB J 7:1045-1051.
32. Olsson H (1989) Reproductive events, occurring in adolescence at the time of development of reproductive organs and at the time of tumour initiation, have a bearing on growth characteristics and reproductive hormone regulation in normal and tumour tissue investigated decades later – a hypothesis. Medical Hypotheses 28:93-97.
33. Olsson H (1990) Reproductive and hormonal factors in relation to cancer occurrence in the breast, prostate, testis, uterine corpus, ovary, uterine cervix, and thyroid gland. In: Nordenskjold B, Bacieira-Coelho A (eds) Cancer and Aging. CRC Press, Boca Raton, pp.110-125.
34. Olsson H, Borg A, Ferno M et al (1991) Her-2/neu and INT2 proto-oncogene amplification in malignant breast tumors in relation to reproductive factors and exposure to exogenous hormones. J Natl Cancer Inst 83:1483-1487.
35. Potter JD, Cerhan JR, Sellers TA et al (1995) Progesterone and estrogen receptors and mammary neoplasia in the Iowa women's health study. How many kinds of breast cancer are there? Cancer Epidemiol Biomarkers Prev 4:319-326.
36. Schildkraut JM, Bastos E, Berchuck A (1997) Relationship between lifetime ovulatory cycles and overexpression of mutant p53 in epithelial ovarian cancer. J Natl Cancer Inst 89:932-938.
37. Malone KE, Daling JR, Weiss NS et al (1996) Family history of breast cancer in relation to reduced mortality in young women with invasive breast cancer. Cancer 78:1417-1425.
38. Marcus JN, Watson P, Page DL et al (1996) Hereditary breast cancer: pathobiology, prognosis, and *BRCA1* and *BRCA2* gene linkage. Cancer 77:697-709.

39. Porter DE, Cohen BB, Wallace MR et al (1994) breast cancer incidence, penetrance and survival in probable carriers of *BRCA1* gene mutation in families linked to *BRCA1* on chromosome 17q12-21. Br J Surg 91:1512-1515.

40. Lakhani SR, Jacquemier J, Sloane JP et al (1998) Multifactorial analysis of differences between sporadic breast cancers and cancers involving *BRCA1* and *BRCA2* mutations. J Natl Cancer Inst 90:1138-1145.

41. Eisinger F, Nogues C (1998) *BRCA1* and medullary breast cancer. Letter J Am Med Ass 280:1227.

42. Malone KE, Daling JR, Ostrander EA (1998) *BRCA1* and medullary breast cancer. Reply to Eisinger letter. J Am Med Ass 280:1127-1128.

43. Rubin SC, Benjamin I, Behbakht K et al (1996) Clinical and pathological features of ovarian cancer in women with germ-line mutations of *BRCA1*. N Engl J Med 335:1413-1416.

44. Swanson CA, Coates RJ, Schoenberg JB et al (1996) Body size and breast cancer risk among women under age 45 years. Am J Epidemiol 143:698-706.

45. Peacock SL, White E, Daling JR et al (1999) Relation between obesity and breast cancer in young women. Am J Epidemiol 149:339-346.

46. Senie RT (1994) Breast cancer prognosis: role of obesity? J Surg Oncology 57:30.

47. Newman SC, Lees AW, Jenkins HJ (1997) The effect of body mass index and oestrogen receptor level on survival of breast cancer patients. Int J Epidemiol 26:484-490.

48. Kroman N, Wohlfahrt J, Andersen KW et al (1997) Time since childbirth and prognosis in primary breast cancer: Population-based study. B Med J 315:851-855.

49. Olson SH, Zauber AG, Tang J et al (1998) Relation of time since last birth and parity to survival of young women with breast cancer. Epidemiology 9:669-671.

50. Olsson H, Borg A, Ferno M et al (1991) Early oral contraceptive use and premenopausal breast cancer – a review of studies performed in southern Sweden. Cancer Detection and Prev 15:265-271.

PART 1. EPIDEMIOLOGY:
BREAST AND PROSTATE CANCER

4

Estrogen Causes Breast Cancer: Increasing Duration of Use of Postmenopausal Hormones Increases the Risk of Breast Cancer

Graham A. Colditz

Introduction

Forty years ago the use of postmenopausal estrogen (E) was advocated to reduce the risk of breast cancer, and early meta-analyses showed no significant relationship between ever use of postmenopausal hormones and risk of breast cancer (BC). However, the vast majority of hormone use at that time was short term, for relief of menopausal symptoms. Today, the long-term use of postmenopausal hormones has been established in an effort to reduce the risk of illnesses associated with aging, such as coronary heart disease, and osteoporotic hip fractures. With this change the clinical question has become, *"Does long-term use of hormone replacement increase risk of BC and, if so, how soon after use has begun does risk increase?"*

Recent epidemiologic studies suggest that the long-term use of E does, in fact, increase BC risk. Furthermore, the combined reanalysis of original data from 51 epidemiologic studies indicates that, for each year a woman uses postmenopausal hormones, her risk of BC increases by 2.3% (1). In this review, I summarize the evidence that endogenous E and replacement hormones are causally related to BC. All epidemiologic studies are considered, and major emphasis is placed on results from systematic review and meta-analyses that address pertinent issues, such as the variation in results among studies.

Reproductive Events and Risk of Breast Cancer

Reproductive events, such as age at menarche, age at first pregnancy, number of pregnancies, and age at menopause play an important role in determining a woman's lifetime risk of BC. These events are markers of exposure to endogenous reproductive hormones and are thought to influence the rate of breast cell growth and the accumulation of DNA damage. In premenopause, late pregnancies are associated with increased risk of BC, and early pregnancies are protective, because the first pregnancy is associated with terminal differentiation of breast cells which is followed by a lengthening of the cell cycle, allowing more time for DNA repair. Moreover, by comparing the reproductive pattern of six or more pregnancies in the developing world to the typical two pregnancies in the developed world, we see that 50% of the international variation in BC rates can be explained by these patterns of childbearing. Early menopause is associated with a reduced risk of BC, as hormone levels drop after menopause. For every one-year increase in age at menopause, the risk of BC increases by 3%.

After menopause, obesity is positively related to reproductive hormone levels, as a biologic function of fat cells is to metabolize androgens to Es. Lean, postmenopausal women have lower E levels and lower age-specific incidence of postmenopausal BC. Obesity is related to risk of BC mortality as well. This is consistent with a role for E as a late promoter of BC. Tamoxifen, which acts as an antiestrogen in the breast, significantly reduces the risk of mortality among women already diagnosed with BC. This serves as evidence for the role of E in facilitating tumor growth.

Breast Cancer Risk and Markers of Hormonal Exposure

Mammographic density and bone density provide insight into BC risk. Denser breasts are associated with higher E levels and higher BC incidence. High bone density also reflects higher levels of E and risk of BC. The prospective study of osteoporotic fractures (2) indicated that bone density in the wrist, hip, and spine has a strong and statistically significant direct relationship with the risk of BC.

Hormone Levels and Breast Cancer Risk

Growing evidence supports a positive relationship between blood levels of Es and risk of BC. The follow-up of the study of osteoporotic hip fractures (3) showed a strong relationship between hormone levels in women not taking postmenopausal hormones and their subsequent risk of BC. Comparing extreme quartiles of E levels, Cauley, Lucas, Kuller, *et al.* (3) observed an RR (relative risk) of 3.2 (95% CI = 1.4-7.0) for women in the highest quartile. Other prospective studies agree with this relationship. The systematic review and quantitative analysis of combined data from prospective studies by Thomas, Reeves, and Key (4) reveals no substantial heterogeneity of results. These authors observed a statistically significant higher risk of BC in women with higher levels of serum estradiol. In a case-control study nested within the Nurses' Health Study (5), researchers revealed an RR of about 3 when women who had used postmenopausal hormones were excluded. Androgens may also be associated with increased risk of BC, though it is likely that they are converted to Es before exerting their biologic action on risk of BC.

Correlates of Use of Postmenopausal Hormones

Biologic correlates, such as the higher reports of hot flashes in women who are lean at menopause, and the lower bone density of women who begin taking postmenopausal hormones, suggest that women who take postmenopausal hormones are at lower risk of BC at time of menopause than women who do not take hormones. This leads to an underestimate of the adverse effects of postmenopausal hormones. In contrast, non-biologic factors, higher socio-economic status and higher rates of mammography, in women who take hormones, result in overestimating the underlying biologic relationship between hormone use and risk of BC.

Sources of bias are often not measured in epidemiologic studies of hormone use and BC risk. Thus, it is possible that there is confounding by indication: The unmeasured correlates of hormone use result in women at lower risk for BC being more likely to take postmenopausal hormones. Confounding by indication leads to a biased estimate of the relationship between hormone use and BC. In addition, women who undergo menopause at an earlier age are more likely to take postmenopausal hormones and to take them for a longer time than women who undergo surgical menopause. Early menopause is associated with a reduced risk of BC. Thus, hormone users are at lower risk of BC than nonusers of the same age group once other risk factors are controlled. Unpublished data from the Nurses' Health Study illustrates the relationship described above. Depending on the category of use of postmenopausal hormones, in women aged 55-59 who had menopause before 47 there is substantial variation in menopause duration. For never users of hormones, the mean time since menopause is 15.2 years; for current users of less than 5 years' duration, it is 16.1 years; and for current users with 5 or more years of use, it is 16.6 years. Variation in time is more extreme in younger age groups. Clearly, in analyses controlling for age at menopause in three categories (< 47 years, 47-52 years, and > 52 years) we have not controlled for age at menopause with sufficient rigor to remove bias in our estimates. Thus, our analyses and those of many other investigators do not give an unbiased estimate of the relationship.

Increasing Risk of Breast Cancer With Longer Duration of Use of Postmenopausal Hormones

Investigators who have conducted meta-analyses of published epidemiologic studies report a positive relationship between duration of hormone use and risk of BC. Steinberg, Smith, Thacker, *et al.* (6) noted that, among U.S. case-control studies published from 1977 to 1991, a positive relationship was observed between duration of hormone use and risk of BC in 11 of 12 studies with community control subjects and in four of nine studies with hospital-based control subjects. Among the prospective studies, an increased risk with increasing duration of use was reported in all four studies.

Investigators at Oxford University (1) undertook a combined reanalysis of original data from 51 epidemiologic studies that included about 52 000 women with BC and 100,000 women without BC. Data from this reanalysis indicate that, for each year of use of postmenopausal hormones, risk of BC increases by 2.3% (95% CI = 1.1%-3.6%; P = 0.0002) and that the findings do not vary significantly between studies. Combined epidemiologic data, therefore, now show a significant increase in the risk of BC with duration of use of postmenopausal hormones. Five or more years of use was associated with an RR of 1.35 (95% CI = 1.21-1.49).

Mechanisms by Which Hormones Can Influence Breast Cancer Risk

In premenopausal women, the proliferative activity of the breast is greatest during the luteal phase of the menstrual cycle. Progesterone may therefore be the major mitogen in the normal breast epithelium of premenopausal women. Evidence in support of this comes from a study of surgically postmenopausal *cynomolgus* macaques (7) that were treated for 30 mo. with either conjugated equine E or a combination therapy of conjugated equine E plus medroxyprogesterone acetate. In that study, combined therapy induced greater breast cell proliferation. However, the proliferation of breast cells *in vitro* has been stimulated by Es and inhibited by progestins. Thus, uncertainty persists as to the role of progestins. Evidence from studies of hormonal carcinogenesis suggests that Es may have dual effects, causing both nongenotoxic cell proliferation and genotoxic effects. Evidence from epidemiologic studies shows a stronger relationship between current use of replacement hormones (typically unopposed E) and risk of BC than is seen for former use of these hormones. This suggests that the major effect of the replacement hormones may be through the promotion of cancer growth rather than through genotoxic effects. The combined reanalysis of epidemiologic studies (1) shows that those who had stopped taking hormones for more than 5 years were not at increased risk compared with nonusers, regardless of how long the women had taken replacement hormones.

Increase in Breast Cancer Risk by Use of Estrogen Alone or Estrogen Plus Progestin

Most epidemiologic studies linking postmenopausal hormones to risk of BC in the United States have focused on the use of unopposed E. Recently, progestins have been added to the regimen to counter the adverse effects of E in developing endometrial cancer. Accumulating evidence, however, does not support the view that combination therapy reduces BC risk. At the cellular level, breast cell division is stimulated by progestins, and investigators (8, 9) report that E plus progestin is associated with a higher BC risk than is E alone.

The Oxford University combined reanalysis (1) of epidemiologic studies found that among women whose duration of current use was greater than 5 years (58 cases), treatment with E plus progestin was associated with a higher risk of BC (RR = 1.53; 95% CI = 0.80-2.92) than the use of unopposed Es (RR = 1.34; 95% CI = 1.12-1.59). The majority of data come from use of cyclic progestin. The recent move to combined continuous therapy has not been evaluated. Epidemiologic evidence, therefore, is not sufficient to determine whether sustained progestin levels can move cells into a phase of reduced division.

Longer Survival Among Women Diagnosed with Breast Cancer While Taking Postmenopausal Hormones than Among Other Breast Cancer Patients

E may induce a less malignant form of endometrial cancer in women taking postmenopausal hormones. Evidence from the American Cancer Society Cancer Prevention Study II (10) suggests Es may have the same effect with regard to BC. In that prospective study, BC mortality during 9 years follow-up was lower among women who had taken Es than among women who had not. This result may reflect better survival among women diagnosed while taking postmenopausal hormones, or it may reflect lower underlying risk of BC in women who have taken hormones.

Criteria for a Causal Relationship

A cause of cancer is a factor that increases the probability that cancer will develop in an individual. Below, I have summarized the evidence according to the Hill (11) criteria (with the exception of analogy, which has little to do with deductive logic) that postmenopausal hormone use and BC is now clearly consistent with a causal relationship.

Strength of Association

On the basis of hormone levels observed among postmenopausal women, the annual increase in the risk of BC after menopause among women taking E alone is 2% per year. The effect of adding postmenopausal hormones is comparable to that of delaying menopause (1). Thus, the association, although not strong by epidemiologic standards, is of the magnitude predicted by the underlying biology. Among current users with 5 or more years of use, the RR was 1.35 (95% CI = 1.21-1.49) compared with never users.

Consistent Relationship

Absence of heterogeneity in results may be used as an indication of consistency. The increase in the risk of BC with increasing duration of use of postmenopausal hormones is reported consistently and, when the combined reanalysis examined for heterogeneity in results among studies, no statistically significant heterogeneity was observed.

Dose-Response Relationship

Evidence comes from two areas to address the issue of a dose-response relationship between postmenopausal hormones and BC. First, the blood level of E related directly to the risk of BC in a dose-response pattern. This pattern was observed in the majority of prospective studies and was substantiated in the combined analysis by Thomas, Reeves, and Key (4). Second, the relationship between increased duration of use of replacement hormones and increased risk reflects a dose-response relationship in which duration of use represents a time-integrated dose (1).

Biologic Mechanism

The presence of estrogen receptors on breast cells, the action of the antiestrogen Tamoxifen in reducing mortality after diagnosis in postmenopausal women, and the relationship between E, progestins, and cell division, all point to a role for E in breast cell growth and division. The presence of higher risk breast mammographic patterns among women who are treated with replacement hormones is further evidence that cell proliferation occurs in response to exogenous hormones.

Specificity

The increase in the risk of cancer among women who take postmenopausal hormones is not limited to BC; it is also observed for endometrial cancer, for which a strong body of evidence supports a hormonal basis for the disease. Thus, like other chronic diseases, the requirement of specificity is not a central consideration for a causal relationship.

Relationship in Time

The epidemiologic data suggest that current use of replacement hormones is associated with the proliferation of cancer cells and that the risk remains elevated 5 or more years after the use of replacement hormones has stopped. Studies based on blood levels of E and bone density indicate that E status among postmenopausal women predicts their future BC risk. The ability to make an earlier prediction of increased risk on the basis of blood levels of E is no doubt due to strong tracking (high correlation over time) of hormone levels among postmenopausal women (12).

Experiment

Clinical trials in which patients are randomly assigned to treatments are considered to be the best strategy to assess the risks and benefits of hormone replacement therapy. To date, no substantial randomized trial has been completed that was designed to quantify the relationship between use of postmenopausal hormones and BC risk. Such evidence is expected to be forthcoming from the Women's Health Initiative where continuous combined E plus progestin has been used. This will not, however, answer questions regarding other forms of postmenopausal hormone therapy.

Coherence of the Evidence

The evidence reviewed above shows a relationship between endogenous hormone levels and the risk of BC. Furthermore, there is a positive relationship between the long-term use of postmenopausal hormones and increased risk of BC. The strong protective effect of early menopause and the relationship between postmenopausal obesity and E levels combine to support the role of Es in the etiology of BC.

Implications for Women Who Take Postmenopausal Hormones

Based on this review, it is evident that postmenopausal hormones cause BC. Given this causal relationship and consistent evidence that hormone replacement reduces the risk of cardiovascular disease, osteoporosis, and other major illnesses, *how do we best present the data so that women can make informed choices? And how do we view this from a public health perspective?* Glasziou and Irwig (13) suggested that one needs to assess the underlying risk and potential benefits of any clinical therapy as it is applied to the individual patient. This would require estimates of heart disease and osteoporosis risk, as well as a risk assessment for BC. To this formula, I believe we must add the individual's fear or concern about the diseases considered, as is recommended for broader risk-benefit or cost-effectiveness considerations where "quality-adjusted" life-years are used as an outcome.

Age-specific mortality from cancer exceeds that from heart disease through age 70 years among women in the United States. The age-adjusted mortality from cancer has been higher than that from heart disease among women since 1990. In 1995, the age-adjusted mortality from heart disease was 104 deaths per 100,000 women; from cancer it was 110 deaths per 100,000 women. In white women, the difference was greater (heart disease, 95; cancer, 109). Other health advantages of postmenopausal hormones relate to the prevention of osteoporosis. The burden of this condition is primarily among older women, placing great demand for prevention strategies that do not increase risk of BC, which has a higher incidence than osteoporotic fractures prior to age 70.

From a public health perspective, we must consider the underlying distribution of risk factors for other chronic conditions. According to the follow-up of women in the Nurses' Health Study (14), those who used postmenopausal hormones for 10 or more years had a 20% reduction in mortality that was statistically significant. However, this benefit was most pronounced among women who were at a higher risk for cardiovascular disease. To achieve a reduction in mortality, some women within the population will pay the price of a BC they otherwise would have not developed. Thus, the action that will benefit public health and the individual's best choice may differ. Further work is needed to improve our understanding and communication of these considerations.

References

1. Breast cancer and hormone replacement therapy. Combined reanalysis of data from 51 epidemiological studies involving 52,705 women with breast cancer and 108,411 women without breast cancer. Collaborative Group on Hormonal Factors in Breast Cancer. (1997) Lancet 350:1047-1059.

2. Cauley JA, Lucas FL, Kuller LH, et al (1996) Bone mineral density and risk of breast cancer in older women: the study of osteoporotic fractures. Study of Osteoporotic Fractures Research Group. J Am Med Ass 276:1404-1408.
3. Cauley J, Lucas F, Kuller L et al (1997) Is bone mineral density a biological marker of a woman's cumulative exposure to estrogen? Presented at a meeting of the American Epidemiological Society, Rochester, MN.
4. Thomas HV, Reeves GK, Key TJ (1997) Endogenous estrogen and postmenopausal breast cancer: a quantitative review. Cancer Causes Control 8:922-928.
5. Hankinson SE, Willet WC, Manson JE et al (1998) Plasma sex steroid hormone levels and risk of breast cancer in postmenopausal women. J Natl Cancer Inst 90:1292-1299.
6. Steinberg KK, Smith SJ, Thacker SB et al (1994) Breast cancer risk and duration of estrogen use: the role of study design in meta-analysis. Epidemiology 5:415-421.
7. Cline JM, Soderqvist G, von Schoultz E (1996) Effects of hormone replacement therapy on the mammary gland of surgically postmenopausal cynomolgus macaques. Am J Obstet Gynecol 174: 93-100.
8. Bergkvist L, Adami HO, Persson I (1989) The risk of breast cancer after estrogen and estrogen-progestin replacement. N Engl J Med 321:293-297.
9. Colditz G, Rosner B (1998) Use of estrogen plus progestin is associated with greater increase in breast cancer risk than estrogen alone. Am J Public Health 147.
10. Willis DB, Calle EE, Miracle-McMahill HL et al (1996) Estrogen replacement therapy and risk of fatal breast cancer in a prospective cohort of postmenopausal women in the United States. Cancer Causes Control 7:449-457.
11. Hill AB (1965) The environment and disease: association or causation? Proc R Soc Med 58:295-300.
12. Hankinson SE, Manson JE, Spiegelman D et al (1995) Reproducibility of plasma hormone levels in postmenopausal women over a 2-3 year period. Cancer Epidemiol Biomarkers Prev 4:649-654.
13. Glasziou PP, Irwig LM (1995) An evidence based approach to individualising treatment. Brit Med Journal 311:1356-1359.
14. Grodstein F, Stampfer MJ, Colditz GA et al (1997) Postmenopausal hormone therapy and mortality. N Engl J Med 336:1769-1775.

5

Frequency of *BRCA2* Mutations in Women with Early Onset Breast Cancer Drawn from a Population-Based Study

Kathleen E. Malone, Janet R. Daling, Nicola M. Suter, Kara Cushing, Thora Jonnasdottir, and Elaine A. Ostrander

Introduction

Most of what has been learned about the autosomal dominant susceptibility genes, *BRCA1* and *BRCA2,* has been derived from studies of high risk families characterized by large numbers of affected women. While ascertainment of such families was necessary for the mapping of *BRCA1* and *BRCA2*, and analysis of high risk families continues to provide critical data about the type and frequency of mutations in rare families with several affected women, these data do not provide information to women drawn from the general population. Many such women who lack a profound family history of breast cancer (BC), both cancer patients and unaffected women, nevertheless they perceive themselves to be at risk of carrying a mutation in one of these genes because of the presence of one or more affected individuals in their family. We have been interested in understanding the role of *BRCA1* and *BRCA2* outside the selected venue of high risk families. Generating data on the frequency of *BRCA1* and *BRCA2* mutations in women with BC drawn from the general population, who have minimal or modest family histories, would provide guidance on the overall impact of these genes within this group, and identify any features that relate to an increased likelihood of carrying a mutation.

Aside from several studies which focused exclusively on women of Ashkenazi Jewish descent (1-3), only two USA studies have addressed the role of *BRCA1* or *BRCA2* in women drawn from the general population (4-6). The work by Langston, et al., (4) and Malone, *et al.* (5) focus on two subgroups of cases drawn from population-based case-control studies of early onset BC in Western Washington. In these studies, 193 women who were diagnosed with BC before age 35 were tested for germline mutations in *BRCA1*. None of the women were selected on the basis of family history status. Twelve (6.2%, 95% CI = 3.2-10.6) were found to have germline *BRCA1* mutations. In addition, 208 women diagnosed before age 45 who had a first-degree family history of BC were tested and 15 (7.2%, 95% CI=4.1-11.6) were found to carry germline mutations in *BRCA1*. Mutation frequency varied in both groups by age and by features of family history. In general, the mutation frequency increased with decreasing age of diagnosis, presence of an ovarian cancer family history, and presence of four or more relatives with BC, particularly, if those relatives were young or had ovarian cancer (OC).

Similar trends were noted by Newman, *et al.* (6) who examined 211 cases, aged 20-74, from a population-based case-control study of invasive BC in central and eastern North Carolina involving both African-American and Caucasian women. Three *BRCA1* disease associated mutations were observed among the 211 cases suggesting (after age-adjustment and race-specific sampling probabilities) that 3.3% of Caucasian women diagnosed in the specified age range were likely to be *BRCA1* carriers (CI = 95%, 0%-7.2%) and 0% in African-American women. The *BRCA1* gene frequency found among women with a family history of BC or OC was 6.6%, and is similar to that observed among comparable groups of women in western Washington.

In this report, we describe analyses of the spectrum and frequency of mutations in *BRCA2* in the same groups of women examined previously. *BRCA2* is a large gene containing 26 coding exons and spanning 10,443 bp (7, 8). As with *BRCA1, BRCA2* mutations do not appear to occur frequently in sporadic tumors (9,10). In most collections of high risk families studied thus far, *BRCA2* is thought to account for about 30% fewer cases of inherited BC then do germline mutations in *BRCA1* (11, 12). The single exception to this is in families of Icelandic origin where a single founder mutation in *BRCA2* has been shown to account for the majority of inherited disease (13). In the following study we address the role of *BRCA2* in two "at risk" groups of women drawn from the general population.

Methods

All subjects selected for this study were drawn from two population-based case-control studies of BC conducted in Western Washington State that have been described previously (14, 15). Cases (women diagnosed with BC) were identified through the Cancer Surveillance System (CSS), a population-based cancer registry which participates in the Surveillance, Epidemiology, and End Results (SEER) Program of the NCI. Controls (similarly aged women without

BC) were identified through random digit dialing. The first study ascertained all incident cases of first primary BC diagnosed January 1, 1983 through April 30, 1990 in Caucasian women born after 1944 who were residents of King, Pierce, and Snohomish counties at diagnosis. Interviews were completed on 845 cases (83.6% of eligible cases) and 961 controls (75.5% of eligible controls). Additional funding allowed for the later collection of blood specimens from 592 cases and a subset of the control women (n=165).

The second study ascertained all incident first primary BC cases diagnosed before age 45 from May 1, 1990 to December 31, 1992 among women of all races residing in the three county area. Interviews were completed on 648 (87.0%) of the eligible cases and 610 (78.7%) of the eligible controls. As part of the original study design and through subsequent blood collection efforts, blood samples were collected from 545 of the cases and 473 of the controls.

In both studies, information regarding potential risk factors for BC was obtained through a structured in-person interview as described previously (5). Data collected included first and second degree family history including the birth year, vital status, death year, history and type of cancer, and laterality (if BC) of all affected relatives. Follow-up contact with all previously interviewed women (or proxies) for updated and extended pedigree information has been initiated as part of an ongoing genetic-epidemiology study. Information on vital status was obtained from the CSS, which conducts systematic long-term follow-up of all cancer patients, and from our ongoing follow-up tracing activities. This study was approved by the Fred Hutchinson Cancer Research Center Institutional Review Board and all study subjects signed an informed consent form prior to participation.

Three groups of women were drawn from the studies described above for the following analysis (1) cases with a first-degree family history of BC (i.e., mother and/or sister affected), (2) cases diagnosed before age 35, regardless of family history status and (3) controls with any first-degree family history of BC. Women with a first-degree family history were selected because their family history could reflect an increased probability of being a carrier of germline mutations in cancer susceptibility genes. Cases diagnosed before age 35 were selected, regardless of their family history, because their earlier onset age might also reflect a greater probability of carrying a mutation.

Molecular Analyses

Genomic DNA was purified from either frozen buffy coats or immortalized lymphoblastoid cell lines. PCR reactions were carried out using conditions described previously (5) using primers that had been described previously by others (16, 17) or novel primers designed to provide redundant coverage of the gene. All variant bands occurring in less then 5% of samples were sequenced using previously described conditions (4).

Statistical Analyses

The Fisher exact test was used to assess differences in age, disease stage, vital status, and family history between women who were and were not tested and to evaluate, among tested women, whether the proportions with mutation varied by age, stage, vital status, and features of family history. Binomial exact 95% confidence intervals (CI) were calculated for the proportions with mutation. P-values and confidence intervals were calculated using Stata statistical software (Stata Corp, College Station, TX).

Table 1. Characteristics of BC cases with first-degree family history of BC: All eligible cases and cases tested for mutations in *BRCA2.*

Characteristic	All eligible cases (n = 297)		Tested cases (n = 225)		P-value[1]
	n	%	n	%	
Age of diagnosis					
21-29	17	(5.7)	13	(5.8)	
30-34	40	(13.5)	29	(12.9)	0.77
35-39	118	(39.7)	87	(38.7)	
40-44	122	(41.1)	96	(42.7)	
Stage of disease					
In-situ	46	(15.5)	35	(15.6)	
Local	149	(50.2)	123	(54.7)	0.01
Regional/distant/ unknown	102	(34.3)	67	(29.8)	
Vital status					
Alive	255	(85.9)	210	(93.3)	<0.001
Deceased	42	(14.1)	15	(6.7)	

[1] P-value for the difference between women who were and were not tested.

Results

BRCA2 mutation status was assessed in 386 women who fell into one or both of two "at risk to carry a mutation" categories: 225 women diagnosed with BC before age 45 who also had a first-degree family history of BC, and 203 women diagnosed before age 35 who were not selected on the basis of family history status. The majority of women were Caucasian (96.6%) with the remainder distributed as follows: 1% African-American, 1.6% Asian/Pacific Islander, 0.3% American Indian/Aleutian, 0.6% other.

In both case groups studied, the proportions tested among women who were eligible did not vary substantively by age of diagnosis or family history (See Tables 1 and 2). As previously described, tested cases were more likely to be alive at last follow-up and were less likely to have been of advanced stage at diagnosis than those unavailable for testing (5). A lag between interviewing and blood collection in the first case-control study accounts for this difference.

Table 2. Characteristics of cases diagnosed with BC before age 35: All eligible cases and cases tested for mutations in *BRCA2*.

Characteristic	All eligible cases (n = 307)		Tested cases (n = 203)		P-value[1]
	n	%	n	%	
Age of diagnosis					
21-29	74	(24.1)	45	(22.2)	**0.32**
30-34	233	(75.9)	158	(77.8)	
Stage of disease					
In-situ	31	(10.1)	27	(13.3)	
Local	151	(49.2)	108	(53.2)	**<0.001**
Regional/distant/unknown	125	(40.7)	68	(33.5)	
Vital status					
Alive	222	(72.3)	179	(88.2)	**<0.001**
Deceased	85	(27.7)	24	(11.8)	
Family history of BC					
None	144	(46.9)	96	(47.3)	
Mother and/or sister affected	57	(18.6)	42	(20.7)	
Aunt and/or grandmother only affected	66	(21.5)	45	(22.2)	**0.09**
Other relative only affected	12	(3.9)	8	(3.9)	
Adopted/unknown	28	(9.1)	12	(5.9)	

1 P-value for the difference between women who were and were not tested.

Distribution and Frequency of Disease-Associated Mutations

Among the 225 cases ages 21-44 with a first-degree family history who were tested, 11 (4.9%, 95% CI = 2.5-8.6) carried germline *BRCA2* mutations (Table 3). Mutation frequency varied considerably with age of diagnosis; it was highest among women under age 30 (15.4% of these women carried a mutation) and lowest in those diagnosed at ages 40-44 (2.1% carried a mutation). Four (21.0%) *BRCA2* mutations were observed in the 19 women who had both a mother and sister with BC. In women with a first-degree family history, mutation frequency did not appreciably increase with the additional presence of an affected second degree relative (6.2% of the women with a first-degree family history who also had an affected aunt and/or grandmother were carriers). We note that no disease-associated mutations were seen in the 71 unaffected controls with a first-degree family history.

BRCA2 mutation frequency was slightly higher in women with one or more first-degree relatives who were diagnosed at younger ages (6.6%), versus those whose affected first-degree relatives had a later age of onset (4.2%). Similar results were seen regarding second degree relatives (data not shown). The number of affected relatives was also important. Mutation frequencies were higher in cases from families with four or more affected members including the proband (10.7%) versus those with fewer affected relatives (3.0%).

Among the 203 women with BC before age 35 who were tested, 7 (3.4%, 95% CI 1.4-7.0) carried a *BRCA2* mutation (Table 4). Of the 45 women aged 21-29, 2 (4.4%) were carriers. Of women aged 30-34, 5 (3.2%) were carriers. In the women under 35, mutation frequency was discernibly greater in those with a first degree family history. Of the 96 cases diagnosed with BC before age 35 who had no family history of BC, none carried a *BRCA2* mutation. Of the 42 cases with BC before age 35 who had a mother and/or sister with BC, 3 (7.1%) had a mutation. Mutation frequencies were lower in those cases under age 35 who only had an aunt and/or grandmother with BC (2.2%). Of four cases diagnosed before age 35 who had both an affected mother and sister, 2 had a *BRCA2* mutation. Similar to our findings in the women with a first-degree family history, mutations were more frequent in cases with one or more first degree relatives who had an earlier onset age (15.0%) than in those whose relatives were all diagnosed at age 45 or later (none). The trend was similar if the diagnosis age of first or second degree relatives was considered (data not shown).

Because OC family history is a significant indicator of *BRCA1* mutation status, both in high risk families as well as in women drawn from the general population, we evaluated its role as an indicator of *BRCA2* carrier status. To maximize precision, we evaluated this question in the entire group of 386 cases tested (Table 5). We note that 89 of the 386 cases tested had neither a family history of BC or OC; none of these women carried a *BRCA2* mutation. Of the 386 cases tested, 245 had a family history of BC only. Of these 13 (5.3%) are *BRCA2* carriers. There were only 7 women who had first or second degree family history of OC but who lacked a family history of BC, and none of these women were carriers. Similarly, of the 33 women who had a family history of both BC and OC, none were *BRCA2* carriers.

We also examined mutation frequency jointly according to the number of family members with BC and the presence/absence of OC in the 386 women (Table 5). The majority of cases (n = 286) had fewer than four family members with BC and no family history of OC. Of these, 7 (2.4%) carried *BRCA2* mutations. Of the 48 cases with 4 or more BC affected family members but no OC affected members, there were 6 (12.5%) *BRCA2* mutations. There were no *BRCA2* mutations in the two groups of women with an OC family history (the two groups being those with fewer than 4 BC affected members and those with 4 or more BC affected members).

Frameshift Mutations

The majority of mutations observed were small insertions or deletions resulting in premature stop codons. Four of 14 frameshifts observed in this study are not listed in the Breast Cancer Information Core (BIC), and thus have not been observed previously. These include small deletions of one to seven base pairs that result in premature stop codons at 3019, 1739, 2845, respectively. There was also a deletion of a single amino acid resulting from a three base pair deletion at nucleotide 4081 resulting in the loss of a lysine at codon 1285 that we current classify as a disease-associated mutation.

Table 3. Distribution of *BRCA2* mutations according to disease characteristics and family history features among BC cases with a first-degree family history of BC.

Characteristics	All tested cases	BRCA2 disease-associated mutations	95% CI[1]	P-Value[2]
	n	n (%)		
All cases with first degree family history	225	11 (4.9)	(2.5, 8.6)	--[4]
Age of diagnosis				
21-29	13	2 (15.4)	(1.9, 45.4)	
30-34	29	1 (3.4)	(0.1, 17.8)	0.10
35-39				
Family history of BC				
Mother and/or sister had BC	225	11 (4.9)	(2.5, 8.6)	--[4]
Both mother and				--[4]
sister had BC	19	4 (21.0)	(6.0, 45.6)	--[4]
Mother had BC	188	11 (5.8)	(3.0, 10.2)	--[4]
Sister had BC	56	4 (7.1)	(2.0, 17.3)	--[4]
Aunt and/or grandmother also had BC	97	6 (6.2)	(2.3, 13.0)	--[4]
Mother/sister had BC < age 45	76	5 (6.6)	(2.2, 14.7)	0.52
Mother/sister had BC ∈ age 45	143	6 (4.2)	(1.6, 8.9)	
1-3 relatives with BC[5]	169	5 (3.0)	(1.0, 6.8)	0.03
> 3 relatives with BC[5]	56	6 (10.7)	(4.0, 21.9)	

1 Confidence interval for the proportion with mutations.
2 P-value for differences in mutation frequency between groups.
3 One-sided 97.5% confidence interval.
4 P-value not presented because there is no comparison or categories are not mutually exclusive.
5 Proband's BC is included.

Table 4. Distribution of *BRCA2* mutations according to disease characteristics and family history among BC cases diagnosed before age 35.

Characteristics	All tested cases	BRCA2 disease-associated mutations	95% CI[1]	P-Value[2]
	n	n (%)		
All cases diagnosed before age 35	203	7 (3.4)	(1.4, 7.0)	--[4]
Age of diagnosis				
21-29	45	2 (4.4)	(0.5, 15.1)	**0.65**
30-34	158	5 (3.2)	(1.0, 7.2)	
Family history of BC				
None	96	0 --	(0.0, 3.8)[3]	
Mother and/or sister had BC	42	3 (7.1)	(1.5, 19.5)	
Aunt and/or grand-mother only had BC	45	1 (2.2)	(0.1, 11.8)	**0.49**
Other relative	8	1 (12.5)	(0.3, 52.6)	
Adopted, family history unknown	12	2 (16.7)	(2.1, 48.4)	
Both mother and sister had BC	4	2 (50.0)	(6.8, 93.2)	--[4]
Mother had BC	33	3 (9.1)	(1.9, 24.3)	--[4]
Sister had BC	13	2 (15.4)	(1.9, 45.4)	--[4]
Mother/sister had BC <45	20	3 (15.0)	(3.2, 37.9)	**0.23**
Mother/sister had BC ∈ age 45	20	0 --	(0.0, 16.8)[3]	
1-3 relatives with BC[5]	189	6 (3.2)	(1.2, 6.8)	**0.40**
> 3 relatives with BC[5]	14	1 (7.1)	(0.2, 33.9)	

[1] Confidence interval for the proportion with mutations.
[2] P-value for differences in mutation frequency between groups.
[3] One-sided 97.5% confidence interval.
[4] P-value not presented because there is no comparison or categories are not mutually exclusive.
[5] Proband's BC is included.

Table 5. Distribution of *BRCA2* mutations among all 386 BC cases tested.

Characteristics	All tested cases	BRCA2 disease-associated mutations	95% CI[1]	P-Value[2]
	n	n (%)		
All cases tested	386	15 (3.9)	(2.2, 6.3)	--[4]
Family history of BC				
At least one relative had BC < age 45	99	5 (5.0))	(1.7, 11.4)	**0.77**
Affected relatives all had BC ∈ age 45	162	7 (4.3)	(1.8, 8.7)	
No. of family members with BC				
1-3	326	9 (2.8)	(1.3, 5.2)	**0.02**
4+	60	6 (10.0)	(3.8, 20.5)	
Family history of BC and OC				
Neither	89	0 --	(0.0, 4.1)[3]	
BC only	245	13 (5.3)	(2.9, 8.9)	**0.08**
OC only	7	0 --	(0.0, 41.0)[3]	
Both BC and OC	33	0 --	(0.0, 10.6)[3]	
No. with BC & presence/absence of OC in relatives				
< 4 BC, no OC	286	7 (2.4)	(1.0, 5.0)	
< 4BC, yes OC	28	0 --	(0.0, 12.3)	**0.02**
4+ BC, no OC	48	6 (12.5)	(4.7, 25.2)	
4+ BC, yes OC	12	0 --	(0.0, 26.5)[3]	

[1] Confidence interval for the proportion with mutations.
[2] P-value for differences in mutation frequency between groups.
[3] One-sided 97.5% confidence interval.
[4] P-value not presented because there is no comparison or categories are not mutually exclusive.
[5] Proband's BC is included.

Missense Changes and Polymorphisms

Several missense changes of unknown significance were also noted in this study. Several of these were observed only in cases and, based upon their position in the gene may be hypothesized to be of functional significance. For instance, two of these, an asparagine to glycine change at amino acid 2811, and a glutamic acid to alanine at amino acid 2856 within the conserved BRCT domain are in regions conserved across the human, mouse and rat sequences. The remaining missense changes are either located outside known functional domains or are not in regions of conserved DNA sequence. There were only two missense changes noted in the control samples; one (threonine to methionine at amino acid 1915) was observed in both cases (23 of 386) and controls (3 of 70) and the other (tryrosine to cysteine at codon 3092) was observed only in a single case in a region of unknown biological significance. Thus, there is no evidence they are disease-associated.

SSCP variants, which are assumed to be common polymorphisms, were observed in several cases. These included changes in DNA sequence which did not change the resulting amino acid, or that were within intron sequences and unlikely to affect splicing of exons. In addition, a nonsense change in two cases and three controls, at base 10204, which generated a stop signal at codon 3326. This change has been noted previously by Mazoyer *et al.* (18) as a polymorphic stop that is not disease-associated.

Discussion

Carrier frequencies derived from studies of high risk families are not easily manipulated to provide risk assessment information to women who lack profound family histories. Estimates of carrier frequency derived from such studies vary widely, due in part to the variation across studies in the numbers of affected members per family, ethnicity, mean age of onset, number of first versus second degree relatives, and presence of other cancers.

Towards the goal of generating relevant estimates of carrier frequency in women not drawn exclusively from high risk families but rather from the general population of all BC cases, we previously screened two defined subgroups of cases drawn from a population based case-control study of early onset BC in Western Washington for germline *BRCA1* mutations (5) and observed that 6.2% (95% CI = 3.2-10.6) of women diagnosed before age 35 years were *BRCA1* carriers. Similarly, 7.2% (95% CI = 4.1-11.6) of women diagnosed before age 45 who had a first degree affected relative were carriers. In both groups of women, mutation frequency was related to age of onset and specifics of family history such as age and number of affected relatives, as well as presence or absence of OC. As predicted from studies of high risk women, we observed that mutation frequency increased with decreasing age of diagnosis, presence of an OC family history, and presence of more than three relatives with BC.

In this report, we expand our studies to focus on the *BRCA2* gene. Our approach is again unique compared to other studies of high risk women; women evaluated here were drawn from two large population-based case-control studies of BC in young women (14, 15). The results are generalizable as an approximation of the *BRCA2* carrier frequency in these two potentially "at risk" groups of cases as they are found in the general population. We report on features of proband or family history which characterize the comparatively lower or higher incidence of *BRCA2* carrier status among the subsets of women studied.

Estimates of expected mutation frequency have been made from studies of selected cohorts of high risk families (19). In the USA, in 53 site-specific BC families originally ascertained for genetic mapping, the frequency of *BRCA1* mutations has been observed to be about twice the frequency of *BRCA2* mutations (11, 12). It is worth noting that a portion of these families were selected based on the presence of an OC family history. In the single largest study of high risk BC families collected irrespective of OC status, a study of 237 BC families, each with at least four cases of BC complied by the Breast Cancer Linkage Consortium, overall disease was linked to *BRCA1* in an estimated 52% of families, and to *BRCA2* in 32% of families, and to neither gene in 16% (20). If the age dependent penetrance of both genes is assumed to be similar, and the families truly selected randomly, this may suggest that the ratio of *BRCA1* to *BRCA2* carriers in the population is about 1.6 to 1. This compares well with observations in our study of young women drawn from the general population, where 6.0% and 3.9% of women overall were *BRCA1* and *BRCA2* positive, proportionately (5, 21). In women diagnosed before the age of 35, these numbers were 5.9% and 3.4%. In women diagnosed before age 45 who had a first degree family history, the numbers were similar, 7.1% and 4.9% respectively. Overall in this study, we observed a 1.53 to 1 ratio of *BRCA1* to *BRCA2* carriers, a result which is consistent with that observed in the study of high risk families. The relative percentages, however, must be taken in light of assumptions about *BRCA2* penetrance. Although the lifetime risk of BC in *BRCA2* carriers is assumed to be similar to that of *BRCA1* carriers, there is some suggestion of lower risk in *BRCA2* carriers who are less than 50 years of age in at least two studies (12, 20). When considering the analysis described in this report, this suggests that in a cohort of young women identified on the basis of a young BC diagnosis the data set may be slightly under represented for *BRCA2* carriers.

When considering the respective contributions of *BRCA1* and *BRCA2* to hereditary BC, USA data are similar with what has been observed elsewhere in the world. A single exception is Iceland, where a single *BRCA2* mutation, 999del5, predominates (22, 23). The population frequency of this mutation is high; it has been observed in 0.6% of the Icelandic population overall, in addition to 7.7% of female BC patients and 40% of males with BC.

Like *BRCA1*, founder mutations for BRCA2 have been described in women of Ashkenazi Jewish descent, with mutations at 6174delT present in about 1-1.5% of Ashkenazi Jewish women and accounting for a significant percentage of hereditary BC among Jewish women (1-3, 24-26). In our analysis of *BRCA1* in this same cohort, six of the 23 women who were observed to carry disease-associated *BRCA1* mutations carried the delAG185 mutation, as well as the associated haplotype, that has been seen in women of Ashkenazi Jewish descent (1, 24, 27, 28). One women carried the 5382insC mutation, which has also been observed in excess in Ashkenazi Jewish women. These data were somewhat surprising given that only about 5% of women from western Washington, in this age group, are of Ashkenazi Jewish descent. Interestingly, we did not see any of the observed *BRCA2* mutations to be more frequent in Ashkenazi Jewish women.

Prior studies of high risk families have suggested that *BRCA2* mutations are related to the occurrence of male BC (16, 29), although the majority of men that apparently harbor *BRCA2* mutations do not go on to get BC. In our population, five of the 386 cases tested reported a family history of male BC, one of whom (20%) was found to carry a *BRCA2* mutation. This is comparable with what has been observed in other studies. In the USA population, only about 14% of men with BC are thought to have disease due to *BRCA2* mutations (29). This is comparable to the 21% that has been observed in Sweden (30). In Iceland, this number rises to 40% (31). Although the rarity of male BC makes it a relatively infrequently occurring indicator for consideration of genetic testing, our finding of a *BRCA2* mutation within the 5 cases with a male relative with BC are consistent with the prior studies.

A correlation between *BRCA2* mutations and OC has been reported previously in some (12, 32) but not all studies (7, 10). In addition, a correlation between the presence of mutations and the likelihood that one will acquire OC has been noted in at least one study, with mutations leading to OC clustered in a region of 3.3 Kb in exon 11 (P = 0.0004) (33). In the results reported here, the risk of OC for women who are *BRCA2* carriers is not comparable to what has been postulated for *BRCA1*. In our previously analysis of this cohort, we showed that 24% of women with both BC and OC family history were *BRCA1* positive, and 14% of women who only an OC family history were BRCA1 positive (5, 21). In this study, we observe that none of the women with either ovarian only or breast OC family history are *BRCA2* positive. Thus while we can not exclude a relationship between *BRCA2* and OC risk, it is not a primary family history feature of the *BRCA2* mutation-positive women identified here.

The above findings must considered in the context of limitations in the sensitivity of all mutational screening strategies. Gel based techniques, like SSCP, can detect over 80% of mutations when carefully done (34, 35). This is aptly demonstrated by Ford *et al.*, who in analyses of 237 families, each with at least four cases of BC, assessed and compared the sensitivity of completely sequencing the coding region of the *BRCA1* gene to the sensitivity of other genomic screening techniques (constant denaturing gel electrophoresis, confirmation sensitive gel electrophoresis, SSCP-heteroduplex analyses, direct screening for deletions and inversions in combination with the protein truncation test, and SSCP alone) and found them to be essentially equivalent for detecting *BRCA1* and *BRCA2* mutations (20). In this study, which utilized SSCP, steps were taken to optimize primers and gel conditions so that even subtle variants could be routinely detected. But in the absence of complete gene sequencing for every women, it must be assumed that some mutations are missed. Most commonly, these will be single base changes leading to either missense or nonsense mutations.

While most nonsense changes leading to production of truncated proteins are thought to be disease associated, the biological significance of most missense changes is unknown. Thus, we are left with examination of functional domains and comparative sequence analysis to determine the likelihood that a given amino acid change is disease associated. In the study described here, we hypothesize that at least two missense changes are disease associated, an asparagine to glycine change at amino acid 2811 and a glutamic acid to alanine at amino acid 2856. Others may exist that went undetected by SSCP.

In addition to the above, mutations affecting expression, splicing or stability of the transcript will not be detected in screens such as the one described. While such mutations are estimated to account for as much as 15-20% of all *BRCA1* mutations (19), their importance with regard to BRC2 has yet to be reported.

Because BC strikes 1 in 8 women in western world at some point in their lives, all women are essentially "at risk" for the disease. The presence of autosomal dominant susceptibility genes which are highly penetrant confers not only excess risk, but also excess anxiety to a population of women already facing a multitude of confusing choices about how their lifestyles and diet affect their reproductive health. As we begin to unravel the role of *BRCA1* and *BRCA2* in BC in women from the general population, we aim to provide women with critical information to be used in making decisions about how best to protect their reproductive health.

References

1. Struewing JP, Abeliovich D, Peretz T et al (1995) The carrier frequency of the *BRCA1* 185delAG mutation is approximately one percent in Ashkenazi Jewish individuals. Nat Genet 11:198-200.
2. Abeliovich D, Kaduri L, Lerer I et al (1997) The founder mutations 185delAG and 5382insC in BRCA1 and 6174delT in BRCA2 appear in 60% of ovarian cancer and 30% of early-onset breast cancer patients among Ashkenazi women. Am J Hum Genet 60:505-514.
3. Fodor FH, Weston A, Bleiweiss IJ et al (1998) Frequency and carrier risk associated with common BRCA1 and BRCA2 mutations in Ashkenazi Jewish breast cancer patients. Am J Hum Genet 63:45-51.
4. Langston AA, Malone KE, Thompson JD et al (1996) *BRCA1* mutations in a population-based sample of young women with breast cancer. N Engl J Med 334:137-142.
5. Malone KE, Daling JR, Thompson JD et al (1998) *BRCA1* mutations and breast cancer in the general population: Analyses in women before age 35 years and in women before age 45 years with first-degree family history. J Am Med Ass 279:922-929.
6. Newman B, Mu H, Butler LM et al (1998) Frequency of breast cancer attributable to *BRCA1* in a population-based series of American women. J Am Med Ass 279:915-921.
7. Wooster R, Neuhausen SL, Mangion J et al (1994) Localization of a breast cancer susceptibility gene, *BRCA2*, to chromosome 13q12-13 Science265: 2088-2090.
8. Tavtigian SV, Simard J, Rommens J et al The complete *BRCA2* gene and mutations in chromosome 13q-linked kindreds. Nat Genet 1996 12:333-337.
9. Teng DH, Bogden R, Mitchell J et al (1996) Low incidence of BRCA2 mutations in breast carcinoma and other cancers. Nat Genet 13:241-244.
10. Takahashi H, Chiu HC, Bandera CA et al (1996) Mutations of the BRCA2 gene in ovarian carcinomas. Cancer Res 56:2738-2741.
11. Serova OM, Mazoyer S, Puget N et al (1997) Mutations in *BRCA1* and *BRCA2* in breast cancer families: Are there more breast cancer-susceptibility genes? Am J Hum Genet 60:486-495.
12. Schubert EL, Lee MK, Mefford HC et al (1997) BRCA2 in American families with four or more cases of breast or ovarian cancer: recurrent and novel mutations, variable expression, penetrance, and the possibility of families whose cancer is not attributable to BRCA1 or BRCA2. Am J Hum Genet 60:1031-1040.

13. Gudmundsson J, Johannesdottir G, Arason A et al (1996) Frequent occurrence of BRCA2 linkage in Icelandic breast cancer families and segregation of a common BRCA2 haplotype. Am J Hum Genet 58:749-756.
14. Daling JR, Malone KE, Voigt LF et al (1994) Risk of breast cancer among young women: Relationship to induced abortion. J Natl Cancer Inst 86:1584-1592.
15. Brinton LA, Daling JR, Liff JM et al (1995) Oral contraceptives and breast cancer risk among younger women. J Natl Cancer Inst 87:827-835.
16. Friedman LS, Gayther SA, Kurosaki T et al (1997) Mutation analysis of *BRCA1* and *BRCA2* in a male breast cancer population. Am J Hum Genet 60:313-319.
17. Kirkpatrick J, Waber P, Hoa-Thai T et al (1997) Infrequency of *BRCA2* alternations in head and neck squamous cell carcinoma. Oncogene 14:2189-2193.
18. Mazoyer S, Dunning AM, Serova O et al (1996) A polymorphic stop codon in *BRCA2*. Nat Genet 14:253-254.
19. Szabo CI, King MC (1997) Population genetics of *BRCA1* and *BRCA2*. Am J Hum Genet 60:1013-1020.
20. Ford D, Easton DF, Stratton M et al (1998) Genetic heterogeneity and penetrance analysis of the *BRCA1* and *BRCA2* genes in breast cancer families. Am J Hum Genet 62:676-689.
21. Malone KE, Daling JR, Neal C et al (Submitted). *BRCA1* and *BRCA2* mutation status in two groups of women perceived to be at-risk.
22. Thorlacius S, Olafsdottir G, Tryggvadottir L et al (1996) A single *BRCA2* mutation in male and female breast cancer families from Iceland with varied cancer phenotypes. Nat Genet 13:117-119.
23. Thorlacius S, Sigurdsson S, Bjarnadottir H et al (1997) Study of a single BRCA2 mutation with high carrier frequency in a small population. Am J Hum Genet 60:1079-1084.
24. Neuhausen S, Gilewski T, Norton L et al (1996) Recurrent BRCA2 6174delT mutations in Ashkenazi Jewish women affected by breast cancer. Nat Genet 13:126-128.
25. Oddoux C, Struewing JP, Clayton CM et al (1996) The carrier frequency of the BRCA2 6174delT mutation among Ashkenazi Jewish individuals is approximately 1%. Nat Genet 14:188-190.
26. Struewing JP, Hartge P, Wacholder S et al (1997) The risk of cancer associated with specific mutations of *BRCA1* and *BRCA2* among Ashkenazi Jews. N Engl J Med 336:1401-1408.

27. Friedman LS, Szabo CI, Ostermeyer EA et al (1995) Novel inherited mutations and variable expressivity of *BRCA1* alleles, including the founder mutation 185delAG in Ashkenazi Jewish families. Am J Hum Genet 57:1284-1297.

28. Tonin P, Serova O, Lenoir G et al (1995) *BRCA1* in Ashkenazi Jewish women. Am J Hum Genet 57:189.

29. Couch FJ, DeShano ML, Erdos MR et al (1997) BRCA1 mutations in women attending clinics that evaluate the risk of breast cancer. N Engl J Med 336:1409-1415.

30. Haraldsson K, Loman N, Zhang QX et al (1998) BRCA2 germ-line mutations are frequent in male breast cancer patients without a family history of the disease. Cancer Res 58:1367-1371

31. Mavraki E, Gray IC, Bishop DT (1997) Germline BRCA2 mutations in men with breast cancer. J Cancer 76:1428-1431.

32. Berman DB, Costalas J, Schultz DC et al (1996) A common mutation in BRCA2 that predisposes to a variety of cancers is found in both Jewish Ashkenazi and non-Jewish individuals. Cancer Res 56:3409-3414.

33. Gayther SA, Mangion J, Russell P et al (1997) Variation of risks of breast and ovarian cancer associated with different germline mutations of the BRCA2 gene. Nat Genet 15:103-105.

34. Sheffield VC, Beck JS, Kwitek AE et al (1993) The sensitivity of Single-Strand Conformation Polymorphism Analysis for the Detection of Single Base Substitutions. Genomics 16:325-332.

35. Jordanova A, Kalaydjieva L, Savov A et al (1997) SSCP analysis: a blind sensitivity trial. Human Mutation 10:65-70.

6

Prostate Cancer, Androgens, and Estrogens

Janet L. Stanford

Introduction

The importance of steroid hormones in the pathogenesis and progression of prostate cancer (PC) has been recognized for many years. The efficacy of orchiectomy and estrogen (E) administration to treat advanced stage PC was first described in 1941 by Huggins and Hodges (1). Subsequent research has led to development of the current therapeutic approaches for complete androgen blockade to treat disseminated disease. Other observations that support the role of hormones, specifically androgens, in relation to PC include the absence of the disease in men castrated before puberty and in men with an inherited deficiency of the enzyme 5α-reductase, which converts testosterone (T) to its active metabolite dihydrotesterone (DHT) in the prostate. Additional evidence from laboratory, clinical, and epidemiological studies confirms the significance of hormones in the development of PC. However, knowledge of the underlying biological and molecular mechanisms whereby androgens and other steroid hormones exert their individual and joint effects in the promotion and progression of PC remains incomplete. This chapter will review evidence that links androgen and E levels with the development of PC and how established risk factors for the disease (age, race, family history) may be related to the hormonal milieu.

Androgens

Androgens are required for the development and maintenance of normal and cancerous prostate tissue (2). T is the most important circulating androgen, with 95% being produced in the testes and a small amount from the adrenal gland (3). There are 3 forms of circulating T: albumin-bound (30-55%), sex hormone binding globulin-bound (SHBG) (45-75%), and free or unbound (2%) (3). Albumin-bound T and free T are the most biologically active forms of the hormone.

Within the prostate, T is converted to its active metabolite, DHT, by the enzyme 5α-reductase (2). DHT affects growth of prostate cells by binding to the androgen receptor (AR) (4), and the DHT-AR complex stimulates the transcription of a cascade of androgen-responsive genes. ARs are present in both epithelial and stromal cells (2). Thus, the androgen responsiveness of the prostate is directly mediated through the interaction of DHT with the AR. Although T can also bind to the AR and stimulate prostate cells, its affinity for the receptor is 4.0- to 5.0- fold lower than that of DHT (5).

Age

There is an interesting relationship between age, PC incidence, and androgen levels. After the age of 40, the age-specific incidence of PC increases substantially (6), but at the same time the levels of total, free, and bioavailable T significantly decline (7-12). In a study of USA military veterans aged 31 to 50 years, Ellis and Nyborg (13) showed that T levels were significantly inversely related to age in both black and white men. Gray, et al. (10) found constant declines of 1.2%/year in free T and 1.0%/year in albumin-bound T in a study of men aged 39-70 years. These investigators also noted that sex hormone-binding globulin (SHBG), which is the major serum carrier of T, increased by 1.2%/year. The net effect of these changes was a constant reduction in total T of 0.4%/year (10).

Race

African-American (AA) and Caucasian-American men have the highest international incidence rates of PC, whereas rates in Asian countries are among the lowest (14). Within the USA, the age-adjusted incidence of and mortality from PC are 60% and 100% higher, respectively, in blacks compared to whites (6). Both genetic background and environmental factors such as dietary fat intake have been hypothesized to explain these racial differences in PC occurrence.

The higher incidence of PC in USA blacks compared to whites may be due to higher T levels, higher 5α-reductase activity, and/or shorter polymorphic CAG repeat lengths in the AR gene (15). In a small study of 40 pregnant women in their first trimester, Henderson, et al. (16) found that serum T levels were 47% higher in black women compared to their white counterparts. These data suggest that black males may be exposed to higher androgen levels in utero. Ross, et al. (17) measured hormone levels in 50 black and 50 white medical students, with a mean age of 20 years in each group. These investigators found that young black men had a 15% higher total T level and a 13% higher free T level than young white men, which they suggested could explain a 2.0-fold difference in PC incidence. Ellis and Nyborg (13) confirmed the higher T levels in blacks compared to whites, and interestingly noted that the magnitude of this difference diminishes with increasing age. These observations support the notion that hormonal exposures during early life may predispose AA men to the development of PC in later years.

Several studies have compared levels of circulating hormones in different racial groups. In an extension of their earlier study, Ross, *et al.* (18) compared hormone levels in young USA black and white men with young (aged 19-23) Japanese men. Blacks had the highest serum T levels, Japanese had intermediate levels, and whites had the lowest levels, although these differences were not significant (18). Two conjugated metabolites of T, androsterone glucuronide and 3α-androstanediol glucuronide (3α-diol G), which are thought to reflect the level of T metabolism and 5α-reductase enzyme activity in the prostate, and SHBG levels were significantly lower in Japanese men compared to whites and blacks. These data suggest that the lower incidence of PC in Japanese men may be due to lower levels of androgen exposure. However, the levels of both androgen metabolites were higher in USA white than black men (18), arguing that these biomarkers do not explain the black/white difference in disease incidence. Another nested case-control study based on 106 patients with incident PC and 106 controls (19) found no association between the level of androsterone glucuronide (adjusted odds ratio, OR=1.2) or 3α-diol G (adjusted OR=1.1) and PC risk.

Levels of total, free, and bioavailable T, DHT, SHBG, and the DHT/T ratio were compared in four different racial groups of healthy older USA men who served as controls for a case-control study of PC (20). Unexpectedly, Japanese and Chinese men had higher levels of total, free and bioavailable T than whites or AA. In addition, Japanese men had the highest DHT and SHBG levels. The DHT/T ratio, which may indirectly reflect 5α-reductase activity, was somewhat lower in Asians than whites or blacks. Based on this observation, Wu, *et al.*(20) suggest that whites and AAs have greater 5α-reductase activity and thus higher intra-prostatic DHT levels compared to Asian-American men.

Family History

Numerous epidemiological studies confirm that a family history of PC in a first-degree relative is associated with 2.0- to 3.0-fold elevations in relative risks. However, only two studies have examined hormone levels in subgroups stratified by family history of PC. Meikle and Stanish (21) found significant intraclass correlations among PC patients (not treated with any form of hormonal therapy) and their brothers in total T (p<0.01) and free T (p<0.05). In addition, fathers and sons had significant intraclass correlations for DHT (p<0.01) and the T/DHT ratio (p<0.05). Overall, however, PC patients, their brothers, and sons had significantly lower levels of total T compared to controls (brothers-in-law) of comparable age. These authors suggest that familial factors markedly affect androgen levels (22). They found no evidence, however, that men with PC and their relatives had higher androgen levels than unrelated controls.

In a large multiethnic case-control study, Whittemore, *et al.* (23) measured androgen levels among controls according to family history of PC in a first-degree relative. Within each racial group evaluated (i.e., Caucasian, AA and Asian American), the median concentrations of total T, free T, bioavailable T, DHT, and the DHT/T ratio were similar in men with compared to men without a family history. The only significant difference observed was in Asian Americans, where SHBG levels were higher in men without a family history (p=0.04). These data do not support the hypothesis that the familial clustering of PC is due to genetically determined differences in androgen levels.

Androgen Levels

Several nested case-control studies have been conducted in which circulating steroid hormone levels were determined from baseline blood samples collected prior to the development of PC (19,24-28). Two studies (19,24) showed no associations with total T or SHBG. The other four studies, which provided relative risk estimates according to levels (i.e., quartiles) of specific androgens, are summarized in Table 1. As shown, the study by Gann, *et al.* (27) observed a significant increase in the odds ratios for PC with increasing levels of total plasma T (p for trend=0.004). Although this is the largest study published to date (222 case-control pairs), only 43% of the 520 PC cases diagnosed in this cohort provided a blood sample sufficient for analysis (150 refused the blood draw and 148 had an inadequate sample volume for analysis). This raises concern about selection bias, which may have affected study results if the distribution of hormone values differed among cases analyzed compared to cases excluded from the analysis. None of these investigations found associations with levels of DHT or 3α-androstanediol glucuronide, an indirect measure of 5α-reductase activity in the prostate. The study by Gann, *et al.* (27) did find significant increases in odds ratios across quartiles of the T/DHT ratio (p for trend=0.02), which may reflect androgen exposure within the prostate. A similar, although not significant, trend related to the T/DHT ratio was observed by Hsing and Comstock (25). In all of these studies, the androgen levels were within the range of normal values.

The availability of androgens is also affected by the level of SHBG, since the fraction of T bound to SHBG is not considered to be biologically active.

Further, there is a positive correlation between total T and SHBG (9, 27). Gann, *et al.* (27) found a significant decline in odds ratios with increasing levels of SHBG (p for trend=0.01). Men in the highest quartile of SHBG experienced a 50% lower risk relative to men in the lowest quartile. T is tightly bound to SHBG, so elevated levels of this binding protein may reduce androgen exposure of the prostate.

Table 1. Odds ratios for PC associated with androgen levels.

Study, year	Hormone[1]	Level 1 (low)	Level 2	Level 3	Level 4 (high)	p for trend
Hsing (25), 93	T	1.0	1.70	2.00	1.50	0.30
Nomura (26), 96		1.0	0.77	0.73	1.03	0.96
Gann (27), 96		1.0	1.41	1.98^2	2.60^2	0.004
Vatten (28), 97		1.0	0.75	0.79	0.83	0.70
Hsing (25), 93	DHT	1.0	0.70	0.80	1.00	0.90
Nomura (26), 96		1.0	0.87	0.74	0.82	0.51
Gann (27), 96		1.0	1.02	0.78	0.71	0.30
Vatten (28), 97		1.0	0.59	0.87	0.83	0.92
Nomura (26), 96	3α-diol G	1.0	0.93	1.20	1.37	0.23
Gann (27), 96		1.0	1.44	1.58	1.60	0.09
Vatten (28), 97		1.0	1.52	1.40	1.10	0.97
Hsing (25), 93	T/DHT ratio	1.0	1.40	1.40	1.70	0.30
Gann (27), 96		1.0	1.68	1.37	2.35^2	0.02
Vatten (28), 97		1.0	1.52	1.40	1.10	0.97

[1] Total T, DHT, 3α-androstanediol glucuronide (3α-diol G).
[2] 95% confidence interval excludes 1.0.

Estrogens

Prior to the development of antiandrogens, synthetic Es were used to treat metastatic PC, with response rates of 70-80% (29). Estrogen receptors (ER) have been found in normal and cancerous prostatic tissue (30, 31) and are primarily located in stromal cells (32). However, prostate epithelial cells have also been shown to contain ER and grow in response to estradiol (E_2) (29). Some animal and *in-vitro* studies indicate that E_2 alone or in combination with androgens may enhance proliferation of prostatic cells and, thereby increasing the risk of PC (29, 33).

There is no consistent association between E levels and age. Unlike the decline with age in circulating T levels, Gray, *et al.* (10) found that serum concentrations of Es (E_2, estrone, estrone sulfate) did not change substantially with advancing age in a cross-sectional study of 1,709 men aged 39-70 years. In another study of 810 men aged 24-90 years, Ferrini and Barrett-Connor (12) found a small decline in total E_2 and a significant decline in bioavailable E_2 with increasing age. In contrast, Baker, *et al.* (7) reported a slight increase in plasma E_2 with advancing age in a study of 466 subjects. In men, E_2 is derived from T through aromatization, and with aging there is an increase in the conversion of T to E_2 (7). Thus, if T levels decline and E_2 levels remain fairly stable or increase slightly as men age, the T to E_2 (T/E_2) ratio would decrease with age. As suggested by Longcope, *et al.* (9) a lower T/E_2 ratio in older men may simply reflect a decline in the concentration of T rather than an increase in E_2. In any case, the relative balance of T to E_2 may be as important in determining PC risk as the absolute levels of these circulating hormones.

Indirect evidence that Es may be important in PC etiology comes from studies of hormonal changes associated with alcohol consumption and men with alcoholic cirrhosis. Hypogonadism and gynecomastia, which are signs of excess E exposure, are frequently observed in men with alcoholic cirrhosis (34, 35). Hormonal abnormalities associated with this disorder include a decrease in plasma T levels and no change or a slight increase in plasma E_2 and estrone concentrations (34), which would result in a lower T/E_2 ratio among alcoholic men. Interest in the possible role of E in the development of PC has focused on whether patients with cirrhosis of the liver experience an excess risk of the disease. In a large autopsy study of men aged 45-90 years conducted by Glantz (35), PC incidence was 3.3% (18/550) in cases dying of cirrhosis compared to 9.1% (59/650) in a randomly selected set of autopsied controls (crude relative risk= 0.36). These data suggest that prolonged exposure to E may actually prevent or delay the development of PC (35).

Direct evidence that Es may be involved in PC comes from epidemiological studies that determined hormone levels in nested case-control studies (Table 2). Two studies found no pattern of risk associated with increasing levels of E_2 or estrone (25,36), based on analyses of 98 case-control pairs in each study. A more recent and larger study by Gann, *et al.* (27) however, found significantly lower relative risks in men with higher levels of circulating E_2. This latter study included 222 case-control pairs and is the largest to date to evaluate E_2 exposure in relation to PC risk. Based on these results, Gann, *et al.* (27) suggest that a low level of circulating E_2 is a risk factor for PC. Overall, the epidemiological data argue that there is a negative association between E_2 levels and risk of PC.

Table 2. Odds ratios for PC associated with E levels.

Study, year	Hormone	Level 1 (low)	Level 2	Level 3	Level 4 (high)	p for trend
Nomura (36), 88	E$_2$	1.0	1.57	0.57		0.32
Hsing (25), 93		1.0	0.90	1.10	1.00	0.90
Gann (27), 96		1.0	0.53[1]	0.40[1]	0.56[1]	0.03
Nomura (36), 88	Estrone	1.0	1.09	0.89		0.79
Hsing (23), 93		1.0	0.80	2.10	0.80	0.60

[1] 95% confidence interval excludes 1.0.

Summary

In summary, most of the evidence regarding the role of androgens and Es in PC etiology is indirect. Limited epidemiological data are available on the potential direct effects of androgens and Es in the development of PC. Observations supporting a role of androgens include the following: 1) androgens are required for the normal growth and maintenance of prostatic tissue; 2) androgens stimulate proliferation of human PC cells *in vitro*; 3) PC regresses after androgen ablation or antiandrogen therapy; 4) androgens induce PC in rodents; 5) men castrated before puberty and men with an inherited deficiency in the 5α-reductase enzyme do not develop PC; and 6) increased levels of circulating androgens (total T and T/DHT ratio) are associated with elevated relative risks of PC. Evidence that Es are involved is based on the following: 1) Es have a palliative effect in advanced stage PC; 2) hyperestrogenic states (cirrhosis) are associated with a reduced relative risk of PC; 3) Es inhibit pituitary secretion of leutinizing hormone, which results in reduced production of T and involution of prostatic epithelial cells; 4) Es act synergistically with androgens to enhance growth of prostatic tumors in animal models; and 5) ERs are present in both epithelial and stromal cells of the prostate. Given these observations, it is apparent that both androgens and Es acting alone, perhaps only at certain concentrations, or in combination are involved in the pathogenesis of PC. Additional epidemiological studies, however, are needed to confirm and expand upon the limited data that are currently available on this topic.

References

1. Huggins C, Hodges CV (1941) The effect of castration, of estrogen and of androgen injection on serum phosphatases in metastatic carcinoma of the prostate. Cancer Res 1:293-297.

2. Cunha GR, Donjacour AA, Cooke PS et al (1987) The endocrinology and developmental biology of the prostate. Endocrine Society 8:338-362.
3. Coffey DS, Isaacs JT (1981) Control of prostate growth. Urology 17:17-24.
4. Coetzee GA, Ross RK (1994) Prostate cancer and the androgen receptor. J Natl Cancer Inst 86:872-873.
5. Wilbert M, Griffin JE, Wilson JD (1983) Characterization of the cytosol androgen receptor of the human prostate. J Clin Endocrin Metab 56:113-119.
6. Stanford JL, Stephenson RA, Coyle LM et al (1998) Prostate Cancer Trends 1973-1995, SEER Program, National Cancer Institute, Bethesda, MD (In press).
7. Baker HWG, Burger HG, de Kretser DM et al (1976) Changes in the pituitary-testicular system with age. Clin Endocrinol 5:349-372.
8. Dai WS, Kuller LH, LaPorte RE et al (1981) The epidemiology of plasma testosterone levels in middle-aged men. Am J Epidemiol 114:804-816.
9. Longcope C, Goldfield SR, Brambilla DJ et al (1990) Androgens, estrogens, and sex hormone-binding globulin in middle-aged men. J Clin Endocrinol Metab 71:1442-1446.
10. Gray A, Feldman HA, McKinlay JB et al (1991) Age, disease, and changing sex hormone levels in middle-aged men: Results of the Massachusetts male aging study. J Clin Endocrinol Metab73:1016-1025.
11. Gray A, Berlin JA, McKinlay JB et al (1991) An examination of research design effects on the association of testosterone and male aging: Results of a meta-analysis. J Clin Epidemiol 44:671-684.
12. Ferrini RL, Barrett-Connor E (1998) Sex hormones and age: A cross-sectional study of testosterone and estradiol and their bioavailable fractions in community-dwelling men. Am J Epidemiol 147:750-754.
13. Ellis L, Nyborg H (1992) Racial/ethnic variations in male testosterone levels: a probable contributor to group differences in health. Steroids 57:72-75.
14. Parkin DM, Whelan SL, Feday J et al eds (1997) Cancer Incidence in Five Continents, Vol. VII, No. 143. IARC Scientific Publications, Lyon.
15. Lopez-Otin C, Diamandis EP (1998) Breast and prostate cancer: An analysis of common epidemiological, genetic, and biochemical features. Endocrine Society 19:365-396.
16. Henderson BE, Bernstein L, Ross RK et al (1988) The early in utero estrogen and testosterone environment of blacks and whites: Potential effects on male offspring. Br J Cancer 57:216-218.
17. Ross R, Bernstein L, Judd H et al (1986) Serum testosterone levels in healthy young black and white men. J Natl Cancer Inst 76:45-48.

18. Ross RK, Bernstein L, Lobo RA et al (1992) 5-alpha-reductase activity and risk of prostate cancer among Japanese and US white and black males. Lancet 339:887-889.
19. Guess HA, Friedman GD, Sadler MC et al (1997) 5α-reductase activity and prostate cancer: A case-control study using stored sera. Cancer Epidemiol Biom Prev 6:21-24.
20. Wu AH, Whittemore AS, Kolonel LN et al (1995) Serum androgens and sex hormone-binding globulins in relation to lifestyle factors in older African-American, Whites, and Asian men in the United States and Canada. Cancer Epidemiol Biom Prev 4:735-741.
21. Meikle AW, Stanish WM (1982) Familial prostatic cancer risk and low testosterone. J Clin Endocrinol Metab 54:1104-1108.
22. Meikle AW, Smith JA, West DW (1985) Familial factors affecting prostatic cancer risk and plasma sex-steroid levels. Prostate 6:121-128.
23. Whittemore AS, Wu AH, Kolonel LN et al (1995) Family history and prostate cancer risk in black, white, and Asian men in the United States and Canada. Am J Epidemiol 141:732-740.
24. Barrett-Connor E, Garland C, McPhillips JB et al (1990) A prospective, population-based study of androstenedione, estrogens, and prostatic cancer. Cancer Res 50:169-173.
25. Hsing AW, Comstock GW (1993) Serological precursors of cancer: Serum hormones and risk of subsequent prostate cancer. Cancer Epidemiol Biomarkers Prev 2:27-32.
26. Nomura AMY, Stemmermann GN, Chyou P-H et al (1996) Serum androgens and prostate cancer. Cancer Epidemiol Biom Prev 5:621-625.
27. Gann PH, Ma J, Hennekens CH et al (1996) Prospective study of sex hormone levels and risk of prostate cancer. J Natl Cancer Inst 88:1118-1126.
28. Vatten LJ, Ursin G, Ross RK et al (1997) Androgens in serum and the risk of prostate cancer: A nested case-control study from the Janus Serum Bank in Norway. Cancer Epidemiol Biom Prev 6:967-969.
29. Carruba G, Miceli MD, Comito L et al (1996) Multiple estrogen function in human prostate cancer cells. Ann NY Acad Sci 784:70-84.
30. Murphy JB, Emmott RC, Hicks LL et al (1980) Estrogen receptors in the human prostate, seminal vesicle, epididymis, testis, and genital skin: A marker for estrogen-responsive tissues? J Clin Endocrin Metab 50:938-947.
31. Ekman P, Barrack ER, Greene GL et al (1983) Estrogen receptors in human prostate: evidence for multiple binding sites. J Clin Endocrin Metab 57:166-176.

32. Chaisiri N, Pierrepoint CG (1980) Examination of the distribution of oestrogen receptor between stromal and epithelial compartments of the canine prostate. Prostate 1:357-366.
33. Wilding G (1992) The importance of steroid hormones in prostate cancer. Cancer Surveys 14:113-130.
34. Gordon GG, Altman K, Southren AL et al (1976) Effect of alcohol (ethanol) administration on sex-hormone metabolism in normal men. N Engl J Med 295:793-797.
35. Glantz GM (1964) Cirrhosis and carcinoma of the prostate gland. J Urology 91:291-293.
36. Nomura A, Heilbrun LK, Stemmermann GN et al (1988) Prediagnostic serum hormones and the risk of prostate cancer. Cancer Res 48:3515-3517.

PART 2. MOLECULAR GENETICS OF HORMONAL CANCERS

Introduction

Breast Cancer Molecular Cytogenetics

Frederic M. Waldman

The development and progression of breast cancer is a multistep process, the result of a series of genetic alterations occurring over the lifetime of a tumor. The search for specific alterations associated with the development and progression of breast tumors involves an intensive analysis of known genes and a search for new ones. Cellular oncogenes or tumor suppressor genes may be modified by gene mutation, rearrangement, amplification, deletion, epigenetic changes (such as methylation), other changes in RNA transcriptional regulation or processing, and post-translational modifications, all leading to altered protein function. Much of the recent work elucidating these various pathways is based on the hypothesis that identification of specific changes which occur in individual breast tumors will result in better predictive markers of clinical behavior and response to therapy.

Despite many years of intensive study, there are few markers which have proved useful in predicting breast cancer behavior. Tumor size, lymph node status, and pathologic grade remain the essential elements for decision making about treatment of individual patients (1-3). Hormone receptor content defines an altered prognosis, but only marginally so (1). A greater value of receptor content is in identifying patients who will respond best to treatment with specific anti-estrogens. The literature is full of reports testifying to the ability of a panoply of markers to predict tumor behavior, but most such candidates are not validated in multivariate analyses, and even the best do not show a consistent effect.

However, as approaches to cancer therapy evolve, and therapeutic choices may potentially be customized to the specific alterations present in an individual tumor, the need for more particular information about each tumor will grow. A large number of specific oncogenes and tumor suppressor genes have been nominated as markers to predict clinical behavior in breast cancer. Recent studies have confirmed common genetic alterations involving c-*myc* on 8q (4), *cyclin D1* (prad1) on 11q (5), *retinoblastoma* on 13q (6), *E-cadherin* on 16q (7-8), *p53* on 17p (7-10), and *erbB-2* (11-12), topoII-α (13), and *nm23* (14), all on 17q. Our own work (15) has led to the identification of candidate oncogenes on 20q, including ZNF217 (16-17). Further CGH and LOH studies in breast cancer have identified regions of altered copy number for which specific genes have not yet been identified, including 1q gain, 3p loss, 8p loss, 8q gain (proximal to c-*myc*), 17q gain (distal to erbB2), and gain of other regions on 20q.

We have used comparative genomic hybridization (CGH) to define sets of chromosomal alterations occurring during tumor progression. Alterations in various grades of ductal carcinoma in situ and their accompanying invasive cancers (in the same patient) have been compared, as have alterations in breast cancer primaries with their own synchronous metastases (18). These studies have shown a surprisingly high degree of similarity between different tumor stages, suggesting that clonal evolution is an early event and that tumors remain relatively clonally stable during further clinical progression. Yet we also have shown that "genetic grade", as defined by the overall number of CGH alterations, was predictive of clinical outcome in node negative tumors (19). Our data suggest that genetic alterations may define the aggressive potential of an individual tumor because they reflect specific sets of genetic changes for each individual patient.

Recently, we and others have begun to extend CGH chromosomal analyses of breast tumor progression by applying array based CGH using DNA chip arrays. The genomic resolution of chromosome based CGH analysis is limited by the condensation of metaphase chromosomes. This limit of resolution can be circumvented by laying down fragments of DNA on a slide so that it is only the size and spacing of the targets which limit the resolution. For DNA analyses, DNA arrays can be generated comprised of cloned DNA targets mapped to regions throughout the genome (20). The human haploid genome of 3×10^9 base pairs can thus be covered at 3 mb resolution with ~1000 targets 100 kb in length. Regions of particular interest can be analyzed with overlapping targets at even higher resolution. By scanning the tumor genome in a large number of tumors at such high resolution, we expect that candidate genes will be sufficiently localized to allow gene identification.

DNA alterations which are biologically relevant will result in significant changes in RNA and protein expression. In fact, if gains and losses of candidate genes are biologically significant, then it is likely that alterations of expression resulting from epigenetic changes should be present in tumors in the absence of copy number alteration. Expression profiling of breast cancers is already underway (21-22). Changes in gene expression which occur during tumor progression are being tested for prognostic and therapeutic relevance.

The current state of molecular genetic analysis of breast tumors is to test whether specific DNA alterations or RNA expression patterns can predict clinical tumor behavior. The goal of these studies is to use this information to help determine the clinical outcome for individual patients. It is expected that particular genetic patterns will be associated with outcome, and that this knowledge will help the patient and physician to decide on their optimal choice of therapy. Some alterations may predict responsiveness to specific types of therapy. As specific gene alterations are identified, their relationships to potential therapeutic interventions will be explored. It is hoped that such studies will produce molecular diagnostic classifications which will be useful for application of gene-based therapies.

References

1. Clark G (1996) Prognostic and predictive factors. In: Harris J, Lippman M, Morrow M, and Hellman S (eds.) Diseases of the breast. Lippencott-Raven Publishers, Philadelphia, pp. 461-486.
2. Page D and Anderson T (1987) Diagnostic histopathology of the breast. Edinburgh: Churchill Living-stone.
3. Harris J, Lippman M, Morrow M et al (1996) Diseases of the breast. Philadelphia: Lippencott-Raven Publishers.
4. Nass SJ and Dickson RB (1997) Defining a role for c-Myc in breast tumorigenesis. Breast Cancer Res Treat 44: 1-22.
5. Courjal F, Louason G, Speiser et al (1996) Cyclin gene amplification and overexpression in breast and ovarian cancers: evidence for the selection of cyclin D1 in breast and cyclin E in ovarian tumors. Int J Cancer 69: 247-253.
6. Band V (1998) The role of retinoblastoma and p53 tumor suppressor pathways in human mammary epithelial cell immortalization. Int J Oncol 12: 499-507.
7. Graff JR, Herman JG, Lapidus et al (1995) E-cadherin expression is silenced by DNA hypermethylation in human breast and prostate carcinomas. Cancer Res 55: 5195-5199.
8. Pierceall WE, Woodard AS, Morrow JS et al (1995) Frequent alterations in E-cadherin and alpha- and beta-catenin expression in human breast cancer cell lines. Oncogene 11: 1319-1326.
9. Bautista S and Theillet C (1997) p53 mutations in breast cancer: incidence and relations to tumor aggressiveness and evolution of the disease. Pathol Biol (Paris) 45: 882-892.
10. Falette N, Paperin MP, Treilleux I et al (1998) Prognostic value of P53 gene mutations in a large series of node- negative breast cancer patients. Cancer Res 58: 1451-1455.
11. Somerville JE, Clarke LA, and Biggart JD (1992) c-erbB-2 overexpression and histological type of in situ and invasive breast carcinoma. J Clin Pathol 45: 16-20.
12. Allred DC, O'Connell P, Fuqua SA et al (1994) Immunohistochemical studies of early breast cancer evolution. Breast Cancer Res Treat 32: 13-18.

13. Lynch BJ, Guinee DG Jr., and Holden JA (1997) Human DNA topoisomerase II-alpha: a new marker of cell proliferation in invasive breast cancer. Hum Pathol 28: 1180-1188.
14. Freije JM, MacDonald NJ, and Steeg PS (1998) Nm23 and tumour metastasis: basic and translational advances. Biochem Soc Symp 63: 261-271.
15. Kallioniemi A, Kallioniemi OP, Sudar D et al (1992) Comparative genomic hybridization for molecular cytogenetic analysis of solid tumors. Science 258: 818-821.
16. Collins C, Rommens JM, Kowbel D et al (1998) Positional cloning of ZNF217 and NABC1: genes amplified at 20q13.2 and overexpressed in breast carcinoma. Proc Natl Acad Sci U S A 95: 8703-8708.
17. Tanner MM, Tirkkonen M, Kallioniemi A et al (1996) Independent amplification and frequent co-amplification of three nonsyntenic regions on the long arm of chromosome 20 in human breast cancer. Cancer Res 56: 3441-3445.
18. Nishizaki T, DeVries S, Chew K et al (1997) Genetic alterations in primary breast cancers and their metastases: direct comparison using modified comparative genomic hybridization. Genes Chromosomes Cancer 19: 267-272.
19. Isola JJ, Kallioniemi OP, Chu LW et al (1995) Genetic aberrations detected by comparative genomic hybridization predict outcome in node-negative breast cancer. Am J Pathol 147: 905-911.
20. Pinkel D, Segraves R, Sudar D et al (1998) High resolution analysis of DNA copy number variation using comparative genomic hybridization to microarrays. Nat Genet 20: 207-211.
21. Pollack JR, Perou CM, Alizadeh AA et al (1999) Genome-wide analysis of DNA copy-number changes using cDNA microarrays. Nat Genet 23:41-46.
22. Perou CM, Jeffrey SS, van de Rijn M et al (1999) Distinctive gene expression patterns in human mammary epithelial cells and breast cancers. Proc Natl Acad Sci U S A 96:9212-9217.

7

Genome Scanning and Tissue Microarrays for the Analysis of Molecular Mechanisms Underlying Hormone Therapy Failure in Prostate Cancer

Lukas Bubendorf, Olli-P. Kallioniemi

Background

Prostate cancer (PC) is the most frequent cancer among men in western countries (1). There is a considerable discrepancy between the prevalence of histological and clinical prostate cancer. More than 30% of all males over fifty have been shown to harbor histological (incidental) PC, but only 9% develop clinical disease during their life-time (2). Therefore, most of the histologically detectable early PCs do not progress to clinically detectable disease. Increased use of the serum PSA assays in screening and early diagnosis has caused a dramatic increase of newly detected prostate cancers during the early 1990's (http://www-seer.ims.nci.nih.gov). Most tumors are now diagnosed at an early stage. However, up to 30% of of the patients still present with locally advanced or metastatic disease at the time of diagnosis (1). PC also remains the second most common cause of cancer deaths in men. This illustrates the inherent lethal nature of this disease, and the fact that advanced PC will remain a significant health problem. Androgen deprivation therapy can initially relieve symptoms in a large proportion of patients with advanced prostate cancer, but long-term cure is rarely achieved because the tumors eventually become hormone- refractory (after a few months or years), and efficient alternative systemic therapies are not yet available.

The molecular mechanisms underlying PC progression during hormonal therapy remain poorly understood. The elucidation of the molecular basis of hormone-refractory PC is crucial for the development improved therapy for patients with advanced PC.

Genome-scale Analysis of Molecular Events Underlying Tumor Progression by CGH and cDNA Microarrays

As a result of the ongoing progress in sequencing of the whole human genome, large-scale surveys of the genome can now be applied to study tumor progression. Tools for genome-wide scanning of DNA sequence copy numbers and differential gene expression have recently become available. These include comparative genomic hybridization (CGH) and cDNA microarrays. CGH is based on the simultaneous hybridization of differentially labeled tumor and control DNA on normal metaphase lymphocyte spreads (3). CGH has been successfully used to identify common genetic alterations in various tumor types (4). CGH is especially helpful in pinpointing chromosomal loci that undergo DNA amplifications. Such regions may highlight genomic sites containing activated oncogenes. Several CGH studies have indicated common chromosomal alterations in PC, including losses of 8p, 13q, 16, and gains of 8q and Xq. High-level amplifications are relatively rare in primary prostate cancer, but are often reported in advanced tumors. For example, amplification of chromosomal region X11.2-12 was seen in 30% of hormone-refractory PCs by CGH) (Figure 1). This was subsequently shown to represent amplification of the androgen receptor (AR) gene by fluorescent in situ hybridization (FISH) (5). AR amplification may enhance the ability of PC to sustain growth even at substantially reduced concentration of androgens which are typical in patients receiving androgen deprivation therapy. The discovery of AR gene amplification provides an example where a genome-wide survey, followed by a focused study at one chromosomal site led to the identification of a novel mechanism of PC progression.

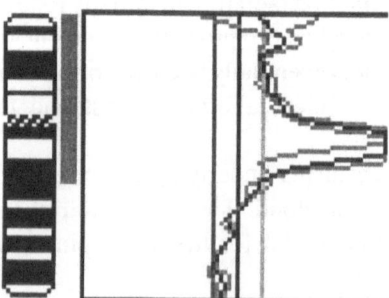

Figure 1. Comparative genomic hybridization (CGH) of a hormone-refractory prostate cancer: CGH-profile of chromosome X showing a high-level amplification of Xq11-12 (androgen receptor).

cDNA microarray technology is a new genome scanning technique, which makes it possible to directly analyze the expression levels of thousands of genes in a tumor at a time (6). Tumor and control RNA are reverse transcribed to cDNA, which is then labeled and hybridized either on filters (radioactive labeling) or on glass slides (fluorescent labeling) which contain an array of thousands of different gene targets (Figure 2). The signal intensity ratio between control and tumor hybridizations is calculated using specialized software for all the thousands of gene targets in the experiment. This technology will significantly increase the ability to study cancer biology by defining gene expression patterns and novel candidate genes.

In our recent cDNA microarray studies, we have used the CWR22 human xenograft system which imitates the progression of PC in patients undergoing androgen deprivation therapy (Figure 3). CWR22 is a serially transplantable tumor which was derived from a Gleason score 9 primary PC with osseous metastasis (7). CWR22 is highly responsive to androgen deprivation and undergoes a marked tumor regression and a decrease of the serum PSA concentration after castration of the mice. About half of the treated animals develop recurrent tumors (CWR22R), which are no longer dependent on androgens and are able to grow in these castrated animals. We utilized cDNA microarrays to explore the differential gene expression patterns between CWR22 and its hormone-refractory CWR22R derivatives to study the molecular mechanisms at this transition between hormone-sensitive and HR PC(8). Using a filter-based cDNA array with 5184 genes or expressed sequence tags (EST's), we found that 172 of these were consistently up-or down regulated in at least 3/4 hormone-refractory CWR22R xenografts as compared with their parental, hormone-sensitive CWR22 tumors. These included novel expressed sequence tags (ESTs) as well as known genes such as insulin-like growth factor binding protein 2, heat shock protein 27, insulin receptor, or NRF1 protein. Genome screening technologies such as cDNA microarrays are also creating new challenges. *How can one prioritize the long lists of possible candidate genes obtained from such experiments and proceed into developing diagnostic, prognostic, and therapeutic approaches?* The follow-up and detailed evaluation of only a fraction of the 172 genes found in our cDNA array experiments would occupy a researcher for several months or years if traditional approaches were pursued. If we want to optimally benefit from this accumulating biological information, we need additional tools and technologies to more effectively translate the findings to clinical applications by screening large numbers of tumors for the expression or copy number of novel genes. The tissue microarray technology was developed to overcome this bottleneck and facilitate the translation of new biological findings to clinical applications (9).

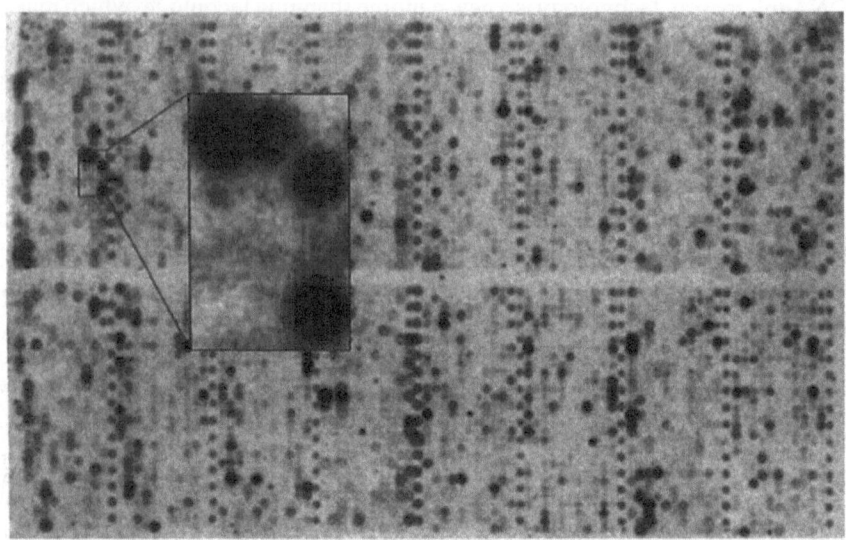

Figure 2. A cDNA microarray experiment providing a gene expression profile of hormone-refractory CWR22R xenograft on a filter-base cDNA microarray (Research Genetics, Inc.) with 5184 transcripts. Spots that are positive indicate the genes expressed in the CWR22R tumors.

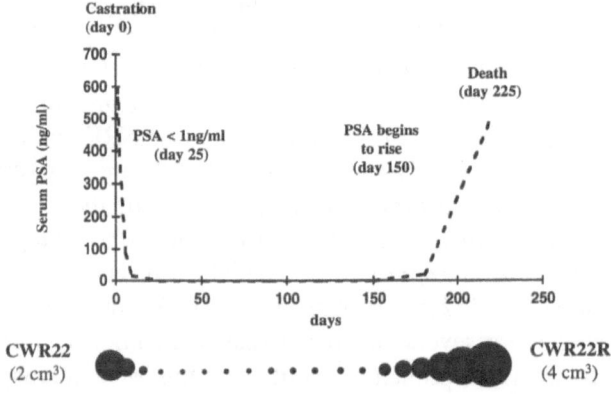

Figure 3. CWR22 xenograft model of hormone-refractory prostate cancer. Human primary, androgen-dependent tumor (CWR22) was implanted in nude mice. After castration, serum of PSA decreased and the tumor regressed. However, CWR22 often recurs as a hormone-refractory tumor (CWR22R), which is androgen-dependent.

Tissue Microarray Technologies for Screening of Hundreds of Tumors at a Time

Tissue microarrays ("tissue chips") are histologic slides containing samples from hundreds of individual tumor specimens (9). The tissue microarray slides can be used for large-scale, massively parallel *in-situ* analysis of DNA by FISH, RNA by mRNA *in-situ* hybridization, and protein by immunohistochemistry. Tissue microarrays are constructed by sampling small cylindrical biopsies from fixed and paraffin-embedded tissues into a new tissue microarray block, which is then cut with a microtome to generate hundreds of tissue array sections.

To construct a tissue microarray, a pathologist first selects the most appropriate regions of each of the tumors to be arrayed by marking representative areas on an Hematoxylin-Eosin (HE) stained slides. A tissue arraying instrument is used to acquire tissue cores from each of the "donor" blocks by a thin-walled needle with an inner diameter of 0.6 mm, held in an X-Y precision guide (Figure 4). The cylindrical sample is retrieved from the selected region in the "donor" tumor and inserted into the "recipient" tissue microarray block with defined array coordinates. After the construction of the tissue microarray block, up to 200 sections can be cut with a microtome from each block. The morphology of all the arrayed tumors can be verified by HE staining of the tissue microarray slides and subsequent sections used for molecular analyses.

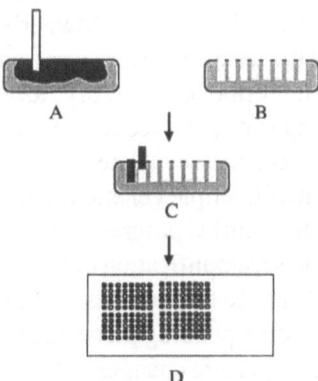

Figure 4. Construction of tissue microarrays: A) Small tissue cores are acquired from a tumor-block ("donor"), on B) an empty paraffin ("recipient") block, they are C) Inserted into holes by a thin-walled needle (0.6 mm). D) Up to 200 sections can be cut with a microtome from each microarray block (not shown).

There are numerous possible applications of tissue microarrays in cancer research. These include analysis of the molecular basis of tumor progression, molecular profiling of large series of tumors with hundreds of biomarkers, validation and prioritization of cDNA microarray data, rapid translation of data from cell line, xenograft, and animal models to human cancer, evaluation of the diagnostic, prognostic, and therapeutic potential of newly-discovered genes and molecules, testing, and optimization of DNA probes and antibodies. Furthermore, the technology provides improved utilization of pathology archives, tissue banks and collaborative tissue resources, including rare and precious tumors or clinical trial materials. The utility of tissue microarrays as a high-throughput tool for molecular pathology has already been demonstrated in a number of studies (8-12). Two examples of PC research will be presented here.

Survey of Gene Amplifications During Prostate Cancer Progression Using Tissue Microarrays

We recently demonstrated that the combination of tissue microarrays with FISH provides a high-throughput tool for analysis of PC development and progression (10). We constructed a PC tissue microarray from 371 formalin-fixed tissue blocks, including benign prostatic hyperplasia (n=32), primary tumors (n=223), as well as both locally recurrent tumors (n=54) and metastases (n=62) from patients with hormone-refractory disease (Figure 5). We used fluorescent probes for five genes, including *AR*, c-*myc*, *cyclin-D1*, *erb-B2*, and n-*myc* together with the corresponding centromeric probes (Vysis, Downer's Grove, Illinois). High-level amplifications of all of the tested loci were very rare (<2%) in primary PC. However, in samples from hormone-refractory locally recurrent or from metastatic deposits, the amplification frequencies were substantially more common for three of the five genes evaluated (Table 1). This supports the hypothesis that accumulation of multiple genetic changes, perhaps as a result of genetic instability, is associated with PC progression. In metastases from patients with hormone-refractory disease, amplification of the *AR* gene was seen in 22%, c-*myc* in 11%, and *cyclin-D1* in 5% of the cases (Figure 6). In specimens from locally recurrent tumors, the corresponding percentages were 23%, 4% and 8%.

Studies of the molecular genetic changes in the metastatic specimens are important, because the distant metastatic sites are primarily responsible for the clinical outcome, and represent the primary targets of systemic therapies. *AR* amplification was equally common in the distant metastatic deposits as in local recurrences. In contrast, c-*myc* was most frequently amplified in metastases, and might therefore be linked to the metastatic capability of PC (10). In addition, we found that also *cyclin-D1* can occasionally be amplified in PC. The biologic and prognostic implication of this newly-discovered amplification in PC remains to be determined. *Erb-B2* and N-*myc* amplifications were never detected at any stage of PC progression, and therefore, they are unlikely to play a significant role in PC.

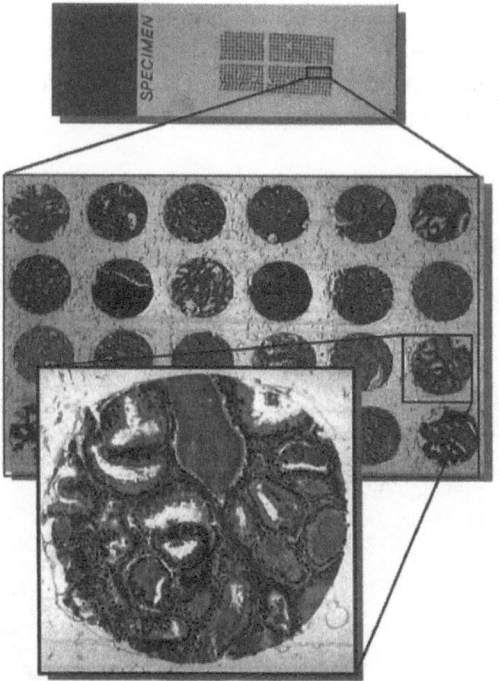

Figure 5. Prostate cancer tissue microarray with 371 specimens from tumors and benign controls (HE-staining).

Table 1. Prevalence of gene amplifications during the progression of prostate cancer by FISH on a prostate tissue microarray containing 371 specimens from different patients. There were no amplifications of *erb-B2* and N-*myc* in any of these specimens.

		Hormone-refractory	
	Primary PRCA	Local Recurrence	Metastasis
AR	2/205 (1.0%)	11/47 (23.4%)	13/59 (22.0%)
c-*myc*	0/168 (0%)	2/47 (4.3%)	5/47 (10.6%)
cyclin-D1	2/172 (1.2%)	3/38 (7.9%)	2/43 (4.7%)

Taken together, in only five experiments, we were able to establish clinical correlations from screening 371 specimens with five gene-specific probes resulting in a total of over 1400 valuable FISH results. If we had applied traditional FISH strategies, this analysis would have been time consuming, laborious, and expensive. In addition, many of the precious original tissue blocks would have been used up in the process of making multiple slides of each tumor for the FISH experiments.

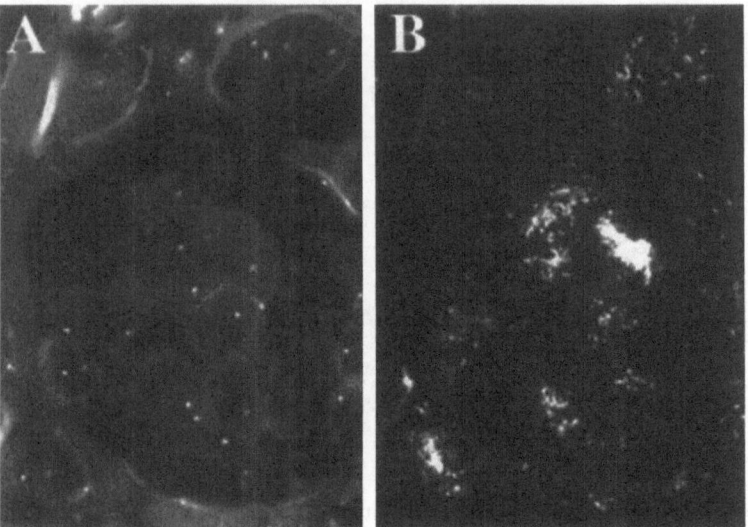

Figure 6. Prostate cancer with AR amplification by FISH on a prostate cancer tissue microarray (x630). A) Two signals are seen in each cell with a reference probe (centromere X). B) A high number of AR signals (>20/cell) are seen after a hybridization with an AR-specific probe.

Combined Utility of cDNA and Tissue Microarray Technology in Prostate Cancer Research

As mentioned above, we screened 5184 prostate-specific cDNAs with cDNA microarrays to find differentially regulated genes between a hormone-sensitive human PC xenograft CWR22, and its hormone-refractory derivative CWR22R (8). We then used 269 clinical specimens on our PC tissue microarray to investigate, whether genes implicated by the DNA chip in this experimental model system are also involved in the progression of clinical PC. cDNA array experiments revealed 37 (0.7%) systematically up- and 135 (2.6%) down-regulated genes in hormone-refractory as compared to untreated, hormone-sensitive xenografts. Insulin-like growth factor binding protein (IGFBP-2) emerged as one of the most highly expressed genes. Tissue microarray analysis showed high levels of IGFBP-2 protein in 100% of hormone-refractory disease, 37% of primary tumors, and in none of the benign prostates (p<0.0001). This implicates IGFBP-2 as a gene involved in the tumor progression not only in the CWR22 model, but also in patients experiencing tumor progression and hormonal therapy failure. This study demonstrates that the combination of cDNA and tumor tissue microarrays is powerful for the rapid identification of novel genes involved in PC progression, as well as for the analysis of their importance in large series of clinical specimens from PC patients.

Conclusion

Genome-scale information on cancer biology is now rapidly increasing. Tissue microarrays provide a powerful tool for the molecular profiling of hundreds of tumors and are likely to significantly facilitate the translation of basic research findings to clinical applications. In PC, these technologies may significantly contribute to a better understanding of cancer progression to a hormone-refractory state, where new therapeutic options are urgently needed.

References

1. Ries LAG, Kosary CL, Hankey BF et al (1998) SEER Cancer Statistics Review, 1973-1995, National Cancer Institute. Bethesda, MD.
2. Scardino PT, Robert WM, Liss AH (1992) Early detection of prostate cancer. Hum Pathol 23:211-222.
3. Kallioniemi A, Kallioniemi OP, Sudar D et al (1992) Comparative genomic hybridization for molecular cytogenetic analysis of solid tumors. Science 258:818-821.
4. Rooney PH, Murray GI, Stevenson DAJ et al (1999) Comparative genomic hybridization and chromosomal instability in solid tumors. Br J Cancer 80:862-873.
5. Visakorpi T, Hyytinen E, Koivisto P et al (1995) In vivo amplification of the androgen receptor gene and progression of human prostate cancer. Nat Genet 9:401-406.
6. Duggan DJ, Bittner M, Chen Y et al (1999) Expression profiling using cDNA microarrays. Nat Genet 21:10-14.
7. Nagabhushan M, Miller CM, Pretlow TP et al (1996) CWR22: the first human prostate cancer xenograft with strongly androgen- dependent and relapsed strains both in vivo and in soft agar. Cancer Res 56:3042-3046.

8. Bubendorf L, Kolmer M, Kononen J et al (in press) Molecular mechanisms of hormone therapy failure in human prostate cancer analyzed by a combination of cDNA and tissue microarrays. J Natl Cancer Inst.
9. Kononen J, Bubendorf L, Kallioniemi A et al (1998) Tissue microarrays for high-throughput molecular profiling of tumor specimens. Nat Med 4:844-847.
10. Bubendorf L, Kononen J, Koivisto P et al (1999) Survey of gene amplifications during prostate cancer progression by high-throughout fluorescence in situ hybridization on tissue microarrays. Cancer Res 59:803-806.
11. Moch H, Schraml P, Bubendorf L et al (1999) High-throughput tissue microarray analysis to evaluate genes uncovered by cDNA microarray screening in renal cell carcinoma. Am J Pathol 154:981-986.
12. Schraml P, Kononen J, Bubendorf L et al (in press) Tissue microarrays for gene amplification surveys in many different tumor types. Clin Cancer Res.

8

Serial Analysis of Gene Expression in Breast Cancer Cells

C. Marcelo Aldaz, Andrzej Bednarek, April Charpentier, Michael MacLeod, Kathleen Hawkins, and Kendra Laflin

Introduction

During the last decades most research in cancer has focused on the study of specific gene alterations in carcinogenesis. Even though progress has been significant, an enormous task lies ahead in order to completely understand the complex pathophysiology of the cancer cell. Due to the considerable research investment in the Human Genome Project, it is estimated that within the next few years we will have access to complete or at least partial sequence information on most of the genes encoded by the human genome. Although this information will be of great value it will not be sufficient to provide a full understanding of a complex disease such as breast cancer (BC). After this, perhaps a more daunting task lies ahead which is to understand how the different genes are altered in the various cancer processes and how complex gene interactions produce a particular outcome. Thus, now it is the time to invest in comprehensive approaches that will create the foundation for the next level of complexity which is to understand how multiple genes interact, and more importantly, to identify which are the key genes involved in producing a particular pathologic outcome. Numerous techniques are under development for the analysis of global gene expression changes in which thousands of gene targets can be assayed simultaneously. One of the most popular approaches relies on the microarraying of specific cDNAs on solid matrices, i.e. glass or membranes (1). A second approach utilizes microchip technology for the synthesis and microarraying of specific oligonucleotides series capable of identifying specific gene targets (2). Both of these approaches require expensive hardware for arraying, scanning, and analysis of the experiments. A third technical approach for the analysis of global gene expression was described a few years ago by Kinzler and Vogelstein (3-5), serial analysis of gene expression (SAGE). This exciting new technique has the potential to revolutionize studies of changes in gene expression. This technique gives a statistical description of the mRNA population present in a cell without prior selection of the genes to be studied. Recently, Kinzler's group demonstrated the utility of applying SAGE for the analysis of human cancer samples, comparing normal colon samples with colon and pancreatic tumor samples and cancer cell lines (5). The data demonstrated the power of SAGE, and also gave a very good idea of the complexity of the problem. The investigators analyzed approximately 300,000 transcripts from 45,000 different genes. They identified 289 transcripts that were expressed at significantly different levels between the colon tumors and normal colon tissue. Of those, 108 transcripts were expressed at higher levels in the colon cancers (average increase, 13 fold). Interestingly, no large differences were found when comparing primary tumors with tumor cell lines. They confirmed that the data collected by SAGE were easily reproduced by Northern analysis with the corresponding probes (5).

The key feature of SAGE is that it is potentially more powerful than other techniques, i.e. differential display, because in the initial step, one obtains both quantitative information on the abundance of each mRNA and a partial sequence. Performing this technique successfully is not trivial, but it can be performed in any laboratory that masters basic molecular biology methodology, and it does not require any special equipment. However, the analysis can be greatly facilitated by access to an automatic DNA sequencer. This approach generates sequence information that allows not only the identification of all the transcripts being expressed in a normal or cancerous cell at any given time, but it also provides quantitative information on the relative abundance of each of the transcripts. This analysis allows the definition of what has recently been termed the cell "transcriptome" by Kinzler, et al. (4).

SAGE has been proven useful in identifying important molecular events in cancer (5). By comparing the expression profiles of aggressive BC cells with those of normal breast epithelial cells, it should be possible to identify genes that may be used as tumor markers with potential impact in BC diagnosis and/or prognosis. Similarly, by comparing the normal mammary gland cell with pre invasive (in-situ) mammary gland carcinoma lesions, it may be also possible to identify marker genes in early tumor detection. Some of these genes may be already known, but, more importantly, this approach also lends itself to the discovery of novel genes.

Among the major objectives of our studies is to create a "database of gene expression changes" in breast carcinogenesis that will constitute the ground work for a variety of possible follow-up studies. Another goal of our work is to use part of the information generated from the SAGE analysis of BC cells with multiple areas of genomic amplification, to identify putative oncogenes that are commonly overexpressed in BC tissues. It is known that one of the most common events in breast carcinogenesis is the overexpression and amplification of oncogenes, growth factors, and growth factor receptors which provide a selective growth advantage and contribute to breast tumor progression (6-8). The identification of such genes may have an impact not only as potential prognostic tools, but they may potentially affect therapeutic modalities as well. In this chapter, we report preliminary results and data validation obtained in the course of optimizing the SAGE methodology in our laboratory.

Summary of SAGE Methodology

The SAGE procedure has previously been described by Velculescu, *et al.* (3). Briefly, polyadenylated RNA is prepared and double stranded cDNA is synthesized using a SuperScript kit (GIBCO). Biotinylated-oligo (dT) is used as primer for first strand synthesis (Figure 1). Step 1. The biotinylated cDNA is digested with an "anchoring" restriction enzyme (AE), NlaIII, that leaves a 3' overhang. The most 3'-fragments are then isolated using streptavidin beads. Step 2. Two linkers, each containing the recognition sequence for a "tagging" restriction enzyme (TE) BsmFI, are ligated onto the Nla III overhangs. This enzyme produces a staggered cut, offset by about 10 base pairs from the recognition sequence (5'-GGGAC). Step 3. Subsequent digestion with BsmFI and blunt end fill-in produces fragments of each cDNA molecule containing unique 14 base pair sequences (including the NlaIII sequence) that provides a "tag" specific to each expressed gene. The abundance of each tag in the population is proportional to the abundance of that mRNA in the original RNA population. Step 4. These tags are then ligated and amplified by PCR. Step 5. Restriction with AE, isolation of ditags, concatenate and clone. The X and O represent nucleotides from different transcripts (Figure 1). Approximately, 40-50 individual "tags" are produced per clone. By sequencing cloned tag concatamers, one can obtain a statistical picture of the relative abundance of the different mRNAs expressed within an individual cell population. Statistical analysis and comparison between different samples is performed following Zhang, *et al.* (5). Presently, we are also using clustering techniques to determine statistical significance and to perform comparative analysis of the data.

Once a database of global gene expression profiles for all experimental groups has been generated it will be necessary to analyze this database to define significant changes in expression of known genes as well as identify novel candidate genes. New genes are entering the GenBank database daily. Therefore updated information is essential when analyzing the SAGE results. The incredible expansiveness of the data collected by performing the SAGE protocol requires effective avenues for analysis and interpretation which we are currently developing. The information presented in figures and tables in this chapter represent only a very small fraction of the data that can be collected upon completion of a SAGE project.

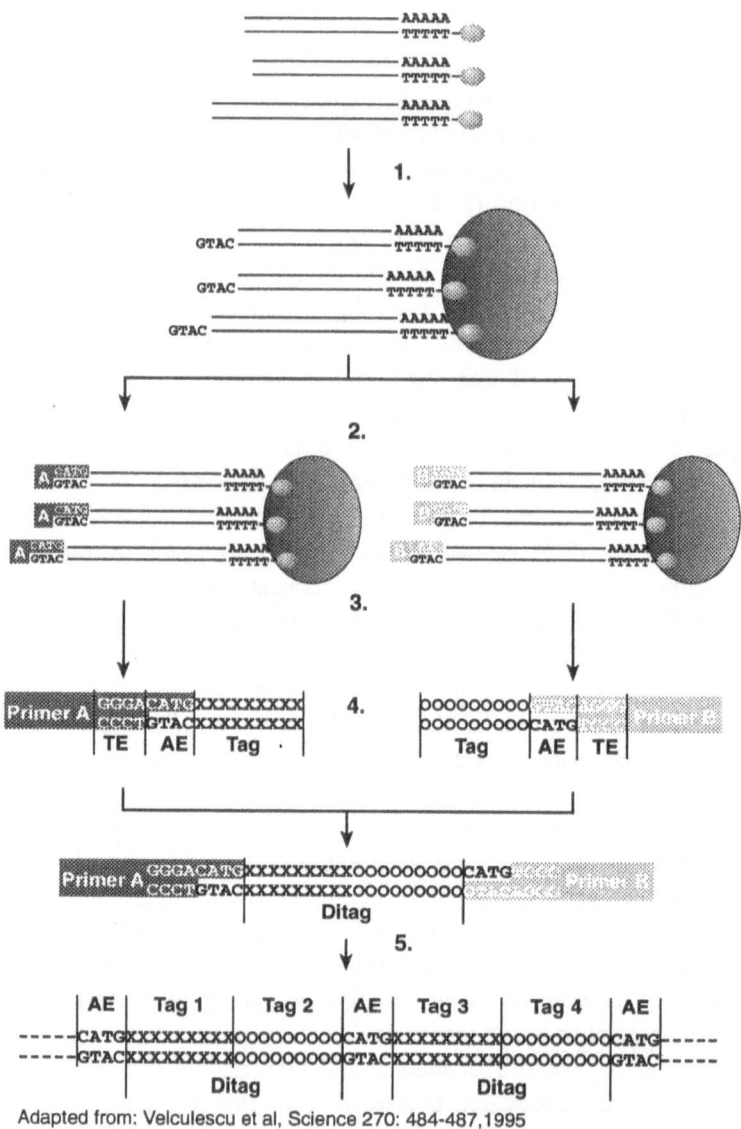

Adapted from: Velculescu et al, Science 270: 484-487,1995

Figure 1. Schematic representation of the SAGE protocol.

The database was created by a SAGE proprietary software developed by the Kinzler and Vogelstein Laboratory Groups at John Hopkins University, School of Medicine, Baltimore MD, which was kindly provided for our studies. The SAGE algorithm creates tag libraries (specific sequences located at the last NlaIII site prior to the poly A tail) using nucleotide sequences from the GenBank database (National Center for Biotechnology Information NCBI).

The SAGE software provides quantitative information on three types of transcripts: 1) Tags identifying known genes, 2) Tags identifying anonymous sequences obtained from the GenBank Est (expressed sequence tags) databases, and 3) Tags identifying transcripts with "no matches" in any of the available databases. This last feature is in itself a very important difference with other techniques for the study of global gene expression, since it allows the potential identification and cloning of novel genes.

We are currently using this exciting and powerful technology in various different projects. Among them we are investigating differences in gene expression between normal human breast epithelial cells and human BC cell lines known to contain various regions of genomic amplification. Our goal is to identify novel overexpressed genes (growth factors, oncogenes or tumor markers) that may be of use in BC diagnosis and or prognosis. We have presently analyzed a total of approximately 60,000 tags, from the MDA-MB 453, SKBR3, and MCF-7 BC cell lines and normal breast epithelial cells, having already identified more than 7,000 different transcripts. As expected the most abundant transcripts are gene products associated with protein synthesis such as the ribosomal proteins typical of cells growing vigorously *in vitro* (3). A representative list of the most abundant ribosomal transcripts found in the various BC lines is shown in Table 1.

Table 1. Relative levels of expression of ribosomal proteins % of total transcripts.

Ribosomal Proteins	MDA453	SKBR32	MCF7 no E₂	MCF7 + E₂
ARPP0	0.05	0.07	0.07	0.06
ARPP1	0.05	0.26	0.38	0.12
ARPP2	0.40	0.13	0.12	0.11
RPL10	0.04	0.18	0.01	0.06
RPL12	0.11	0.15	0.50	0.46
RPL13	0.17	0.16	0.56	0.43
RPL13A	0.13	0.31	0.61	0.51
RPL14	0.05	0.04	0	0
RPL17	0.12	0.07	0.2	0.28
RPL18	0.01	0.07	0.04	0.06
RPL18A	0.18	0.34	0.57	0.65
RPL19	0.05	1.16	0.04	0.10

Table 1. Relative levels of expression of ribosomal proteins % of total transcripts (continued).

Ribosomal Proteins	MDA453	SKBR32	MCF7 no E₂	MCF7 + E₂
RPL21	0.10	0.30	0.91	0.74
RPL23	0.10	0.14	0.24	0.27
RPL23a	0.02	0.26	0.06	0.06
RPL26	0.01	0.08	0.03	0.12
RPL27	0	0.10	0.09	0.13
RPL27a	0.06	0.49	0.39	0.13
RPL28	0.18	0.25	0.44	0.16
RPL35A	0.04	0.12	0.08	0.15
RPL37	0.03	0.14	0.12	0.04
RPL37a	0.23	0.24	0.89	0.72
RPL38	0.09	0.20	0.01	0.01
RPL39	0	0.06	0.22	0.13
RPL4	0.15	0.06	0.13	0.28
RPL41	0.19	0.59	1.13	1.42
RPL5	0.03	0.06	0.01	0
RPL6	0.02	0.10	0.04	0.12
RPL7	0.02	0.07	0	0
RPL8	0.10	0.13	0.34	0.34
RPL9	0.02	0.07	0.17	0.18
RPS10	0	0.08	0.02	0.09
RPS11	0.01	0.02	0.01	0.03
RPS12	0.16	0.63	0.18	0.12
RPS13	0	0.18	0.01	0.02
RPS16	0.04	0.38	0.05	0.11
RPS17	0.01	0.04	0.01	0.02
RPS18	0.16	0.33	0.23	0.61
RPS19	0.11	0.68	1.03	0.51
RPS20	0.01	0.09	0.03	0.01
RPS24	0.05	0.21	0.30	0.53
RPS25	0.08	0.14	0.24	0.27
RPS26	0.06	0.12	0.20	0.05
RPS27	0.13	0.48	0.91	0.74
RPS28	0.14	0.20	0.18	0.17
RPS29	0.17	0.57	0.86	0.33
RPS3	0.08	0.20	0.25	0.24
RPS3a	0.02	0.19	0.61	0.68
RPS4X	0.09	0.26	0.46	0.21
RPS5	0.09	0.19	0.02	0.10
RPS6	0.02	0.15	0.04	0.12
RPS7	0	0.08	0.04	0.06
RPS8	0.08	0.28	0.46	0.18
Homolog of RP	0.08	0.16	0.08	0.12

Table 2. Most abundant transcripts of human breast cancer cells (excluding ribosomal protein).

MDA453	%	SKBR3	%	MCF7	%
Apoferritin H chain	0.4	Cyclophilin	0.7	K8	1.8
Laminin	0.4	ESTs	0.7	NO MATCH	1.1
Laminin receptor	0.4	K8	0.7	MLC3	0.9
Aldolase A	0.3	Cathepsin D	0.5	GAPDH	0.8
EF1α	0.3	Laminin-b p	0.4	Many ESTs	0.8
Cofilin	0.3	NADH:ubiqu oxidored	0.4	K18	0.7
K8	0.2	Ubiquitin-Uba80	0.4	Interferon-induced GIP3	0.7
NO MATCH	0.2	UBE2A (Ubiq.conjued enz)	0.3	EF2	0.6
Prothymosin α	0.2	K7	0.3	NRAS	0.5
Cyclophilin	0.2	Clusterin prec	0.3	Translat contr Tumor protein	0.4
K7	0.2	EF1-α	0.3	HMG-17	0.4
AA583999 EST-prost.	0.2	Cofilin	0.3	Cofilin	0.4
MIF	0.2	K19	0.3	Laminin receptor	0.3
G6PDH	0.2	Thymosin β10	0.3	HSP27	0.3
Laminin- b p	0.2	Laminin receptor	0.2	Cyclophilin	0.3
NO MATCH	0.2	Transl control tumor protein	0.2	CD24 signal transd.?	0.3
ATM	0.1	K18	0.2	S100A10 (Calpactin I)	0.3
γ-Actin	0.1	NO MATCH	0.2	AA583999 EST (prost.)	0.3
STRL22	0.1	Prolif.assoc(PAGA)	0.2	EF1-β	0.2
Filamin (Actin-b p)	0.1	S100A10 (Calpactin I)	0.2	NPM1	0.2
MLC3	0.1	ESTs	0.2	Retinoic acid ind RIG-E	0.2
Ca^{++} dep protease	0.1	GAPDAH	0.2	Apoferritin H chain	0.2
Nuc. p68 protein	0.1	β2-Microglob	0.2	EF1-α	0.2
S100A10 (calpactin)	0.1	α-Enolase	0.2	GTPase (rhoC)	0.2
α-Tubulin	0.1	Nuclear protein SDK3	0.2	XAPC7 (proteos.sub)	0.2

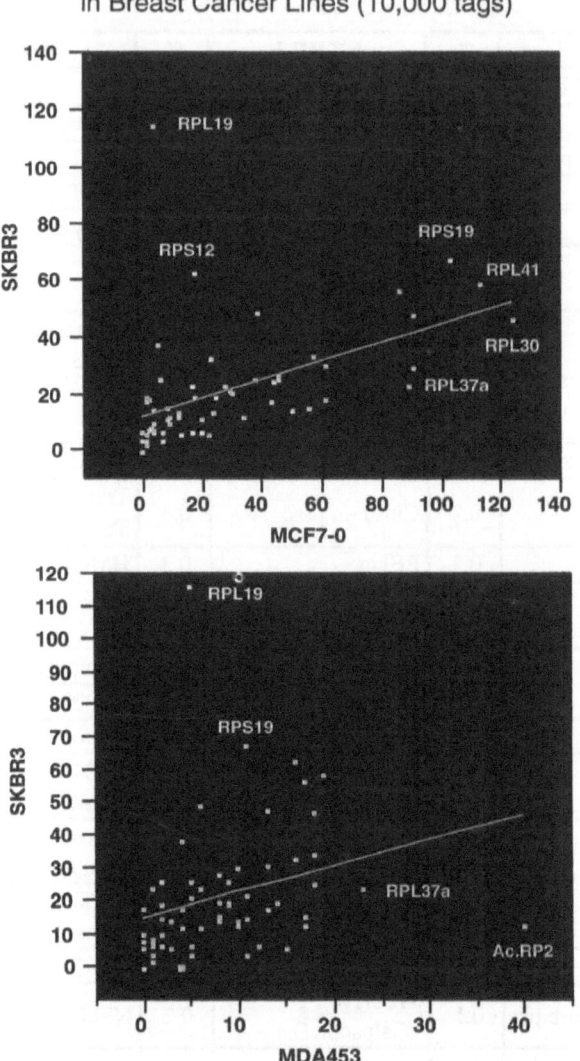

Figure 2. SAGE Analysis of ribosomal proteins in BC lines (10,000 tags). Scattergrams comparing levels of expression of the various ribosomal proteins, (expressed as number of tags) detected by SAGE in BC lines as described in Table 1. Note the complete lack of correlation between the different cell lines in the relative levels of expression of these highly expressed proteins.

Although the number of transcripts (tags) shown is relatively small, we can roughly estimate the number of copies per cell of each to the transcripts based on a total estimate of 300,000 total transcripts/cell (4). In Table 2, we show the most abundant mRNAs (excluding ribosomal proteins) found in the three BC lines under analysis. We have already identified numerous interesting overexpressed genes such as laminin, its receptors, and laminin binding proteins, all commonly overexpressed in all BC lines. Figure 2 illustrates a comparative analysis of the levels of expression of the various ribosomal proteins in the different BC lines.

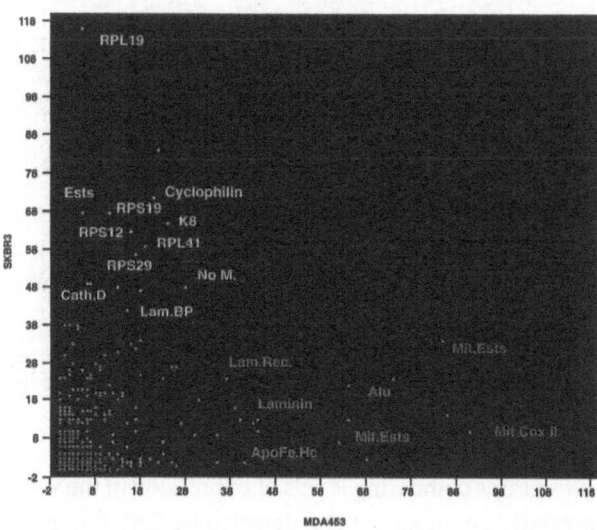

Figure 3. Scattergram comparing levels of expression of all transcripts (expressed as number of tags) detected by SAGE in BC lines SKBR3 and MDA453 at the 10,000 tag level. No correlation can be observed in the levels of expression of highly abundant proteins when comparing both cell lines.

Figure 3 illustrates a comparison, at the 10,000 tag level, of all transcripts expressed in BC lines SKBR3 vs. MDA453. This scattergram displays the name of some of the most abundant transcripts in each of the cell lines. Both data illustrate the significant heterogeneity between different BC lines, with no correlation on the levels of transcript expression. Figure 4, on the other hand, demonstrates the reproducibility of SAGE by comparing the expression level of various ribosomal proteins in two independently processed samples of the same cell line, the estrogen receptor positive MCF7 BC line, with or without estradiol (E_2) treatment. As can be observed in the scattergram, in spite of the E_2 treatment, the correlation between both samples is overall very good, r square = 0.78.

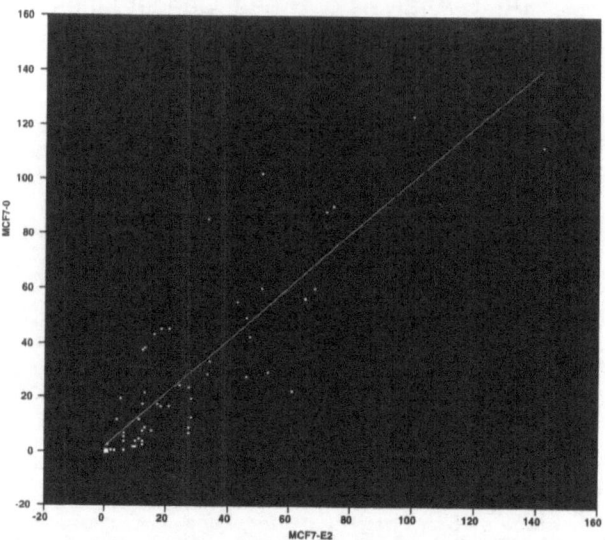

Figure 4. Scattergrams comparing levels of expression of the various ribosomal proteins, (expressed as number of tags) detected by SAGE in the same BC line, MCF7 before (MCF7-0) and after E_2 treatment (MCF7-E_2). In contrast with the findings displayed in Figures 2 and 3, note the very good correlation observed in the levels of expression of these highly abundant proteins (r square = 0.78).

Conclusions

Present day advances in gene expression technology are starting to allow researchers to define global changes in gene expression for specific tissue and cell targets. This constitutes just a glimpse into the next level of genomic complexity which will be of critical importance in the post Human Genome

Project era. Technologies such as SAGE and microarray technologies are at the cutting edge of this new undertaking. The ability to understand the detailed mechanisms of tumor progression, from the very early stages of carcinogenesis through metastasis, will allow researchers to identify key components and interactions of the malignant pathway. The knowledge obtained by defining global and specific alterations in gene transcription of premalignant and malignant cells, will allow researchers to focus on gene targets that will better serve as diagnostic and prognostic tools. Ultimately, it would be ideal to achieve a very precise matching of treatment to individual tumors profiles. A logical additional consequence will be the design of more rationale therapeutic approaches.

Acknowledgment

This work was supported in part by NIEHS grant ES07784 and the Susan G. Komen Breast Cancer Foundation.

References
1.   DeRisi J, Penland L, Brown PO et al (1996) Use of a cDNA microarray to analyse gene expression patterns in human cancer. Nature Gen 14:457-460.
2.   Lockhart DJ, Dong H, Byrne MC et al (1996) Expression monitoring by hybridization to high-density oligonucleotide arrays. Nature Biotechnol 14:1675-1680.
3.   Velculescu VE, Zhang L, Vogelstein B et al (1995) Serial analysis of gene expression. Science 270:484-487.
4.   Velculescu VE, Zhang L, Zhou W et al (1997) Characterization of the yeast transcriptome. Cell 88:243-251.
5.   Zhang L, Zhou W, Velculescu VE et al (1997) Gene expression profiles in normal and cancer cells. Science 276:1268-1272.
6.   Slamon DJ, Clark GM, Wong SG et al (1987) Human breast cancer: correlation of relapse and survival with amplification of the HER-2/neu oncogene. Science 235:177-182.
7.   Kraus MH, Popescu NC, Amsbaugh SC et al (1987) Overexpression of the EGF receptor-related proto-oncogene erbB-2 in human mammary tumor cell lines by different molecular mechanisms. EMBO J 6:605-610.
8.   Brenner A and Aldaz CM (1997) The Genetics of Sporadic Breast Cancer. In: Aldaz CM, Gould M, McLachlan J et al (eds) Etiology of Breast and Gynecological Cancer, Progress in Clinical and Biological Research. Wiley Liss, New York, pp. 396:63-82.

9

The Effects of Triphenylethylene Antiestrogens on Parameters of Multistage Hepatocarcinogenesis in the Rat

Yvonne P. Dragan, Emile Nuwaysir, Linda Sargent, Dong-Hui Li, V. Craig Jordan, and Henry C. Pitot

Carcinogenesis is a multi-stage (1, 2), multi-step (3, 4), and multi-pathway (5) process. Certain chemicals may modulate this process at any step in a genetic and/or epigenetic manner. In animals, the stages of initiation, promotion, and progression can be operationally demonstrated (1, 2). The rat liver has been extensively analyzed as a multistage model system for analysis of the stage(s) at which a compound can act to modify the carcinogenic process (6).

Agents with an antiestrogenic action have been developed for the therapy and prevention of breast cancer and potentially for treatment or prevention of osteoporosis and heart disease (7, 8). The development of Tamoxifen (TAM) more than three decades ago and its use by Jordan (9) as an inhibitor of the chemical induction of breast cancer in rats paved the way for its place as the endocrine agent of choice in all stages of human breast cancer and, more recently, in its use as a chemopreventive in women at high risk of developing this disease. Today, a number of analogs are being tested in both the laboratory and the clinic for potential therapeutic and chemopreventive applications. The chemical structure of several of the antiestrogens currently being tested in the clinic are provided in Figure 1.

Because of the extensive clinical use of TAM and now several of its related triphenylethylene antiestrogens, potential chronic toxicities have been extensively investigated in rodents, as is done with all drugs developed for potential human use. This paper briefly reviews acute and chronic toxic effects that may contribute to the potential carcinogenic use of these chemicals in vivo.

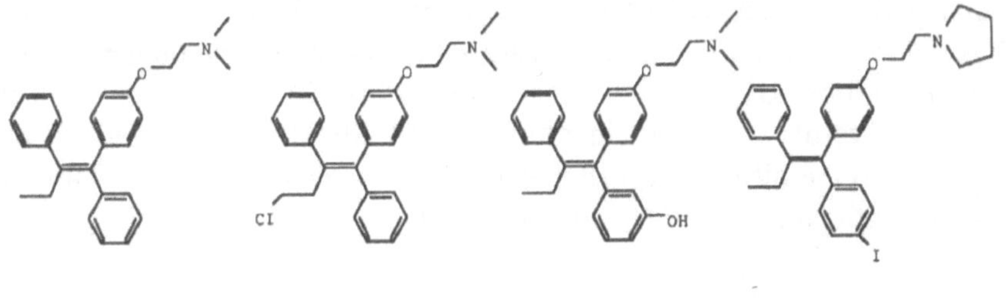

Tamoxifen   Toremifene   Droloxifene   Idoxifene

Figure 1. Structures of tamoxifen and several related, clinically relevant antiestrogens.

Initiation

Recently, TAM has been shown to induce liver tumors in rats (10, 11). Single-dose administration to rats has not been demonstrated convincingly to produce an initiating action in a two-stage model of rat hepatocarcinogenesis (12) which is in concert with the lack of mutagenicity in standard tests (13, 14). However, several studies indicate that chronic administration of TAM has an initiating action in such liver carcinogenesis models (15-17). Studies with acute administration of TAM have indicated that DNA adducts can be detected in the liver after its administration (14,18-20). In addition, similar studies have indicated that DNA adducts and modifications accumulate with protracted TAM administration. Furthermore, studies by Carthew, et al. (17) indicate that TAM is a cumulative genotoxin in these in vivo models. Both acute and chronic administration of toremifene can result in DNA adduct formation, but a lower number of adducts are detected in the rat liver after toremifene administration than has been observed with TAM (21). Toremifene and several other antiestrogens have been developed to have a more rapid clearance than observed with TAM in order to limit the spectrum and severity of potential chronic side effects (8). While a lower adduct burden has been observed with toremifene than with TAM, structural alerts imply a genotoxic potential for toremifene as well (22). Importantly, peroxidative metabolism of both TAM and toremifene results in DNA damage and protein adduct formation (23). In addition, a number of studies indicate that toremifene, similar to TAM, can induce micronuclei and aneuploidy in appropriate test systems (21, 24-28). Droloxifene (3-hydroxy TAM) is rapidly glucuronidated and cleared from the body and does not result in detectable DNA adducts (26). Similarly, idoxifene is not as readily metabolized as is TAM and may lack the ability to induce DNA adducts. However, pyrrolidino TAM readily forms DNA adducts, indicating that idoxifene has the potential for their formation (26). Figure 2 indicates that acute administration (14 days) of TAM results in the formation of several detectable DNA adducts, which increase in intensity with more chronic administration (18 mo.). In addition, to these more polar adducts described by our group (Li et al., unpublished results) and other investigators (18-20), DNA modifications, due potentially to the differential metabolism of endogenous substances, also are increased with prolonged TAM administration.

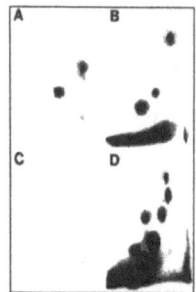 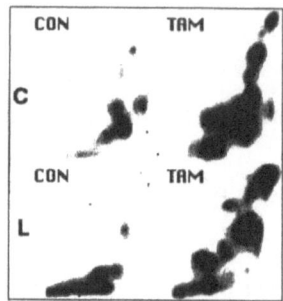

Figure 2. Chromatograms from [^{32}P]-postlabeling analysis of liver from control female Sprague-Dawley rats and rats treated for 14 days (A) or 18 mo. (B) with TAM. Panels labeled A and B correspond to more polar DNA modifications that correspond with the label C in panel B (Li *et al.* unpublished results).

The metabolism of TAM to reactive species that can bind to both protein and DNA probably underlies the carcinogenic potential of TAM and several related compounds for the rat liver (14, 18-20). Several metabolites of TAM and related compounds result in the generation of electrophilic derivatives capable of binding to DNA. At least two pathways for generation of reactive intermediates have been proposed for TAM (29, 30). One pathway, which may account for adduct generation, is that of α-hydroxylation with consequent esterification by sulfation or acetylation, resulting in a very reactive compound (31). The second pathway has not been characterized, and several hypotheses exist including formation of a quinone methide (32), a 3,4 catechol formed by 3,4 epoxidation (33), or a metabolite derived from metabolite E or 4-hydroxy TAM (34). The pathway responsible for the metabolic generation of the TAM electrophile may be CYP3A or CYP2C (27, 33, 35), although other potential pathways (e.g. a peroxidative one in the uterus) may exist (23, 27, 36, 37). The metabolic activation of TAM is likely to be concentration- and tissue- (and potentially species-) specific.

Several findings indicate a biological activity of TAM-treated tissue generally indicative of a mutagenic potential. For example, mutations in the p53 gene have been detected in liver neoplasms from TAM-treated rats (38), and likewise mutations in Ki-ras have been associated with endometrial neoplasms in humans treated with TAM (39). Recently, a mutagenic action of TAM has been demonstrated in Fischer lacI transgenic rats administered TAM (40, 41). In vitro studies on templates containing TAM-adducted bases have demonstrated a mutagenic potential for TAM-derived DNA adducts (42). These findings demonstrate the importance of identifying promutagenic derivatives of TAM, the metabolic pathways responsible for their generation, including both tissue and species specificity and the specific preneoplastic lesions resulting from initiation by the triphenylethylene antiestrogen.

Promotion

Estrogenic agents are effective tumor promoters for the rat and human liver (43, 44). Interestingly, TAM administration can inhibit the estrogen-induced hepatic tumor promotion observed in rats treated with a two-stage, initiation-promotion protocol (45, 46). This action of TAM is due to its competitive antagonism of estrogen at the estrogen receptor and results in a decrease in the estradiol-induced cell proliferation of hepatocytes (47). However, administration of TAM in combination with an estrogenic agent can result in an additive effect on promotion, and under certain circumstances TAM alone can be shown to have a promoting action in the rat liver. One study demonstrated that TAM is a more effective promoting agent in the Fischer rat than in the Sprague-Dawley rat (47). Other studies have shown that TAM is more carcinogenic in the Wistar and Lewis rat strains than in the Fischer strain (17). These latter studies have been attributed to differences in apoptosis and cell proliferation as a consequence of TAM administration to these strains (17). The observed strain difference in parameters associated with TAM-induced hepatic tumor promotion, coupled with the potential importance of TAM as a promoting agent for human endometrial cancer development, indicate the relevance of determining the mechanism of tumor promotion by TAM in these tissues. Several studies have indicated effective promotion of DEN-induced altered hepatic foci in the rat liver by TAM (16, 17, 21, 48-50). The dose-dependent promotion as a consequence of dose administered and serum level achieved is given in Figure 3. In addition, the incidence of neoplasms in TAM-treated Fischer rats administered TAM in relation to serum and liver levels achieved after 18 mo. of TAM administration may be seen in Table 1.

Table 1. Hepatic tumor incidence and corresponding serum and liver levels in female Fischer rats administered TAM for 18 mo.[+]

TAM (ppm in diet)	Serum (ng/ml)	Liver (mcg/g)	NN	HCC
0	--	--	16/22	0/22
250	249 ± 164	23.9 ± 3.2	13/15	1/15
500	644 ± 194	34.2 ± 4.7	15/15	8/15

[+]Female rats were fed an AIN-based semi-synthetic diet to which 0, 250, or 500 ppm TAM was admixed. The rats were sacrificed after 18 mo. of TAM administration, and the liver histopathology was assessed. Serum and liver concentrations of TAM were determined by HPLC analysis. The serum and liver concentrations are the average and standard error for all rats in each treatment group. NN, hepatic neoplastic nodules; HCC, hepatocellular carcinoma. The incidence of each pathology is indicated. (For further details see reference 21).

Progression

TAM is structurally related to diethylstilbesterol (DES), a known carcinogen. The induction of aneuploidy by DES has been correlated with its carcinogenic action (51). Several studies have indicated that progression of cancer development is characterized by an evolving karyotypic instability and aneuploidy (52-54). To this end, Syrian hamster embryo (SHE) cells have been used to demonstrate that the carcinogenic action of DES is primarily due to its ability to induce aneuploidy (51, 55). Studies in the MCL-5 lymphoblastoid cell line indicate that TAM, toremifene, and their 4-hydroxy derivatives can induce micronuclei in these cells, indicating that either numerical chromosomal changes or spindle disruption was induced (27). In cells lacking metabolic activity, the 4-hydroxy metabolites but not the parent compounds were able to induce aneuploidy. Both TAM and toremifene can induce clastogenesis in this system, but aneuploidy is observed only with further metabolism to the 4-hydroxy derivative. TAM has also been demonstrated to induce aneuploidy in a Syrian hamster embryo cell system in the absence of an exogenous metabolizing system (28). Interestingly, droloxifene, which has a hydroxyl group at the 3 position, does not transform SHE cells, whereas the 4-hydroxy metabolite of TAM does transform these cells (28). Acute administration of TAM to female Fischer rats resulted in a markedly increased incidence of aneuploidy coupled with microscopic evidence of spindle disruption (25, 56). These studies were extended to include toremifene and the 4-hydroxy derivatives of both TAM and toremifene in rats. These studies confirmed the acute effects of TAM (25) and demonstrated a chronic effect of both TAM and toremifene (24). Several studies have indicated that DES induces aneuploidy through disruption of tubulin organization, which may result in chromosomal non-disjunction and hence aneuploidy (28, 53, 57).The generation of protein adducts between TAM and chromosomal or spindle-related proteins may also contribute to the induction aneuploidy (58). Alternatively, the altered phosphorylation status of spindle or chromosome-associated proteins may contribute to the observed aneuploidy.

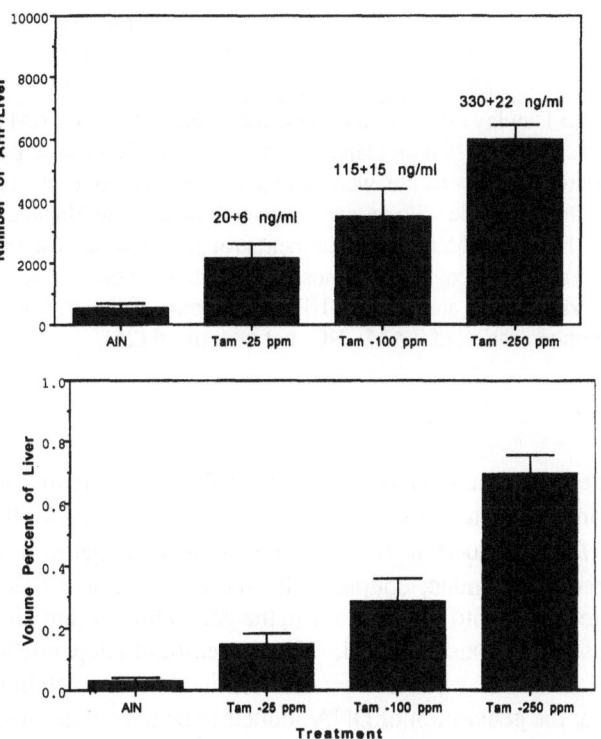

Figure 3. Dose-dependent promotion of altered hepatic foci in female Fischer rats initiated with 10 mg diethylnitrosamine 2 weeks prior to beginning treatment with TAM admixed in the diet.

In support of this latter hypothesis, TAM is known to induce a G1 block in breast cancer cells (59) and to inhibit regenerative hyperplasia in the liver. This is indicative of the induction of a G1 block which may result in aneuploidy. Disruption of the tightly coordinated processes of spindle formation and chromosomal integrity can result in aneuploidy (53, 57). The stage of progression is characterized by evolving karyotypic instability (2), and thus the clastogenic effect of several triphenylethylene antiestrogens indicates their potential for activity in inducing and/or enhancing the stage of progression. Such an effect, coupled with their obvious tumor promoting activity and formation of DNA adducts, suggests that at least TAM may be classified as a complete carcinogen.

Table 2. Acute effects of Tamoxifen on hepatic aneuploidy[+]

Dose (mg/kg)	Aneuploidy (%)	Serum (ng/ml)	Liver (mcg/g)
0	3 ± 3	–	–
0.3	71 ± 8	NQ	0.1 ± 0.01
3.0	70 ± 5	7.4 ± 1.5	0.5 ± 0.07
35.0	85 ± 7	58 ± 34	3.4 ± 0.20

[+]Female Sprague-Dawley rats were administered a single dose of TAM or the solvent trioctanoin and sacrificed 24 hours later. At sacrifice, the livers were perfused in situ and single hepatocyte suspensions were obtained. The hepatocytes were placed into culture, stimulated to divide with epidermal growth factor, and blocked in metaphase with colcemid. For each of 5 rats per treatment group, 100 metaphase spreads of good morphology were analyzed for chromosome number. Serum and liver samples collected at sacrifice were analyzed by HPLC and compared with standard curves to ascertain the concentration of TAM. NQ, not quantified (25).

Discussion

The carcinogenic action of TAM for rat liver suggests a potential for the risk of secondary cancers in humans with chronic exposure to TAM therapy. The induction of DNA adducts in rat liver and the promutagenic action of TAM administration in lacI mice, coupled with the evidence that incorporation of TAM-adducted bases into DNA results in the generation of mutations, indicates that TAM has a genotoxic potential. The concentration dependence and tissue specificity of this action has not been determined. The metabolic pathways responsible for the generation of DNA adducts need to be determined in human tissues at clinically relevant doses. The requirement to use higher doses in rodents to achieve the therapeutic level needed in the human may result in a greater tissue accumulation in the rodent with its higher metabolic rate than in the human at comparable serum levels.

The perturbation of hormonal action by TAM and related compounds may contribute to the promotion of certain neoplasms in animals and of endometrial tumors in humans. The intrinsic estrogenicity of TAM and related compounds probably contributes to their ability to support the growth of rat liver and human endometrial tissue. These triphenylethylene antiestrogens are able to effect proliferation, apoptosis, and differentiative status of responsive tissues. In addition, TAM and related compounds can alter cell cycle kinetics and hence may lead to aneuploidy, loss of chromosomal integrity, and altered spindle assembly or function.

In extrapolating the observed carcinogenicity of TAM in rat liver to humans, the similarities and differences in these two models from a physiologic and metabolic point of view need to be considered. Administration of TAM at high dose by gavage in oil results in a higher peak and cumulative dose than lower dose administration to patients. Frank malignancy has been observed in the rat liver after 2 years of daily administration of 5 mg or more of TAM per day but not with 2.8 mg TAM/kg/day. Patients receiving 20 mg per day of TAM for therapeutic or preventative measures are exposed to approximately 0.3-0.4 mg/kg/day. In addition, the constellation and concentration of phase 1 and phase 2 metabolizing enzymes differ between species and even within tissues of the same species. In patients, an increased incidence of endometrial carcinomas has been reported with an increased level of TAM administration (60). This has been previously described for unopposed estrogen use in general (61). The potential for carcinogenicity with TAM will thus reflect the specificity of metabolism, and the cell proliferative, apoptotic, and DNA repair capacity of the cell types at risk.

References

1. Hennings H, Glick AB, Greenhalgh DA et al (1993) Critical aspects of initiation, promotion, and progression in multistage epidermal carcinogenesis. Proc Soc Exp Biol Med 202:1–8.
2. Dragan YP, Sargent L, Xu YD et al (1993) The initiation-promotion-progression model of rat hepatocarcinogenesis. Proc Soc Exp Biol Med 202:16–24.
3. Fearon ER, Vogelstein, B (1990) A genetic model for colorectal tumorigenesis. Cell 61:759-767.
4. Harris CC (1996) Tumor suppressor genes: at the crossroads of molecular carcinogenesis, molecular epidemiology, and human risk assessment. Prev Med 25:10–12.
5. Nowell PC (1994) Cytogenetic approaches to human cancer genes. FASEB J. 8:408–413.
6. Goldsworthy TL, Hanigan MH, Pitot HC (1986) Models of hepatocarcinogenesis in the rat – contrasts and comparisons. CRC Crit Rev Toxicol 17: 61–89.
7. Lerner LJ, Jordan VC (1990) Development of antiestrogens and their use in breast cancer: Eighth Cain Memorial Award Lecture. Cancer Res 50: 4177–4189.
8. Tonetti DA, Jordan VC (1997) Targeted antiestrogens. Prog Clin Biol Res 396:245–255.
9. Jordan VC (1976) Effect of tamoxifen (ICI 46,474) on initiation and growth of DMBA-induced rat mammary carcinomata. Eur J Cancer 12:419–424.
10. Greaves P, Goonetilleke R, Nunn G et al (1993) Two-year carcinogenicity study of tamoxifen in Alderley Park Wistar-derived rats. Cancer Res 53: 3919–3924.

11. Williams GM, Iatropoulos MJ, Djordjevic MV et al (1993) The triphenylethylene drug tamoxifen is a strong liver carcinogen in the rat. Carcinogenesis 14:315–317.

12. Dragan Y, Xu Y, Pitot HC (1991) Tumor promotion as a target for estrogen/antiestrogen effects in rat hepatocarcinogenesis. Prev Med 20: 15–26.

13. Tucker M, Adam H, Patterson J (1984) Tamoxifen. In: Lawrence D, McLean A, Weatherall M (eds) Safety testing of new drugs. Academic Press, Orlando, FL, pp. 125–161.

14. International Agency for Research on Cancer. Tamoxifen. IARC Monographs (1996) 66:274–365.

15. Ghia M, Mereto E (1989) Induction and promotion of γ-glutamyltranspeptidase-positive foci in the livers of female rats treated with ethinyl estradiol, clomiphene, tamoxifen and their associations. Cancer Lett 46:195–202.

16. Williams G, Iatropoulos M, Karlsson S (1997) Initiating activity of the anti-estrogen tamoxifen, but not toremifene in rat liver. Carcinogenesis 18: 2247–2253.

17. Carthew P, Martin E, White I et al (1995) Tamoxifen induces short-term cumulative DNA damage and liver tumors in rats: promotion by phenobarbital. Cancer Res 55:544–547.

18. Tannenbaum S (1997) Comparative metabolism of tamoxifen and DNA adduct formation and in vitro studies on genotoxicity. Semin Oncol 24: s81–s86.

19. Busch H (1997) Adducts and tamoxifen. Semin Oncol 24: s98–s104.

20. Han X, Liehr JG (1992) Induction of covalent DNA adducts in rodents by tamoxifen. Cancer Res 52: 1360–1363.

21. Li D, Dragan Y, Jordan VC et al (1997) Effects of chronic administration of tamoxifen and toremifene on DNA adducts in rat liver, kidney, and uterus. Cancer Res 57:1438–1441.

22. Cunningham A, Klopman G, Rosenkranz H (1996) A study of the structural basis of the carcinogenicity of tamoxifen, toremifene, and their metabolites. Mutat Res 349:85–94.

23. Davies A, Martin E, Jones R et al (1995) Peroxidase activation of tamoxifen and toremifene resulting in DNA damage and covalently bound protein adducts. Carcinogenesis 16:539–545.

24. Styles J, Davies A, Davies R et al (1997) Clastogenic and aneugenic effects of tamoxifen and some of its analogs in hepatocytes from dosed rats and in human lymphoblastoid cells transfected with human P450 cDNAs (MCL-5 cells). Carcinogenesis 18:303–313.

25. Sargent L, Dragan Y, Bahnub N et al (1996) Induction of hepatic aneuploidy in vivo by tamoxifen, toremifene, and idoxifene in female Sprague-Dawley rats. Carcinogenesis 17: 1051–1056.
26. White INH, de Matteis F, Davies A et al (1992) Genotoxic potential of tamoxifen and analogues in female Fischer F244/n rats, DBA/2 and C57BL/6 mice and human MCL-5 cells. Carcinogenesis 13:2197–2203.
27. Styles J, Davies A, Lim C et al (1994) Genotoxicity of tamoxifen, tamoxifen epoxide, and toremifene in human lymphoblastoid cell containing human cytochrome P450s. Carcinogenesis 15:5–9.
28. Metzler M, Schiffmann D (1991) Structural requirements for the in vitro transformation of Syrian hamster embryo cells by stilbene estrogens and triphenylethylene-type antiestrogens. Am J Clin Oncol 14 (suppl 2):30–35.
29. Randerath K, Moorthy B, Mabon N et al (1994) Tamoxifen: evidence by ^{32}P-postlabeling and use of metabolic inhibitors for two distinct pathways leading to mouse hepatic DNA adduct formation and identification of 4-hydroxytamoxifen as a proximate metabolite. Carcinogenesis 15:2087–2094.
30. Randerath K, Moorthy B, Mabon N et al (1994) Tamoxifen: evidence by ^{32}P-postlabeling and use of metabolic inhibitors for two distinct pathways leading to mouse hepatic DNA adduct formation and identification of 4-hydroxytamoxifen as a proximate metabolite. Carcinogenesis 15, 2087–2094.
31. Phillips D, Carmichael P, Hewer A et al (1996) Activation of tamoxifen and its metabolite α-hydroxytamoxifen to DNA binding products: comparisons between human, rat, and mouse hepatocytes. Carcinogenesis 17:89–94.
32. Marques MM, Beland FA (1997) Identification of tamoxifen-DNA adducts formed by 4-hydroxytamoxifen quinone methide. Carcinogenesis 18: 1949–1954.
33. Dehal SS, Kupfer D (1995) Evidence that the catechol 3,4-dihydroxy-tamoxifen is a proximate intermediate to the reactive species binding covalently to proteins. Cancer Res 56:1283-1290.
34. Pathak D, Pangracz K, Bodell W (1996) Activation of 4-hydroxy tamoxifen and the tamoxifen derivative Metabolite E by uterine peroxidases to form DNA adducts: comparison with DNA adducts formed in the uterus of Sprague-Dawley rats treated with tamoxifen. Carcinogenesis 17:1785–1790.
35. Mani C, Pearce R, Parkinson A et al (1994) Involvement of cytochrome P4503A in catalysis of tamoxifen activation and covalent binding to rat and human liver microsomes. Carcinogenesis 15:2715–2720.
36. White I, Martin E, Mauthe R et al (1997) Comparisons of the binding of [^{14}C] radiolabeled tamoxifen or toremifene to rat DNA using accelerator mass spectrometry. Chem-Biol Interact 106:149–160.

37. Mani C, Kupfer D (1991) Cytochrome P450 mediated activation and irreversible binding of the antiestrogen tamoxifen to proteins in rat and human liver; possible involvement of flavin-containing monooxygenases in tamoxifen activation. Cancer Res 51:6052–6058.
38. Vancutsem P, Lazarus P, Williams G (1994) Frequent and specific mutations of the rat p53 gene in hepatocarcinomas induced by tamoxifen. Cancer Res 54:3864–3867.
39. Barakat R, O'Connor B, Banerjee D et al (1995) Mutation of c-Ki-ras in tamoxifen associated endometrial carcinoma. Proc Am Assoc Cancer Res 36:186 (1106A).
40. Davies R, Oreffo V, Martin E et al (1997) Tamoxifen causes gene mutations in the livers of lambda/lacI transgenic rats. Cancer Res 57:1288–1293.
41. Davies R, Oreffo V, Bayliss S et al (1996) Mutational spectra of tamoxifen-induced mutations in the livers of lacI transgenic rats. Environ Mol Mutag 28:430–433.
42. Shibutani S, Dasaradhi L (1997) Miscoding potential of tamoxifen-derived DNA adducts: α-(N^2-deoxyguanosinyl)tamoxifen. Biochemistry 36 13010–13017.
43. Yager JD, Yager R (1980) Oral contraceptive steroids as promoters of hepatocarcinogenesis in female Sprague-Dawley rats. Cancer Res 40: 3680–3685.
44. Edmondson HA, Henderson B, Benton B (1976) Liver-cell adenomas associated with use of oral contraceptives. N Engl J Med 294:470–472.
45. Mishkin SY, Farber E, Ho RK et al (1983) Evidence for the hormone dependency of hepatic hyperplastic nodules: inhibition dependency of malignant transformation after endogenous β estradiol and tamoxifen. Hepatology 3:308–316.
46. Kohigashi K, Fukuda Y, Imura H (1988) Inhibitory effect of tamoxifen on DES-promoted hepatic tumorigenesis in male rats and its possible mechanism of action. Gann 79:1335–1339.
47. Francavilla A, Polimeno L, DiLeo A et al (1989) The effect of estrogen and tamoxifen on hepatocyte proliferation in vivo and in vitro. Hepatology 9: 614–620.
48. Yager J, Roebuck B, Paluszcyk T et al (1986) Effects of ethinyl estradiol and tamoxifen on liver DNA turnover and new synthesis and appearance of gamma glutamyl transpeptidase positive foci in female rats. Carcinogenesis 7:2007–2014.
49. Dragan YP, Fahey S, Street K et al (1994) Studies of tamoxifen as a promoter of hepatocarcinogenesis in female Fischer F344 rats. Breast Cancer Res Treat 31:11–25.

50. Kim D, Han S, Ahn B et al (1996) Promotion potential of tamoxifen on hepatocarcinogenesis in female SD or F344 rats initiated with diethylnitrosamine. Cancer Lett 104:13–19.
51. Tsutsi T, Maizumi H, McLachlan J et al (1983) Aneuploidy induction and cell transformation by diethylstilbestrol: a possible chromosomal mechanism in carcinogenesis. Cancer Res 43:3814–3821.
52. Nowell PC (1994) Cytogenetic approaches to human cancer genes. FASEB J. 8:408–413.
53. Oshimura M, Barrett JC (1986) Chemically induced aneuploidy in mammalian cells: Mechanisms and biological significance in cancer. Environ Mutag 8:129–159.
54. Aldaz C, Conti C, Klein-Szanto A et al (1987) Progressive dysplasia and aneuploidy are hallmarks of mouse skin papillomas: relevance to malignancy. Proc Natl Acad Sci USA 84:2029–2032.
55. McLachlan J, Wong A, Degen G et al (1982) Morphologic and neoplastic transformation of Syrian hamster embryo fibroblasts by diethylstilbesterol and its analogs. Cancer Res 42:3040–3045.
56. Sargent L, Dragan Y, Bahnub N, et al (1994) Tamoxifen induces hepatic aneuploidy and mitotic spindle disruptions after a single in vivo administration to female Sprague-Dawley rats. Cancer Res 54:3357–3360.
57. Liang J, Brinkley B (1985) Chemical probes and possible targets for the induction of aneuploidy. Basic Life Sci 36:491–505.
58. Epe B, Hegler J, Metzler M (1987) Site specific covalent binding of stilbene-type and steroidal estrogens to tubulin following metabolic activation in vitro. Carcinogenesis 8:1271–1275.
59. Musgrove E, Wakeling A, Sutherland R (1989) Points of action of estrogen antagonists and a calmodulin antagonist within the MCF-7 human breast cancer cell cycle. Cancer Res 49:2398–2404.
60. Fisher B, Costantino JP, Redmond CK et al (1994) Endometrial cancer in tamoxifen-treated breast cancer patients: Findings from the National Surgical Adjuvant Breast and Bowel Project (NSABP) B-14. J Natl Cancer Inst 86:527–537.
61. Barrett-Connor E (1992) Hormone replacement and cancer. Br Med Bull 48:345–355.

PART 3. ESTROGEN RECEPTOR INTERACTIONS

Introduction

The Curious Pharmacology
of the Antiestrogens

Elwood V. Jensen

Background

Since the advent of Tamoxifen (TAM) (1), the first of the triphenylethylene-related antiestrogens to be tolerated on long term administration, antiestrogen treatment has essentially replaced endocrine ablation as first line therapy for advanced breast cancer (BC) of the hormone-dependent kind (2). These so-called type I agents show curious pharmacological behavior. Depending on species, tissue, and concentration, these compounds, and their active metabolites, can act either as agonists or antagonists (3). In human BC cells in culture, low levels of such agents enhance cell growth, while higher concentrations inhibit this stimulation as well as that induced by 17β-estradiol (E_2) (4-5). Type II or "pure" antiestrogens also have been developed, which show only antagonism. These are steroid derivatives and include ICI 182780 (6) and RU 58668 (7). Both types of antiestrogen compete with E_2 for its binding to the estrogen receptor (ER), but thereafter their interaction pathways have been thought to differ. However, we have shown that, unlike E_2, the two types of antiestrogen share the ability both to interact with a second binding site in the ER and to induce the exposure of an occult antigenic determinant for a particular monoclonal antibody.

The question of how the same compound can act either as agonist or antagonist presents a challenge. Our demonstration of an additional, antagonist-specific binding site in the ER molecule, and of the presence in some species of a substance that can limit antagonist concentration, provides a reasonable explanation for the species and concentration differences in the agonist/antagonist properties of TAM and related agents.

Epitope Exposure

After TAM therapy for BC became established, several laboratories reported that tumor specimens from such patients, or from animals receiving TAM , showed higher values for ER content when analyzed by immunoassay than by ligand-binding assay. It was then found that direct addition of TAM to a BC cytosol likewise increased the immunoassay result (8). Systematic study of this phenomenon demonstrated that TAM and related type I antiestrogens, but not E_2, react with the ER to expose an additional epitope for the particular monoclonal antibody used as the enzyme-labeled marker in the Abbott immunoassay procedure (9). A similar action was later observed with type II antiestrogens (10). Because the immunoassay is carried out with ER saturated with a large excess of E_2, it was proposed (9) that this phenomenon results from reaction of the antiestrogen with an ER site not recognized by the hormone.

Antagonist-specific Binding

Evidence for an additional binding site in the ER was provided by measuring the binding capacity of cytosol from MCF-7 BC cells for 4-OH-TAM (H-TAM) and RU 58668 as compared to that for E_2 as indicated by the greater size of the 8S sedimentation peak seen in sucrose gradients (10). That this secondary binding is to the ER protein itself and not to ER-associated proteins (RAPs) or to some other 8S component of the cytosol is indicated by the fact that the additional binding is also seen in high-salt gradients, where RAPs are dissociated, and that the entire sedimentation peak can be shifted on the gradient by addition of an ER-specific antibody (11).

Two-site Model for Antiestrogen Action

The fact that type I and type II antiestrogens are similar in showing secondary binding and in increasing receptor immunoreactivity suggests a unified model for explaining hitherto puzzling effects of concentration on the agonist vs antagonist properties of these agents (10). On the basis of competition studies, it was shown that H-TAM has a high affinity for the ER equal to (12) or greater than (13) that of E_2, whereas RU 58668 shows only one-fifth the affinity of the hormone (7). If the binding of type I agents to secondary sites is weaker than to primary, at low levels of antiestrogen, only primary sites will be filled (as with all concentrations of E_2 which does not recognize secondary sites), and this results in the agonism observed (4-5). At higher concentrations of H-TAM, secondary sites also are filled, leading to antagonism no matter what ligand is in the primary site. With type II agents, binding to the primary site is weaker than that of E_2, the affinities for primary and secondary sites may be comparable, so that both become filled concurrently and the agonist structure (only the primary site is occupied) is never formed. Comparison of the total binding of H-TAM and of RU 58668 with that of E_2 at various concentrations gives results consistent with this model (10).

Species Variation in Agonist vs Antagonist Actions of Tamoxifen

While TAM shows mixed agonist/antagonist action in the rat and human, it is a pure agonist in the mouse and guinea pig (3, 14). Unlike human BC cells and rat uterus, guinea pig uterus was found to contain a macromolecule that binds H-TAM but not E_2 (10). The complex of this substance with $[^3H]$-H-TAM is readily detected on a sucrose gradients, where it sediments more slowly than the ER. The affinity of H-TAM for this substance is less than for primary binding to the receptor, but it is present in substantial amounts. Thus, once primary binding is saturated, excess H-TAM is taken up by this macromolecule to keep its free concentration below that required for secondary binding. As a result, guinea pig ER shows neither secondary binding nor the epitope exposure that appears to depend on secondary binding.

Recently we have found that the type II agent, RU 58668, also reacts with the antiestrogen-binding substance in guinea pig uterus, but with a lower affinity than that of H-TAM. Mouse uterus also contains the more slowly sedimenting substance and, as expected, H-TAM does not induce immunoenhancement with ER from the mouse. These observations are consistent with the concept that TAM acts as a pure agonist in the mouse and guinea pig because their tissues contain an "antiestrogen buffer" that limits the concentration of free antiestrogen.

Summary

A model for antiestrogen action is proposed that ascribes agonist activity to the occupancy of the E_2-binding site in the ER, and agonist activity to interaction with a secondary, antagonist-specific site. On the basis of a reasonable assumption for the relative binding affinities for the two sites, this model can explain how, in the same cells, type I antiestrogens can act as agonists at low concentration and antagonists at higher levels, while type II agents show only antagonism. The presence of a component that limits the level of free antistrogen explains why, in some species, TAM acts only as an agonist. Reaction of antiestrogen with the secondary site causes a conformational change in the ER that exposes an occult epitope for a particular monoclonal antibody, leading to an increased value in the conventional immunoassay. This phenomenon may provide a simple means for identifying abnormal ER in those human BCs that do not respond to antiestrogen therapy.

References

1. Harper MJK, Walpole AL (1967) A new derivative of triphenylethylene: effect on implantation and mode of action in rats. J Reprod Fertil 13:101-119.
2. Jordan VC, Murphy CS (1990) Endocrine pharmacology of antiestrogens as antitumor agents. Endocr Rev 11:578-610.
3. Jordan VC (1984) Biochemical pharmacology of antiestrogen action. Pharmacol Rev 36:245-276.
4. Katzenellenbogen BS, Kendra KL, Norman MJ et al (1987) Proliferation hormonal responsiveness, and estrogen receptor content of MCF-7 human breast cancer cells grown in the short-term and long-term absence of estrogen. Cancer Res 47:4355-4360.
5. Poulin R, Merand Y, Porier D et al (1989) Antiestrogenic properties of keoxifene, *trans*-4-hydroxytamoxifen, and ICI 164384, a new steroidal anti-estrogen, in ZR-75.1 human breast cancer cells. Breast Cancer Res Treat 14:65-76.
6. Wakeling AE, Dukes M, Bowler J (1991) A potent specific pure antioestrogen with clinical potential. Cancer Res 51:3867-3873.
7. Van de Velde P, Nique F, Bouchoux F et al (1994) RU 58 668, a new pure antiestrogen inducing a regression of human mammary carcinoma implanted in nude mice. J Steroid Biochem 48:187-196.
8. Kiang DT, Kollander R, Schulstrom S et al (1987) Modulation of estrogen receptor (ER) from tamoxifen in human breast cancer. Proc Am Assoc Cancer Res 28:234.
9. Martin PM, Berthois Y, Jensen EV (1988) Binding of antiestrogens exposes an occult antigenic determinant in the human estrogen receptor. Proc Natl Acad Sci USA 85:2533-2537.
10. Hedden A, Müller V, Jensen EV (1995) A new interpretation of antiestrogen action. Ann NY Acad Sci 761:109-120.
11. Jensen EV (1996) Steroid hormones, receptors and antagonists. Ann NY Acad Sci 784:1-17.
12. Eckert RL, Katzenellenbogen BS (1982) Physical properties of estrogen receptor complexes in MCF-7 hunan breast cancer cells. J Biol Chem 257:8840-8846.

13. Tate AC, Greene GL, DeSombre ER et al (1984) Differences between estrogen- and antiestrogen-estrogen receptor complexes from human breast tumors identified with an antibody raised against the estrogen receptor. Cancer Res 44:1012-1018.
14. Furr BJA, Jordan VC (1984) The pharmacology and clinical uses of tamoxifen. Pharmacol Ther 25:127-205.

10

Estrogen Receptor-β: An Important Player in Estrogen Action

Jan-Åke Gustafsson

The recent discovery of a second estrogen receptor (ER-β) (1) has opened up a new dimension in the field of estrogen action. The previous concept of one single estrogen receptor (ER) mediating all effects of estrogenic hormones led to severe limitations in our understanding of estrogen action, for instance with reference to tissue specific hormonal effects. The entrance of a new ER with slightly different ligand binding specificity than the "old" receptor (ER-α) combined with varying ratios between ER-α and ER-β in different tissues has stimulated attempts to develop tissue specific estrogenic or antiestrogenic drugs. This type of research is obviously of immense importance from the point of view of hormone replacement therapy of postmenopausal women where previous treatments have been associated with an increased risk for endometrial as well as mammary carcinoma. Accordingly, a tremendous interest in ER-β is obvious from both academic and commercially oriented research groups as our knowledge in this field increases rapidly.

The human ER-β is localized on chromosome 14 as opposed to ER-α which is situated on chromosome 6. Interestingly, the more specific site of ER-β on chromosome 14, 14q22-23, appears to be in the same area on the chromosome where researchers are now looking for Alzheimer-related genes (2). This may or may not be of significance in view of the emerging concept that estrogens have an alleviating and/or preventive effect on the development of Alzheimer's disease. Furthermore, ER-β seems to exist as several isoforms. Since most of currently available information refers to ER-β mRNA species and levels, it is too early to make statements concerning which form or forms are the predominant ones at the protein level. Nevertheless, it would appear as if there exists at least one major short form of 485 amino acids with the apparent MW on SDS gels of 55 kDa, as well as a major longer form of 530 amino acids (in the human) or 548 amino acids (in rat) with apparent MW's on SDS gels of about 60 kDa. Western blotting experiments carried out in our laboratory (Margaret Warner, unpublished observations) utilizing antibodies recognizing both the long and the short form of ER-β indicate that these isoforms occur at different ratios in different tissues. The significance of this finding is not clear at the present time since experiments comparing the transactivation efficiency of the short and the long form, respectively, in cells with ERE-dependent reporter genes have failed to reveal any different potency between the two species. On the other hand, it is quite conceivable that the short and long forms may indeed have different biological activity on other response elements, however, more work is needed to settle this issue. In addition to the short and the long form, there are several other ER-β isoforms that have been described, for instance, a variant with an 18 amino acid insert in the ligand binding domain that drastically changes the ER-β ligand binding characteristics (3).

The tissue distribution of ER-β, which has mainly been studied at the mRNA level employing both Northern blotting techniques as well as *in-situ* hybridization, indicates that ER-β predominates over ER-α in many tissues such as bone, urogenital tract, CV system, as well as the CNS (2, 4). In the ovaries, ER-β constitutes about 90 % of the total pool of ER and is mainly concentrated in the granulosa cells whereas ERα is mainly present in the stroma. Also, in the lung, ER-β appears to predominate whereas the liver seems to contain almost exclusively ER-α. There are also indications that the immune system is particularly rich in ER-β. In both the uterus and the mammary gland, on the other hand, ER-α is the major ER but ER-β also seems to play an important role in these tissues and the ratio ER-α/ER-β appears to change during different physiological states of the mammary gland. Overall it would appear as if ER-β may well represent the quantitatively predominant ER in the body, and perhaps it could be suggested that ER-α is mainly involved in regulation of reproductive functions, whereas ER-β appears to be the major mediator of nonreproductive aspects of estrogen action. Obviously, this speculation represents a gross oversimplification and there are probably many exceptions to this tentative rule.

Within a particular tissue containing both ER-α and ER-β, there appears to be cells which contain only ER-α or ER-β, while there are others that contain both ERs. In these cases, heterodimerization of ER-α and ER-β is probably an important event (5). Studies in our laboratory indicate that ER-β is the dominant partner in the ERα/ER-β heterodimer, determining the overall sensitivity to estrogens and antiestrogens. For instance, the heterodimer is less sensitive to estradiol (E$_2$) than the ER-α homodimer, thereby displaying similar characteristics as the ER-β homodimer. Similarly, the heterodimer is more sensitive to tamoxifen (TAM) than the ER-α homodimer, again assuming the characteristics of ER-β homodimer in this regard. Obviously, these findings may be of great clinical significance in terms of breast cancer (BC) treatment where the ER-α/ER-β ratio in BC cells may determine the sensitivity to antiestrogens. Clearly, one of the most important and immediate potential clinical implications of the finding of ER-β is in BC treatment, particularly in view of the fact that currently available ER assay kits do not seem to detect ER-β. It appears essential to complement the current tests with ER-β assays in order to increase the quality of ER-based predictions of patients' sensitivities to alternative treatments.

With reference to the biological function of ER-β, only speculations can be offered at this point in time. It is of interest that ER-β often appears to be expressed in rapidly replicating cells. As indicated above, the granulosa cells in rat ovarian follicles are rich in ER-β, particularly during the first half of the estrus cycle (6). Towards the end of the cycle when the replication of granulosa cells winds down following the gonadotropin surge, ER-β mRNA is rapidly down regulated. Interestingly, ER-β mRNA levels are increased up to 80-fold in smooth muscle cells surrounding the vessel lumen following denudation of the endothelial layer of the vessel by a balloon technique (7). It is well known that smooth muscle cell replication in vessels can be inhibited by estrogen and ER-β may be a major mediator of this effect.

However, it is also conceivable that ER-β may have yet other functions in these rapidly replicating cells. A third example is the intestinal mucosa, particularly the large intestine, where ER-β is intensely expressed in a cell type undergoing continuous replication. The notion that ER-β may have some kind of protective function in these cases is further substantiated by the demonstration that ER-β, via an AP1-like antioxidant response element, may regulate expression of quinone reductase, an enzyme implied in control of reactive oxygen species and free radicals (8, 9). Indeed, this response which is elicited by TAM may well represent an important aspect of the therapeutic effect of TAM in BC treatment. In may be predicted that also other enzyme activities participating in the cascade of responses following antioxidant treatment, such as superoxide dismutase, glutathione transferase, glutathione peroxidase, etc., may be turned on following activation of ER-β by an appropriate antioxidant. In this context, it is of interest that estrogens, particularly phytoestrogens, as well as antiestrogens such as TAM have been described as antioxidants. Accordingly, it may be suggested that an important function of ER-β is to protect rapidly replicating cells from unwanted effects of free radicals that are generated at a higher frequency in replicating cells than in resting cells.

Interestingly, some support for this notion is given in the phenotype of the recently generated ER-β knockout animals (10). In these mice, the ovarian phenotype is characterized by a high degree of anovulation with distended follicles with difficulties to extrude the ovum. Accordingly, the ER-β -/- female mice are most often infertile. This particular ovarian phenotype appears to be quite similar to the one seen in mice with deleted superoxide dismutase gene, perhaps reflecting the end result of insufficient coping with free radical stress in granulosa cells during follicular maturation. Again, these notions obviously need to be tested rigorously.

In mice less than three mo. old, no histological abnormalities were found in the prostates of ER-β -/- males. However, in older -/- males the epithelium and stroma of prostatic ductules showed signs of hyperplasia. Likewise, whereas younger ER-β -/males (less than three mo. old) appeared to have a normal urogenital tract, testis and epididymis, older ER-β -/- males showed two types of abnormalities. In one type, the bladder wall including the epithelium and muscle layer was hyperplastic, resulting in increased folding of the mucosa. In the other type, the bladder wall was extremely thin, possibly as result of long term distension of the bladder. The latter finding was in agreement with the frequent finding of a very distended bladder in both female and male -/- mice older than three mo. of age. Preliminary observations indicate that these mice have increased urinary volume. Possibly, the thickened bladder wall seen in some -/- mice might develop as a reaction to the continuous tension of the bladder wall resulting from the large urinary volumes. It is interesting to speculate that the exclusive occurrence of ER-β in the paraventricular nucleus containing oxytocin and vasopressin synthesizing neurons might indicate an obligatory ER-β regulation of vasopressin synthesis and secretion from the paraventricular nucleus into the neurohypothalamus. Accordingly when ER-β gene is deleted, secretion of vasopressin is severely reduced, thus leading to a phenotype of diabetes insipidus. Again this finding needs to be confirmed by many more experiments including studies on levels of vasopressin in the paraventricular nucleus of ER-β -/- mice.

Acknowledgments

This work was supported by grants from the Swedish Cancer Society, Nutek and KaroBio AB.

References

1. Kuiper GGJM, Enmark E, Pelto-Huikko M et al (1996) Cloning of a novel estrogen receptor expressed in rat prostate and ovary. Proc Nati Acad Sci 93:5925-5930.
2. Enmark E, Pelto-Huikko M, Grandien K et al (1997) Human estrogen receptor β gene structure, chromosomal localization, expression pattern. J Clin Endocrinol Metab 82:4258-4265.
3. Chu S, Fuller P (1997) identification of a splice variant of the rat estrogen receptor beta gene. Molecular and Cellular Endocrinology 132:195-199.
4. Kuiper GGJM, Carlquist M, Gustafsson J-Å (1998) Estrogen is a male and female hormone. Science & Medicine 5:36-45.

5. Pettersson K, Grandien K, Kuiper GGJM (1997) Mouse estrogen receptor B forms estrogen response element binding heterodimers with estrogen receptor f3. Mol Endocrinol 11:1486-1496.
6. Byers M, Kuiper GGJM, Gustafsson J-Å et al (1997) Estrogen receptors MRNA expression in rat ovary: Down-regulation by gonadotropins. Mol Endocrinol 11:172-182.
7. Lindner V, Kim SK, Karas RH et al (1998) Increased expression of estrogen receptors MRNA in male blood vessels after vascular injury. Circ Res 83: 224-229.
8. Paech K, Webb P, Kuiper GGJM (1997) Differential transactivation properties of the estrogen receptor isotypes (α, β): Estrogen-like effects with antiestrogens and antiestrogen effects with estrogen. Science 277:1508-1510.
9. Montano MM, Jaiswal AK, Katzenelienbogen BS (1998) Transcriptional regulation of the human quinone reductase gene by antiestrogen-liganded estrogen receptors and estrogen receptor-β. J of Biol Chem 39:25443-25449.
10. Krege JH, Hodgin JB, Couse JF et al (1998) Generation and reproductive phenotypes of mice lacking estrogen receptor β. Proc Natl Acad Sci USA 95:15677-15682.

11

Estrogen Receptor-mediated Genomic Instability in the Syrian Hamster Kidney: A Critical Event in Hormonal Oncogenesis

Jonathan J. Li, S. John Weroha, Marilyn Cansler, and Sara Antonia Li

Introduction

Perhaps one of the most unique early hormonal events in estrogen (E) oncogenesis is the elicitation of genomic instability as a consequence of estrogen receptor (ER-α)-mediated cell proliferation. The focus of the studies presented herein is to provide evidence for this contention, and for a multi-stage sequence of events leading to tumor development, employing the Syrian hamster E-induced and -dependent renal neoplasm model.

Renal Tumor Cell of Origin

The development basis for renal tumors arising in the Syrian hamster after chronic E treatment is the finding that the urogenital and reproductive tracts are derived from the same embryonic germinal ridge (1). It is evident that the interstitial renal "stem" cells of the Syrian hamster kidney have carried over genes that are expressed and responsive to Es (2). In contrast, the Turkish hamster, which does not develop renal tumors following prolonged E treatment, does not express ER-α and PR in its interstitial cells and therefore unlikely to respond to E (Li SA, Coe J, Li JJ, unpublished data). Typical early tumorous lesions, emerging after 3.5- to 4.5-mo. of E treatment, consist of nests of small crowded cells with hyperchromatic nuclei and scant cytoplasm (Figure 1). Invariably, these cells are found in the interstitium, between tubules, and are generally separated by small amounts of connective tissue. The earliest tumorous lesions are frequently associated with small blood vessels. Large, well-established renal tumors are composed of two distinct cell populations, a poorly differentiated "primitive" small cell component that, evidently, is more

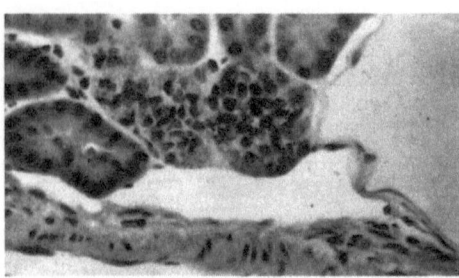

Figure 1. Typical early renal interstitial tumorous lesion (arrow), after 4.3-mo. E treatment of a male Syrian hamster. The small cells comprising the lesion appear crowded with scant cytoplasm and hyperchromatic nuclei (H&E x450).

differentiated and highly epithelial (4, 5). A mixture of these cell components appear as a gradient from small to large cells in established renal tumors.

Estrogen Receptor-α

Previously, we characterized the hamster kidney and renal tumor ER-α by competitive binding, sucrose gradient, and Scatchard plot analyses (6-10). Herein, employing ER-α specific antibodies (ERID5-DAKO, and C-311-Santa Cruz), the hamster renal ER-α was localized in paraffin kidney sections (Figure 2A, B), and assessed in cytoplasmic fractions by Western blot analysis (MC-20-Santa Cruz).

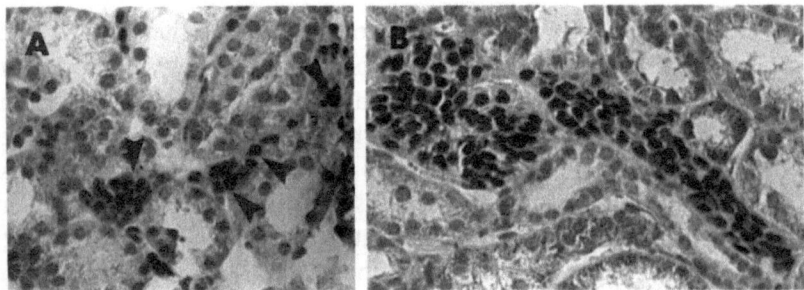

Figure 2. Immunohistochemical detection of ER-α expression in castrated male Syrian hamster kidneys. A. 3.5-mo. untreated control cortical tubule cells (arrows) exhibit weak ER-α nuclear staining (200x). B. 5.0-mo. E-treated hamster kidney, ER$^+$ cells in a moderate size renal tumor foci (200x).

Faint nuclear ER-α protein (data not shown) was detected in untreated hamster kidney proximal tubular cells consistent with our previous biochemical data (6). The ER-α protein was localized in renal interstitial cells and nascent tumorous foci at 3.5- to 4.5-mo. in E-treated castrated hamsters (Figure 2A, B). However, the faint ER-α staining seen in normal proximal tubules was down regulated in estrogenized hamsters. There was co-localization of both E and progesterone receptors (PR) in interstitial "stem" cells. A 64-KDa ER-α protein was detected in 6.0-mo. E-treated kidneys, renal tumors, and uterine hamster samples. The increased intensity of ER-α and PR (data not shown) protein staining in nascent renal tumorous lesions, and in small and large kidney tumor foci, provides compelling evidence that ER-α plays a central role in E-induced oncogenesis in the hamster kidney, and further lends credence to the belief that a subset of kidney interstitial cells are the cells of origin of E-induced tumor development.

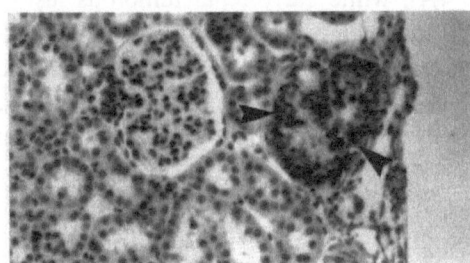

F i g u r e   3.   P C N A immunohistochemical staining of estrogen-induced early renal tumor foci derived from a hamster treated for 4.0-mo. Note the large population of PCNA-positive tumorous cells (arrowheads) compared to adjacent uninvolved renal cells.

Renal Interstitial Cell Proliferation

Cell proliferation, mediated by ER-α in a subset of interstitial renal cells, is a prerequisite for aneuploidy. After 1 mo. of E treatment, the outer and middle cortical regions exhibited no appreciable difference in PCNA labeling compared to age-matched untreated control kidneys (11). However, at this time interval, interstitial renal cells in the corticomedullary junction showed a modest 1.6-fold rise in PCNA-labeled interstitial cells. Relative to their corresponding castrated, age-matched, untreated groups, the corticomedullary junction region exhibited a marked rise of 3.0-, 6.0-, and 6.5-fold in S-phase PCNA-labeled interstitial renal cells after 3.0, 4.0, and 5.0 mo. of E treatment, respectively. A modest rise in PCNA-labeled interstitial renal cells was evident in the adjacent middle cortical region after 4.0 and 5.0 mo. of E treatment (11). The significant increase in S-phase PCNA-labeled renal cells in the corticomedullary junction of the hamster kidney between 4.0 and 5.0 mo. of E treatment was largely confined to nascent and early renal tumorous foci which appeared during these time periods (Figure 3). These data provide strong evidence that E, acting via ER-α on a subset of interstitial renal cells, elicits a proliferative response, thus setting conditions for subsequent genomic destabilization.

Nuclear Image Cytometry: Evidence for Aneuploidy

When compared to flow cytometry, the advantages of NIC are that it is a more sensitive method for assessing aneuploidy since individual cells can be morphologically identified (12-14). Moreover, ploidy assessment can be readily done in either very small early pre-malignant or malignant lesions present in tissue sections. Therefore, NIC was used to analyze Feulgen-stained sections of kidneys from untreated, castrated, age-matched hamsters, early renal tumorous foci from 3.0 mo, and frank renal tumors derived from 6.0 to 8.0 mo. E-treated castrated male hamsters. As anticipated, untreated kidneys exhibited a normal diploid frequency, n = 44 (Figure 4A), while early renal tumorous lesions examined between 3.5 to 5.0 mo. of E treatment were all highly aneuploid (85-100%). The aneuploid frequency of large well-established kidney tumor foci was also substantial (90-100%), (Figure 4C). These data clearly indicate that genomic instability is an early event in E-induced renal oncogenesis in the Syrian hamster.

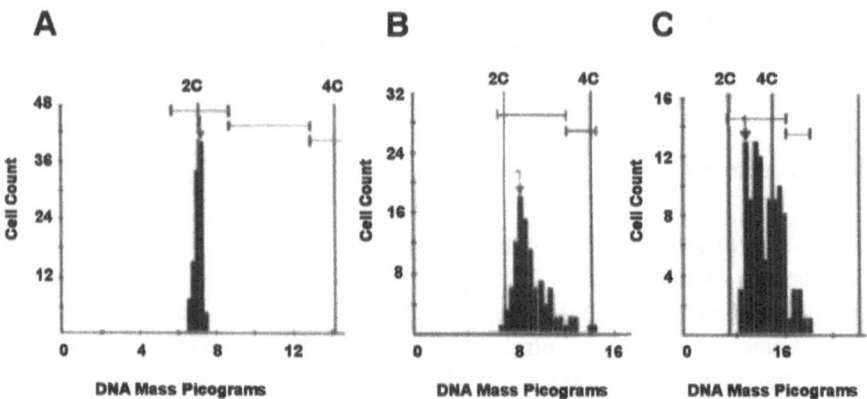

Figure 4. Representative NIC histogram from **A.** 3.5-mo. untreated hamster kidney; DNA index 0.99 - Diploid, 100%. **B.** Early tumorous lesions, 4.0 mo. DES-treated; DNA index 1.21 - Aneuploid, 94%. **C.** Well-established kidney tumor foci, 6.0 mo. DES treated; DNA index 1.78, Aneuploid - 91%.

Karyotypic Analysis

Karyotypic analysis was performed in thirty individual primary renal neoplasms derived from either castrated diethylstilbesterol (DES)- or 17β-E_2-treated hamsters. Both Es induced renal tumors which exhibited a number of nonrandom and random numerical chromosomal changes (3), consistent with the NIC data described previously. In the renal tumors examined, chromosomal gains (e.g., trisomies and tetrasomies) were found in chromosomes 1, 2, 3 (6), 11, (13), 16, 20, and 21. The numerical chromosomal changes cited were common to both DES and 17β-E_2-induced kidney tumors. A representative renal tumor karyotype is shown in Figure 5. Chromosome number alterations indicated in parentheses, 6 and 13, were either consistent or recurrent in renal tumors induced after either E treatment. Hamster kidneys obtained from DES-treated animals for 3.0 and 5.0 mo. also exhibited consistent gains in chromosomes 21, and 20 and 21, respectively (3). Consistent and recurrent losses were also seen in chromosomes 8 and 20 in renal neoplasms induced with either E. Taken together, the NIC and karyotypic data, strongly implicate genomic instability as a primary event in E-induced hamster renal oncogenesis.

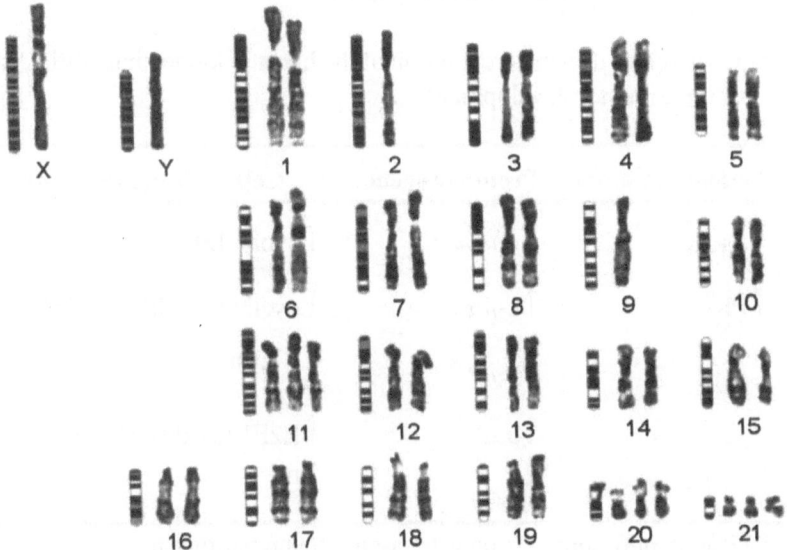

Figure 5. Representative G-banded karyotype of metaphase chromosomes from an E-induced renal tumor. Note consistent trisomies in chromosomes 11, 20, 21.

Deregulation of Gene and Protein Expression

The overexpression of E-mediated early response nuclear proto-oncogenes (c-*myc*, c-*fos*, and c-*jun*) and their protein products during E-induced renal oncogenesis has been reported by us (3, 15). It was observed, also that c-*myc*, but not c-*fos*, was amplified 2.0-4.0-fold in 67% of the primary renal tumors studied (3). Using fluorescence *in-situ* hybridization, the hamster c-*myc* gene was localized in chromosome 6 qb (3). Interestingly, chromosome 6 exhibited a high frequency of trisomies and tetrasomies in 5.0-mo. E-treated hamster kidneys and in primary renal neoplasms. These data are summarized in Table 1. Recent evidence, employing a variety of murine cell lines, indicate that c-*myc* and MYC protein overexpression alone can induce genomic instability (16, 17). A number of possible mechanisms for MYC-induced generation of aneuploidy have been proposed (16, 18-20). MYC may contribute to oncogenesis via a dominant mutator effect by abrogating checkpoints during G_1/S transition. Also, MYC may reduce transcription or inhibit the function of gene products responsible for regulating cell cycle transit. Finally, the abbreviated G_1 resulting from MYC-induced acceleration through this cell cycle phase, may itself be mutagenic. Therefore, MYC overexpression itself may play a singular role in solely E-induced tumorigenic processes.

Table 1. Estrogen-driven deregulation of the hamster kidney interstitial "stem" cells leading to tumor development.

Steroid receptors	Proto-oncogenes	Cell cycle components
↑ ER-α	↑ c-*myc* *	↑ cyclin D1
↑ PR	↑ c-*fos*	↑ cyclin E (50kDa → 35kDa)
	↑ c-*jun*	↑ p27^{kip1}
	↑ *p53*	↑ E2F1 (62kDa → 57kDa)
	↑ *WT1*	

* Gene amplification: Trisomy, tetrasomy at chromosome 6

In early renal tumor foci and established kidney tumors, Liao, *et al* (21) have provided compelling evidence that the cell cycle is deregulated. Protein levels of cyclin D1, a 35-kDa cyclin E variant, and Rb were elevated in renal neoplasms (Table 1). Interestingly, the predominance of the 35-kDa cyclin E protein has also been observed in various human breast cancer cell lines and in primary breast cancer specimens (22, 23). It has been suggested that the deregulation of this protein may be involved in cell transformation, loss of growth control, and possibly functions as an oncogene (22). Moreover, both RNA and protein levels of p27[kip], a cyclin-dependent kinase inhibitor, were found to be substantially elevated in early and frank renal tumors when compared with adjacent normal renal tissue and kidneys of untreated age-matched hamsters (21). It is deemed significant that the enhanced p27 expression occurs in early proliferating interstitial renal tumorous lesions.

Finally, well-established renal neoplasms exhibited a 57 kDa-E2F1 protein variant and a decline in the level of the 62 kDa-E2F1 native form. These data demonstrate an unusual deregulation of the cell cycle during renal oncogenesis and in kidney tumors. It would be highly pertinent to determine whether the deregulation of the cell cycle described herein contributes to the destabilization of the cellular genome in susceptible interstitial cells.

Concluding Remarks

Since only very low serum and renal tissue levels of 17β-E_2 (low ng/pg) are necessary to elicit high incidences of renal tumors in hamsters (24), it is evident that at these low 17β-E_2 concentrations, hormonal activity would predominate. The cause of the genomic destabilization as a consequence of E-driven proliferation of renal interstitial "stem" cells is presently unclear. One possibility may be that a subset of interstitial stem cells, which normally would be destined for the reproductive tract, but ectopically located in the kidney, becomes "inherently" genomic unstable. However, this event does not occur unless the cells are exposed to E. Alternatively, under constant E exposure, normal proliferative responses to E may become progressively deregulated leading to inappropriate gene responses in susceptible cells. These possibilities are unlikely to be mutually exclusive.

References

1. Kirkman H (1959) Estrogen-induced tumors of the kidney in Syrian hamsters. J Natl Cancer Inst Monogr 1:1-59.
2. Coe JE, Cieplak W, Hadlow WJ et al (1997) Female protein, amyloidosis, and hormonal carcinogenesis in Turkish hamster: Differences from Syrian hamster.Am J Physiol 273:R934-941.
3. Li JJ, Hou X, Banerjee, SK et al (1999) Overexpression and amplification of c-myc in the Syrian hamster kidney during estrogen carcinogenesis: A probable critical role in neoplastic transformation. Cancer Res 59:2340-2346.

4. Gonzalez A, Oberley TD, Li JJ (1989) Morphological and immunohistochemical studies of the estrogen-induced Syrian hamster renal tumor: Probable cell os origin. Cancer Res 49:1020-1028).

5. Oberley TD, Gonzalez A, Lauchner et al (1991) Characterization of early lesions in estrogen-induced renal tumors in the Syrian hamster. Cancer Res 51:1922-1929.

6. Li JJ, Talley, DJ, Li SA et al (1974) An estrogen binding protein in the renal cytosol of the intact, castrated, and estrogenized golden hamsters. Endocrinol 95:1134-1141.

7. Li JJ, Talley DJ, Li SA et al (1976) Receptor characteristics of specific estrogen binding in the renal adenocarcinoma of the golden hamster. Cancer Res 36:1127-1132.

8. Li JJ, Li SA and Cuthbertson (1979) Nuclear retention of all steroid hormone receptor classes in the hamster renal carcinoma. Cancer Res 39:2647-2651.

9. Li JJ and Li SA (1984) Estrogen-induced tumorigenesis in the Syrian hamster: Roles for hormonal and carcinogenic activities. Arch Toxicol 55:110-118.

10. Li JJ, Li SA, Oberley TD et al (1995) Carcinogenic activities of various steroidal and nonsteroidal estrogens in the hamster kidney: Relation to hormonal activity and cell proliferation. Cancer Res 55:4347-4351.

11. Li JJ, Gonzalez A, Banerjee S et al (1993) Estrogen carcinogenesis in the hamster kidney: Role of cytotoxicity and cell proliferation. Environ Health Perspect 101(suppl 5):259-264.

12. Peiro G, Lerma E, Climent MA et al (1997) Prognostic value of S-phase fraction in lymph node-negative breast cancer by image and flow cytometric analysis. Mod Pathol 10:216-222.

13. Alanen KA, Lintu M, Joensuu H (1997) Image cytometry of breast carcinomas that are DNA diploid by flow cytometry. Time to revisit the concept of DNA diploidy? Anal Quant Cyto Histol 20:178-186.

14. Spyratos F, Briffod M (1997) DNA ploidy and S-phase fraction by image and flow cytometry in breast cancer fine-needle cytopunctures. Mol Pathol 10(6):556-563.

15. Hou X, Li JJ, Chen WB et al (1996) Estrogen-induced protooncogene and suppressor gene expression in the hamster kidney: Significance for estrogen carcinogenesis. Cancer Res 56:2616-2620.

16. Felsher DW, Bishop M (1999) Transient excess of MYC activity can elicit genomic instability and tumorigenesis. Proc Natl Acad Sci USA 96:3940-3944.

17. Yin XY, Grove L, Datta NS et al (1999) c-myc overexpression and p53 loss cooperate to promote genomic instability. Oncogene 18:1177-1184.

18. Marhin WW, Chen S, Facchini LM et al (1997) Myc represses the growth arrest gene gadd45. Oncogene 14:2825-2834.
19. Lengauer G, Kinzler KW, Vogelstein B (1997) Genetic instability in colorectal cancers. Nature 386:623-627.
20. Paulovich AG, Toczyski DP, Hartwell LH (1997) When checkpoints fail. Cell 88:315-321.
21. Liao DJ, Hou X, Li SA et al (2000) Elevation of p27^{kip}, altered cyclins and cdks activities, and aberrant E2F1 expression in nascent and frank estrogen-induced renal neoplasia in the Syrian hamster. Carcinogenesis, in press.
22. Keyomarsi K, Pardee AB (1993) Redundant cyclin overexpression and gene amplification in breast cancer cells. Proc Natl Acad Sci USA 90:1112-1116.
23. Keyomarsi K, O'Leary N, Molnar G et al (1994) Cyclin E, a potential prognostic marker for breast cancer. Cancer Res 34:380-385.
24. Li SA, Xue Y, Xie Q et al (1994) Serum and tissue levels of estradiol during estrogen-induced renal tumorigenesis in the Syrian hamster. J Steroid Biochem Molec Biol. 48:283-286.

PART 4.
ESTROGEN/PROGESTERONE - BREAST CANCER

Introduction

Breast Cancer Prevention with Estrogen and Progesterone: Mimicking the Protective Effect of Pregnancy

Satyabrata Nandi, Raphael C. Guzman, Jason Yang,
Lakshmanaswamy Rajkumar, and Gudmundur Thordarson

Breast cancer (BC) is a complex disease with genetic, environmental, and socioeconomic factors playing a role. Although the etiology of BC is unknown, there are known risk factors. Among these risk factors are early age at menarche, late age at menopause, post-menopausal obesity, hormone replacement therapy, and alcohol consumption (1, 2). Taken together, the risk factors for BC all suggest that the cumulative lifetime exposure to ovarian hormones is the most important factor in breast carcinogenesis (3). Hormonal prevention strategies that are being developed for women are based on reducing the exposure to ovarian hormones, thus lowering the proliferation of the breast epithelial cells and inhibiting the promotion to BC (4).

Women who have a full-term pregnancy during their teens have a significantly reduced life-time risk of developing BC compared to nulliparous women (5). The protective effect of pregnancy is of major consequence in the consideration of means for the prevention of BC since it is natural and the effect occurs in women of all backgrounds. The development of procedures that would mimic the protective effect of pregnancy in nulliparous females would be of major importance in the prevention of BC. In the accompanying chapter, we briefly summarize our attempts in mimicking the protective effect of pregnancy against BC in nulliparous rats.

Model System Studies

Rats and mice that undergo a pregnancy, before or soon after carcinogen exposure, have a greatly reduced susceptibility to mammary gland carcinogenesis as compared with virgin animals and are used as experimental models (6-8). The mechanisms for the protective effect of pregnancy have not been defined. The most widely accepted explanation is the one put forth by the Russo's (8-9), that the protective effect is due to the pregnancy-induced differentiation of the target structures for carcinogenesis, the terminal end buds and terminal ducts, that show high proliferation, to lobuloalveolar structures that have a low level of proliferation. In essence, pregnancy causes the removal of a population of cells that are highly susceptible to BC. In addition, following pregnancy, the mammary cells have an enhanced capability for DNA repair (8). Pregnancy has also been found to cause the reduction of blood levels of mammogenic hormones in women and rats, and a decrease in the receptors for epithelial growth factor (EGF) and estrogen (ER) in the mammary glands of parous rats. This reduction in mammogenic hormonal environment and decrease in mammogenic hormone receptors might explain the refractoriness to mammary carcinogenesis (10-11). Administration of exogenous hormones has also been used to induce protection from mammary carcinogenesis in rats. Also protective are treatments with human chorionic gonadotropins and combinations of 17β-estradiol (E_2) and progesterone (P) either prior to or following treatment with chemical carcinogens (9, 12-15).   Again, the most accepted explanation for the induction of refractoriness to mammary carcinogenesis is that either the mammary target cells for cancer induction are differentiated to a non-susceptible state or lost, or the preneoplastic cells following carcinogen treatment are differentiated following lactogenic hormone treatment.

Mimicking the Protective Effects of Pregnancy against Mammary Gland Cancer

Pregnancy results in the morphological and biochemical differentiation of the mammary gland in preparation for lactation. However, pregnancy is a complex physiological process involving many hormonal and tissue interactions. Mimicking this complex phenomena is not feasible. We hypothesized that, it might be possible to induce a pregnancy-like morphogenesis to lobuloalveolar-alveolar structures and lactogenesis in the mammary glands of young virgin rats, by short-term administration of various unrelated exogenous differentiating agents. Differentiation induced by these agents, followed by involution after cessation of treatment, might result in a refractoriness similar to that induced by pregnancy. This will lend support to the Russos' hypothesis (8-9) explaining the protective effect of pregnancy from subsequent mammary carcinogenesis.

To test our hypothesis, we used perphenazine, a dopamine receptor antagonist, and the natural steroid hormones E_2 and P, as the differentiating agents to be tested for efficacy to induce refractoriness to mammary carcinogenesis. Perphenazine causes the acute release of prolactin from the anterior pituitary by blocking the inhibitory influence of dopamine from the hypothalamus (16). This excessive stimulation by prolactin results in the proliferation and differentiation of mammary epithelial cells to a near lactational state after a short period of treatment. E_2 and P are mammogenic steroids.

Three-week treatment with either perphenazine or $E_2 + P$ induced a high level of proliferation and lobuloalveolar- alveolar differentiation in the mammary glands of the treated rats. Milk-like secretion was visible in the mammary glands. Peripheral plasma E_2 concentrations of perphenazine-treated rats were comparable to those of young virgin controls. $E_2 + P$-treated rats had elevated E_2 levels compared to non-pregnant controls, but the levels were lower than the peak levels found in pregnant rats. P levels in perphenazine-treated rats were elevated and comparable to peak levels in pregnant rats. Plasma P levels in $E_2 + P$-treated rats were approximately doubled those detected in non-pregnant controls.

The effect of treatment with perphenazine and/or $E_2 + P$ on mammary carcinogenesis was then undertaken. Virgin Lewis rats, seven-week old, were treated with a single injection of N-methylnitrosourea (MNU). Two weeks after carcinogen treatment, these rats were treated for three weeks with perphenazine and/or $E_2 + P$. Tumor incidence was recorded until the animals reached 43 weeks of age. The results from these and additional experiments have been recently reported (17) and are summarized below.

From the control rats treated only with MNU, 90% (2.3 cancers/rat) developed mammary cancers, while 73% (1.3 cancers/rat) of the rats treated with perphenazine developed mammary cancers, however, there was a decrease in the multiplicity of cancers as compared with controls. Treatment with either a combination of perphenazine and $E_2 + P$ or $E_2 + P$ highly protected the rats from mammary carcinogenesis. BC occurred in 16% of the rats (0.16 cancers/rat) treated with perphenazine and $E_2 + P$. BCs were detected only in 9% (0.1 cancers/rat) of the rats treated with $E_2 + P$ during the 36 weeks of observation following MNU treatment. Rats treated with $E_2 + P$ experienced a 96% reduction in BCs compared with controls. The effect of $E_2 + P$ treatment on the reduction of mammary cancers in rats was repeated in four different experiments. These rats developed 93% fewer BCs compared with controls.

The effect of either E_2 or P given singly was tested to determine their role in inducing protection from mammary carcinogenesis. During the nine mo.-period of observation, 100% of the control rats developed BC (2.9 cancers/rat). Treatment with E_2, but not P alone, provided protection from mammary carcinogenesis. Of the rats treated with E_2 alone, 38% developed BC (0.5 cancers/rat). In contrast, 100% of the rats treated with P developed BCs (3.6 cancers/rat).

Assays of plasma levels of E_2 and P indicate that, with perphenazine treatment, only P was increased to pregnancy levels, while there was no increase in E_2 levels compared to untreated virgin rats. Treatment with $E_2 + P$ resulted in moderate levels lower than peak values seen in pregnancy, yet these levels were highly protective against mammary carcinogenesis (17, 18). The experiments in which E_2 or P were administered singly also suggest that, the pregnancy levels of E_2 were the most significant in inducing protection from mammary carcinogenesis.

Our current studies provide convincing evidence that, in young nulliparous rats, a short treatment period of sustained, elevated pregnancy levels of E_2 and P, but not perphenazine, is highly effective in protecting them against mammary carcinogenesis following exposure to high concentrations of MNU. Since both treatments with perphenazine or with E_2 and P result in pregnancy-like growth and differentiation of the mammary gland, these findings also suggest that differentiation and involution are insufficient to induce parity associated refractoriness to mammary carcinogenesis. We still do not know the mechanism that allows the E_2 + P treatment to be so effective against MNU-induced BC. On the basis of past and current studies (10-11, 19-21), we speculate that such treatment results in either a permanent reduction of the systemic hormonal environment involved in tumor promotion/progression, and/or a reduced sensitivity of the mammary epithelial cells to proliferation by mammogenic hormones.

The treatment with E_2 + P, for a short period of time, for the prevention of BC, provides a simple method which uses natural hormones at physiological (pregnancy) levels. Whether a similar strategy could ultimately be used for the prevention of BC in women can only be speculated at this time.

Acknowledgments

This work was supported by grants CA 05388 and CA 62598 awarded by the National Institutes of Health, Department of Health and Human Services.

References

1. Kelsey JL, Gammon MD, John EM (1993) Reproductive factors and breast cancer. Epidemiol Rev 15: 36-47.
2. Henderson BE, Ross RK, Pike MC (1993) Hormonal chemoprevention of cancer in women. Science 259: 633-638.
3. Feigelson HS, Henderson BE (1996) Estrogen and breast cancer. Carcinogenesis 17: 2279-2284.
4. Pike MC, Spicer DV (1993) The chemoprevention of breast cancer by reducing sex steroid exposure. J Cell Biochem 17G: 26-36.
5. MacMahon B, Cole P, Brown J (1973) Etiology of human breast cancer: a review. J Natl Cancer Inst 50: 21-42.
6. Moon RC (1969) Relationship between previous reproductive history and chemically induced mammary cancer in rats. Int J Cancer 4: 312-317.

7. Welsch CW (1985) Host factors affecting the growth of carcinogen-induced rat mammary carcinomas: a review and tribute to Charles Brenton Huggins. Cancer Res 45: 3415-3445.
8. Russo I, Russo J (1996) Mammary gland neoplasia in long-term rodent studies. Envir Health Persp 104: 938-967.
9. Russo J, Russo I (1987) Biological and molecular bases of mammary carcinogenesis. Lab Investig 57: 112-137.
10. Musey VC, Collins DC, Musey PI et al (1987) Long-term effect of a first pregnancy on the secretion of prolactin. New Eng J Med 316: 229-234.
11. Thordarson G, Jin E, Guzman RC et al (1995) Refractoriness to mammary tumorigenesis in parous rats: is it caused by persistent changes in the hormonal environment or permanent biochemical alterations in the mammary epithelia? Carcinogenesis 16: 28472853.
12. Huggins C, Moon RC, Morii S (1962) Extinction of experimental mammary cancer. I. Estradiol 17β and progesterone. Proc Natl Acad Sci USA 48:379-386.
13. McCormick GM, Moon RC (1973) Effect of increasing doses of estrogen and progesterone on mammary carcinogenesis in the rat. Europ J Cancer 9:483-486.
14. Grubbs CJ, Juliana MM, Whitaker LM (1988) Short-term hormone treatment as a chemopreventive method against mammary cancer initiation. Anticancer Res 8: 113-117.
15. Sivaraman L, Stephens LC, Markaverich BM et al (1998) Hormone-induced refractoriness to mammary carcinogenesis in Wistar-Furth rats. Carcinogenesis 19: 1573-1581.
16. Ben DM (1968) Mechanism of induction of mammary differentiation in Sprague-Dawley female rats by perphenazine. Endocr 83: 1217-1223.
17. Guzman RC, Yang J, Rajkumar L et al (1999) Hormonal prevention of breast cancer: Mimicking the protective effect of pregnancy. Proc Natl Acad Sci USA 96: 2520-2525.
18. Numan M (1994) Maternal behavior. In: Knobil E, Neill JD (eds) The Physiology of Reproduction, Second Edition. Raven Press Ltd ,New York, pp. 221-302.
19. Abrams TJ, Guzman RC, Hirokawa Y et al (1997) Refractoriness of parous rats to mammary carcinogenesis is overcome by treatment with ovarian hormones. Proc Am Assoc Cancer Res 38: 297.
20. Abrams TJ, Guzman RC, Swanson SM et al (1998) Changes in the parous rat mammary gland environment are involved in parity-associated protection against mammary cancer. Anticancer Res 18: 415-422.
21. Yang J, Yoshizawa K, Nandi S et al (1999) Protective effects of pregnancy and lactation against N-methyl-N-nitrosourea-induced mammary carcinomas in female Lewis rats. Carcinogenesis 20: 623-628.

12

The Dual Role of Estrogens and Cathepsin D in Invasion and Metastasis

Henri Rochefort

Introduction

It is well established that estrogens (Es) stimulate the growth of estrogen receptor (ER)-positive breast cancers (1, 2) even though the mechanism of this mitogenic activity is still being debated (Sutherland, this book). Before stimulating cell proliferation, Es regulate a number of genes via interaction of the ER with estrogen responsive elements and different co-activators. Among these gene products (3-4), our laboratory has been particularly engaged in studying the induction of cathepsin D (cath-D) by Es and growth factors. Cath-D is induced by estrogen in ER-positive breast and ovarian cancer cell lines (5- 6) and is also constitutively overexpressed in ER-negative breast cancers (3). There is further dysfunction of the pro-enzyme which is secreted in excess instead of being targeted to the lysosomes (7). The high level of cath-D in primary breast cancer (BC) is associated with an increased risk of further metastasis, as shown by several independent clinical studies (8), including a meta-analysis on node-negative BCs (9) and a recent study of the Rotterdam Cancer Center on 2810 patients (10). On the basis of the proteolytic activity of this marker, it was tempting to propose that, as for other proteases, increased expression and secretion of this protease could facilitate an escape of tumor cells through the basement membrane. Another prediction was that estrogen, inducing this protease, could also facilitate invasion (Figure 1). However, our experimental data did not support this prediction. Herein, the role of cath-D on metastasis, specifically, does cath-D facilitate invasion or proliferation, and the possible role of Es on invasion and motility will be discussed.

Overexpression of Human Cath-D by Transfection Increases the Number of Tumor Cells Rather than Their Invasive Properties

The natural overexpression of cath-D in aggressive BC, as observed in several clinical studies (8-10), is not only a parameter, but also appears to be one of the factors responsible for further development of metastasis, as shown by transfecting cath-D cDNA in tumor cell lines (3Y1-Ad12) expressing low levels of endogeneous cath-D (11).

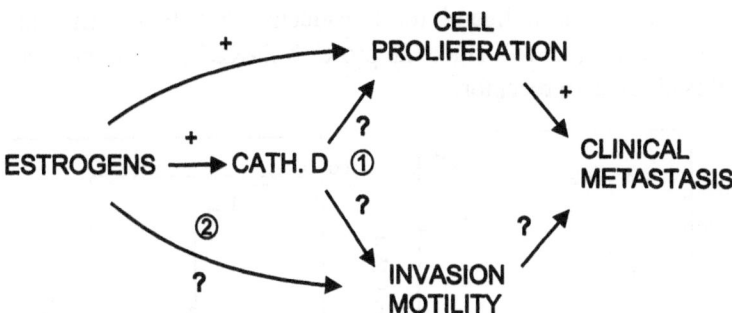

Figure 1. Estrogens stimulate both cell proliferation and the expression of cath-D, a lysosomal protease. However, the effect of estrogen on invasion and metastasis is not clear. An attempt has been made to answer two questions. *Does cath-D stimulate invasion or only cell proliferation?* and *What is the effect of Es on tumor cell motility and invasion?*

To assess the potential role of cath-D in cancer metastasis, Garcia, *et al.* (11), stably transfected an expression vector of human pro-cath-D, or a control vector alone, into a rat tumorigenic cell line (3Y1-Ad12) which does not secrete cath-D *in vitro*. The metastatic potential of cath-D-expressing clones was compared to that of control clones in athymic mice. Four cath-D clones isolated from two independent transfection experiments grew at higher density in culture (Figure 2) and displayed a higher metastatic potential than four corresponding control clones. The incidence and size of gross liver metastases were significantly increased in mice injected with cath-D clones. This was the first evidence that cath-D overexpression decreases the time required for metastases to appear.

In an attempt to determine whether the facilitation of liver metastasis by cath-D involved its proteolytic activity, the maturation of pro-cath-D was prevented by inserting a KDEL endoplasmic reticulum retention signal at the C-terminal of the coding sequence (12). Mice injected with six different KDEL clones developed metastases with the same incidence as those injected with control clones. A control KDAS peptide inserted at the same position did not affect cath-D maturation and its metastatic effect. The metastatic potential of cath-D was totally inactivated by modification of two amino acids (KDEL *vs* KDAS) in the protein structure. This strongly supports a direct and specific · effect of cath-D on the metastatic process and excludes artifacts due to transfection or the selection procedure. The major consequence of pro-cath-D retention in the endoplasmic reticulum was to prevent both its intracellular maturation and its stimulatory effect on experimental metastasis, suggesting its role as a protease. However, the results of this study did not exclude a potential role of pro-cath-D as a ligand for transducing signals via an alternative membrane receptor (13-15), since the pro-cath-D-KDEL might be inactivated to bind this alternative receptor.

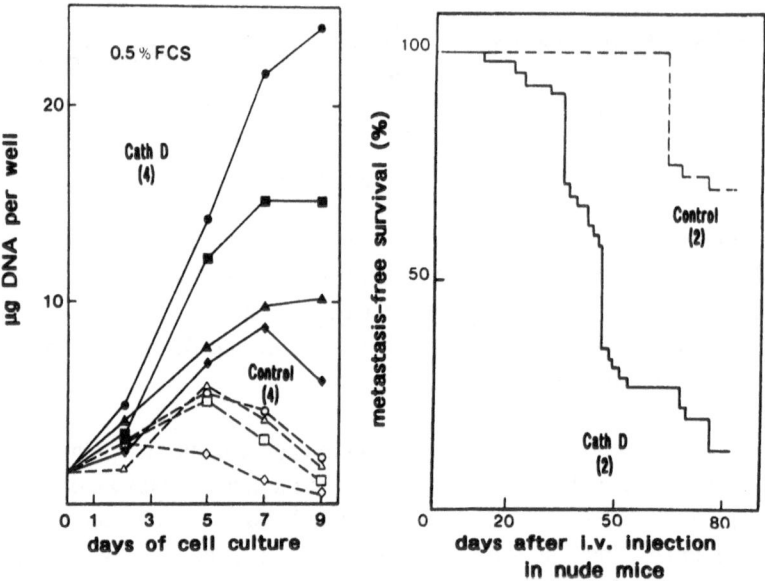

Figure 2. Transfection of human pro-cath-D into a rat tumor cell (3YAd12) stimulates cell growth at confluence in low-serum culture conditions (left panel) and increases the rate of appearance of liver metastasis in nude mice (right panel). The number of different cath-D and control (vector alone) clones is indicated in brackets. Reprinted and summarized from results of ref. 11, by permission of the editor.

Recently and independently, using a retroviral approach, Sawyers' group (16) showed that cath-D-overexpression increased soft agar colony formation of NIH3T3 cells and the progression of LNCAP human prostate cancer.

Most proteases are believed to play a role in degrading the basement membrane following secretion and extracellular activation (17). Cancer cells can then cross the basement membrane border to invade the stroma and extravasate in blood. However, it is unlikely that this is the major role of cath-D in metastasis as opposed to neutral proteases. Maturation of the enzyme appears to be required in the rat tumor cell model. Maturation also occurs *in vivo* in primary BCs since separate assays of pro-cath-D and total cath-D, using different monoclonal antibodies, showed that the tumor contained only 4 to 6% of pro-cath-D (18) while metastatic BC cell lines secrete *in vitro* up to 50% of the precursor (7). However, the mechanism in the rat tumor model may differ from that of human tumors. Overall, the overexpressed and secreted enzyme could act as a protease after its activation on membranes or as a ligand on membrane receptors before its activation (Figure 3). The action could take place extracellularly, as suggested by the high hypersecretion of this proenzyme, or intracellularly following or not its endocytosis via membrane receptors. At present, it is difficult to exclude any of these mechanisms, which are also not exclusive. Moreover, according to conditions observed *in vivo* in tumors (particularly pH and oxygenation), the importance of one mechanism or the other could vary (19).

Overall, most results indicate that cath-D overexpression increases cell proliferation, increases cell growth at confluence, and decreases cell-cell contact inhibition by degrading secreted growth inhibitors (20). We have no current experimental evidence of increased invasion through an extracellular matrix such as Matrigel (Garcia, M. and Derocq, D., unpublished data). Therefore, cath-D, contrary to other proteases, seems to act more as a mitogen than as a protease, allowing cancer cells to cross the basement membrane. The initial results obtained in our laboratory on the 52 kDa protein before its identification as pro-cath-D (21), as well as results of other laboratories (22), also indicate that cath-D may act more on cell proliferation than on cell invasion.

Since Es increase both cell proliferation of ER-positive cancer cells and induce cath-D (a protease), the next question was to determine whether Es stimulate tumor cell invasion.

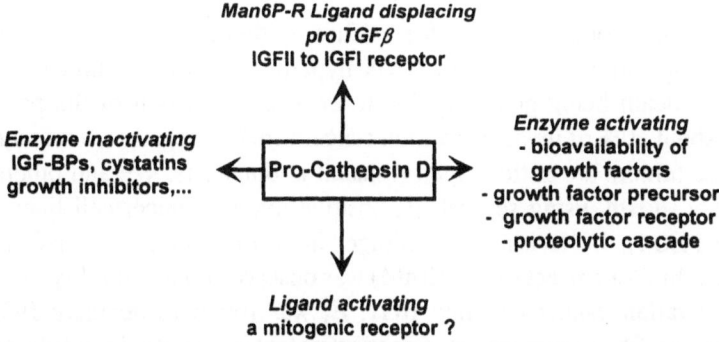

Figure 3. Simplified representation of the different mechanisms by which pro-cath-D overexpression could result in stimulating tumor cell proliferation. Cath-D could act as a ligand (without activation at neutral pH) or as a protease (following its activation at acidic pH) on different substrates.

Estrogens Decrease the Invasiveness and Motility of Breast and Ovarian Cancer Cells Via the ER

The first indication on the effect of estradiol (E_2) on invasion was obtained through studies of BC MDA-MB231 clones stably transfected with the ERα (23). In this system, E_2 was shown to decrease the number of experimental lung metastases in nude mice when the MDA-MB231 cell line stably transfected with ERα (two clones) was injected IV to the mice. Moreover, E_2 also decreased the invasive ability of these two clones through Matrigel in the transwell two-chamber system. A similar inhibitory effect of E_2 was observed in the 3Y1-Ad12 cell line stably transfected with ER-α (24). Interestingly, no effect of E_2 was observed in MDA-MB231 control cell lines transfected with the vector only, indicating that ER-β which might be expressed in this cell line (at least at the RNA level) could not trigger this inhibitory effect. However, since in these transfected models, E_2 also decreased cell proliferation, in contrast to wild-type ER-positive BC cell lines (MCF7 or T47D cells), this inhibitory effect of E_2 could have been artefactual, even though the ER-α level was similar in transfected MDA-MB231 clones and in wild-type MCF7 cells. Therefore, the effect of E_2 on invasion and motility of several ER-positive breast and ovarian cancer cell lines whose growth was stimulated by Es was studied in short culture conditions in which cell proliferation was not observed.

Estrogens Inhibit the Motility of ER-positive Ovarian Cancer Cells. This Effect May Be Mediated by Fibulin-1, a Secreted Extracellular Matrix Protein

Ovarian cancers originate from the surface epithelium of ovaries which are mostly ER-positive. They develop via hyperplasia into carcinomas of poor prognosis, death being generally due to extensive invasion of the peritoneal cavity. About 50% of invasive ovarian cancers are ER-negative, but contrary to BCs these tumors are antiestrogen resistant at diagnosis. We and others have previously shown, using several ER-positive ovarian cancer cell lines (BG1, SKOV3, PEO4), that E_2 is a strong mitogen in ovarian cancers as in BCs (5, 25). A strong inhibitory effect of E_2 (10 nM) was observed on the motility of the ER-positive ovarian cancer cell line BG1. E_2 was found to decrease BG1 cell motility when fibronectin was used as an attractant in haptotoxis and chemotaxis tests, regardless of whether fibronectin was adsorbed on the filter or added in solution in the lower compartment (26). Since in this cell line E_2 also induces fibulin-1, an extracellular matrix secreted protein which strongly interacts with fibronectin (27, 28), we also tested the effect of purified fibulin-1 in this system.

An excess of pure fibulin-1 incubated with fibronectin was found to dose-dependently inhibit the motility of BG1 cells induced by fibronectin (26). This correlation suggests that, at least in ovarian cancer, estrogen-induced fibulin-1 might play a role in the E_2-induced inhibition of epithelial cancer cell motility by conditioning the surrounding extracellular matrix to inhibit fibronectin activity.

Estrogens Also Inhibit the Motility and Invasiveness of ER-positive Breast Cancers

In the *in-vitro* system described above, ER-positive BC cell lines are clearly less invasive and motile than ER-negative BC cell lines (Figure 1c). Using non-synchronized MCF7 cells, ER-α immunostaining with the 1D5 monoclonal antibody (from Dako) revealed that, after 6 h, migration through Transwell chamber filters with fibronectin as an attractant, the percentage of ER-positive MCF7 cells migrating under the filter was 2.0-fold lower than that of MCF7 cells remaining on the top of the filter. This decreased percentage of ER-positive cells having migrated was also observed in T47D and ZR75-1 cell lines (29-30). These results suggest that ER-negative cells are more motile than ER-positive cells in the same cell lines with heterogeneous ER expression, in agreement with previous studies (31-32).

The effects of E_2 and antiestrogens were also investigated on MCF7 cells using a standard Matrigel assay as described by Albini, *et al.* (33). E_2 significantly inhibited invasion regardless of whether cells were treated for 2 or 7 days (30). By contrast, in this test, hydroxytamoxifen or ICI 164,184 alone stimulated invasion as compared to E_2-treated cells. Therefore, in all ER-positive cell lines that we have studied, E_2 displayed a dual effect, i.e. stimulating cell proliferation but inhibiting tumor cell invasion.

ER Transfection Into ER-negative Breast Cancer Cell Lines to Study the Mechanism by Which ER Inhibits Cancer Cell Motility and Invasion

Interestingly, the effect of E_2-activated ER on cell motility and invasion through Matrigel was similar in ER-negative cancer cells stably transfected with the wild-type ER-α than in ER-positive cancer cells. A comparison of the effects of E_2 on different parameters of BC cells in MCF7 and in MDA-MB231 cancer cells stably transfected with ER-α, and containing similar ER concentrations as in MCF7 cells (23), led us to conclude that, while E_2 has reverse effects on cell proliferation (i.e. stimulation in MCF7 cells, inhibition in MDA-MB231 cells), it has the same activity on *in vitro* invasion through Matrigel in both cell lines

(Fig. 4). The mechanism by which estrogen inhibits cancer cell motility and invasion, and the ER-α domain and amino acid sequence required to mediate this effect are now being studied (29). The mechanism by which activated ERα has reverse effects on cell proliferation in ER-positive BC cells and in ER-negative BC cells is not the purpose of the present review. This point is currently being investigated in several laboratories (including ours), and may be due to a different cross-talk of ER with AP1 transcription factors (34-35), since the ER facilitates AP1 activity in MCF7 cells and other ER-positive cells, but inhibits this activity in ER-negative cancer cells. However, other mechanisms can not be excluded.

Effect of Estradiol	MCF7 cell	MDA-MB231 ER+ (2 clones)
Estrogen Receptor sites/cells	50,000	-40,000 -20,000
in vitro : Cell prolif.	↗	↘
: Matrigel invasion	↘	↘
In vivo : Tumor growth	↗	→
: Lung Metastasis (iv)	N.D.	↘

Figure 4. A comparison of the effects of E_2 in MCF7 cells (ER-positive) and in MDA-MB231 cells (two stable ER-α transfectants) on four tumor progression parameters. The ER concentration was similar in MDA-MB231 clones and MCF7 cells, indicating that the growth inhibitory effect of E_2 in these clones could not be due to artefactual non-specific squelching. Lung metastases were measured after intraveinous injection of cancer cells in the tail of nude mice. The same inhibitory effect of E_2 on invasion and motility was observed in the MDA-MB231 transfected cells (23) and in the wild-type ER-positive MCF7 cells (30). N.D., not determined. Modified from ref. 30, by permission of the editor.

Estrogen and Estrogen Receptor(s) *In Vivo*: Are They Good or Bad?

This is a difficult question since Es stimulate cell proliferation but appear to inhibit cell invasion. There have been few other studies on the effect of estrogen and antiestrogen on cell invasion and they are not all consistent. Bracke, *et al.* (36), studying invasiveness and aggregation of MCF7 cells, reported an inhibitory effect of antiestrogens via E.-cadherin. Albini, *et al.* (33), indicated that E_2 stimulated invasion of transfected MCF7 cells through Matrigel. By contrast, in agreement with our results, E_2 has been shown to decrease motility of vascular smooth muscle cells in a Boyden chamber (37). The extrapolation of data obtained with established cell lines in culture to the *in-vivo* situation may be hazardous. On one hand, estrogen can modulate the growth and invasiveness of tumor cells by acting on cells other than tumor cells, such as cells involved in angiogenesis, immunological defense, etc. Paracrine regulation is also ignored by this reductionist approach. Moreover, metastasis are the result of different steps including invasion, attachment, motility, and growth ability in distant sites, and this latter step might be predominant *in vivo* (38). In addition, in BC, the hormone responsiveness and ER content of distant metastases often vary according to their site, suggesting that the protective effect of ER on the invasive process may also vary according to the colonization site. Overall, different points favor a protective role of the activated ER on distant invasion. Clinical results of hormone replacement therapy for menopause indicate a slight increase of BC incidence in women treated by Es, but these cancers have a better prognosis (less N+ and M+ tumors) (39). Since the studies of McGuire, *et al.* (40), it is known that ER+ BCs have an initial better prognosis than ER- BCs (40). This protective effect of ER might be operational at early steps of BC since patients with high grade (comedo type) ductal *in-situ* BCs, which generally contain less ER than low grade (non-comedo type) tumors (41, 42) have a higher risk of developing invasive BCs. The mechanism involved in this dual effect of estrogen (stimulating cancer cell proliferation and inhibiting tumor cell invasion) is unknown. Different pathways and ER domains might be involved. Whether ER-β behaves as ER-α in this respect is unknown. It is tempting to consider that the inhibitory effect of E_2 on invasion could be mediated by estrogen-induced proteins, which in turn inhibit cell motility. We suggest that one candidate in ovarian cancer cells could be fibulin-1, which is able to neutralize the haptotactic and chemotactic activities of fibronectin (26). Other mechanisms might be operational in BC cell lines, within which fibulin-1 is only expressed at very low level. Induction of a protease inhibitor such as α1-antichymotrypsin (43) is one possibility, but there are other candidate genes such as maspin (44). Irrespective of the mechanism involved, it should be pointed out that many growth factors are both mitogenic and motogenic, whereas Es are mitogenic and anti-motogenic. This could be a clue for defining the transduction pathway involved in the motogenic inhibitory effect of Es.

Starting from cath-D, an estrogen-induced protease, we have now come to the conclusion that both cath-D and Es are mostly involved in stimulating tumor cell proliferation. Unexpectedly, E_2 via its receptor, also strongly decrease tumor cell invasion. This dual effect of estrogen may have practical consequences concerning the prevention of invasive breast and ovarian cancers and the broad use of estrogen replacement therapy for menopause. Further studies aimed at determining the different molecular pathways involved in these effects should subsequently help to decrease the incidence and mortality of estrogen responsive cancers.

Acknowledgements

This work was supported by the «Institut National de la Santé et de la Recherche Médicale», the «Faculté de Medecine de Montpellier», the «Association pour la Recherche sur le Cancer», the «Groupement des Entreprises Françaises dans la Lutte Contre le Cancer», and the «Ligue Nationale Française Contre le Cancer». We are grateful to Prof. Pierre Chambon (Illkirch, France) for the gift of ER plasmids, to Dr. W.S. Argraves (Charleston, SC, USA) for fibulin-1 studies, to our colleagues at the INSERM Unit 148 who are quoted in the references, and to Edith Moreno for the preparation of this manuscript.

References

1. Dickson RB, McManaway ME, Lippman M (1986) Estrogen-induced factors of breast cancer cells partially replace estrogen to promote tumor growth. Science 232:1540-1544.
2. Chalbos D, Vignon F, Keydar I et al (1982) Estrogens stimulate cell proliferation and induce secretory proteins in a human breast cancer cell line (T47D). J. Clin. Endocrin Metab 55:276-283.
3. Rochefort H, Cavaillès V, Augereau P et al (1989) Overexpression and hormonal regulation of pro-cathepsin D in mammary and endometrial cancer. J Steroid Biochem 32:177-182.
4. Rio MC, Bellocq JP, Gairard B et al (1987) Specific expression of the pS2 gene in subclasses of breast cancers in comparison with expression of the estrogen and progesterone receptors and the oncogene ERB2. Proc Natl Acad Sci USA 84:9243-9247.
5. Cavaillès V, Augereau P, Rochefort H (1993) Cathepsin D gene is controlled by a mixed promoter and estrogens stimulate only TATA dependent transcription in breast cancer cells. Proc Natl Acad Sci USA 90:203-207.
6. Galtier-Dereure F, Capony F, Maudelonde T et al (1992) Estradiol stimulates cell growth and secretion of pro-cathepsin D and 120 kDa protein in the human ovarian cancer cell line BG-1. J. Clin. Endocrinol. Metab 75:1497-1502.

7. Capony F, Rougeot C, Montcourrier P et al (1989) Increased secretion, altered processing, and glycosylation of pro-cathepsin D in human mammary cancer cells. Cancer Res 49:3904-3909.

8. Rochefort H (1992) Cathepsin D in breast cancer: a tissue marker associated with metastasis. Eur J Cancer 28A:1780-1783.

9. Ferrandina G, Scambia G, Bardelli F et al (1997) Relationship between cathepsin-D content and disease-free survival in node-negative breast cancer patients: a meta-analysis. Br J Cancer 76:661-666.

10. Foekens JA, Look MP, Bolt-de Vries J et al (1999) Cathepsin D in primary breast cancer: prognostic evaluation involving 2810 patients. Br J Cancer, 79:300-307.

11. Garcia D, Derocq D, Pujol P et al (1990) Overexpression of transfected cathepsin D in transformed cells increases their malignant phenotype and metastatic potency. Oncogene 5:1809-1814.

12. Liaudet E, Garcia M, Rochefort H (1994) Cathepsin D maturation and its stimulatory effect on metastasis are prevented by addition of KDEL retention signal. Oncogene 9:1145-1154.

13. Capony F, Braulke T, Rougeot C et al (1994) Specific mannose-6-phosphate receptor-independent sorting of pro-cathepsin D in breast cancer cells. Exp Cell Res 215:154-163.

14. Fusek M, Vetvicka V (1994) Mitogenic function of human procathepsin D: the role of the propeptide. Biochem J 303:775-780.

15. Laurent V, Farnoud MR, Lucas A et al (1998) Endocytosis of pro-cathepsin D into breast cancer cells is mostly independent of mannose-6-phosphate receptors. J. Cell Sci 111(Pt 17):2539-2549.

16. Wu X, Craft N, Raitano A et al (1998) Functional expression cloning identifies cathepsin D as a candidate gene for prostate cancer progression. Abstract n#878, 89th Annual Meeting of the American Association for Cancer Research, March 28-April 1, New Orleans (LA, USA).

17. Liotta LA, Steeg PS, Stetler-Stevenson WG (1991) Cancer metastasis and angiogenesis: an imbalance of positive and negative regulation. Cell 64:327-336.

18. Brouillet JP, Spyratos F, Hacene K et al (1993) Immunoradiometric assay of pro-cathepsin D in breast cancer cytosol: Relative prognostic value versus total cathepsin D. Eur J Cancer 29A:1248-1251.

19. Rochefort H, Liaudet E, Garcia M (1996) Alterations and role of human cathepsin D in cancer metastasis. In: Ossowski L., Mira y Lopez R, editors. Enzyme & Protein. Karger:Basel 49:106-116.

20. Liaudet E, Derocq D, Rochefort H et al (1995) Transfected cathepsin D stimulates high density cancer cell growth by inactivating secreted growth inhibitors. Cell Growth Differ 6:1045-1052.

21. Vignon F, Capony F, Chambon M et al (1986) Autocrine growth stimulation of the MCF7 breast cancer cells by the estrogen-regulated 52K protein. Endocrinology 118:1537-1545.
22. Johnson MD, Torri JA, Lippman ME et al (1993) The role of cathepsin D in the invasiveness of human breast cancer cells. Cancer Res 53:873-877.
23. Garcia M, Derocq D, Freiss G et al (1992) Activation of estrogen receptor transfected in a receptor negative breast cancer cell line decreases the metastatic and invasive potential of the cells. Proc Natl Acad Sci USA 89:11538-11542.
24. Garcia M, Derocq D, Platet N (1997) Both estradiol and tamoxifen decrease proliferation and invasiveness of cancer cells transfected with a mutated estrogen receptor. J. Steroid Biochem. Mol Biol 61:11-17.
25. Langdon SP, Hirst GL, Miller EP et al (1994) The regulation of growth and protein expression by estrogen in vitro: a study of 8 human ovarian carcinoma cell lines. J. Steroid Biochem. Mol Biol 50:131-135.
26. Hayashido Y, Lucas A, Rougeot C et al (1998) Estradiol and Fibulin-1 inhibit motility of human ovarian and breast cancer cells induced by fibronectin. Int J Cancer 75:654-658.
27. Argraves WS, Tran H, Burgess WH et al (1990) Fibulin is an extracellular matrix and plasma glycoprotein with repeated domain structure. J Cell Biol 111:3155-3164.
28. Clinton G, Rougeot C, Derancourt J et al (1996) Estrogens increase the expression of fibulin-1, an extracellular matrix protein, secreted by human ovarian cancer cells. Proc Nat Acad Sci USA 93:316-320.
29. Platet N, Derocq D, Cunat S et al Inhibition of *in vitro* invasiveness of human breast cancer cells by transfected estrogen receptor before and after its activation by estrogen. In preparation.
30. Rochefort H, Platet N, Hayashido Y et al (1998) Estrogen receptor mediated inhibition of cancer cell invasion and motility: an overview. J Ster Biochem Mol Biol 65:163-168.
31. Price JE, Polyzos A, Zhang RD et al (1990) Tumorigenicity and metastasis of human breast carcinoma cell lines in nude mice. Cancer Res 50:717-721.
32. Thompson EW, Paik S, Brünner N et al (1992) Association of increased basement membrane-invasiveness with absence of estrogen receptor and expression of vimentin in human breast cancer cell lines. J Cell Physiol 150:534-544.
33. Albini A, Graf J, Kitten GT et al (1986) 17β-estradiol regulates and v-Ha-*ras* transfection constitutively enhances MCF7 breast cancer cell interactions with basement membrane. Proc Natl Acad Sci USA 83:8182-8186.

34. Philips A, Chalbos D, Rochefort H (1993) Estradiol increases and antiestrogens antagonize the growth factor-induced activator protein-1 activity in MCF7 breast cancer cells, without affecting c-*fos* and c-*jun* synthesis. J Biol Chem 268:14103-14108.
35. Philips A, Teyssier C, Galtier F et al (1998) FRA-1 expression level modulates regulation of AP-1 activity by estradiol in breast cancer cells. Mol Endocrinol 12:973-985.
36. Bracke ME, Charlier C, Bruyneel EA et al (1994) Tamoxifen restores the E-cadherin function in human breast cancer MCF-7/6 cells and suppresses their invasive phenotype. Cancer Res 54:4607-4609.
37. Kolodgie FD, Jacob A, Wilson PS et al (1996) Estradiol attenuates directed migration of vascular smooth muscle cells *in vitro*. Am J Pathol 148:969-976.
38. Chambers AF, MacDonald IC, Schmidt EE et al (1995) Steps in tumor metastasis: new concepts from intravital video-microscopy. Cancer Metastasis Rev 14:279-301.
39. Collaborative group on hormonal factors in breast cancer, Breast cancer and hormone replacement therapy: collaborative reanalysis of data from 51 epidemiological studies of 52 705 women with breast cancer and 108 411 women without breast cancer. The Lancet 1997; 350:1047-1059.
40. McGuire WL (1978) Hormone receptors: their role in predicting prognosis and response to endocrine therapy. Semin Oncol 5:2428-433.
41. Holland PA, Knox WF, Potten CS et al (1997) Assessment of hormone dependence of comedo ductal carcinoma in situ of the breast. J Natl Cancer Inst 14:1059-1065.
42. Roger P et al Cathepsin D and ERα level in 170 human pre-invasive breast tumors by semi-quantitative immunohistochemistry. In preparation.
43. Massot O, Baskevitch PP, Capony F et al (1985) Estradiol increases the production of 1-antichymotrypsin in MCF7 and T47D human breast cancer cell lines. Mol Cell Endocrinol 42:207-214.
44. Sheng S, Carey J, Seftor EA et al (1996) Maspin acts at the cell membrane to inhibit invasion and motility of mammary and prostatic cancer cells. Proc Natl Acad Sci USA 93:11669-674.

13

Estrogen-induced Breast Cancer in Female ACI Rats

Sara Antonia Li, Joshua DeZhong Liao, and Jonathan J. Li

Introduction

It has become increasingly evident that neither physical (i.e. ionizing radiation) nor environmental agents (carcinogens, xeno-estrogens) can appreciably account for the gradual and persistent rise in breast cancer (BC) incidence since 1940. In the USA, it is estimated that 1:8 women will develop BC over their lifetime (1-3). It is now realized that estrogens (Es) and progesterone (P), to some extent, are critically involved in the etiology, promotion, and progression of human BC. Most, if not all, of the major risk factors associated with invasive sporadic BC, which comprises 90 to 95% of BCs, are associated with sex hormones, particularly Es. Well-established BC risk factors include: Early age at menarche, late age at menopause, nulliparity, late age at first pregnancy, obesity, and hormone replacement therapy (4-7). Even weaker indirect risk factors for BC, such as dietary fat and alcohol intake, appear to be associated with increase E levels (8, 9).

It is well known that various strains of mice and rats, both females and males, are highly susceptible to E carcinogenesis in their mammary glands (MG) (10-17). The lack of sex difference in the ability of Es to induce mammary gland tumors (MGTs) in rats reflects what has been reported in humans. The strongest risk factor for BC in men, although relatively rare, is Kleinfelter's syndrome, a condition resulting from an inheritance of an extra X chromosome, resulting in testicular dysfunction and gynecomastia (18). Therefore, it is evident that Es play a significant role in the development of BC in both males and females.

Tumor Incidence

Early studies have clearly demonstrated that high MGT incidences (80-100%) may be induced in ACI rats (11, 12), and in both Noble and Long Evans rats (65-90%), of both sexes, by either natural or synthetic Es (11-13). The Sprague Dawley and Wistar-Wag strains elicit between 36-45% MGT incidences after E treatment (14). Generally, E-induction of MGTs requires prolonged latency periods (8.0 - 15.0 mo.). However, high MGT incidences may be effected in the ACI rat in only 5.0 - 6.0 mo. following chronic 17β-estradiol (E$_2$) administration at low serum concentrations (12, 19). Employing a single E-pellet implant (3 mg E$_2$ + 17 mg cholesterol), consistently high MGT incidences were also observed in this rat strain by us. Interestingly, in those rat strains (i.e., Wistar-Wag, Noble) requiring prolonged E exposure for tumor induction, the latency period for MGT induction can be substantially reduced (6.0 mo.) by the concomitant administration of either progesterone or androgen (15-17).

Histologic Evaluation of ACI Mammary Tumors

The normal intact virgin female ACI rat MG largely consists of ducts embedded within fat fads (Figure 1A). No benign or malignant lesions have ever been reported in MGs of untreated rats. After 3.5- and 4.5-mo. of either E$_2$ or diethylstilbesterol (DES) treatment, intraductal epithelial hyperplasias are abundant (Figures 1B, C). Commonly, these epithelial hyperplasias occurred in terminal ductal units, and attained moderate thickness (3-4 cells). Focal atypical dysplastic lesions (FADLs), typically seen nested within epithelial hyperplasias, were the most distinctive morphological findings observed after 3.5 to 4.5 mo. of treatment (Figures 1B, C). The nuclei of FADLs appeared more hyperchomatic when compared to the nuclei of hyperplastic cells. The majority of E-induced ACI rat MGTs have been classified as ductal carcinomas (Figure 1D). Some MGTs also exhibit papillary or cribiform patterns. Mitoses are seen in most of the intraductal carcinomas. A few intraductal carcinoma foci contained microscopic invasion characterized as small tongues of cell groups penetrating the surrounding stroma and eliciting a desmoplastic reaction.

Generally, normal intact cycling virgin MG sections displayed uniform S-phase PCNA-positive epithelial cells (Figure 2A). After 3.0- to 5.0-mo. of E-treatment, more intense PCNA-staining was observed in hyperplastic mammary epithelial cells (Figure 2B). FADLs, nested within MG epithelial hyperplasias, showed an even more uniform S-phase PCNA labeling pattern of even greater staining intensity, indicating a further rise in proliferative activity (Figure 2B).

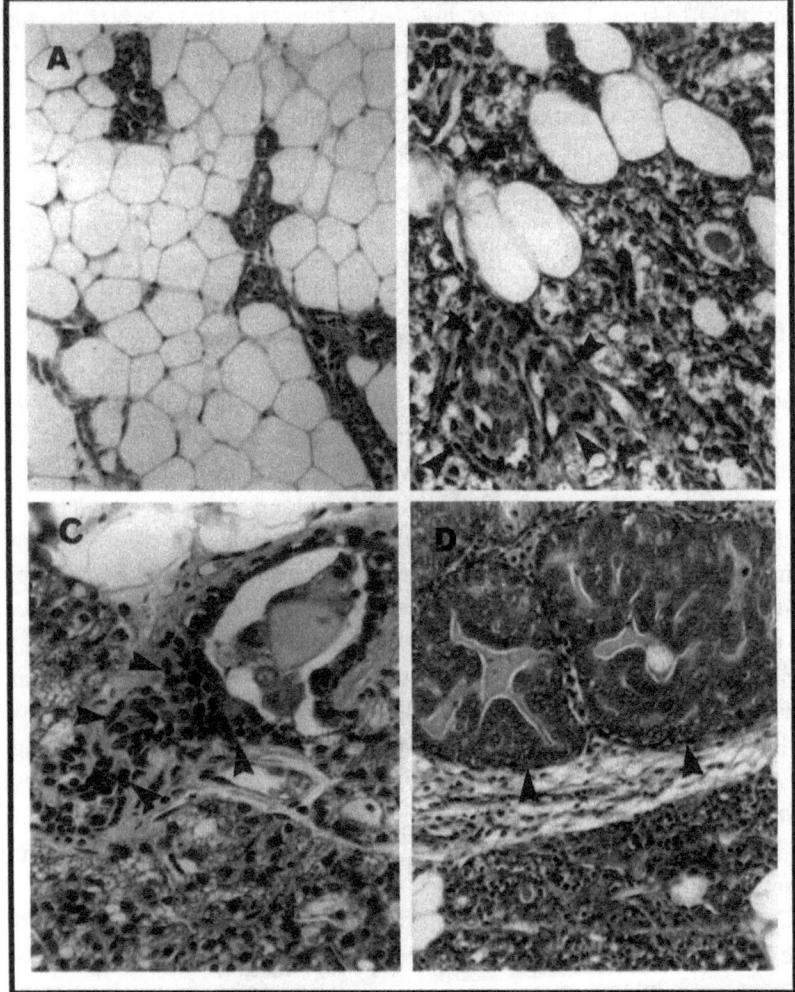

Figure 1. H&E stained tissue samples **A.** Normal MG from untreated ACI rat
(3.5 mo.) consisting of adipose tissue, terminal ducts, ductules, and acini (x200).
B & C. FADL's from 3.5- and 4.5 mo. E_2-treated ACI rats, respectively. Note
FADLs (arrows) nested within surrounding hyperplastic cells (x200, x400). **D.**
MGT (arrows) from a 6.0-mo. E_2-treated rat (x200).

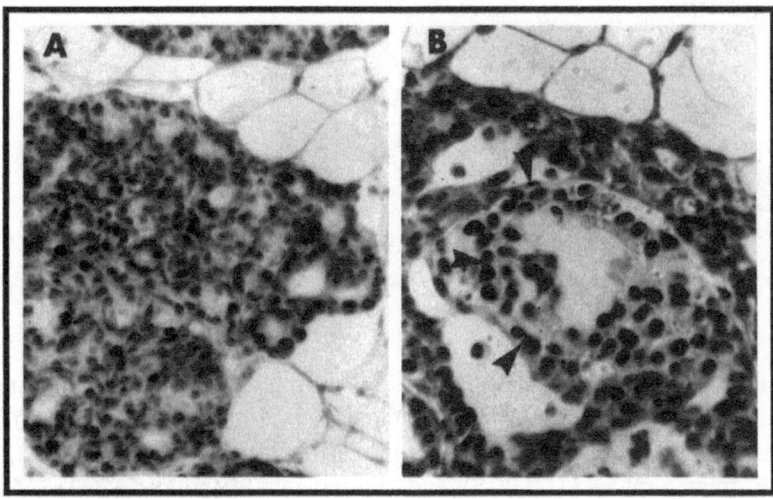

Figure 2. PCNA-labeling from formalin-fixed tissue sections. **A.** Untreated virgin female MG (x200). **B.** MG FADL (arrows) from a 4.5 mo. E_2-treated female ACI rat (x400).

Estrogen and Progesterone Receptors

Estrogen Receptor α (ER-α) In addition to the 66-kDa ER-α, likely the full-length ER-α form (20), the female ACI E_2-treated uterus exhibited two truncated forms of the ER, 56- and 54-kDa (Figure 3). In the mouse uterus, it is now evident that the native form of the ER-α has a molecular weight of 65-66 kDa (21). The untreated ACI MG exhibited two faint ER isoforms, 66- and 56-kDa, while the 3.0-mo. E_2-treated MG showed three, 66-, 58-, and 54-kDa. Similarly, the E_2-induced MGT exhibited the 58- and the 54-kDa isoforms present in the E_2-treated MG, but, in contrast to all the other MG tissues examined, and additional 47-kDa isoform was also present. Employing either the respective ER-α blocking peptide or pre-immune serum, no nonspecific ER-α protein bands were visualized. The presence of the 47-kDa isoform in the MGTs, and the absence of the 66-kDa full-length ER in E_2-treated MGs and MGTs may have particular significance. It has been suggested that ER-α isoforms may differentially affect signaling mechanisms, and thus, gene activities within target tissues (21, 22). Therefore, the induction of these isoforms in E_2-treated MGs and MGTs may alter mitogenic signaling responses leading to a differential enhanced growth responses that differ from those seen in the E_2-stimulated uterus.

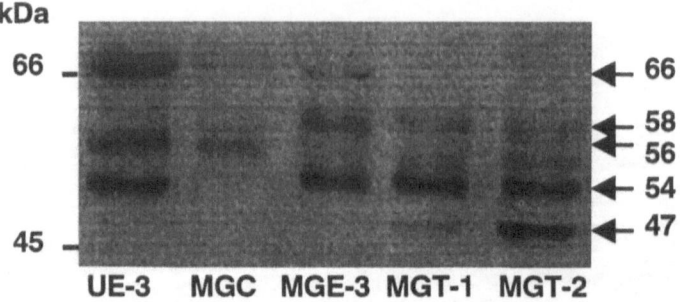

Figure 3. Western blot analysis of ER-α during E$_2$ treatment, using a rabbit polyclonal ERα antibody (MC-20, Santa Cruz). Protein aliquots (20 μg) from 3.0-mo. E$_2$-treated rat uterus (UE-3), untreated age-matched MG (MGC), 3.0-mo. E$_2$-treated rat MG (MGE-3), and two separate E$_2$-induced MGTs (MGT-1 and -2). The numbers at the left of the blot indicate the ~kDa value of pre-stained standards ran along with the samples. The right arrows represent the calculated ~kDa of the ER-α isoforms detected.

Estrogen Receptor β (ER-β). Our initial studies with ER-β were performed at the same antibody concentration used to detect ER-α (1:3000). At such concentration, we did not detect any ER-β [specific rabbit polyclonal anti-mouse ER-β antibody (Y19, Santa Cruz) reactive to mouse and rat] in ACI rat MGs from either untreated or E$_2$-treated rats, or in MGT samples. Recently, however, when the antibody concentration was doubled, a weak 60-kDa ER-β was found in the MGT. The respective ER-β blocking peptide eliminated this band, as well as a strong ER-β signal observed in rat prostate, serving as a positive control (data not shown). Although these data indicate ER-β may be present in the ACI rat MGT, evidently, it is present at significantly lower concentrations than ER-α.

Progesterone Receptor (PR). PR isoforms were assessed in the ACI MG and MGT using a rabbit polyclonal human anti-PR antibody (C-19, Santa Cruz), reactive to both mouse and rat (Figure 4). As previously reported in other rat strains, the E$_2$-treated ACI uterus exhibited two isoforms of the PR, B and A, while the untreated ACI MG expressed only PR-A. The E$_2$-treated-MG and the E$_2$-induced MGTs exhibited the three PR isoforms. Interestingly, PR-B in the MGTs appears as a doublet, similar to that observed in normal human endometrium (23). PR-A and PR-B isoforms have differential ability to activate transcription, and PR-A can act as a repressor of PR-B as well as of ER-α (24, 25). The PR-C isoform has been show in human breast tumor cells (25).

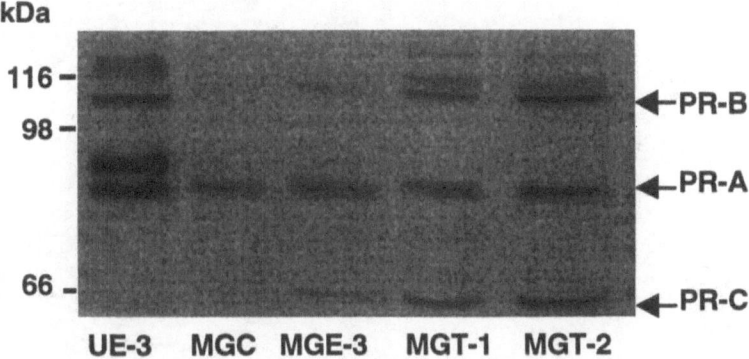

Figure 4. Western blot analysis of PR during E_2 treatment, using a rabbit polyclonal PR antibody (C-19, Santa Cruz). Protein aliquots (15 μg) from 3.0-mo. E_2-treated uterus (UE-3), age-matched untreated 3.0-mo.-old MG (MGC). 3.0-mo. E_2-treated MG (MGE-3), and two separate MGTs (MGT-1 and -2). The numbers at the left of the blot indicate the ~kDa value of pre-stained standards ran along with the samples. The right arrows represent the PR isoforms detected, their respective ~kDa values were: PR-B 110, PR-A 90, PR-C 64.

Immunohistochemical of ER-α and PR

Specific ER-α localization in paraffin-embedded sections of untreated virgin MGs and E-induced primary MGTs was made. ER-α staining of moderate intensity was found in most ductal MG epithelial cells (Figure 5A). Some stromal cells also showed weak to moderate nuclear ER-α staining. Following E treatment, 2.0- to 3.0-mo., the hyperplastic ductal epithelial cells displayed increased nuclear ER-α staining (data not shown). Essentially, all frank MGTs exhibited intense nuclear ER-α staining activity (Figure 5B). No ER-α positive cells were observed in serial MGT sections when the ER-α antibody was replaced with rabbit IgG, or neutralized by concomitant incubation with its respective ER-α blocking peptide.

MGTs induced by Es in ACI rats also exhibited strong nuclear PR positive staining (Figure 5C). In contrast, adjacent hyperplastic MG cells showed only moderate nuclear PR staining. Similarly, no PR positive cells were detected in similar MGT sections in the presence of PR blocking peptide, or when the PR antibody was replaced with rabbit IgG (Figure 5D).

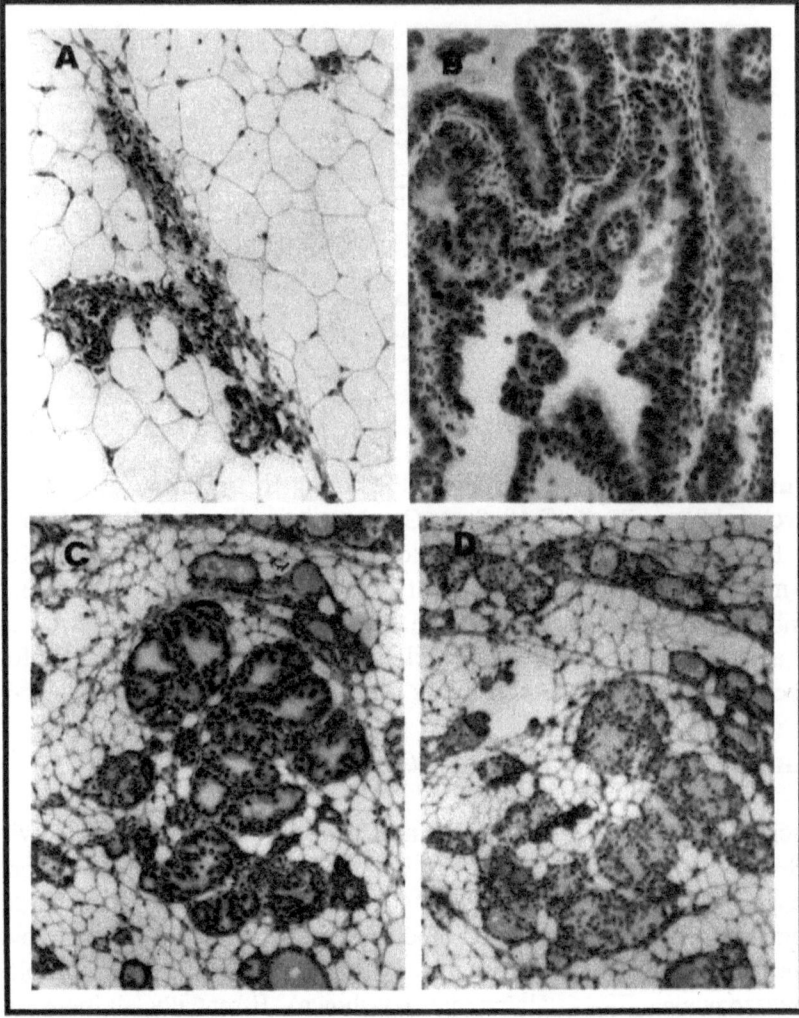

Figure 5. ER-α staining in a 4.0-mo untreated age-matched (**A**) and an E₂-treated ACI rat MG (**B**). **A.** Most epithelial cells in terminal ducts and many stromal cells exhibit weak to moderate ER-α nuclear staining (x200). **B.** Epithelial cells of a FADL (arrows) showing stronger ER-α nuclear staining compared to hyperplastic cells in adjacent tissue (x400). PR staining of a MGT (6.0 mo. E₂-treated ACI rat) in the absence (**C**) and in the presence of PR blocking peptide (**D**). **C.** Note the presence of nuclear PR staining in most MGT cells and its absence in hyperplastic MG cells (x400). **D.** Note the loss of nuclear PR staining in tumor cells (x400).

High Aneuploid Frequencies in Early FADL and Frank ACI and Noble Rat Mammary Tumors

The detection of high aneuploid frequencies in early renal tumorous lesions and in frank tumors induced solely by Es in Syrian hamsters (26, 27) has led us to study the ploidy status using nuclear image cytometry (NIC) of MGTs induced by Es alone in ACI and Noble rats.

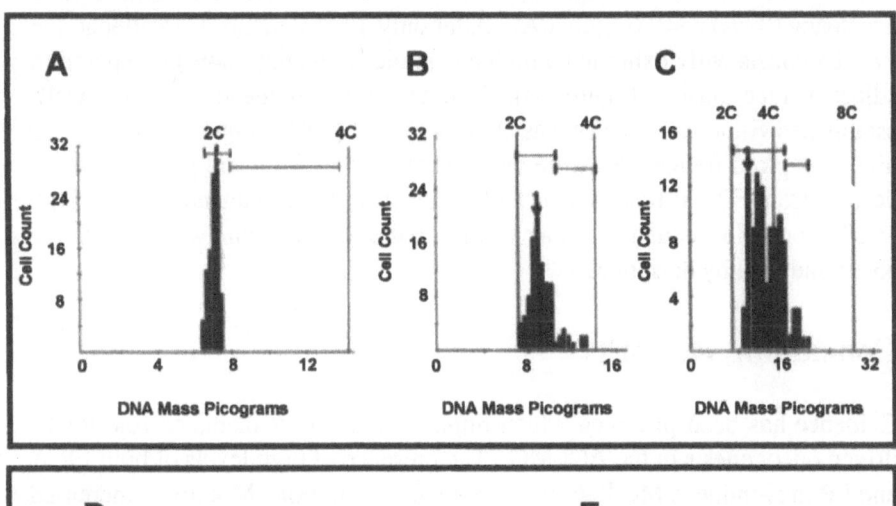

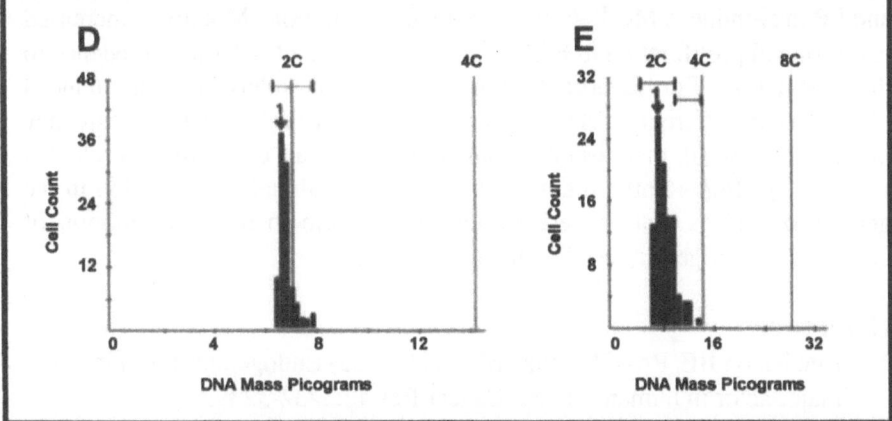

Figure 6. Representative NIC of Feulgen-stained MG sections from female ACI (A-C) and male Noble rats (D, E). A total of 100 cells/section were counted. **A.** MG from a 3.5-mo. untreated rat, 100% diploid cells. **B.** FADL from a 5.0-mo. E_2-treated rat, 88% aneuploid cells. **C.** Primary MGT from a 6.0-mo. E_2-treated rat, 91% aneuploid cells. **D.** MG from a 4.0-mo. untreated rat, 100% diploid cells. **E.** Primary MGT from a 6.0-mo. E_2 + testosterone propionate-treated rat, 89% aneuploid.

NIC is a more sensitive technique for assessing aneuploidy, when compared to flow cytometry, because tumor cells can be morphologically distinguished from normal cells, epithelial as well as stromal (28, 29). Moreover, assessment using NIC can be readily determined in either microscopic early pre-malignant or malignant lesions in tissue sections. NIC of Feulgen-stained sections of MGs from untreated, age-matched female ACI rats, 3.5-5.0 mo. of E-treated, and established E-induced MGTs were assessed for their aneuploid frequency (Figure 6A-C). As anticipated, normal MGs exhibited a normal diploid frequency (99%) n=42 (Figure 6A). After only 3.5-5.0 mo. of E-treatment, the FADLs consistently exhibited a high aneuploid frequency (84%) compared to adjacent hyperplasias (Figure 6B). The aneuploid frequency of large, well-established E-induced MGTs was slightly higher (90%) (Figure 6C). Similar high aneuploid frequencies were also observed in FADLs and primary MGTs derived from E + TP-treated male Noble rats (21). These data indicate that high MGT aneuploid frequency is not confined to the ACI rat strain when MGTs are solely induced by hormones.

Concluding Remarks

Evidence has been provided which implicates an ER-α-mediated role for E-driven oncogenesis in the ACI MG. The presence of high levels of both ER-α and PR in E-induced MGTs is consistent with this notion. Moreover, increased levels of cell proliferation in FADLs and in E-induced MGTs lend credence to this postulation. Furthermore, for the very first time, solely hormone-induced MGTs in two different rat strains have been shown to exhibit a high frequency of aneuploidy (30), that resembles human ductal breast cancer in this relevant aspect (31). Importantly, these results provide a rationale for E action in the genesis of MGTs that exceeds its established role in tumor promotion of chemical carcinogen-induced mammary tumors.

References
1. Henderson BE, Ross RK, Pike MC et al (1982) Endogenous hormones as a major actor in human cancer. Cancer Res 42:3232-3239.
2. Li JJ, Li SA (1998) Breast cancer: Evidence for xenoestrogen involvement in altering its incidence and risk. J Pure Appl Chem 70:1713-1723.
3. Harris JR, Lippman, ME, Veronesi U et al (1992) Breast cancer. N Engl J Med 327:319-328.
4. Colditz, GA, Stampfer MJ, Willet WC et al (1992) Type of postmenopausal hormone use and risk of breast cancer: 12-year follow up from the Nurse's Health Study. Cancer Causes Cont 3:433-438.

5.   Hoover R, Glass A., Finkle WD et al (1981) Conjugated estrogens and breast cancer risk in women. J Natl Cancer Inst 67:815-820.

6.   Brinton LA, Schairer C (1993) Estrogen replacement therapy and breast cancer risk. Epidemiol Rev 15:66-79.

7.   Toniolo P, Pasternack BS, Shore R et al (1991) Endogenous hormones and breast cancer: A prospective case-control study. Breast Cancer Res Treat 18:S23-S26.

8.   Wu AH, Pike MC, Stram DO (1999) Meta-analysis: Dietary fat intake, serum estrogen levels and risk of breast cancer. J Natl Cancer Inst 91:529-534.

9.   Howe G, Rohan T, Decarli A et al (1991) The association between alcohol and breast cancer risk: Evidence for the combined analysis of six dietary case-control studies. Inter J Cancer 47:707-710.

10. Lacassagne MA (1932) Apparition de cancers de la mammelle chez la souris mal, soumiseades injections de foliculine. CR Acad Sci (Paris) 19:630-632.

11. Cutts JH, Noble RL (1964) Estrone-induced mammary tumors in the rat. I. Induction and behavior of tumors. Cancer Res 24:1116-1130.

12. Holtzman S, Stone JP, Shellabarger CJ (1981) Synergism of estrogens and x-rays in mammary carcinogenesis in female ACI rats. J Natl Cancer Inst 67:455-459.

13. Nelson, WO (1944) The induction of mammary carcinoma in the rat. Yale J Biol Med 17:217-228.

14. Blankenstein MA, Broerse JJ, de Vries JB et al (1977) The effect of subcutaneous administration of oestrogens on plasma oestrogen levels and tumour incidence in female rats. Europ J Cancer 13:1437-1443.

15. Hannouche N, Samperez S, Riviere M-R et al (1982) Estrogen and progesterone receptors in mammary tumors induced in rats by simultaneous administration of 17β-estradiol and progesterone. J Steroid Biochem 17:415-419.

16. Liao D-Z, Pantazis CG, Hou X et al (1998) Promotion of estrogen-induced mammary gland carcinogenesis by androgen in the male Noble rat: Probable mediation by steroid receptor. Carcinogenesis 19:2173-2180.

17. Xie B, Tsao SW, Wong YC (1999) Sex hormone-induced mammary carcinogenesis in female Noble rats: The role of androgens. Carcinogenesis 20:1597-1606.

18. Thomas DB, Jimenez LM, McTiernan et al (1992) Breast cancer in men: Risk factors with hormonal implications. Am J Epidemiol 135:734-748.

19. Shull JD, Spady TJ, Snyder MC et al (1997) Ovary-intact, but not ovariectomized female ACI rats treated with 17β-estradiol rapidly develop mammary carcinoma. Carcinogenesis 18:1595-1601.

20. Kraus WE, Katzenellenbogen BS (1993) Regulation of progesterone receptor gene expression and growth in the rat uterus: Modulation of estrogen actions by progesterone and sex hormone antagonists. Endocrinology 122:2371-2879.

21. Horigone T, Ogata F, Golding TS et al (1988) Estradiol-stimulated proteolytic cleavage of the estrogen receptor in the mouse uterus. Endocrinology 123:2540-2548.

22. Hu C, Salman MH, Needleman DS et al (1996) Expression of estrogen receptor variants in normal and neoplastic human uterus. Mutation Res 118:173-179.

23. Feil PD, Clarke CL, Satyarswaroop PG (1988) Progestin-mediated changes in progesterone receptor forms in the normal human endometrium. Endocrinology 123:2506-2513.

24. Chalbos D, Galtier F (1994) Differential effect of forms A and B of the human progesterone receptor on estradiol-dependent transcription. J Biol Chem 269:23007-23012.

25. Natraj U, Richards JS (1993) Hormonal regulation, localization, and functional activity of the progesterone receptor in granulosa cells of rat pre-ovulatory follicles. Endocrinology 133:761-769.

26. Li JJ, Gonzalez A, Banerjee S et al (1993) Estrogen carcinogenesis in the hamster kidney: Role of cytotoxicity and cell proliferation. Environ Health Perspect 101 (Suppl 5):259-264.

27. Li JJ, Hou X, Banerjee SK et al (1999) Overexpression and amplification of c-myc in the Syrian hamster kidney during estrogen carcinogenesis: A probable critical role in neoplastic transformation. Cancer Res 59:2340-2346.

28. Peiro G, Lerma E, Climent MA et al (1997) Prognostic value of S-phase fraction in lymph node-negative breast cancer by image and flow cytometric analysis. Mod Pathol 10:216-222.

29. Spyratos F, Briffod M (1997) DNA ploidy and S-phase fraction by image and flow cytometry in breast cancer fine-needle cytopunctures. Mol Pathol 10:556-563.

30. Li SA, Weroha JS, Liao DZ et al (1999) Deregulation of the cell cycle in the estrogen-induced ACI rat mammary carcinoma: Possible mechanism leading to genomic instability. Proc Amer Assoc Cancer Res 40 (Abst):4072.

31. Rzymowska J (1997) AgNOR counts and their combination with flow cytometric analyses and clinical parameters is a prognostic indicator in breast carcinoma. Tumori 83:938-942.

14

A Transgenic Mouse Model for Mammary Carcinogenesis

Kristen L. Murphey and Jeffrey M. Rosen

Introduction

Tumorigenesis is a multistage process involving multiple genetic aberrations. Advances in transgenic and knockout technologies make it possible to genetically engineer mice to mimic the individual steps in this process, in order to better understand events contributing to cancer progression at the molecular level. Specifically, mouse models prone to genetic instability have been generated that may be useful to screen for early molecular events involved in hormonal carcinogenesis.

p53 is the most commonly mutated gene in human cancers, with approximately 40% of tumors displaying some alteration in the p53 locus. Unlike deletion or nonsense mutations observed in other tumor-suppressor genes, most p53 alterations are missense mutations resulting in the expression of a functionally altered protein (1). Such p53 mutations may result not only in a loss of wild-type function, but also in the generation of dominant-negative and gain-of-function mutants (2). Specific p53 mutations, including those at codon 175, have been associated with a poor prognosis in breast cancer (BC) patients, and also with primary resistance to chemotherapy (3). This is one of five "hotspot" codons present in the sequence-specific DNA binding domain of p53 that represent ~20% of all p53 mutations reported (1). Class II mutations, such as those at codon 175, affect residues crucial for maintenance of the correct orientation of the DNA-binding surface of non-contiguous loops and helices (4). The unique properties of certain p53 mutants may reflect their selective activation of specific DNA targets (2, 5) and/or participation in novel protein-protein interactions (6).

The development of both p53 knockout and p53 mutant transgenic mice has greatly facilitated studies of the role of p53 in carcinogenesis and tumor progression (7). By crossing p53 null mice with lines of transgenic mice overexpressing specific oncogenes, it has been possible to gain new insights into the mechanisms by which different signal transduction pathways interact with p53 to affect tumorigenesis (8). However, p53 knockout mice have some limitations for experiments designed to determine the role of p53 in mammary tumorigenesis, as these mice frequently die from lymphomas and sarcomas prior to mammary tumor development (9). Consequently, mice containing a mutant p53 transgene targeted specifically to the mammary gland have been generated for these studies. The 175R-H mutation is the second most-frequent p53 mutation observed in BC, accounting for approximately 6% of those reported to date (1). In order to study the role of the murine-equivalent 172 R-H mutant p53 protein in mammary tumorigenesis, a genomic minigene construct containing this mutation was targeted specifically to the mammary gland of transgenic mice using the whey acidic protein (WAP) promoter.

The WAP-p53 172R-H Transgenic Model

The 172 R-H transgenic mice exhibit a negligible level of spontaneous tumorigenesis (10-11). Transgene expression alone does not alter normal mammary development at the gross histological level, and as assessed through the analysis of apoptosis during involution and proliferation during pregnancy. The mutant protein also does not alter the expression levels of p21, MDM2, proliferative cell nuclear antigen (PCNA), or several other genes known to be regulated directly by wild-type p53 at the transcriptional level (11). To determine whether the presence of the transgene predisposed these mice to mammary tumorigenesis, they were given pituitary isografts to stimulate transgene expression and treated with the carcinogen, dimethylbenz(a)anthracene (DMBA). Tumors arising in carcinogen-treated nontransgenic (FVB) and transgenic mice were analyzed to determine the mechanisms by which this mutant p53 might promote tumorigenesis in the mammary gland.

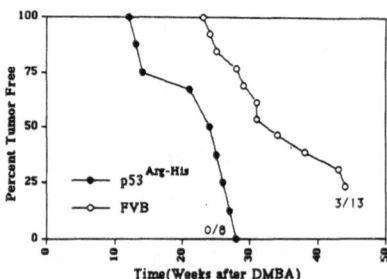

Figure 1. Overexpression of p53 172R-H decreases the latency of DMBA-induced mammary tumors. One hundred percent of transgenic mice developed tumors by week 28 post-DMBA treatment, while only 85% of FVB nontransgenic mice developed tumors by week 45. The fractions at the bottom of the curves are the number of tumor-free animals divided by the total number of animals in the group.

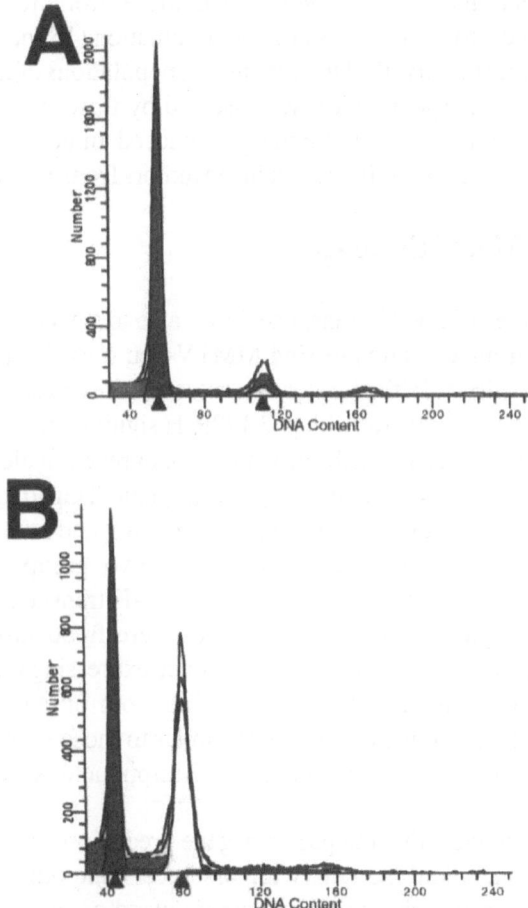

Figure 2. Flow cytometric analyses of DMBA-induced tumors from nontransgenic (A) and p53 172R-H transgenic (B) mice. The large light-colored peak in panel B represents an aneuploid population of cells that is not seen in the tumor in panel A.

Carcinogen Susceptibility and Tumor Analysis

The 172 R-H transgenic mice developed tumors more rapidly than controls (Figure 1), and exhibited a greater tumor burden (11). Apoptosis and cell proliferation in tumors from transgenic and nontransgenic mice were compared, but no significant differences were found (11). Loss of p53 function has been shown in the choroid plexus to influence tumorigenesis primarily through the inhibition of apoptosis (12), but this does not appear to be the case in the mammary gland. However, tumor cell nuclei from the transgenic mice were in most cases larger and more irregular than those from tumors arising in nontransgenic mice. Since p53 loss (13-14) or mutation (15) has been shown to result in genomic instability, the DNA content of populations of tumor cells from transgenic and nontransgenic mice was assessed by flow cytometry. Aberrant ploidy was more often seen in carcinogen-induced tumors from transgenic animals (Figure 2) than in carcinogen-induced tumors from control animals (11).

Bitransgenic Model Systems

Mice carrying the 172 R-H transgene have also been crossed in separate experiments with mice overexpressing MMTV-neu (*erb-B2*) (10), WAP-*des*-IGF-1, or WAP-TGF-α. In the former two crosses, co-expression of the growth factor receptor or growth factor with p53 172R-H significantly decreased tumor latency relative to that seen with the growth factor or receptor alone. In the TGF-α cross, both the bitransgenic and single transgenic TGF-α mice developed tumors with a mean latency of approximately 100 days, and because of this short latency no significant difference between the two groups was observed. Mammary tumors from mice expressing the 172 R-H transgene in conjunction with any of these growth factors or receptors were frequently aneuploid, as assessed by flow cytometry, but tumors from mice expressing only the *neu, des*-IGF-1, or TGF-α transgene were not. Tumors from bitransgenic mice also contained large irregular nuclei (Figure 3) similar to those seen in tumors from the DMBA-treated transgenic mice (10, and Murphy and Rosen, unpublished observations).

These results suggest that the p53 transgene predisposes female mice to the development of aneuploid mammary tumors once some other initiating event (*i.e.*, oncogene co-expression in the mammary gland or carcinogen treatment) has taken place. Since the expression of the p53 172R-H transgene alone resulted in very few spontaneous tumors in mice less than a year old, while accelerating tumorigenesis caused by both carcinogen treatment and oncogene expression, this appears to be an excellent model system in which to study early events in mammary tumorigenesis, including those involved in hormonal carcinogenesis. Furthermore, although most advanced-stage human BCs are aneuploid, mammary tumors generated in most mouse model systems to date have been uniformly diploid, which limits the utility of these models. This is the first mouse model system to our knowledge that consistently generates aneuploid tumors similar to grade 3, high S phase, hormone-independent human BCs. Patients with these types of tumors usually have the poorest prognosis.

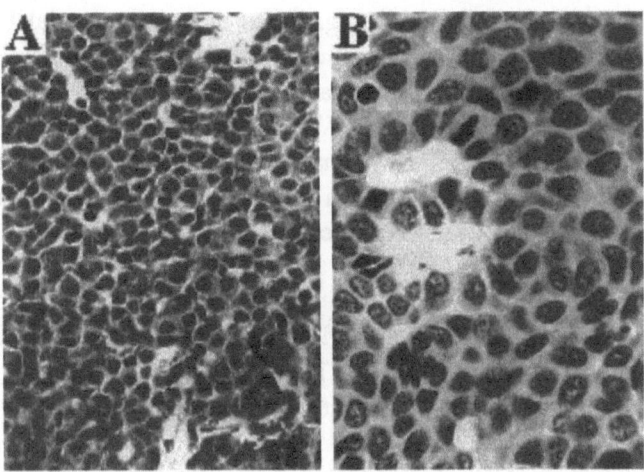

Figure 3. Large pleiomorphic nuclei in mammary tumors from mice co-expressing *neu* and p53 172R-H (B). These nuclei were not seen in tumors from mice only expressing *neu* (A).

p53 172R-H as a Gain-of-Function Mutant

The 172R-H p53 can act as a dominant-negative mutant in that it can interact with wild-type p53, but is no longer capable of specific DNA binding. This mutant, therefore, loses many of the direct transcriptional properties of wild-type p53, but, in addition, appears to confer novel functions indicating that it is a gain-of-function mutant. For example, it is capable of stimulating expression of MDR-CAT, a human multidrug resistance (MDR-1) gene promoter-CAT construct, in p53-null cells, in a manner reversible by co-transfection of wild-type p53 (16). When the 172R-H mutant was transfected into p53-null Saos-2 cells, it conferred a growth advantage. Injection of a cell line expressing this mutant p53 protein into nude mice resulted in tumorigenesis, which was not seen with the parental p53-null cells (2). This mutant protein was also able to cooperate in co-transfection experiments with activated H-*ras* in the transformation of rat embryo fibroblasts.

As suggested by the results obtained from several different experimental models, this p53 mutant protein has profound gain-of-function effects at the level of genomic stability. The absence of wild-type p53 is known to contribute to aberrant centrosomal duplication (13). Centrosomal hypertrophy has been implicated in at least two processes that adversely affect prognosis in cancer patients: 1) loss of cell polarity and tissue organization, and 2) an increased occurrence of multipolar mitoses, which predisposes to the development of aneuploidy since it affects the proper segregation of genetic material. High-grade human mammary adenocarcinomas often have centrosomes that are amplified in number, display aberrant structural characteristics, and have increased microtubule nucleating capacity (17). When the 172R-H mutant was targeted to skin and centrosomal duplication was analyzed, skin samples from the transgenic mice showed far more centrosomes than did skin from p53-null or nontransgenic mice (18). Preliminary results indicate that mammary tumors from both the WAP-172R-H/TGF-α bitransgenics and WAP-TGF-α single transgenics demonstrate marked centrosome abnormalities, although no aberrant ploidy was seen in tumors from the TGF-α single transgenics (Murphy, B. Kolle, and Rosen, unpublished observations). This unexpected finding suggests that centrosomal dysregulation is a necessary, but not sufficient prerequisite for the later development of aneuploidy.

Recently, it has been suggested that at least some genomic instability is the result of failures in the DNA repair pathway. Wild-type p53 has been reported to interact with both BRCA1 and RAD51, and the latter protein can interact with BRCA2. Thus, this multiprotein complex may play an important role in DNA repair (19-20), and it is conceivable that the 172R-H mutant p53 protein may, therefore, be promoting genomic instability at least partially through disrupting the normal function of this complex in DNA repair. Furthermore, cells containing this p53 mutation exhibit a dominant gain-of-function defect in spindle (G2/M) checkpoint control. When incubated with colcemid, a spindle assembly inhibitor, cells containing wild-type p53 arrest with 4n DNA content, but cells containing this p53 mutant can re-enter S phase and subsequently become polyploid (21).

Potential Gain-of-Function Mechanisms

As p53 is a multifunctional protein, the p53 gain-of-function mutants may lose the ability to regulate transcription of certain target genes involved in cell cycle control and apoptosis, like p21 or Bax, that require direct DNA binding, but still retain other functions that require protein-protein interactions. The latter may fall into several categories. First, interactions with other transcription factors or co-activators could lead to transcriptional activation from novel promoters. It has recently been reported that p53 participates in transcriptional induction of the *GADD45* gene through an interaction with WT-1 bound to an Egr-1 site on the GADD45 promoter, but not as a result of direct DNA binding by p53 (Figure 4) (22). Second, nonsequence-specific interactions of the p53 carboxy-terminus with single-stranded DNA or RNA could affect gene regulation. For example, recently, it has also been reported that p53 mutants can induce *c-myc* gene expression through an interaction between the carboxy-terminal region of p53, which possesses a single-stranded DNA and RNA binding activity, and a region located at the exon 1/intron 1 boundary of *c-myc* (23) (Figure 4). This interaction may overcome the block to transcriptional elongation known to occur in the *c-myc* gene. Finally, nontranscriptional interactions such as those already known to exist between wild-type p53 and centrosome elements/microtubules (24) could affect mitotic fidelity and genomic stability in early tumor development. These mechanisms may account for the apparent "gain-of function" and predisposition to genomic instability that have been observed not only in transgenic mice overexpressing WAP-172R-H p53, but also in cell culture systems.

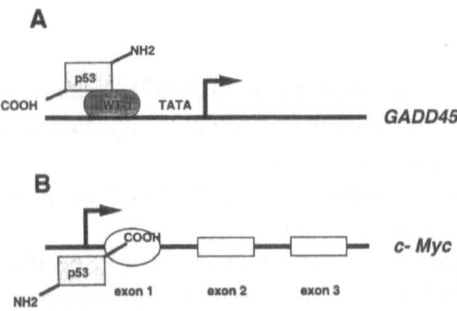

Figure 4. Potential models for indirect gene regulation by p53 mutants lacking sequence-specific DNA-binding capability. In A, transcription from the GADD45 promoter is induced as a result of the interaction between p53 and GADD45 promoter-bound WT-1 (22). In B, interaction between the nonspecific single-stranded DNA- and RNA-binding C-terminal region of p53 and a region at the exon 1/intron 1 boundary of the *c-myc* gene induces *c-myc* gene expression (23).

Conclusions

Cancer initiation and progression are complex processes involving many genetic and epigenetic factors. One of the goals of the National Cancer Institute is the development of improved models to help elucidate the mechanisms underlying these processes and to test new diagnostic and therapeutic regimens. Therefore, the WAP-p53 172R-H transgenic model developed in our laboratory is unique in that it consistently produces tumors characteristic of high-grade breast adenocarcinomas. This model should serve as an excellent system to study the mechanisms responsible for genetic instability and may help identify those factors that promote tumor progression and metastasis. Finally, because mammary gland abnormalities are rarely observed in the absence of carcinogen treatment or oncogene co-expression, this model should facilitate the identification of earlier genetic lesions that may occur as a result of hormonal carcinogenesis.

Acknowledgements

This research was supported by grant CA16303 from the National Institutes of Health. K.L.M. was supported in part by Cell and Molecular Biology Interdisciplinary Program training grant GM08231. The authors would like to thank Dr. Baolin Li, who initiated the p53 transgenic mouse studies, and Dr. Arch Perkins, Yale University, for the erbB2/p53 bigenic mouse studies.

References

1. Hainaut P, Soussi T, Shomer B et al (1997) Database of p53 gene somatic mutations in human tumors and cell lines; updated compilation and future prospects. Nucleic Acids Res 25:151-157.
2. Dittmer D, Pati S, Zambetti G et al (1993) Gain of function mutations in p53. Nature Genetics 4:42-46.
3. Aas T, Borresen AL, Geisler S et al (1996) Specific p53 mutations are associated with de novo resistance to doxorubicin in breast cancer patients. Nature Med 2:811-814.
4. Cho Y, Gornia S, Jeffrey PD et al (1994) Crystal structure of a p53 tumor suppressor-DNA complex: Understanding tumorigenic mutations. Science 265:346-355.
5. Thukral SK, Lu Y, Blain GC et al (1995) Discrimination of DNA binding sites by mutant p53 proteins. Mol Cell Biol 15:5196-5202.
6. Chen Y, Chen PL, and Lee WH (1994) Hot-spot p53 mutants interact specifically with two cellular proteins during progression of the cell cycle. Mol Cell Biol 14:6764-6772.
7. Donehower L (1996) Effects of p53 mutation on tumor progression: recent insights from mouse mammary tumor models. Biochim Biophys Acta 1242:171-176.
8. Donehower LA, Godley LA, Aldaz CM et al (1995) Deficiency of p53 accelerates mammary tumorigenesis in Wnt-1 transgenic mice and promotes chromosomal instability. Genes & Dev 9:882-895.
9. Donehower LA, Harvey M, Slagle BL et al (1992) Mice deficient for p53 are developmentally normal but susceptible to spontaneous tumours. Nature 356:215-221.

10. Li B, Rosen JM, McMenamin-Blano J et al (1997) Neu/erbB-2 cooperates with p53 172H during mammary tumorigenesis in transgenic mice. Mol Cell Biol 17(6):3155-3163.
11. Li B, Murphy KL, Laucirica R et al (1998) A transgenic mouse model for mammary carcinogenesis. Oncogene 16:997-1007.
12. Symonds H, Krall L, Remington L et al (1994) p53-dependent apoptosis suppresses tumor growth and progression in vivo. Cell 78:703-713.
13. Fukasawa K, Choi T, Kuriyam R et al (1996) Abnormal centrosome amplification in the absence of p53. Science 271:1744-1747.
14. Cross SM, Sanchez CA, Morgan CA et al (1995) A p53-dependent mouse spindle checkpoint. Science 267:1363-1356.
15. Liu PK, Krause E, Wu TA et al (1996) Analysis of genomic instability in Li-Fraumeni fibroblasts with germline p53 mutations. Oncogene 2267-2278.
16. Chin K, Ueda K, Pastan J et al· (1992) Modulation of activity of the promoter of the human MDR1 gene by ras and p53. Science 255:459-462.
17. Lingle WL, Lutz WH, Ingle JN et al (1998) Centrosome hypertrophy in human breast tumors:Implications for genomic stability and cell polarity. Proc Natl Acad Sci USA 95:2950-2955.
18. Wang XJ, Greenhalgh DA, Jiang A et al (1998) Expression of a p53 mutant in the epidermis of transgenic mice accelerates chemical carcinogenesis. Oncogene 17:35-45.
19. Patel KJ, Vu VP, Lee H et al (1998) Involvement of BRCA2 in DNA repair. Mol Cell 1:347-357.
20. Zhang H, Somasundaram K, Peng Y et al (1998) BRCA1 physically associates with p53 and stimulates its transcriptional activity. Oncogene 16:1713-1721.
21. Gualberto A, Aldape K, Kozakiewicz K et al (1998) An oncogenic form of p53 confers a dominant, gain-of-function phenotype that disrupts spindle checkpoint control. Proc Natl Acad Sci USA 95(9):5166-5171.
22. Zhan Q, Chen IT, Antinore MJ et al (1998) Tumor suppressor p53 can participate in transcriptional induction of the GADD45 promoter in the absence of direct DNA binding. Mol.Cell.Biol 18(5):2768-2778.
23. Frazier MW, He X, Wang J et al (1998) Activation of c-myc gene expression by tumor-derived p53 mutants requires a discrete c-terminal domain. Mol.Cell.Biol 18(7):3735-3743.
24. Brown CR, Doxsey SJ, White E et al (1994) Both viral (adenovirus E1B) and cellular (hsp70, p53) components interact with centrosomes. J Cell Physiol 160:47-60.

PART 5. CELL CYCLE, CELL PROLIFERATION

Introduction

Receptor Tyrosine Kinases and the Effects of Ovarian Steroids on Cell Proliferation

Richard P. DiAugustine, Diane M. Klotz, and R. Gregg Richards

Numerous epidemiologic and laboratory studies support the concept that ovarian steroid hormones can significantly affect cancer risk in target organs such as the mammary gland and uterus. The relatively high incidence of cancers in these organs has prompted investigation of pathways used by the ovarian steroids to regulate cell growth. The speakers for this session have made significant contributions to our knowledge of cognate receptors and cell cycle regulatory proteins that mediate the proliferative actions of ovarian steroids. Below, I shall describe some of the progress that has been made in the study of hormonally-responsive receptor tyrosine kinases that may link ovarian steroid ligand/receptor complexes with the cell cycle machinery.

It is conceptually appealing to consider that one or more growth factors and their cognate receptors function to mediate the proliferative action of estrogens (Es) in the uterus. Polypeptide growth factors, such as EGF, stimulate proliferation of uterine epithelial cells (1) and the transcripts for many of these growth factors are elevated *in vivo* in response to ovarian hormones (2-3). This increase in the bioavailability of a growth factor may be an event that converges steroid receptor activation with growth regulatory pathways. An alternative view is that Es stimulate proliferation by a more direct action on the cyclins, e.g. cyclin D1, and their associated kinases; in support of this view, an E-responsive *cis*-acting element is present in the promoter region of the cyclin D1 gene (4).

In order to identify uterine growth factor pathways that are activated *in vivo* in response to Es, our laboratory analyzed uterine extracts from ovariectomized mice for receptor tyrosine kinases (RTK) and related substrates. In a limited survey of these kinases, we found that the insulin-like growth factor-1 receptor (IGF-1R) and the insulin receptor substrate-1 (IRS-1), a docking protein, exhibited increased tyrosine (Tyr) phosphorylation within 6 hours following treatment with estradiol (E_2); this response did not occur with progesterone (P), 5α-dihydrotestosterone, or dexamethasone (5). These data are in accord with earlier reports demonstrating that E_2 rapidly stimulates rat uterine IGF-1 mRNA levels (6) and that the chicken IGF-1 gene promoter is controlled by E_2 through a pathway involving fos, jun, and the DNA-binding domain of the E receptor (7).

The direct or indirect interaction of the E receptor with an AP-1 motif in the 5Õ-flanking region of the IGF-1 gene may represent one mechanism by which the ovarian steroids activate mitogenic growth factor pathways; progestins and glucocorticoids may attenuate E action at the level of the AP-1 response element (8).

To further define the signaling proteins assembled by hormonally-activated uterine IGF-1R, we analyzed immunoprecipitates of this receptor for selected docking and Src-homology-2 (SH2) proteins. The presence of a docking protein in a receptor complex expands the potential for divergent signals to originate from a single RTK. The docking proteins IRS-1 and IRS-2 were present in IGF-1R precipitates from E_2-treated mice; phosphatidylinositol (PI) 3-kinase activity and its regulatory subunit (p85) were also complexed with the receptor (9). Because immunodepletion of IRS-1 from extracts markedly reduced the amount of PI3-kinase associated with IGF-1R, it is likely that this enzyme does not bind directly to IGF-1R, but, instead, binds to IRS-1, which has multiple binding sites for p85 (10). Previous studies have linked PI3-kinase to mitogenesis (11) or inhibition of apoptosis (12), and we are now interested in determining whether signals that emanate from the IGF-1R/IRS/PI3-kinase complex contribute to these or other biological endpoints. To address this issue, we are currently investigating aspects of E action in the uterus that are compromised in IGF-1 (13) or IRS-1 (14) nullizygous, as well as IGF-1$^{m/m}$, mice (15).

As a means of conferring specificity to hormonal action, we should expect that the different ovarian hormones will activate distinct growth factor pathways. In this regard, we noted above that P, unlike E_2, does not activate the uterine IGF-1R pathway. However, we recently observed that P does increase Tyr phosphorylation of uterine EGF receptor (EGFR, erbB-1) (unpublished observation). EGFR is not activated by E_2 in the mouse uterus (5), and uterine transplants from EGFR nullizygous mice maintained in the renal capsule of female nude mice still undergo epithelial cell DNA synthesis in response to E_2 (16). The P_4-induced Tyr phosphorylation of EGFR probably occurs as a result of increased EGFR-ligand synthesis. In support of this notion, P_4 can rapidly increase amphiregulin mRNA in the uterine epithelium (17). The temporal expression pattern of amphiregulin mRNA during the murine estrous cycle is also in accord with a role for P in regulating gene expression of this growth factor (17). Furthermore, E_2 suppresses both the P-induced expression of amphiregulin (17) and EGFR Tyr phosphorylation (unpublished observation). Therefore, it is important to determine whether the signaling cascade that occurs in response to P-stimulation of EGFR Tyr phosphorylation accounts for the capacity of this hormone to attenuate the proliferative effects of E_2 on the uterine epithelium.

E_2 is considered to act directly on the mammary gland to stimulate ductal development (18). Previous reports provided indirect evidence that EGFR is important for this event (19-20). A more recent study utilized two mutant mouse models to resolve the importance of this RTK in mouse mammary gland development. The glands from EGFR nullizygous or wild-type mice were implanted under the renal capsule of female nude mice. Under these conditions, the glands from wild-type mice established a ductal tree by thirty days; however, the glands from EGFR nullizygous mice remained as rudimentary structures (21).

Mammary gland morphogenesis was also examined in spontaneous mutant waved-2 mice, which have impaired EGFR kinase activity as a result of a point mutation (Val743Gly) in the kinase domain (22). Whole mounts of the inguinal mammary glands from these mutant mice at 36 days of age revealed fewer branching structures with terminal end buds and less extension of the ducts into the fat pad when compared to glands from age-matched, wild-type controls (21). However, the mammary ducts of both control and waved-2 mice reached the limits of the fat pad by 100 days of age.

To complement the above studies, EGFR and other members of the erbB family were analyzed in extracts of normal mammary glands undergoing ductal morphogenesis. Tyr phosphorylation of EGFR was variable during this period of mammary development but coincided with that of erbB-2. Moreover, treatment of mice with EGF stimulated Tyr phosphorylation of both EGFR and erbB-2 (21). These cumulative findings suggest that the EGFR is essential for mammary development and functions *in vivo* as a heterodimer with erbB-2.

Conclusions

We were prompted to identify RTKs regulated by ovarian steroids in normal target organs since hormonal carcinogenesis may originate by perturbation of these same pathways. The importance of maintaining the microenvironment of the cell-normal or -neoplastic is a critical factor in accurately determining the qualitative and quantitative responses to ovarian steroid hormones.

It is well known that polypeptide growth factors stimulate cells *in vitro* to progress through the checkpoints of the cell cycle. If we consider this with the fact that ovarian steroids can regulate growth factor gene expression, then ligand bioavailability becomes an important variable in determining what receptor pathways are activated by these steroids. In contrast, the expression of receptor tyrosine kinases, their docking and adapter proteins, and other proximal signaling components that function prior to the G1 cyclins/cyclin-dependent kinases is likely more constant in the quiescent cell.

It is not unreasonable to expect that more than one RTK pathway will be activated in a cell in response to Es or progestins and not all of these RTKs will directly stimulate the proliferative machinery. Ovarian hormone responsive cells in the uterus and mammary gland are highly organized and adhesive units within the organ. One of the actions of ovarian hormones may include modulation of the cell-cell adhesion system, such as the §-catenin/E-cadherin proteins, which may have a permissive role in the capacity of cells to proliferate. The findings reported above should encourage the combined use of normal and mutant mouse models to identify RTK pathways activated by ovarian steroids, and to understand the function of these RTKs in hormone-regulated cell proliferation or other responses.

References

1. Toomoka Y, DiAugustine RP, McLachlan JA (1986) Proliferation of mouse uterine epithelial cells in vitro. Endocrinology 118:10111-1018.
2. Nelson KG, Takahashi T, Lee DC et al (1992) Transforming growth factor α is a potential mediator of estrogen action in the mouse uterus. Endocrinology 131:1657-1664.
3. DiAugustine RP, Petrusz P, Bell GI et al (1988) Influence of estrogens on mouse uterine epidermal growth factor precursor protein and messenger ribonucleic acid. Endocrinology 122:2355-2363.
4. Tam SW, Theodoras AM, Shay JW et al (1990) Differential expression and regulation of Cyclin D1 protein in normal and tumor human cells: association with Cdk4 is required for Cyclin D1 function in G1 progression. Oncogene 9:2663-2674.
5. Richards RG, DiAugustine RP, Petrusz P et al (1996) Estradiol stimulates tyrosine phosphorylation of the insulin-like growth factor-1 receptor and insulin receptor substrate-1 in the uterus. Proc Natl Acad Sci USA 93:12002-12007.
6. Murphy LJ, Murphy LC, Friesen HG (1987) Estrogen induces insulin-like growth factor-1 expression in the rat uterus. Mol Endocrinol 1:445-450.
7. Umayahara Y, Kawamori R, Watada H et al (1994) Estrogen regulation of the insulin-like growth factor-1 gene transcription involves an AP-1 enhancer. J Biol Chem 269:16433-16442.
8. Uht RM, Anderson CM, Webb P et al (1997) Transcriptional activities of estrogen and glucocorticoid receptors are functionally integrated at the AP-1 response element. Endocrinology 138:2900-2908.
9. Richards RG, Walker MP, Sebastian J et al (1998) Insulin-like growth factor-1 (IGF-1) receptor-insulin receptor substrate complexes in the uterus. Altered signaling response to estradiol in the IGF-1$^{m/m}$ mouse. J Biol Chem 273:11962-11969.
10. White M (1998) The IRS-signaling system: A network of docking proteins that mediate insulin action. Mol Cell Biochem 182:3-11.

11. Valius M, Kazlauskas A (1993) Phospholipase C-gamma and phosphatidylinositol 3 kinase are the downstream mediators of the PDGF receptors mitogenic signal. Cell 73:321-334.

12. Yao R, Cooper GM (1995) Requirement for phosphatidylinositol-3 kinase in the prevention of apoptosis by nerve growth factor. Science 267:2003-2006.

13. Liu J-P, Baker J, Perkins AS et al (1993) Mice carrying null mutations of the genes encoding insulin-like growth factor (*Igf1*) and type 1 IGF receptor (*Igf1r*). Cell 75:59-72.

14. Tamemoto H, Kadowaki T, Tobe K et al (1994) Insulin resistance and growth retardation in mice lacking insulin receptor substrate-1. Nature 372:182-186.

15. Lembo G, Rockman HA, Hunter JJ et al (1996) Elevated blood pressure and enhanced myocardial contractility in mice with severe IGF-1 deficiency. J Clin Invest 98:2648-2655.

16. Hom YK, Young P, Wiesen JF et al (1998) Uterine and vaginal organ growth requires epidermal growth factor receptor signaling from stroma. Endocrinology 139:913-921.

17. Das SK, Chakraborty I, Paria BC et al (1995) Amphiregulin is an implantation-specific and progesterone-regulated gene in the mouse uterus. Mol Endocrinol 9:691-705.

18. Daniel CW, Silberstein GB, Strickland P (1987) Direct action of 17β-estradiol on mouse mammary ducts analyzed by sustained release implants and steroid autoradiography. Cancer Res 47:6052-6057.

19. Coleman S, Silberstein GB, Daniel CW (1988) Ductal morphogenesis in the mouse mammary gland: evidence supporting a role for epidermal growth factor. Dev Biol 127:304-315.

20. Snedeker SM, Brown CF, DiAugustine RP (1991) Expression and functional properties of transforming growth factor-a and epidermal growth factor during mouse mammary gland ductal morphogenesis. Proc Natl Acad Sci USA 88:276-280.

21. Sebastian J, Richards RG, Walker MP et al (1998) Activation and function of the epidermal growth factor receptor and erbB-2 during mammary gland morphogenesis. Cell Growth Diff 9:777-785.

22. Luetteke NC, Qui TH, Pfeiffer RL (1994) The mouse waved-2 phenotype results from a point mutation in the EGF receptor tyrosine kinase. Genes Dev 8:399-413.

15

Transcriptional Control of Cell Cycle Progression by Estrogenic Hormones: Regulation of Human Cyclin D1 Gene Promoter Activity by Estrogen Receptor-α

Valeria Belsito Petrizzi, Luigi Cicatiello, Lucia Altucci, Raffaele Addeo, Raphaelle Borgo, Massimo Cancemi, Massimo Ancora, Juan Leyva, Francesco Bresciani, and Alessandro Weisz

Introduction

Estrogens (Es) are mitogens for breast and uterine epithelial cells, where they exert also a tumor-promoting action that appears to be directly linked to their growth promoting effects (1-3). Although during recent years the general bases of estrogen receptor (ER) action, in particular the role of these nuclear proteins on regulation of gene transcription, have been elucidated (4), the mechanisms that underlie E control of cell proliferation still remain largely unclear, mainly due to our relatively poor knowledge of the effects of these steroids on the cell cycle regulatory pathways. In eukaryotic cells, these pathways have been found to consist of an orderly sequence of genetic and biochemical processes, controlled by extracellular mitogens as well as oncogenes, that are required for and allow completion of the different tasks leading to cell cycle progression and cell division. They include both growth regulatory or primary events, and growth regulated processes, consequent to the effects evoked in the cell by the primary events (5-6). The evident analogy of these pathways with the general mechanism of action of Es in target cells (7) raises the possibility that cell cycle regulatory (or 'master') genes and gene products could be target of the ER s and mediate their growth promoting actions. A better understanding of the molecular basis of the mitogenic activity of Es will be greatly fostered by the identification of such cell cycle regulatory genes and molecules, and by the subsequent elucidation of their functional interactions with the hormone and its receptors.

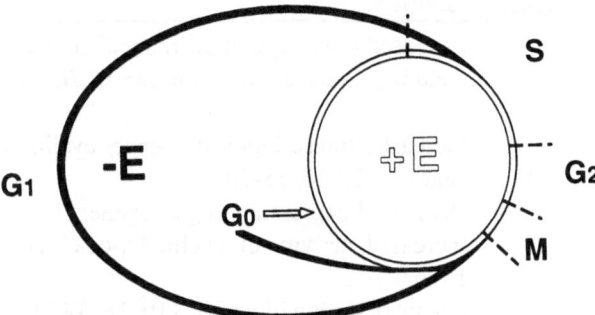

Figure 1. Effects of E on cell cycle kinetics in growth-responsive target cells. E deprivation (-E) induces elongation of the G_1 transition time, accompanied by exit of hormone-dependent cells from the cycle to G_0, resulting in reduced cell proliferation kinetics. On the contrary, stimulation with E (+E) is rapidly followed by recruitment of quiescent cells into the cycle, acceleration of G_1 kinetics and G_1-S transition rate, resulting in efficient cell cycle completion and accelerated growth.

Estrogen Control of Cell Cycle Regulatory Pathways

The mitogenic activity of Es has been best characterized in rodent uterus, ovary, and mammary gland *in vivo* and in ER-positive human breast cancer cells in culture. In both cases, E deprivation or antiestrogen treatment is followed by a reduction of cell proliferation kinetics, resulting from hormone-dependent cells exiting from the proliferative compartment to G_0, mainly occurring in normal cells *in vivo*, and from a reduction of the cell cycle progression rate, predominantly at the G_1 phase, in cycling cells (Figure 1). Stimulation of E-deprived cells with a mitogenic dose of E is followed by synchronous resumption of cell cycle progression, resulting in a first wave of DNA synthesis and cell duplication, generally observable within the first 24-36 hrs of hormone stimulation, followed by sustained cell proliferation, that can be readily reversed at any time by E withdrawal or by antiestrogens. Kinetic analysis of cell cycle parameters and phase-specific markers expression indicates that in most cases the mitogenic response evoked by the hormone occurs without any considerable delay, and it is the result of the recruitment of quiescent cells in cycle, accompanied by a considerable shortening of the G_1 transition time in cycling cells (Figure 1).

Table 1. Cell cycle regulatory events detectable in hormone responsive human breast cancer and rodent mammary gland, uterine and granulosa cells following stimulation with a mitogenic dose of E.

Time[1]	Cell cycle	Events
10^1-10^2	($G_0 \rightarrow$ early G_1)	Increased transcription of 'immediate-early' genes, including c-*fos*, c-*jun*, *jun B*, *jun D*, *JE*, etc. (1, 8-9)
10^2-10^3	(G_1)	Increased transcription of c-*myc*, cyclin D_1, D_2, & D_3 genes (1, 10-16, 18-20)
		Decreased expression of *gas-1* gene[2] (17)
		Increased activity of cyclin D_1-cdk4 complexes (10, 18-20)
		Phosphorylation of p105^{Rb} (10, 16, 18-20)
		Increased expression of cyclin E gene (11, 16, 18, 20)
	(G_1-S)	Increased activity of cyclin E-cdk2 complexes (19-20)
		Increased activity of cdk5[2] and 6 (11)
		Hyper-phosphorylation of p105^{Rb} (10, 16, 18-20)
>10^3	(S)	Increased expression of cyclin A gene (11, 16, 20)
		Increased activity of cyclin A-cdk complexes (19)
	(G_2)	Increased expression of cyclin B1 gene (14, 16, 18-21)

[1] Minutes of exposure to E of hormone-deprived, G_0/early G_1-arrested cells

[2] Detected only in rat ovary granulosa cells and/or uterus

These experimental evidences, pointing to a direct role of Es in cell cycle control, led the way to the quest for the intracellular effectors of this hormonal action. This was made possible by the considerable expansion of our knowledge on the basic cell cycle regulatory machinery in higher eukaryotes that occurred during the most recent years, in particular by the identification of genes whose products exert a determining role in the control of each phase of the cell cycle (5-6). As reported in Table 1, the results of these studies provided conclusive evidences of timed and direct effects of Es on the activity of cell cycle regulatory pathways. These include, in particular: (1) rapid activation of a number of 'immediate-early' genes, coincident with recruitment of quiescent cells into the cycle (1, 8-9); (2) transient enhancement of c-*myc* protooncogene transcription during early G_1 progression, accompanied by a longer lasting activation of D-type cyclin genes with accumulation in E-stimulated cells of the corresponding proteins, assembly of active cyclin D-cdk (cyclin-dependent protein kinase) 4 and 6 complexes and initial phosphorylation of the retinoblastoma gene product (p105^{Rb}; 1, 10-16, 18-20); (3) accumulation of cyclin E mRNA and protein during late G$_1$ and activation of cyclin E-cdk2 complexes, with further p105^{Rb} phosphorylation (10-16, 18-20), that is enhanced by the sequestering of cdk inhibitors by the intracellular accumulation of E-induced, enzymatically inactive cyclin D1-cdk2 complexes (19-20); (4) activation of A and B1 cyclin genes during the S phase and in late S-G$_2$, respectively, with activation of cyclin A-cdk complexes and maximal p105^{Rb} phosphorylation (11, 16, 19-21).

While some of these events are likely to be a secondary cellular response to the hormone, representing the activity of the so-called 'cell cycle clock' (a cascade of biochemical and gene regulation processes that once set in motion functions in a mitogen-independent fashion to perform the multiple tasks required for a correct and orderly completion of the latter phases of the cell cycle), these results support the view that Es act directly on a limited set of primary cell cycle regulatory targets to exert their growth-promoting activity. Indeed, few such targets have been identified, to include 'immediate-early' genes, such as c-*fos*, c-*jun* and *JE*, as well as c-*myc*, that are endowed with estrogen response elements (EREs) or ERE-like sequences and thus might respond directly to ligand-activated ER s (1).

The Cyclin D1 Gene is a Direct Target of the Estrogen Receptor-α

The best known regulators of G$_1$ progression in mammalian cells are represented by the three D-type cyclins (D1-3), whose concentration in the cell increases characteristically during progression through G$_1$. They act predominantly by associating with, and thereby regulating, the catalytic subunits of cdk4 and 6, and show considerable structural and functional homologies with each other. D-type cyclins and their cdk partners are essential to drive cell cycle progression to and beyond a restriction point in late G$_1$ that checks S-phase entry (6). D1 is the best characterized of these G$_1$ cyclins, for it is widely expressed in different cell types and exerts a central regulatory role not only in normal but also in cancerous cell proliferation. Expression of this cyclin is induced by mitogens from mid-G$_1$ on, as part of the 'delayed-early' response, while its over-expression was found to determine acceleration of G$_1$ completion in different cell types. Moreover, microinjection in G$_1$ cells of anti-D1 antibodies, expression of anti-sense D1 mRNA or inactivation of the gene in mice interfere with S phase entry and severely hamper *in-vitro* mitogen-induced cell proliferation.

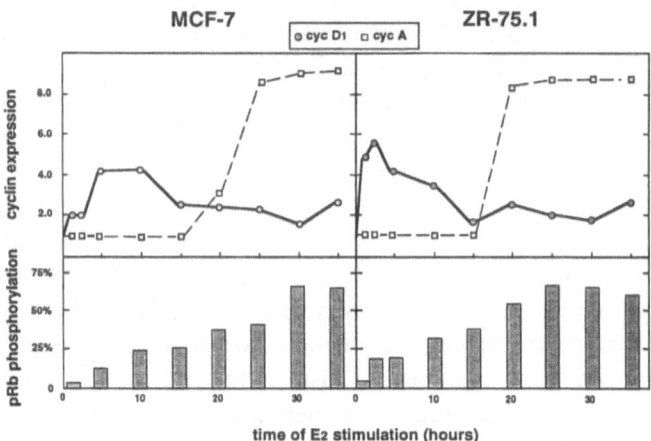

Figure 2. 17β-estradiol rapidly induces cyclin D1 accumulation, followed by cell cycle progression (here marked by accumulation of the S phase marker cyclin A and by progressive pRb hyper-phosphorylation), in estrogen-responsive human breast cancer cells previously arrested in early G_1 by hormone deprivation and (MCF-7 cells only) inhibition of serum mitogen-responsive signal transduction pathways (9).

Interestingly, the mammary gland of D1-deficient mice fails to respond to ovarian steroids, suggesting that this protein is likely to be involved in stimulation of mammary gland growth by sex steroids. Several cdk catalytic subunits associate with D1, namely cdk2, 4, 5, and 6, but assembly of this cyclin into an holoenzyme with cdk4 and 6 is particularly important for its function as a positive regulator of G_1. Targets of the D1-cdk complexes include p105^{Rb} and other pRb-related proteins, that are inactivated by phosphorylation, and thereby relieve the cell from their inhibitory actions.

Analysis of cyclin D1 expression during E stimulation of hormone responsive cells in culture shows that the intercellular concentration of this protein is controlled by these steroids. As shown in Figure 2, when hormone-deprived human breast cancer MCF-7 or ZR-75.1 cells are exposed to a mitogenic dose of 17β-estradiol (E_2) this cyclin readily accumulates in both cell lines. Expression of the protein follows a complex pattern, as it start to increase within the first 2 h of stimulation, to reach a peak level after 5 to 10 h and decrease thereafter to a value that remains 2- to 3-fold higher than that of un-stimulated cells. This results in the assembly of active cyclin D1-cdk complexes with the consequent initial phosphorylation of p105^{Rb} at specific sites (10, 19-20). The antiestrogens trans 4-OH-tamoxifen and ICI 182,780, that inhibit the mitogenic effects of E by blocking ER activity, antagonize hormone-dependent cyclin D1 accumulation and G_1 progression in E-stimulated human breast cancer cells (10, 16), further establishing a functional link between this cyclin and the mitogenic action of Es.

The increase in cyclin D1 expression was studied in detailed and found to be mediated by transcriptional activation of the corresponding gene (*hCCND1*:10). When a recombinant plasmid including the promoter region of this gene, including about 3.0 Kb of 5'-flanking DNA and linked to a luciferase reporter gene, pD1D-2966 (22), is transfected in human breast cancer ZR-75.1 cells, its transcription is clearly stimulated by E_2 (Figure 3), indicating the presence of E-responsive *cis*-acting regulatory DNA element(s) in the *CCND1* gene promoter region. This same result was obtained following stable transfection of the same reporter gene in MCF-7 cells (10). At least one of these elements can be mapped in the 5'-flank on the gene between positions -1720 and -742, by comparing the response to E treatment of the reporter pD1D-1720 with that of pD1D-742, that lacks any significant response to the hormone (Figure 3). By comparison, the response to E of an ERE-containing test gene (ERE-luc, including a perfectly palindromic ERE cloned upstream of the HSV-Tk gene promoter) is also shown in Figure 3; this appears to be comparable to that of the cyclin D1 gene promoter, although more pronounced and longer lasting (data not shown).

Sequence analysis of the -1720/-743 E responsive DNA region of the cyclin D1 gene failed to show similarities with known ER -responsive cis-acting regulatory elements, in particular EREs or ERE-like sequences, with the notable exception of an AP-1 site, that binds a transcription factor complex controlled by Es in breast cancer cells (1). However, site directed mutagenesis of this AP-1 site failed to prevent the reporter gene's response to E_2 (data not shown), suggesting that in this case the AP-1 complex is not mediating this hormonal effect.

In order to verify the possibility that the ERα, the only ER subtype expressed in MCF-7 and ZR-75.1 cells, might be directly involved in the transcriptional response of the *hCCND1* gene to Es, further transfection experiments were performed in the ER-negative breast epithelial MCF-10A cells. While the pD1D-1720 reporter was unresponsive to E_2 when transfected in this cell line (data not shown), its transcription was activated by E_2 to an extent comparable to that observed in MCF-7 or ZR-75.1 cells upon co-transfection of the expression vector HEG0, encoding wt ER-α (23), (Figure 4).

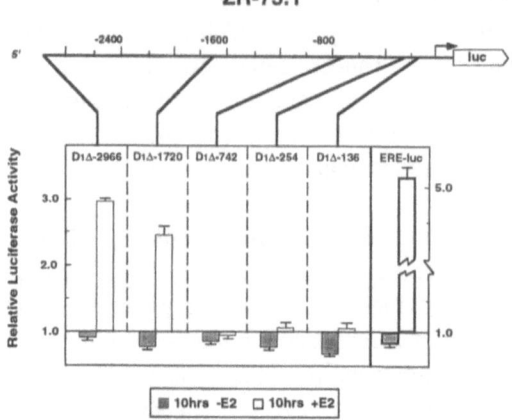

Figure 3. Mapping of an E-responsive region in the human cyclin D1 gene promoter. The indicated luciferase reporter genes, each including variable length of 5'-flanking DNA region, were transiently transfected in ZR-75.1 cells and tested for their response to E. The data represent reporter gene activity in the presence of $5 \times 10^{-8} M E_2$ (+ E_2), compared to that of untreated (- E_2) controls.

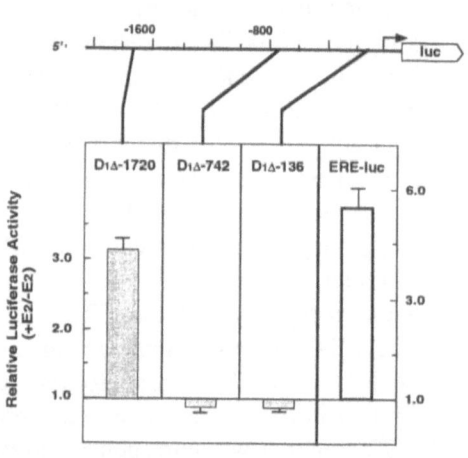

Figure 4. Ligand-activated ERα stimulates human cyclin D1 gene promoter activity. Human breast epithelial MCF-10A cells were transiently transfected with the indicated cyclin D1 promoter-luciferase reporter genes and an expression vector (HEG0) encoding wt human ER-α. The data represent reporter gene activity following cell stimulation with 5×10^{-8} M E_2 for 12 h (+E_2), compared to that detectable in cells transfected with the same plasmids but not stimulated with the hormone (-E_2).

Deletion of the region located between 1720 and 743 (mutant pD1D-742) even in this case prevents activation of the promoter by the hormone, suggesting the possibility that the element(s) involved in the response to E of the transfected gene promoter in ER positive MCF-7 and ZR-75.1 cells and in ER-complemented MCF-10A cells coincide. These results support the following conclusions: (1) ligand-activated ER-α appears to act directly on the cyclin D1 gene promoter through an hormone-responsive region located between positions 1720 and 743; (2) since MCF-10A cells constitutively expressing the ER-α subtype do not grow in response to Es, failing to show any significant cell cycle activation in response to the hormone (24), the response of the transfected cyclin D1 gene promoter to E is not secondary to cell cycle activation but a primary gene response to the hormone.

The response of the human *CCND1* gene to various classes of mitogens, active oncogenes and components of mitogen-responsive signal transduction pathways have been extensively studied in different cell types. This led to the identification of multiple mitogen-responsive elements in the promoter region of this gene (Figure 5). Herber, *et al.* (22), first reported that multiple cis-acting elements, located within the first Kbp upstream of the transcription startsite, are responsible for activation of this gene promoter by serum and c-*jun*, including also the closely spaced AP-1 and mitogen-inducible elements (MIE) and a cAMP-response element (CRE). Subsequently, the AP-1 site was found to be involved in this promoter activation by c-*jun* and active *Ha-ras* (25), angiotensin II and Erk2 MAP kinase (26) and, at least in part, by transforming growth factor α (TGF-α) (27).

The main target of the intracellular signal transduction pathways activated by TGF-α, however, appears to be the Egr site of the gene (27). Finally, a cluster of Sp1 sites found close to the capsite of the gene is mediating the transcriptional response to nerve growth factor (28) and, in combination with the E2F site located immediately upstream, to active c-*ErbB2/Neu* oncogene (29), while a least two promoter-near c-Ets sites are mediating gene activation by epidermal growth factor and p41^{Erk} MAP kinase (25).

Preliminary results of deletion and site-specific mutagenesis of the 1720/743 DNA region indicate that still un-characterized transacting enhancer factors are involved in the transcriptional response of this promoter to E during G_1, all binding to the same DNA sequence and acting in concert with ER-α. The composite E-responsive DNA element of the *hCCND1* gene, that we defined Estrogen-Responsive G_1 Element (ERGE), appears thus to be unique between those found to mediate the transcriptional effects of these steroids, since it is active predominantly during G_1 via the combined actions of ligand-activated ER and multiple transacting factors.

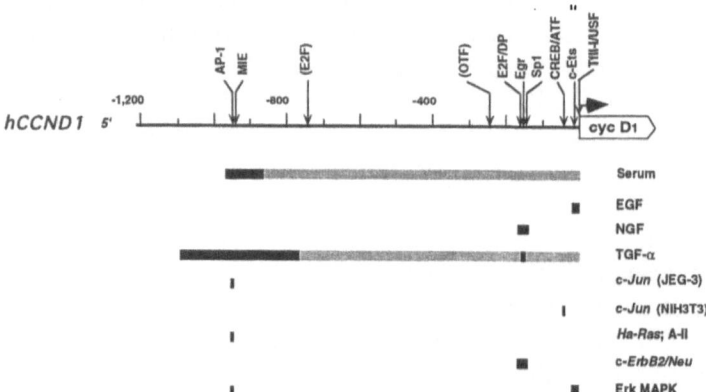

Figure 5. Mitogen-, oncogene- and MAP kinase-inducible elements identified in the human cyclin D1 gene promoter region. For details and references see the text. A-II: angiotensin II; EGF: epidermal growth factor; NGF: nerve growth factor; TGF: transforming growth factor; MAPK: mitogen-activated protein kinase.

EGF and TGF-α are mitogenic for human breast cancer cells, and E-stimulated cells secrete these growth factor in the medium (30). This led to the hypothesis that these and other hormone-induced polypeptide growth factors (estromedins) could be mediating the mitogenic activity of Es. However, as shown here, the E-responsive region of the cyclin D1 gene do not co-localize with the EGF and TGF-α responsive regions, and the transcriptional response of both chromosomal and transfected D1 gene occurs very rapidly after E stimulation. Thus, based on these observations, it appears unlikely that activation of this cell cycle regulator by Es be mediated by accumulation of hormone-induced growth factors in the culture medium.

Activation of the Cyclin D1 Gene Promoter by Estrogens in Human Breast Cancer Cells do not Requires Active Erk-1 and -2 Mitogen-activated Protein Kinases

Recently, Migliaccio, *et al.* (31) reported that Erk-2 activity can be stimulated by Es in human breast cancer cells, suggesting that this protein kinase could be part of the mitogenic pathway of these steroids in cancer cells. Although it has been shown that efficient stimulation of cell cycle progression by E_2 in G_1-arrested MCF-7 cells can occur independently of Erk-1 and -2 MAP kinases activity (9, 16, 32), this interesting possibility remains to be fully verified. For this reason, we expressed dominant interfering Erk MAP kinase mutants (33-34) in ZR-75.1 cells and tested their effects on the response of the cyclin D1 gene promoter to E. Results show that inhibition of Erk-1 and -2 MAP kinases does not prevent cyclin D1 promoter activation by E. As shown in Figure 6, expression of dominant negative mutants of either kinase does not affect activation of the pD1D-1720 reporter by E_2 in ZR-75.1 cells. Both Erk mutants, in fact, determine a dose-dependent reduction of the basal transcriptional activity of the reporter, but the relative extent of E-induced activation remains unmodified in all cases. On the contrary, the same MAP kinase dominant interfering mutants are fully effective in inhibiting EGF-mediated activation in MCF-10A cells, that are highly responsive to this growth factor, as the decrease in basal promoter activity in the presence of either dn Erk mutant parallel was found to accompany in this case a clear inhibition of the transcriptional enhancement induced by EGF (data not shown).

Essentially similar results have been observed upon interference with Erk-1 and -2 activity by over-expression of two Erk-inactivating MAPK phosphatases in ZR-75.1 or MCF-10A cells (16). Even in this case, a reduction in basal promoter activity did not interfere with E-mediated activation of the reporter, but completely abolished EGF-mediated induction.

As activation of these Erk MAP kinases is thought to be a crucial step in the mitogenic response of epithelial cells to polypeptide growth factors, these data further support the notion that Es exert their growth-promoting activity in human breast cancer cells *in vitro* by a growth factor-independent mechanism.

Conclusions

Given the central role of cyclin D1 in cell cycle control during the pre-replicative phase, and its oncogenic potential in a wide range of cell types including also breast epithelial cells, the findings described here support the view that Es, through their nuclear receptors, are fully capable of stimulating directly G_1 progression in growth-responsive cells by controlling the cell division cycle, at least in part, through timed activation of key regulatory gene networks. Accordingly, Es should be classified as true mitogens, since they can stimulate directly target cell proliferation. This is in contradiction with the hypothesis, predominant for some time, that the mitogenic activity of Es is mediated exclusively by autocrine growth factors released by hormone-stimulated cells. However, several other physiological roles for E-induced growth factors can be foreseen. They could act *in vivo* as paracrine mitogens, helping to coordinate growth of E-responsive and -unresponsive cells, such as for example those in the stromal and vascular compartments that are needed to support proliferating epithelia. In addition, they may complement in an autocrine fashion E action, for example by contributing to full activation of the ER through its phosphorylation. Finally, they may be necessary to edit the differentiated phenotype of E-responsive growing cells, determining their functional maturation. These hypotheses do not exclude that growth factors can regulate growth of E-responsive cells in the absence of E, as seen in several instances. In fact, cell proliferation can be controlled by different extracellular signals via multiple intracellular pathways, not necessarily mutually exclusive in a given cell type. It is conceivable that growth factors can interplay with, or even substitute for, E in the mitogenic stimulation of hormone-responsive cells, depending upon the physiological setting.

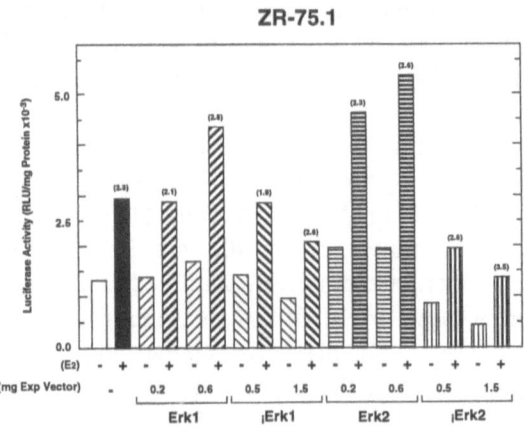

Figure 6. E activation of the human cyclin D1 gene promoter occurs independently of Erk-1 and -2 MAP kinases activity. Cells were transiently transfected with the reporter pD1D-1720 (see Figure 4), without or with the indicated amounts of expression vectors, before stimulation with 5×10^{-8} M E_2 for 12 h. Erk1 and Erk2: expression vectors encoding wt X. Laevis Erk1 and rat Erk2 MAP kinases, respectively; iErk1 and iERK2: encoding the corresponding kinase-defective dn mutants Erk1K>M and Erk2K>R (33-34).

Summary

Es are potent mitogens for a subset of their target cells, where they exert a central role in cancer promotion and progression. Analysis of the effect of these steroids on cell cycle regulatory molecular pathways led to the identification of a number of key components of these pathways that are direct target of regulation by E, including the G_1 cyclins D1-3, cyclin-dependent protein kinases. Transcription of the human cyclin D1 gene is enhanced by E through functional interaction of hormone-activated ER-α

with a DNA element that is distinct from previously characterized mitogen- and oncogene-responsive elements of this gene. Furthermore, E activation of cyclin D1 gene transcription does not appear to be mediated by the Erk-1 and -2 MAP kinases cascade in human breast cancer cells. These findings indicate that the mitogenic activity of E involves the direct control by ligand-activated nuclear ERs of a subset of cell cycle 'master' genes, that in turn drive the cascade of hormone induced intracellular events leading to DNA replication and cell division.

Acknowledgements

Work supported by the European Community (Biomed 2 Program: Contract BMH4.CT98.3433), the Italian Association for Cancer Research (A.I.R.C.), the National Research Council of Italy (Contract 9704417CT14) and the Second University of Naples (quota parte co-finanziamento 1997). R. B. is a fellow of Association pour la Recherche contre le Cancer (France).
Also, the authors acknowledge M. Beato (I.M.T., Marburg, Germany), P. Chambon (I.G.B.M.C., Strasbourg, France), A. Gutierrez-Hartmann (U. of Colorado, Denver, U.S.A.) and M. Kortenjann (U. of Nottingham, U.K.) for providing recombinant DNA clones and for helpful comments and suggestions.

References

1. Weisz A, Bresciani F (1993) Estrogen regulation of protooncogenes coding for nuclear proteins. CRC Critical Rev. Oncogenesis 4:361-388.
2. Henderson BE, Ross R, Bernstein L (1988) Estrogens as a cause of human cancer. Cancer Res 48:246-253.
3. Moolgavkar S (1986) Hormones and multistage carcinogenesis. Cancer Surv 5:635-648.
4. Weisz A (1998) Estrogen regulated genes. In: Oettel M and Schillinger E (eds) Handbook of experimental pharmacology: estrogens and antiestrogens. Springer Verlag, Heidelberg, pp. 135 (In press).
5. Muller R, Mumberg D, Lucibello FC (1993) Signals and genes in the control of cell-cycle progression. Biochim Biophys Acta 1155:151-179.
6. Grana X, Reddy EP (1995) Cell cycle control in mammalian cells: role of cyclins, cyclin-dependent kinases, growth suppressor genes and cyclin-dependent kinase inhibitors. Oncogene 11:211-219.
7. Dean DM, Sanders MM (1996) Ten years after: reclassification of steroid-responsive genes, Mol. Endocrinol. 10:1489.
8. Cicatiello L, Sica V, Bresciani F et al (1993) Identification of a specific pattern of 'immediate-early' gene activation induced by estrogen during mitogenic stimulation of rat uterine cells. Receptor 3:17-30.

9. Bonapace IM, Addeo R, Altucci L et al (1996) 17b-estradiol overcomes a G_1 block induced by HMG-CoA reductase inhibitors and fosters cell cycle progression without inducing ERK-1 and -2 MAP kinase activation. Oncogene 12:753-763.

10. Altucci L, Addeo R, Cicatiello L et al (1996) 17b-estradiol induces cyclin D1 gene transcription, $p36^{D1}$-$p34^{cdk4}$ complex activation and $p105^{Rb}$ phosphorylation during mitogenic stimulation of G_1-arrested human breast cancer cells. Oncogene 12:2315-2324.

11. Altucci L, Addeo R, Cicatiello L et al (1997) Estrogen induces early and timed activation of cyclin-dependent kinases 4, 5 and 6 and increases cyclin messenger ribonucleic acid expression in rat uterus. Endocrinology 138:978-984.

12. Said TK, Conneely OM, Medina D et al (1997) Progesterone, in addition to estrogen, induces cyclin D1 expression in the murine epithelial cells in vivo. Endocrinology 138:3833-3939.

13. Geum D, Sun W, Paik SK et al (1997) Estrogen-induced cyclin D1 and D3 gene expression during mouse uterine cell proliferation in vivo: differential induction mechanism of cyclin D1 and D3. Mol Reprod Dev 46:450-458.

14. Zhang Z, Laping J, Glasser S et al (1998) Mediators of estrogen-stimulated mitosis in rat uterine luminal epithelium. Endocrinology 139:961-966.

15. Robker RL, Richards JS (1998) Hormone-induced proliferation and differentiation of granulosa cells: a coordinate balance of the cell cycle regulators cyclin D2 and $p27^{Kip1}$. Mol Endocrinol 12:924-940.

16. Cicatiello L, Addeo R, Altucci L et al (1998) Estrogen control of G_1 progression and G_1/S transition in hormone-responsive human breast cancer cells: Stepwise activation of the cyclin-dependent cell cycle control pathway by 17b-estradiol requires persistent nuclear estrogen receptor activation. Submitted for publication.

17. Ferrero M, Cairo G (1993) Estrogen-regulated expression of a growth arrest specific gene (gas-1) in rat uterus. Cell Biol Int 17:857-862.

18. Foster JS, Wimalasena J (1996) Estrogen regulates activity of cyclin-dependent kinases and retinoblastoma protein phosphorylation in breast cancer cells. Mol Endocrinol 10:488-498.

19. Planas-Silva M, Weinberg RA (1997) Estrogen-dependent cyclin E-cdk2 activation through p21 redistribution, Mol Cell Biol 17:4059-4069.

20. Prall OWJ, Sarcevic B, Musgrove EA et al (1997) Estrogen-induced activation of cdk4 and cdk2 during G_1-S phase progression is accompanied by increased cyclin D1 expression and decreased cyclin-dependent kinase inhibitor association with cyclin E-cdk2. J Biol Chem 272:10882-10894.

21. Thomas T, Thomas TJ (1994) Regulation of cyclin B1 by estradiol and polyamines in MCF-7 breast cancer cells. Cancer Res 54:1077-1084.
22. Herber B, Truss M, Beato M et al (1994) Inducible regulatory elements in the human cyclin D1 promoter. Oncogene 9:1295-1304.
23. Ponglikitmongkol M, Green S, Chambon P (1988) Genomic organization of the human oestrogen receptor gene. EMBO J 7:3385-3388.
24. Hong J, Shah NN, Thomas TJ et al (1998) Differential effects of estradiol and its analogs on cyclin D1 and cdk4 expression in estrogen receptor positive MCF-7 and estrogen receptor-transfected MCF-10AEwt5 cells. Oncol Rep 5:1025-1033.
25. Albanese C, Johnson J, Watanabe G et al (1995) Transforming p21^{ras} mutants and c-Ets-2 activate the cyclin D1 promoter through distinguishable regions. J Biol Chem 270:23589-23597.
26. Watanabe G, Lee RJ, Albanese C et al (1996) Angiotensin II activation of cyclin D1-dependent kinase activity. J Biol Chem 271:22570-22577.
27. Yan Y-X, Nakagawa H, Lee M-H et al (1997) Transforming growth factor-a enhances cyclin D1 transcription through the binding of early growth responsive protein to a cis-regulatory element in the cyclin D1 promoter. J Biol Chem 272:33181-33190.
28. Yan GZ, Ziff EB (1997) Nerve growth factor induces transcription of the p21 WAF/CIP1 and cyclin D1 genes in PC12 cells by activating the Sp1 transcription factor. J Neurosci 17:6122-6132.
29. Lee RJ, Watanabe G, Albanese C et al (1998) Regulation of cyclin D1 by the Neu, c-erbB2, proto-oncogene. Proc Am Assoc Cancer Res 39: 253 and 1730.
30. Davidson NE, Lippman ME (1989) The role of estrogens in growth regulation of breast cancer. CRC Critical Rev. Oncogenesis 1:89-111.
31. Migliaccio A, Di Domenico M, Castoria G et al (1996) Tyrosine kinase/ p21^{ras} /MAP-kinase pathway activation by estradiol-receptor complex in MCF-7 cells. EMBO J 15:1292-1300.
32. Lukas J, Bartkova J, Bartek J (1996) Convergence of mitogenic signalling cascades from diverse classes of receptors at the cyclinD-cyclin-dependent kinase-pRb-controlled G$_1$ checkpoint. Mol Cell Biol 16:6917-6925.
33. Conrad KE, Oberwetter JM, Vaillancourt R et al (1994) Identification of the functional components of the ras signalling pathway regulating pituitary cell-specific gene expression. Mol Cell Biol 14:1553-1565.
34. Kortenjann M, Thomae O, Shaw PE (1994) Inhibition of v-raf-dependent c-fos expression and transformation by a kinase-defective mutant of the mitogen-activated protein kinase Erk2. Mol Cell Biol 14:4815-4824.

16

Estrogen Regulation of Cell Cycle Progression

Owen W.J. Prall, Eileen M. Rogan, Elizabeth A. Musgrove,
Colin K.W. Watts, and Robert L. Sutherland

Introduction

Estrogens (Es) are essential for the normal development and physiological function of the female reproductive tract and secondary sex organs including the mammary gland. The development and progression of cancer in adult E target tissues is also dependent on E which has led to the effective use of E antagonists, particularly tamoxifen, in the treatment and potential prevention of breast cancer. The involvement of E in these major physiological and pathological processes is thought to be mediated via the potent mitogenic activity of Es. While these properties of Es have been long appreciated, it is only recently that the links between E action and the cell cycle machinery have begun to be dissected.

Cell Cycle Progression

Early studies on cell proliferation in the rodent uterus and mammary gland *in vivo* demonstrated that E increases the proportion of cells synthesizing DNA by recruiting non-cycling cells into the cell cycle and reducing the duration of G_1 phase in already cycling cells. Further experiments to test the effect of E added at different stages of the cell cycle using breast cancer cells synchronized at the G_1/S boundary or at G_2/M indicated that the sensitive cells were in early G_1 phase, immediately following mitosis [reviewed in reference (1)]. These conclusions are in agreement with data demonstrating that breast cancer cells arrest in G_0/G_1 following antiestrogen treatment (2). More precise mapping of the point of antiestrogen action within G_1 phase using cells synchronized by mitotic selection identified a window of sensitivity in early to mid-G_1 phase (3). Together these data (Figure 1) are compatible with a model whereby Es and antiestrogens, through their interactions with the estrogen receptor (ER), regulate the transcription of genes that control key cell cycle transitions in G_1 and perhaps G_0 phase. Our recent studies have focused on E regulation of the function of those cyclin-dependent kinases (Cdks) that control progression through G_1 phase of the cell cycle.

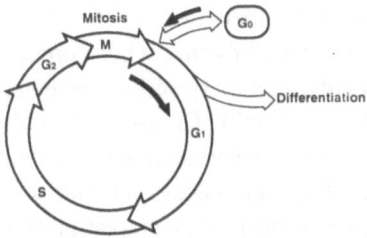

Figure 1. Cell cycle phase-specific effects of Es. The four phases of the cell cycle: G_1, S, G_2 and M are illustrated. Cells can leave the cell cycle and enter a resting or G_0 phase which allows re-entry into the cell cycle. Alternatively, cells can exit the cell cycle to enter an irreversible program of differentiation. The major sites of E action in promoting cell proliferation are identified by the solid arrows.

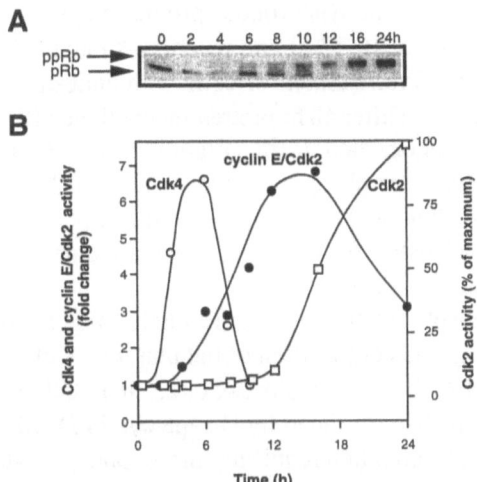

Figure 2. Effect of estradiol on pRb phosphorylation and Cdk activity. MCF-7 cells pretreated with the antiestrogen, ICI 182780, for 48 hr were treated with 17β estradiol at 0 hr. A. Cell lysates were harvested at the times indicated and blotted for pRb: ppRb represents the hyperphosphorylated form and pRb the hypophosphorylated form. B. The kinase activity of Cdk4, cyclin E and Cdk2 immunoprecipitates was determined by phosphorylation of *in vitro* substrates.

Cyclin/Cdk Expression and Function

Progress through G_1 phase requires inactivation of the retinoblastoma (pRb) protein by phosphorylation and the consequent release of a number of transcription factors including members of the E2F family. These transcription factors then activate the expression of genes whose products are required for S phase progression (4). Phosphorylation of pRb is mediated by the action of the G_1 phase Cdks (Cdk4, Cdk6 and Cdk2). Control of G_1 Cdk activity is achieved by several mechanisms including: transcriptional activation of D-type cyclins and cyclin E, the rate-limiting regulatory subunits of the G_1 cyclin-Cdk complexes (Cdk4/6 and Cdk2, respectively); activation and inactivation of these enzyme complexes by phosphorylation/dephosphorylation events; and the abundance and action of two families of Cdk inhibitors (5). Modulation at any of these levels can regulate pRb phosphorylation and hence G_1 phase progression.

The effect of E on these families of regulatory molecules was investigated in an *in vitro* model of E-induced cell cycle progression. In this model, E-responsive MCF-7 breast cancer cells were arrested in G_0/G_1 phase by pretreatment with the pure antiestrogen ICI 182780 for 48 hr. Addition of 17β estradiol resulted in the semi-synchronous progression of cells through G_1 and into S phase, beginning at 10-12 hr and reaching a maximal 60% of cells in S phase at 21-24 hr (1). Pretreatment of cells with antiestrogens inhibited pRb phosphorylation such that after 48 hr pretreatment all the pRb was in the growth inhibitory, hypophosphorylated form (Figure 2A). By 6 hr following E treatment less mobile, hyperphosphorylated forms of pRb were apparent. This shift continued until 12 hr, when cells were entering S phase and all the pRb was in the hyperphosphorylated form, a situation maintained until 24 hr when S phase was maximal.

Since these phosphorylation events are likely to be mediated by Cdks we measured the activity and composition of the major G_1 Cdk complexes in these cells i.e. cyclin D1-Cdk4 and cyclin E-Cdk2. It is believed that the initial phosphorylation of pRb is mediated by D-type cyclin D-Cdk4/6 complexes in mid-G_1 phase with full activation requiring further phosphorylation by cyclin E-Cdk2 complexes later in G_1 near the G_1-S interface. Data presented in Figure 2B demonstrate that Cdk4 activity was markedly increased by 4 hr and was maximal at 6 hr coincident with the first increases in pRb phosphorylation; thereafter Cdk4 activity declined. Cyclin E-Cdk2 activity began to increase at 4 hr and was significantly increased at 6 hr. However, maximum activity was not reached until 12-16 hr coincident with maximal accumulation of hyperphosphorylated pRb and entry into S phase. Cyclin E complexes constitute only a minority of total Cdk2 activity which is predominantly due to cyclin A-Cdk2. Consequently major changes in total Cdk2 activity were only observed subsequent to 12 hr when cyclin A expression was markedly increased as cells entered S phase (1).

Further analysis of cyclin and Cdk gene expression demonstrated that cyclin D1 levels were increased at 4 hr and remained elevated until cells entered S phase at 12 hr while Cdk4 levels increased 2-fold between 12 and 24 hr (1). Analysis of the composition of cyclin D1-associated complexes provided support for the view that an E-induced increase in cyclin D1 gene expression is the predominant determinant of active cyclin D1-Cdk4 complexes. In marked contrast, the level of expression of cyclin E and Cdk2 changed little over the 24 hr time course and the composition of cyclin E complexes including cyclin E, Cdk2 and the inhibitors p21 and p27, remained constant during the first 10 hr of E treatment (1). Thus, in contrast to the situation with Cdk4 complexes, there was no discernible change in the composition of the cyclin E-Cdk2 enzyme complexes at a time when the activity of the complexes was rapidly increasing i.e. between 4 and 12 hr. The mechanistic basis for this effect was investigated further.

Activation of Cyclin E-Cdk2 Complexes

Separation of the cyclin E-Cdk2 complexes by gel filtration chromatography indicated that E treatment was associated with the formation of high molecular weight, high specific activity complexes (Figure 3). These complexes constituted a minority of the cyclin E-Cdk2 protein but a majority of the activity. This increased activity, which was associated with a shift in Cdk2 to the enzymatically active, threonine 160-phosphorylated form, was accounted for by the relative deficiency of the Cdk inhibitors p21 and p27 in the high molecular weight complexes (Figure 3). Thus although no changes in complex composition were apparent on analysis of whole cell lysates, separation of such lysates revealed different forms of the enzyme complex with markedly different composition and activity. These data are consistent with a mechanism of activation of cyclin E-Cdk2 involving both reduced Cdk inhibitor association and consequent phosphorylation of Cdk2 at threonine 160 by the Cdk-activating kinase. Such a conclusion implicates redistribution of p21 and p27, rather than regulation of the levels of these proteins, as a critical event in the early mitogenic response to E. A predominant role for p21 in this effect is suggested by the demonstration that E treatment relieves an inhibitory activity toward cyclin E-Cdk2, and that this inhibitory activity is depleted by p21, not p27 immunodepletion or precipitation (1, 6).

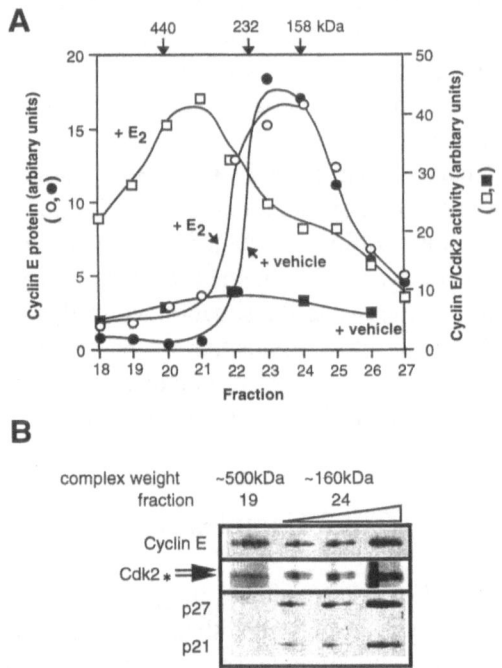

Figure 3. Cyclin E-Cdk2 activation is accompanied by loss of Cdk inhibitor association and Cdk2 Thr-160 phosphorylation. Cell lysates were prepared 8 hr after estrogen (E$_2$) or vehicle treatment and fractioned on a Superose 12 gel filtration column. A. Fractions were Western blotted for cyclin E or assayed for cyclin E-Cdk2 activity. B. Cyclin E immunoprecipitates from fractions 19 and 24 (E$_2$ lysate) were analysed for cyclin E, Cdk2, p21 and p27. Various quantities of the cyclin E immunoprecipitate from fraction 24 were analysed to permit comparison of inhibitor ratios at equivalent cyclin E levels with fraction 19. The asterisk marks the more mobile form of active Cdk2 phosphorylated on Thr-160.

Role of c-*myc*

Regulation of expression of the proto-oncogene c-*myc* is among the earliest detectable responses to Es and antiestrogens. c-*myc* is necessary for G$_1$ to S phase progression in several cell types including breast cancer cells where antisense oligonucleotides inhibit E-stimulated cell proliferation (7). Furthermore, recent data provide evidence for a role for c-*myc* in the activation of cyclin E-Cdk2 (8). Consequently, we investigated whether the rapid activation of this enzyme complex following E treatment might be mediated, at least in part, by c-*myc*.

To provide further insight into the activation of cyclin E-Cdk2 we constructed MCF-7 cells expressing either c-*myc* or cyclin D1 under the control of an inducible promoter (9). Similar to the situation following E treatment, expression of c-*myc* or cyclin D1 was sufficient to activate cyclin E-Cdk2 by promoting the formation of high molecular weight, high specific activity complexes lacking the Cdk inhibitor p21. c-*myc* expression was not accompanied by increased cyclin D1 expression or Cdk4 activation, nor was cyclin D1 induction accompanied by increases in c-*myc* expression. Together these results suggest that E upregulates separate c-*myc* and cyclin D1 pathways, which then converge on the activation of cyclin E-Cdk2.

A major question remaining unanswered is the mechanistic basis for the distribution of the p21 Cdk inhibitor between the active and inactive cyclin E-Cdk2 complexes. One potential explanation is that E-induced accumulation of cyclin D1-Cdk4 complexes sequesters p21 thereby reducing its association with cyclin E-Cdk2 (6). Alternatively, E may alter the properties of p21, reducing its ability to bind to the complex, perhaps as a result of increased c-*myc* expression. A similar mechanism has been proposed to account for c-*myc*-mediated activation of cyclin E-Cdk2 in fibroblasts, involving prevention of the association between the Cdk inhibitor p27 and cyclin E-Cdk2 (10). Recent evidence that the pRB-related proteins, p107 and p130, can compete with p21 for cyclin-Cdk binding raises the possibility that these proteins may be recruited to the cyclin E-Cdk2 complex following E treatment, contributing to the increased apparent molecular weight of the complex and the decreased association with p21. This is supported by our recent evidence that immunodepletion of p130 from lysates of E treated cells abolishes the formation of the high molecular weight active complexes (9).

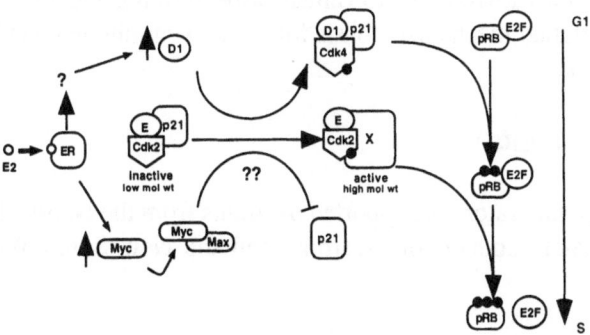

Figure 4. A model of E effects on molecules regulating G1 phase progression.

Conclusions

Es exert potent mitogenic effects on ER-positive mammary epithelial cells which are mediated predominantly in the G_1 phase of the cell cycle. The recent development of a powerful *in vitro* model, wherein breast cancer cells are growth-arrested with a pure antiestrogen and the cell cycle progression reinitiated with E, has facilitated dissection of some early molecular events in E action (1). A schematic representation of current knowledge developed from this model and the results of others is present in Figure 4. This indicates that the mitogenic effects of E appear to be mediated by at least two apparently distinct pathways of which c-*myc* and cyclin D1, respectively, are the key regulators. Transcriptional activation of c-*myc* is rapid and thought to be directly mediated via interaction with the ER. In contrast, E stimulation of cyclin D1 expression requires the *de novo* synthesis of, as yet unidentified, intermediary proteins. Increased expression of cyclin D1 leads to formation of active complexes with Cdk4 and phosphorylation of pRB.

The net result of E-induced c-*myc* or cyclin D1 expression is early activation of the cyclin E-Cdk2 holoenzyme by the formation of high molecular weight cyclin E-Cdk2 complexes deficient in the Cdk inhibitor p21. This process appears to involve redistribution of p21 away from a small proportion of the total cellular cyclin E-Cdk2 complexes. Two potential mechanisms have been invoked to account for this redistribution involving sequestration by cyclin D1-Cdk4 or an as yet undefined c-*myc*-induced process. Subsequently, the cyclin E-Cdk2 complexes acquire a higher molecular weight (presumably due to association with p130 and unidentified protein(s) labeled "X" in Fig. 4) and high specific catalytic activity. Phosphorylation of pRB is a primary target of cyclin E-Cdk2 activity, resulting in the well documented release of E2F transcription factors necessary for DNA synthesis, and progression from G_1 to S phase of the cell cycle.

Further studies are required to validate aspects of this model with an aim to providing a detailed mechanistic basis for the known mitogenic effects of E in its target tissues.

Acknowledgments

Research in the laboratory is supported by grants from the National Health and Medical Research Council of Australia and the New South Wales Cancer Council.

References

1. Prall OWJ, Sarcevic B, Musgrove EA et al (1997) Estrogen-induced activation of Cdk4 and Cdk2 during G_1-S phase progression is accompanied by increased cyclin D1 expression and decreased cyclin-dependent kinase inhibitor association with cyclin E/Cdk2. J Biol Chem 272:10882-10894.

2. Sutherland RL, Hall RE and Taylor IW (1983) Cell proliferation kinetics of MCF-7 human mammary carcinoma cells in culture and effects of tamoxifen on exponentially growing and plateau-phase cells. Cancer Res 43:3998-4006.

3. Taylor IW, Hodson PJ, Green MD et al (1983) Effects of tamoxifen on cell cycle progression of synchronous MCF-7 human mammary carcinoma cells. Cancer Res 43:4007-4010.

4. Weinberg RA (1995) The retinoblastoma protein and cell cycle control. Cell 81:323-330.

5. Morgan DO (1995) Principles of Cdk regulation. Nature 374:131-134.

6. Planas-Silva MD and Weinberg RA (1997) Estrogen-dependent cyclin E-cdk2 activation through p21 redistribution. Mol Cell Biol 17:4059-4069.

7. Watson PH, Pon RT and Shiu RP (1991) Inhibition of c-myc expression by phosphorothioate antisense oligonucleotide identifies a critical role for c-myc in the growth of human breast cancer. Cancer Res 51:3996-4000.

8. Steiner P, Philipp A, Lukas J et al (1995) Identification of a myc-dependent step during the formation of active G1 cyclin-cdk complexes. EMBO Journal 14:4814-4826.

9. Prall OWJ, Rogan EM, Musgrove EA et al (1998) c-myc or cyclin D1 mimics estrogen effects on cyclin E-Cdk2 activation and cell cycle reentry. Mol Cell Biol 18:4499-4508.

10. Perez-Roger I, Solomon DL, Sewing A et al (1997) Myc activation of cyclin E/Cdk2 kinase involves induction of cyclin E gene transcription and inhibition of p27(Kip 1) binding to newly formed complexes. Oncogene 14:2373-2381.

PART 6. ONCOGENES/TUMOR SUPPRESSOR GENES

17

Estrogen and c-*myc* Protooncogene Actions in Human Breast Cancer

R.P.C. Shiu, D. Dubik, M. Venditti, J. Sparling, B. Iwasiow, and P.H. Watson

Introduction

It has been said that all breast cancers (BC) begin as estrogen (E)-responsive/-dependent entities. In initial diagnosis, however, close to 60% of the BCs have already progressed to an E independent state. Given time, virtually all BCs become E-independent, that is, they have circumvented the need for E. These hormone-independent tumors may or may not retain their estrogen receptors (ER) (1).

The molecular mechanism underlying the emergence of hormone independency in BC is not well understood, but is likely to involve the constitutive expression of critical cellular genes whose expression is initially stimulated by E at an earlier stage of the cancer when it is E- responsive. In our laboratory, we have been primarily focussed on the role that the c-*myc* protooncogene plays in the progression of BC from the E-dependent to the hormone-independent state.

The impetus to study the involvement of c-*myc* gene in E action in BC was provided by the observation that the growth of c-*myc*-induced mammary tumors in transgenic mice were E independent (2-3). Therefore, these transgenic mouse studies suggested that c-*myc* protooncogene is an important factor determining E responsiveness in BC.

We initiated our studies using a pair of human BC cell lines: MCF-7, an ER-positive (ER$^+$) and -responsive cell line, and MDA-MB-231, an ER-negative (ER$^-$) and -independent cell line. The growth of the ER$^+$-MCF-7 was substantially reduced when charcoal-stripped serum was used, due to the depletion of most of the steroidal hormones from the culture medium. Addition of antiestrogenic compounds such as Tamoxifen (TAM), or the pure antiestrogens ICI 164,384 and ICI 182,780, further diminished growth. The addition of 17β-estradiol (E$_2$) restored cell growth. The ER$^-$-MDA-MB-231 cells, on the other hand, were totally refractory to the effects of E$_2$ or TAM (4).

The pattern of c-*myc* protooncogene expression mirrors that of cell growth. That is, in ER$^+$-MCF-7 cells, TAM suppressed and E$_2$ stimulated c-*myc* expression. In the E-independent, ER$^-$-MDA-MB-231 cells, the expression of c-*myc* was high and constitutive, and affected neither by E$_2$ nor TAM (4).

It is important to note that c-*myc* expression is essential for cell proliferation in both the hormone-dependent and -independent BC cells, because the abolition of c-*myc* expression using antisense oligonucleotides reduced the growth of both ER$^+$-MCF-7 and ER$^-$-MDA-MB-231 cells (5). However, this experiment using antisense c-*myc* oligonucleotides did not yield any insight into whether c-*myc* expression alone was sufficient to confer cell growth in the absence of E.

Recalling that in the hormone-independent cell line ER$^-$-MDA-MB-231, c-*myc* expression is constitutively high, then one may ask whether *is this due to an enhanced rate of transcription of the c-myc gene?* Nuclear run-on experiments indicated that c-*myc* transcription in the ER$^-$-MDA-MB-231 nuclei was similar to that of ER$^+$-MCF-7 nuclei from cells maintained in the absence of E$_2$. Yet, the level of accumulated c-*myc* mRNA in the ER$^-$-MDA-MB-231 cells was much higher than that present in the ER$^+$-MCF-7 cells. These data suggest that the increased level of c-*myc* mRNA in the ER$^-$-MDA-MB-231 was regulated post-transcriptionally. Messenger RNA stability studies showed that the c-*myc* mRNA in ER$^-$-MDA-MB-231 (t2 = 1 hr) was 3-4 times more stable than that of ER$^+$-MCF-7 cells (t2 = 15 min) (6). Thus, it appears that an increase mRNA stability may be one mechanism used by E-independent cells to achieve the elevation of c-*myc* mRNA. Therefore, it is possible that the progression of BC, during hormonal progression from E-dependency to -independency, involves alteration of cellular proteins that regulate c-*myc* mRNA degradation. In view of the recent identification of mRNA- destabilizing and -stabilizing proteins that bind c-*myc* mRNA (7-8), it is speculated that hormone progression involves altered expression of c-*myc* mRNA binding proteins. This hypothesis remains to be tested.

With respect to the molecular mechanism underlying the activation of c-*myc* gene expression by E in hormone-responsive BC cells, transient transfection expression studies were performed using chimeric DNA constructs consisting of varying lengths of the 5'-promoter sequences of the human c-*myc* gene coupled to a reporter gene (e.g. CAT). These analyses have led to the conclusion that a 120 bp upstream of the major c-*myc* promoter, P2, is capable of conferring E$_2$ response (9). This 120 bp region contains an ERE-half site that is separated by ~20 bp from a Sp1 binding site. This configuration is similar to that found in the 5'-promoter regions of several known E-response genes such as creatine kinase B and Hsp 27 (10-11). It has been demonstrated that Sp1 binding to the ER facilitates its binding to the ERE-half site on the Hsp 27 promoter. This protein-protein interaction between Sp1 and ER is apparently sufficient to allow stable binding to the promoter and to effect gene activation. Therefore, it appears that the same mechanism may be used for the activation of the c-*myc* promoter, by way of an association between ER and Sp1 (12).

Based on the above observations, a working model for E activation of BC growth is proposed (Figure 1). In this model, E activates, via binding to its receptors, a host of cellular genes, one of which is the c-*myc* protooncogene. The c-MYC protein, being a transcriptional factor, in turn switches on (or off) downstream genes. These whole host of E-regulated genes are responsible for inducing cell proliferation and other relevant biological consequences that are likely to include tumor cell invasion and metastasis. It is also conceivable that, under certain circumstances (e.g. exposure to chemotherapeutic agents and other "stress" factors), the elevated c-*myc* expression can promote program cell death (apoptosis) in BC cells, similar to the situations reported for hemopoietic cells and fibroblasts (13).

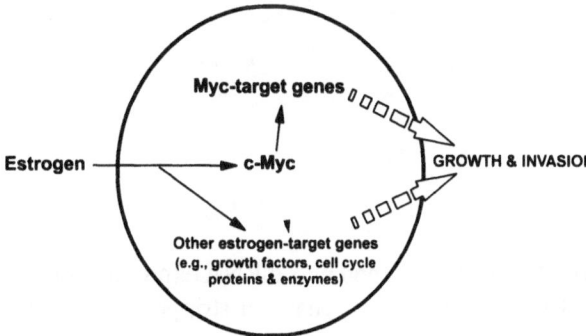

Figure 1. Proposed mechanisms of E action and c-*myc* protooncogene in human BC.

To understand the full extent of the biological actions of c-*myc* requires a detailed analysis of the many cellular regulators that affect it. Mainly through its basic region/helix-loop-helix/leucine zipper domain, the c-MYC protein has been shown to dimerize with a host of cellular proteins (14) resulting in the formation of a variety of heterodimers containing c-MYC. Many of these heterodimeric complexes are believed to have important functions in the transactivation and repression of gene activities. The best known c-MYC-binding protein is MAX. The c-MYC activity is dependent on its association with its partner protein, MAX (15). It is the MYC-MAX dimer that transactivates target genes through binding to enhancer elements called E-boxes. In addition to dimerization with c-MYC, MAX also forms dimers with several known proteins that include the MAD (16) and MXI1 (17) families. These latter proteins essentially compete with c-MYC for MAX. Because of the inability of

MAX-MXI1 and MAX-MAD dimers to transactivate genes, the association of MXI1 and MAD with MAX essentially reduces or prevents the formation of MYC-MAX dimers, and thus reducing the activity of c-MYC. Therefore, the activity of c-MYC protein is highly dependent on the status of these MYC-regulators.

In view of the fact that c-MYC is an E regulated protein, it would be of interest to examine if MAX, MAD, and MXI1 are similarly regulated by E_2. When ER$^+$-MCF-7 cells were treated with E_2, there was a significant increase in *max* mRNA concomitant with an increase in c-*myc* mRNA (Figure 2). Furthermore, the expression of both c-*myc* and *max* was inhibited by the antiestrogens, ICI 182,780 and TAM. The expression of *mxi1* and *mad*, however, was not affected by E_2 or antiestrogens.

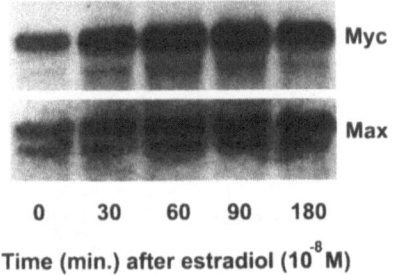

Figure 2. E stimulation of c-*myc* and *max* mRNA expression in the ER$^+$-MCF-7 cells maintained in the presence of charcoal-stripped fetal bovine serum. E_2 treatment was 90 minutes.

Evidence that c-*myc* and *max* are E target genes was also obtained for human breast tumors *in vivo*. In this study, a panel of 45 primary breast tumors were assayed for ER content, and mRNAs for c-*myc, max, mxi1,* and *mad* were semi-quantitated by RT-PCR. There was a significant correlation between ER contents with c-*myc* ($P<0.002$) and *max* ($P<0.02$) mRNA levels, but not with *mxi1* and *,ad* mRNA levels. These data add further support to the findings using the ER$^+$-MCF-7 cell line. In the course of studying this panel of breast tumors, it was found that 4/45 tumors contained a 4-5-fold amplification of the c-*myc* gene, as assessed by Southern blot analysis of genomic DNA extracted from the tumors.

Therefore, our studies indicate that at least three mechanisms can lead to an elevated expression of the c-*myc* protooncogene in human BC: (1) up-regulation of transcription by E, (2) increased c-*myc* mRNA stability; and (3) c-*myc* gene amplification. A given population of BC cells may possess two (or more) of these mechanisms.

There are still a number of important issues regulating c-*myc* actions in BC cells that need to be addressed. For example, (1) *to what extent does c-myc contribute towards E's overall biological effects?* (2) *is it possible to separate those E regulated biological and genetic events that are independent of c-myc and those that are direct consequences of c-myc expression?* (3) *what are the c-myc target genes in BC?* Answers to some of these questions could only be derived from experiments in which we can manipulate the expression, and therefore, the activity of c-*myc* alone in BC. Those trophic factors such as E and growth factors known to activate c-*myc* expression are unsuitable because they activate a whole array of cellular events in addition to c-*myc* expression. To circumvent this difficulty, we have developed a BC cell model in which only the c-*myc* expression can be manipulated. A series of ER$^+$-MCF-7 clones were made that contain the stable integration and expression of the reverse-tetracycline transcriptional activator (rtTA) plasmid (18), in addition to a plasmid containing the c-*myc* cDNA driven by the tet-operator promoter. An example is ER$^+$-MCF-7 clone 35, this clone retains E responsiveness. The endogenous c-*myc* gene was activated by E$_2$ and was totally inhibited by the antiestrogen ICI 182,780. Addition of doxycycline (DOX), an analog of tetracycline, to the ICI 182,780 inhibited the cells effectively, and stimulated the expression of the transfected c-*myc* gene to a level comparable to that seen in cells grown in the presence of E. Furthermore, this DOX-inducible c-*myc* produces a biologically active c-MYC protein capable of transacting an EBox-luciferase chimeric construct that was transiently transfected. In preliminary experiments, we were able to show that, in the presence of fetal bovine serum and E, the growth of ER$^+$-MCF-7 clone 35 was completely inhibited by ICI 182,780, and DOX addition was able to partially reverse the inhibition by the antiestrogen. Over a seven-day growth assay, DOX + ICI 182,780 achieved 5 times more cells than ICI alone, but 5 times less cells than uninhibited cells (DOX alone). These data indicate that c-*myc* expression alone was sufficient to promote cell growth and confer resistance to antiestrogens. However, it was also clear that c-*myc* expression alone cannot completely replace E$_2$ in achieving optimal cell growth.

In any event, our c-*myc*-inducible ER$^+$-MCF-7 cell model should provide a powerful tool to dissect the mechanisms of action of E in hormone-responsible BC. As well, this novel cell model allows the identification of potential c-*myc* target genes (14, 19) that may be important for hormone-dependent BC proliferation. Such knowledge may be the key to our understanding of the emergence of hormone-independent BCs which are primarily responsible for the failure of hormonal therapy.

References

1. McGuire WL, Lippman ME, Osborne CK et al (1987) Resistance to endocrine therapy. A panel discussion. Breast Cancer Res Treat 9:165-173.
2. Sinn E, Muller W, Pattengale P et al (1987) Coexpression of MMTV/v-Ha-ras and MMTV/c-myc genes in transgenic mice: synergistic action of oncogenes in vivo. Cell 49:465-475.
3. Schöenenberger CA (1988) Targeted c-myc gene expression in mammary glands of transgenic mice induces mammary tumours with constitutive milk protein gene transcription. EMBO J 7:169-175.
4. Dubik D, Dembinski TC, Shiu RPC (1987) Stimulation of c-myc oncogene expression associated with estrogen-induced proliferation of human breast cancer cells. Cancer Res 47:6517-6521.
5. Watson PH, Pon R, Shiu RPC (1991) Inhibition of c-myc expression by phosphorothioate antisense oligodeoxynucleotides identifies a critical role for c-myc in the growth of human breast cancer. Cancer Res 51:3996-4000.
6. Dubik D, Shiu RPC (1988) Transcriptional regulation of c-myc oncogene expression by estrogen in hormone-responsive human breast cancer cells. J Biol Chem 263:12705-12708.
7. Lafon I, Carballes F, Brewer G et al (1998) Developmental expression of AUF1 and HuR, two c-myc mRNA binding proteins. Oncogene 16:3413-3421.
8. Leeds P, Kren BT, Boylan JM et al (1997) Developmental regulation of CRD-BP, an RNA-binding protein that stabilizes c-myc mRNA *in vitro*. Oncogene 14:1279-1286.
9. Dubik D, Shiu RPC (1992) Mechanism of estrogen activation of c-myc oncogene expression. Oncogene 7:1587-1594.
10. Wu-Peng XS, Pugliese TE, Dickerman HW et al (1992) Delineation of sites mediating estrogen regulation of the rat creatine kinase B gene. Mol Endocrinol 6:231-240.
11. Porter W, Saville B, Hoivik D et al (1997) Functional synergy between the transcription factor Sp1 and the estrogen receptor. Mol Endocrinol 11:1569-1580.
12. Dubik D, Watson PH, Shiu RPC. (1994) Estrogen, c-myc, and breast cancer. In: Khan SA, Stancel GM (eds) Protooncogenes and Growth Factors in Steroid Hormone Induced Growth and Differentiation. CRC Press, Florida, pp. 175-186.
13. Thompson EB (1998) The many roles of c-myc in apoptosis. Annu Rev Physiol 60:575-600.
14. Facchini LM, Penn LZ (1998) The molecular role of myc in growth and transformation: recent discoveries lead to new insights. FASEB J 12:633-651.

15. Kretzner L, Blackwood E, Eisenman RN (1992) Transcriptional activities of the Myc and Max proteins in mammalian cells. Curr Topics Microbiol Immunol 182:435-443.
16. Ayer E, Kretzner L, Eisenman RN (1993) Mad: a heterodimeric partner for Max that antagonizes Myc transcriptional activity. Cell 72:211-222.
17. Zervos A, Gyuris J, Brent R (1993) Mxil, a protein that specifically interacts with Max to bind Myc-Max recognition sites. Cell 72:223-232.
18. Gossen M, Freundlieb S, Bender G et al (1995) Transcriptional activation by tetracyclines in mammalian cells. Science 268:1766-1769.
19. Grandori C, Eisenman RN (1997) Myc target genes. Trends Biochem Sci 22:177-181.

18

Steroid Hormone Regulation of Vascular Endothelial Growth Factor (VEGF) Production: A Potential Step in Hormonal Carcinogenesis

Salman M. Hyder, Holly L. Boettger-Tong, Sari Mäkelä, and George M. Stancel

Introduction

The provision of a sufficient nutrient supply is a basic requirement for the growth, replication, and performance of differentiated function of all cells. In mammalian tissues the supply of nutrients is regulated largely by the vascular system, and some of the most dramatic changes in the mammalian vasculature occur in the female reproductive tract. These include both the growth of blood vessels such as that observed in the primate endometrium during the menstrual cycle, as well as changes in vascular permeability that regulate the transit of water, small molecules, and proteins from vessels to the intracellular space. In the physiological setting, these vascular effects are regulated largely by the cyclical secretion of ovarian steroid hormones, and these events can be mimicked experimentally by the administration of exogenous estrogens (E) and progestins. Understanding the underlying mechanisms by which steroid hormones regulate vascular events has received considerable attention, since these changes are likely essential for normal endometrial growth and successful implantation.

Historically, the rodent uterus provided a major experimental system for studying the effects of Es on the uterine vasculature. Shortly after the isolation of Es, Astwood observed that injection of these hormones produced massive uterine hyperemia. This change occurred very rapidly and was maximum by 2-3 hours after hormone treatment. Numerous investigators working in this system established that Es increased capillary permeability to water, as well as small molecular weight nutrients such as glucose and amino acids, and plasma proteins as large as albumin. These changes were so dramatic that the uterine interstitial fluid after hormone administration came to resemble "plasma more than an ultra filtrate." These events occur primarily in the stromal layer, and a rapid and massive stromal edema remains a hallmark effect of Es in the rodent uterus. Early investigators recognized that these vascular events correlated well with the tissue hypertrophy and hyperplasia which occur at slightly later times, and blockade of early vascular changes (e.g., with glucocorticoid treatment) blunts subsequent growth responses. Thus, in the early 1950's, endocrine physiologists had postulated that early vascular changes produced by Es played an important role in hormone-mediated growth and cell proliferation. A comprehensive review of early work in this area has been provided by Spaziani (1).

Because of the perceived importance of vascular changes in the uterus, a substantial effort was directed to define the underlying mechanisms. Most early work in this area focused on the action of steroids on the possible regulation of the uterine vasculature by neurogenic mechanisms, since the uterus has autonomic innervation by humoral agents such as histamine and kinins (1). Studies in the 1960's also established that E treatment produces changes in the fenestrations or pores of uterine vessels through which particles and proteins exit the plasma and enter the interstitial fluid (1). Despite a very large number of studies, however, a clear picture of the underlying mechanisms has not emerged, due in large part to an insufficient understanding of the molecular events that regulate capillary growth and permeability.

More recently, it has become clear that the growth of new blood vessels from existing capillaries (angiogenesis), and capillary permeability are regulated in large part by peptide growth factors, such as vascular endothelial growth factor (VEGF). VEGF has two distinct activities: (a) stimulates angiogenesis by virtue of its mitogenic actions on vascular endothelial cells, and (b) causes an increase in vascular permeability (2). Because of its effects on vascular permeability, it is also referred to as vascular permeability factor (VPF) or VEGF/VPF. The earliest experimental evidence for the involvement of VEGF in the regulation of capillary growth and function in the uterus was provided by Cullinan-Bove and Koos in the rat (3), and Charnock-Jones, et al. (4) in the human. These initial reports stimulated our interest in the regulation of VEGF by steroid hormones in normal tissues as well as hormone-responsive tumors.

Control of Uterine VEGF Expression by Estrogens

In our initial studies, we treated immature female rats with 17β-estradiol (E$_2$) for various times, and analyzed uterine RNA for the level of VEGF transcripts by Northern blot analysis. The results of such experiments are shown in Figure 1.

ESTRADIOL INDUCTION OF VEGF

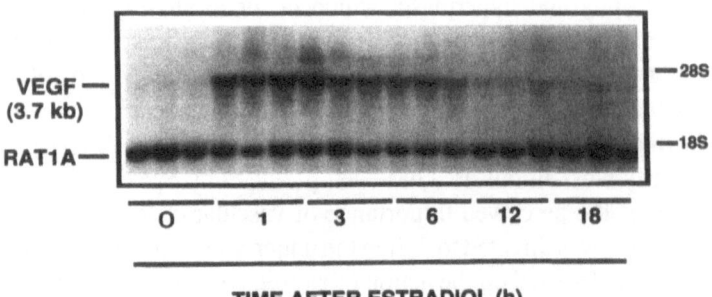

TIME AFTER ESTRADIOL (h)

VEGF INDUCTION IN RAT UTERUS

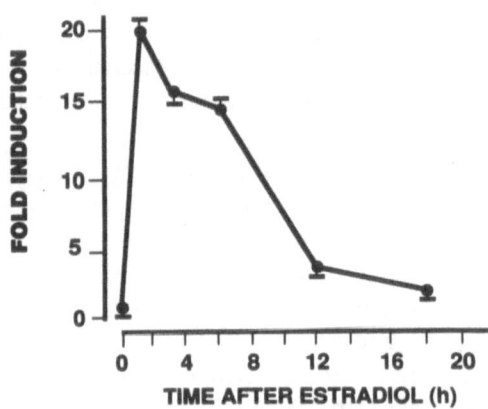

TIME AFTER ESTRADIOL (h)

Figure 1. Time-dependent induction of VEGF in the rat uterus by E_2. *A,* ovariectomized rats were treated with E_2 (40 mg/kg) for the periods indicated. Uteri were removed and RNA was isolated. Each lane contains 20 mg RNA from pooled tissue of three animals. Each time point was analyzed in triplicate. The Rat 1 A transcript was used as an internal standard. *B,* bands representing 3.7-kb VEGF mRNA were scanned with a laser densitometer and corrected for internal variation using the Rat 1 A signal. The mean values (n = 3) are expressed as fold induction above the vehicle-treated controls, the bars represent the SE. Reprinted by permission from the authors (5).

These studies confirmed Cullinan-Bove and Koos (3) findings, and illustrate that E induce a massive increase in VEGF expression that is maximum within 1 h, and remains elevated for at least 6 h. Thus, this time course is consistent with a role for VEGF in the E-induced changes in uterine vascular permeability observed in earlier studies in this system (1). This effect of E is specific since neither glucocorticoids nor androgens produced this action (5). A number of splice variants of VEGF are known to exist, and we demonstrated, by RT-PCR analysis of uterine RNA, that the increase seen in Figure 1 represents changes in transcripts coding for at least 3 variants: $VEGF_{188}$, $VEGF_{164}$, and $VEGF_{120}$ (5).

A number of observations suggest that the induction of VEGF by Es is, at least in part, a direct transcriptional response. Consistent with such mechanism, the induction of VEGF is blocked by actinomycin D (*ACT D*), but not by puromycin (*PURO*), as illustrated in Figure 2.

INFLUENCE OF METABOLIC INHIBITORS ON VEGF INDUCTION

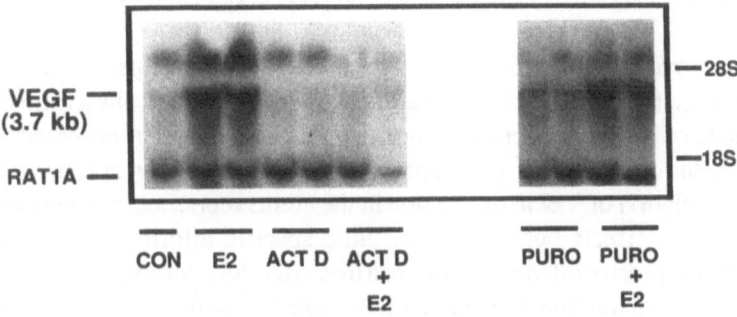

Figure 2. Effect *ACT D* and *PURO* on VEGF induction. Animals were treated with *ACT D* 3 h before E_2 treatment, and again at the time of E_2 treatment. Animals (three per sample) were killed 3 h after the E_2 injection, uterine RNA was prepared followed by Northern blot analysis. For the *PURO* studies, animals received 100 mg/kg of the inhibitor, 30 min prior to the E_2 treatment. The animals were killed 3 h later, and uterine RNA was prepared. Each lane represents pooled RNA from three different animals. *CON*, control. Reprinted by permission from the authors (5).

In addition, the dose/response curve for VEGF induction is similar to that for other E receptor (ER)-mediated events in the uterus (5). Based upon these results, we have initiated a search for an E response element(s) in the VEGF gene. To date, we have identified at least two sequences, one in the 3'-region and the other in the 5'-region of the gene which bind purified human ER (unpublished observations). Interestingly, both sequences bind both, ER-α and the more recently discovered ER-β. Our current efforts in this area are directed toward determining whether these sequences, alone or in combination with other elements, confer functional E-inducibility to reporter constructs in transfection studies.

Another indication that VEGF-induction occurs via the classical ER pathway is that the pure antiestrogen, ICI 182,780, blocks increased production of the growth factor transcript by E (6). Interestingly, however, the blockade of VEGF induction by the ICI compound displays a different dose/response curve than that observed for inhibition of other responses, such as the E-induction of the protooncogene c-*fos* (6). This indicates that this antiestrogen selectively blocks the induction of other uterine genes relative to VEGF, suggesting differences in the mechanism by which Es induce this growth factor and other genes. At present, we do not understand the molecular basis for this selectivity, but it may be due to differences in hormone response elements, co-activators, or co-repressors involved in ER-induction of different genes.

Effects of Progestins on Uterine VEGF Expression

Cullinan-Bove and Koos (3) originally showed that progestins increase VEGF expression in the immature rat uterus, and we confirmed their observations. The magnitude of VEGF induction by progestins is less than that observed by Es, however, the onset of the induction is also slower. It thus appears that the overall regulation of VEGF expression in the uterus represents an interplay of E and progestin effects but, at present, little specific information is available regarding the precise interaction between these steroids. An understanding of the physiological interactions between Es and progestins in the regulation of uterine VEGF expression will probably require similar studies in mature animals, however, the hormone interactions in that setting may be quite different than those observed in the immature rat model.

Induction of VEGF Expression by Tamoxifen

Figure 3 illustrates the induction of VEGF mRNA by Tamoxifen (TAM) in the rat uterus. The magnitude of VEGF induction (20-fold) was similar to that observed after E_2 treatment, but interestingly, the TAM time course was somewhat slower. At present, we do not know whether this fluctuation was due to differences in the rate of absorption or distribution of these compounds, or whether the induction seen after TAM treatment was due to its metabolism to a more active compound. In previous studies, we have shown that 4-OH-TAM is a more potent inducer of VEGF expression than the parent compound (7).

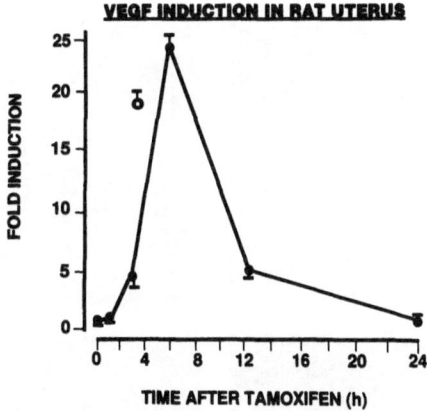

Figure 3. Time-dependent induction of VEGF in the rat uterus by TAM. Ovariectomized rats were treated with TAM (1 mg/kg) for the times indicated. Uteri were removed, RNA was isolated and analyzed for VEGF mRNA levels by Northern analysis as in Figure 1. The 3.7-kb VEGF mRNA was scanned with a laser densitometer and corrected for internal variations using Rat 1 A values. The open circles represents E_2-induced VEGF message at 3 h. The mean values (n = 3) are expressed as fold induction above vehicle treated controls, and the bars represent SE. Reprinted by permission from the authors (5).

Given that both E and TAM induce VEGF expression in the rat uterus, we examined the cellular pattern of this response following treatment with both agents. The results of such studies are shown in Figure 4, and indicate that both compounds induce an identical pattern of VEGF induction. In both cases, VEGF expression was limited to the stroma, and within this tissue layer, transcript levels appear to exhibit a differential distribution, higher in areas nearest to the lumen. However, careful examination of data obtained with [^{35}S]-labeled probes (Figure 4), and from similar studies using digoxigenin-labeled probes, which allow better definition of cell types by hematoxylin and eosin staining (unpublished observations), indicated that luminal and glandular epithelial cells were completely devoid of VEGF expression following E or TAM treatment. This cellular pattern of VEGF expression was consistent with previous findings indicating that vascular changes in the uterus are most prominent in the stroma.

In contrast to our findings that TAM stimulates VEGF production in the uterus, others have observed that this drug and other antiestrogens exhibit antiangiogenic activity in a different experimental system, the chick egg chorioallantoic membrane assay (7). Given this observation, we sought to determine whether the effect of TAM on VEGF expression that we observed in the uterus was unique to this compound, or whether it was common to other antiestrogens of the triphenylethylene class.

244 S.M. Hyder, et al.

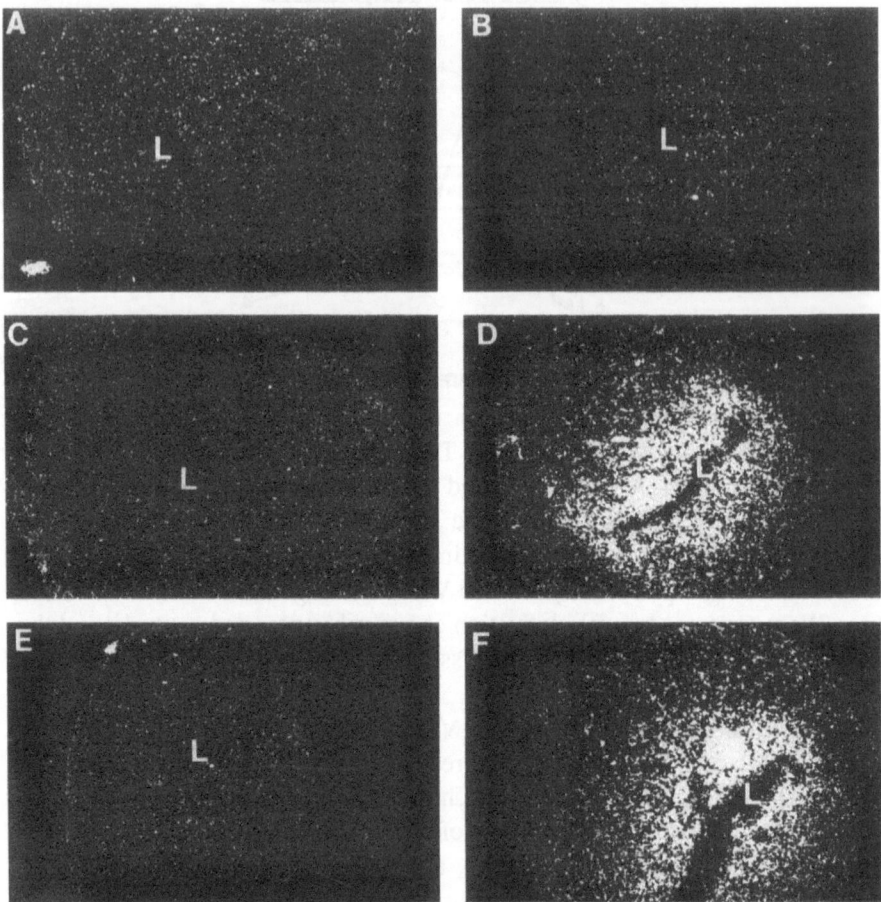

Figure 4. *In-situ* hybridization of VEGF expression in the rat uterus by E$_2$ and TAM. Sections shown in *A, C,* and *E* were treated with a sense probe. *A,* vehicle-treated control; *C,* E$_2$-treated sample (3 h); *E,* TAM-treated sample (6 h). Sections *B, D,* and *F* were treated with antisense VEGF probe. *D* and *F,* corresponding E$_2$-treated (3 h) and TAM-treated (6 h) samples, respectively. *B,* vehicle-treated control, *L,* lumen of the uterus. The signal obtained was mainly in the stromal compartment just beneath the luminal epithelial cell layer. Reprinted by permission from the authors (5).

This study indicated that TAM, 4-OH-TAM, nafoxidine, and clomiphene produce a similar induction of VEGF expression in the rat uterus (7), even though these compounds are antiangiogenic in the chick egg chorioallantoic membrane assay. These data indicate that the effects of antiestrogens on angiogenic factors are tissue specific and may involve multiple mechanisms (7).

Steroid Regulation of VEGF in Human Breast Cancer Cells

Our initial studies focused on the regulation of VEGF expression by steroids and antihormones in normal uterine tissue in the rat model. However, it is quite clear that angiogenesis plays an important role in the growth and metastasis of many types of cancer, including BC (8). For example, tumors may not grow past a certain size unless the density of micro vessels in their vicinity increases, and the density of blood vessels near a tumor can influence its ability to metastasize. It is also known that, the production of angiogenic factors such as VEGF is high in many human breast tumors, and that, in general, there is an inverse relationship between the level of VEGF expression in a patient's tumor and her overall prognosis. In addition, at least one recent study demonstrated the induction of VEGF expression in the 7,12-dimethylbenz(a)anthracene (DMBA)-induced rat mammary tumors by Es (9). Given these observations and the clear effect of steroid hormones on BC, we decided to extend our studies on E and progestin regulation of VEGF to human BC cells.

To initially investigate the effects of progestins, we used human T47-D BC cells which express high levels of the progesterone receptor (PR). These studies illustrated that progesterone causes a 3-4 fold induction of VEGF protein secretion into the cell growth medium (Figure 5). This effect was specific for progesterone and interestingly, neither E or the synthetic E DES increased VEGF secretion in these cells which do contain ER. Other experiments revealed that medroxyprogesterone acetate and a variety of synthetic progestins used for contraception and hormone replacement therapy cause similar increases in VEGF secretion. Thus, this appears to be a generalized effect of progestins, both endogenous and synthetic. It is also important to note that, this effect occurs at physiological levels of progesterone, with increases in VEGF secretion observed at a dose range of 0.1 to 10 nM (10). Not all PR containing cell lines display increased VEGF induction in response to progestins, however, as we have not observed this effect in MCF-7, ZR-75, MDA-MB-231 cells, or the Ishikawa endometrial carcinoma cell line (10). This clearly indicates that regulation of VEGF expression by Es and progestins is tissue and cell type specific.

The mechanism of progestin regulation of VEGF expression is not unequivocally established, but appears most likely to represent a direct PR-mediated transcriptional event. This is suggested by the blockade of progesterone induction by the antagonist RU-486 (Figure 5), and the dose response relationship for VEGF induction (10). More importantly, we have shown in transfection studies that the 5'-flanking region of the rat VEGF gene confers progestin inducibility to reporters in HeLa cells co-transfected with human PR, and preliminary studies have also shown that progestins increase the level of VEGF mRNA in T-47D cells (unpublished observations).

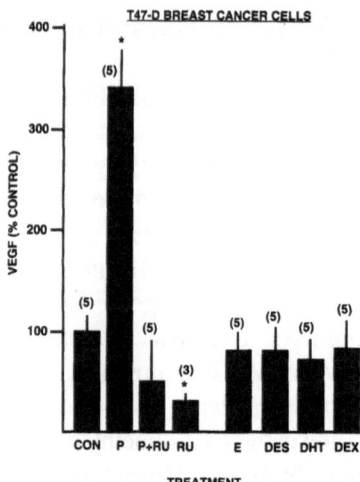

Figure 5. Progesterone increases VEGF in culture media from T47-D cells. Cells were treated with various steroids (10^{-8} M) for 18 h. RU-486 was used at 10^{-6} M. Media were harvested for ELISA analysis of VEGF protein. Values were calculated as pg VEGF/mg total cellular protein, and expressed as a percentage of the control for the number of determinations indicated. *, Values significantly different from control ($p < 0.01$). CON, control; P, progesterone; *E*, estradiol; *DES*, diethylstilbesterol; *DEX*, dexamethasone; *DHT*; dihydroxytestosterone. Reprinted by permission from the authors (10).

As noted above, we have not yet observed an induction of VEGF protein or mRNA expression by Es in any of the human BC cell lines we have studied in vitro (T-47D, MCF-7, ZR-75, or MDA-MB-231). This is in contrast to the studies of Brodie, *et al.* (9), who have shown that Es increase VEGF expression in DMBA-induced rat tumors *in vivo*. This may indicate that E control of the VEGF gene in BC is specific for DMBA or other rodent tumors, and does not occur in human BCs. Alternatively, it may indicate that the effect observed in the rat model *in vivo* represents a paracrine effect of Es rather than a direct action on the tumor cells, or that Es induce VEGF expression in BCs via a mechanism that involves interactions with another factor(s) that was not present in our cell culture experiments. Because of the potentially important role of VEGF in human BCs, we are continuing studies to distinguish between these various possibilities.

Discussion

The transient increase in VEGF expression in the rat uterus is maximal within 1 h after hormone treatment, and is the most rapid example of mRNA induction in the uterus that we are aware of. By way of comparison, induction of other "immediate early genes" induced in this system (e.g., c-*fos*, c-*jun*, and c-*myc*), is typically maximal after 2-3 h of E treatment. Thus, the rapid VEGF induction in the uterus is consistent with the rapid changes in vascular permeability seen in this system, which are some of the fastest changes that occur following E treatment (1). The primarily stromal pattern of VEGF expression is also consistent with a role to mediate E-induced changes in vascular permeability, since the stroma has the highest density of blood vessels in the uterus, and this tissue layer exhibits massive edema after E treatment. It also seems likely that an increased nutrient supply from the perilumenal vasculature would be required to support E-induced proliferation of the epithelium lining the lumen. E-induced production of stromal VEGF expression may represent a very fundamental type of stromal-epithelial interaction that may play an important role in the *in vivo* responses of the epithelial cells during the estrus cycle.

It is important to note that while the subregion of the stroma, closest to the uterine lumen, is the main site of micro vessel growth in the rat uterus, the perilumenal region of the stroma is also a major site of blood vessel growth that occurs during decidualization, following embryo-attachment to the uterine wall. The site of implantation in rodents is characterized by local edema and increased vascular permeability which are also consistent with a role of VEGF in preparing the uterus for the attachment of the blastocyst. Charnock-Jones, *et al.* (4) have clearly demonstrated that the human uterus also expresses several forms of VEGF. As in the immature rat, they also observed that VEGF expression occurs in stromal cells, and a region of stroma, the functionalis layer of the endometrium, is the major site of angiogenesis during postmenstruation/regeneration of the primate endometrium. Thus, regulation of VEGF in the stroma may have some similarities in the two systems. In addition, however, they noted some expression of VEGF in vascular smooth muscle, the myometrium, the glandular epithelium, and infiltrating leukocytes. Since their studies were performed with tissue from cycling women, it may be important to determine whether similar changes are seen in comparable cells during the estrus cycle in mature rats.

Collectively, the studies described herein and others strongly suggest a role for VEGF in the response of normal uterine tissue to steroid hormones. It seems likely that these effects encompass both short-term changes in vascular permeability and longer changes in vascular regeneration, especially in primates. Since Charnock-Jones, *et al.* (4) did not observe expression of basic FGF, the other major angiogenic factor in mammals, it may be in fact that VEGF is the primary regulator of angiogenesis, and a key regulator of vascular permeability in the normal uterus.

These studies also raise the issue of whether VEGF plays a role in uterine cancer. It is becoming increasingly clear that tumors require an increased nutrient supply as they grow past the microscopic size, and that many tumors secrete angiogenic factors such as VEGF to foster growth of new capillaries to supply their nutrient needs (8). In the uterus, it has been clear for many years that Es increase the incidence of endometrial carcinoma, and more recent studies have also shown an increased incidence of uterine cancer in women receiving TAM treatment (6). Others have also shown that a number of human endometrial cancer cell lines (Ishikawa, HEC 1-A, and HEC 1-B) express VEGF (4). Collectively, these studies raise the possibility that the effects of Es on endometrial cancer may in part involve increases in VEGF production. E-induced increases in VEGF expression and the resultant angiogenesis could also play a role in metastatic endometrial cancer cells, since an increase in vessel density near a tumor would be expected to enhance this process. While these are potentially important concerns for hormonal carcinogenesis, it is well established that Es have an etiological role in uterine cancer, and this role has long been thought to involve hormonal effects on the production of peptide growth factors.

Our studies on the induction of VEGF production in human BC cells by progestins, however, provide a new conceptual basis for a potential role of these hormones in hormonal carcinogenesis. Our findings suggest the possibility of a particularly insidious interaction between the two hormones. Es could have a primary role in the initial carcinogenic event in breast cells. This could occur via their proliferative effects and/or by other actions such as genotoxicity caused by reactive metabolites or free radicals formed during redox cycling associated with the biotransformation of endogenous or therapeutic Es. Then, progestins may exert a separate action to enhance angiogenesis via stimulation of initiated cells to produce VEGF and direct capillary growth specifically to the developing tumor. This type of mechanism has obvious implications in the etiology of primary breast tumors for the subset of cancer cells that may express VEGF in response to progestins.

In addition, these observations also have potentially important implications for the endocrine therapy of BC. On the one hand, progestin agonists, such as high doses of megestrol acetate, have been used in clinical studies to treat certain tumors with some efficacy. However, if this compound induces VEGF levels in a subset of tumor cells, such as we observed in T47-D cells, it could exacerbate the disease in those patients. Antiprogestins have also been found to suppress the growth of some BCs, and we have shown that the antiprogestin RU-486 completely blocks the induction of VEGF by progesterone in T47-D cells. This may suggest that part of the anti-cancer activity observed to date with antiprogestins is due to blockade of angiogenesis, and raises the possibility of combining antiprogestin and antiestrogen therapy to treat BC. If antiestrogens suppress an E-stimulated increase in peptide growth factors that are mitogenic for the BC cells, and antiprogestins decrease the nutrient supply of tumors via an antiangiogenic activity, combination therapy might prove highly efficacious to stop both the proliferation and metastasis of BC cells. In theory, this may lead to a synergistic action of the two classes of drugs for BC treatment.

References

1. Spaziani E (1975) Accessory reproductive organs in mammals: control of cell and tissue transport by sex hormones. Pharmacol Rev 27:207-286.
2. Ferrara N, Davissmyth T (1997) The biology of vascular endothelial growth factor. Endocrine Rev 18:4-25.
3. Cullinan-Bove K, Koos RD (1993) Vascular endothelial growth factor/vascular permeability factor expression in the rat uterus: rapid stimulation by estrogen correlates with estrogen-induced increases in uterine caterpillary permeability and growth. Endocrinology 133:829-837.
4. Charnock-Jones DS, Sharkey AM, Rajput-Williams J et al (1993) Identification and localization of alternately spliced mRNAs for vascular endothelial growth factor in human uterus and estrogen regulation in endometrial carcinoma cell lines. Biol of Reprod 48:1120-1128.
5. Hyder SM, Stancel GM, Chiappetta C et al (1996) Uterine expression of vascular endothelial growth factor is increased by estradiol and tamoxifen. Cancer Res 39:54-3960.
6. Hyder SM, Chiappetta C, Murthy L et al (1997) Selective inhibition of estrogen-regulated gene expression *in vivo* by the pure antiestrogen ICI 182,789. Cancer Res 57:2547-2549.
7. Hyder SM, Chiappetta, Stancel GM (1997) Triphenylethylene antiestrogens induce uterine vascular endothelial growth factor expression via their partial estrogen agonist activity. Cancer Lett 120:165-171.
8. Claffey KP, Robinson GS (1996) Regulation of vegf/vpf expression in tumor cells-consequences for tumor growth and metastasis. Cancer Metastasis 15:165-176.
9. Nakamura J, Savino A, Lu Q et al (1996) Estrogen regulates vascular endothelial growth permeability factor expression in 7,12-dimethylbenz(*a*)anthracene-induced rat mammary tumors. Endocrinology 137:5589-5596.
10. Hyder SM, Murthy L, Stancel GM (1998) Progestin regulation of vascular endothelial growth factor in human breast cancer cells. Cancer Res 58:392-395.

19

A TGF-β/Estrogen-inducible Early Gene (TIEG): A Candidate Tumor Suppressor or Cell Cycle Regulator?

Thomas C. Spelsberg, Malayannan Subramaniam, Katrina M. Waters, Theresa E. Hefferan, David J. Rickard, and Gregory G. Reinholz

Introduction

This laboratory has identified and partially characterized a transforming growth factor-β (TGF-β) inducible early gene (TIEG) which encodes a 3-Zn finger transcription factor-like protein which is expressed in a variety of human cell types, and shown to be rapidly induced by estrogen (E_2) and TGF-β in several cell types, including human osteoblasts, the bone forming cells on the skeleton (1-4). E_2 and TGF-β represent two important regulators of cell proliferation, differentiation, and gene transcription in normal and transformed bone cells as well as other cell types. This chapter presents a brief overview of the properties of this gene and its coded protein, which are members of the 3-Zn finger family of transcription factors. The data show that this protein is a nuclear protein, possibly a nuclear transcription factor, involved in the TGF-β and E_2-signaling pathway in processes related to cell cycle regulation, tumor suppressor function, and/or apoptosis.

TGF-β Regulation of Bone Cell Processes

TGF-ß is thought to play an important role in human bone cell physiology (1). It is highly concentrated in bone, produced by both normal human bone forming osteoblasts (hOB), and bone resorbing osteoclasts (OC), and has major effects on hOB and OC activities (1, 2). The production and activation of TGF-ß is regulated by E_2, parathyroid hormone, glucocorticoids, and other important bone regulatory agents including TGF-ß itself (3-5). It is known to have multiple effects on bone specific genes in cultured osteoblastic cells. TGF-ß has been shown to increase type I collagen, osteopontin, and alkaline phosphatase synthesis (6), and to decrease osteocalcin synthesis in osteoblasts in culture. The regulation of most of these genes by TGF-ß has been measured after 18-24 h of the growth factor treatment.

Rapid Induction of TIEG by TGF-β in Normal Human Osteoblasts

A novel, TGF-ß inducible, early gene (TIEG) in normal human fetal osteoblasts (hFOB) has been identified using differential display PCR (1). Using this differentially expressed cDNA fragment of TIEG to screen a hOB cDNA library, a near-full length cDNA for this gene was isolated. As shown in Figure 1, Panel A, Northern blot analyses show that the steady state levels of the 3.5-kb TIEG mRNA increased within 30 minutes treatment of hFOB cells, and reached a maximum of 10-fold above control levels at 120 minutes post-treatment (1). This regulation was independent of new protein synthesis.

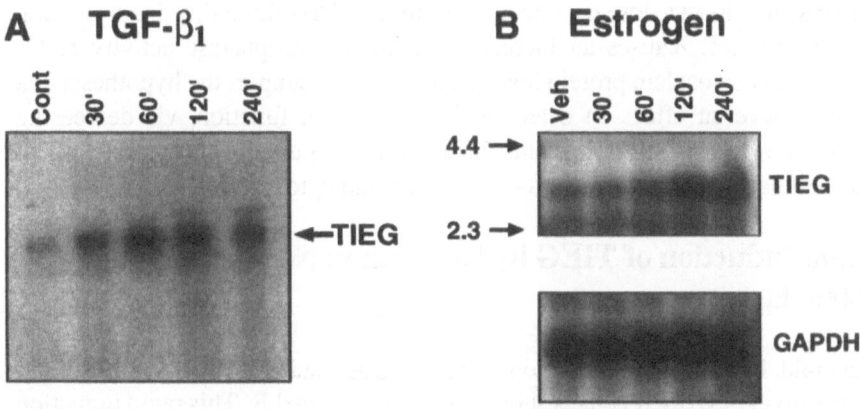

Figure 1. Induction of TIEG. Northern blot analyses of the TIEG mRNA steady state levels of TGF-β (Panel A) and E_2 (Panel B) treated normal human osteoblast cells in culture (h). Reprinted with permission, Panel A, Subramania, *et al.* (2), and Panel B, Tau, *et al.* (3).

Rapid Induction of TIEG and Pancreatic Epithelial Cells in Culture

We have also shown that TIEG is expressed in exocrine pancreatic epithelial cells (4). The gene is expressed in both acinar and ductular epithelial cell populations from the exocrine pancreas. In this system as well, the expression of TIEG is rapidly induced by TGF-β as an early response gene in human pancreatic epithelial cell lines in culture. Since TGF-β and its receptors are reported growth inhibitions in pancreatic carcinoma cells, TIEG may serve in this capacity, as a participant in the TGF-β mediated growth inhibition in these cells.

Estrogen Regulation of Bone Cell Processes

E_2, another important regulator of bone metabolism, has been used clinically to prevent bone loss and reduce fracture risk in post-menopausal women (7). The discovery of estrogen receptors (ER) in osteoblasts (8, 9), identified them as potential target cells for E_2. Other studies have reported that E_2 increases the production of cytokines and growth factors as well as their binding proteins by human osteoblasts, including interleukin-6 (IL-6), insulin-like growth factor-1 (IGF-1), IGF binding proteins, and TGF-β. Indeed, one of the main end points of E_2 action in osteoblasts is the induction of TGF-ß production (7, 10).

Recent studies in our laboratory have shown that during the stage of rapid cell proliferation, E_2 treatment of hFOB/ER9 cells (hFOB cells stably transfected with ER) results in a dose dependent inhibition of [^{3}H]-thymidine incorporation (11). Further, E_2 causes an increase in alkaline phosphatase activity and a decrease in osteocalcin protein levels. These results support the hypothesis that E_2 does have an effect on osteoblastic growth and function, via decreasing hFOB/ER9 cell proliferation and differentially regulating the production of extracellular matrix proteins, growth factors, and cytokines.

Rapid Induction of TIEG by Estrogen in Normal Human Osteoblasts

The rapid, but transient, induction of TIEG steady-state mRNA levels by E_2 in ER positive, hFOB/ER cells is shown in Figure 1, Panel B. This rapid induction appears to be ER- and steroid dose-dependent, but protein synthesis independent. An antagonism between E_2 and PTH, which occurs in skeletal tissues, is shown to rapidly concur with TIEG mRNA expression. The rapid E_2-induced increase in TIEG expression is followed by an E_2-induced inhibition of DNA synthesis in the hFOB/ER cells. Antiestrogens block not only the induction of TIEG mRNA levels, but also the inhibition of cell proliferation.

Cytokine Specific Induction of TIEG

Figure 2 shows Northern blot analyses supporting that the induction of TIEG mRNA steady state levels in normal human osteoblasts is cytokine specific. Of nine cytokines examined, only TGF-β and its family member, EGF, induce TIEG mRNA steady state levels. In similar studies using members of the TGF-β family, TGF-$β_1$, $β_2$, and $β_3$ as well as BMP-2, were shown to induce TIEG mRNA and protein levels in these cells.

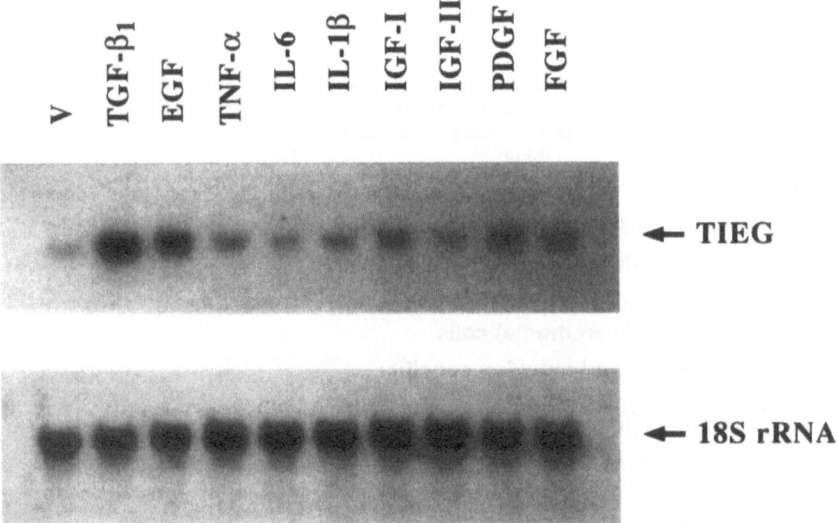

Figure 2. Northern blot analyses of the TIEG mRNA steady state levels in the cytokine treated normal human osteoblast cells (hFOB). The abscissa lists the cytokines used to treat the hFOB cells. Reprinted with permission from Subramaniam, *et al.* (1).

Protein Structure and Nuclear Localization of TIEG Protein

As depicted in Figure 3, predicted computer sequence analyses indicates that TIEG mRNA encodes for a 480 amino acid protein. The TIEG protein contains three Zn finger motifs, with homologies to the Krüppel family of Zn finger transcription factors. It contains several proline-rich src homology-3 (SH3) binding domains at the C-terminal end, and is homologous in this region to the Zn finger-containing transcription factor family of genes. Using TIEG specific polyclonal antibody and immunoprecipitation methods in hFOB cells, we have now demonstrated that TIEG encodes a 72 kDa protein whose levels are transiently increased as early as 2 h of TGF-ß treatment. As shown in Figure 4, polarized confocal microscopic analysis of human keratinocytes cells shows a cytoplasmic/perinuclear localization of TIEG protein in untreated cells in culture. Interestingly, when the cells are treated with E_2 or TGF-β or its metabolic product in these cells, H_2O_2 for 2 h, a nuclear translocation of the TIEG protein is observed (2, 3).

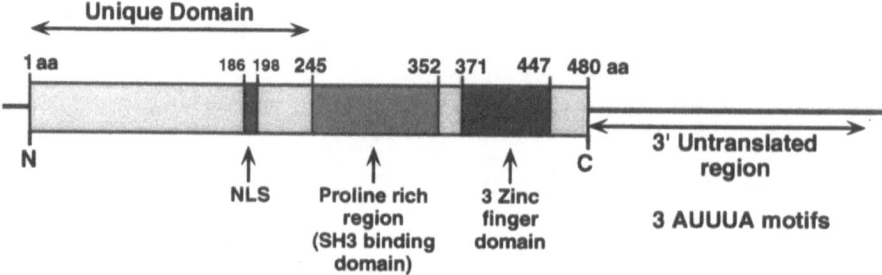

- **Member of the 3 zinc finger transcription factor family**
- **Expression is tissue and cell-type specific**
- **Regulated by E$_2$, TGF-β, and BMP's in human osteoblastic (pancreatic and carcinoma) cells**
- **Induction is GF and cytokine specific**
- **Colocalizes in human chromosome 8q 22.2, with leukemia and osteopetrosis genes**
- **TIEG protein is perinuclear, but nuclear translocated when cells treated with estrogens or TGF-β**

Figure 3. Structure of TIEG protein. Model of the structure of TIEG protein including functional domains.

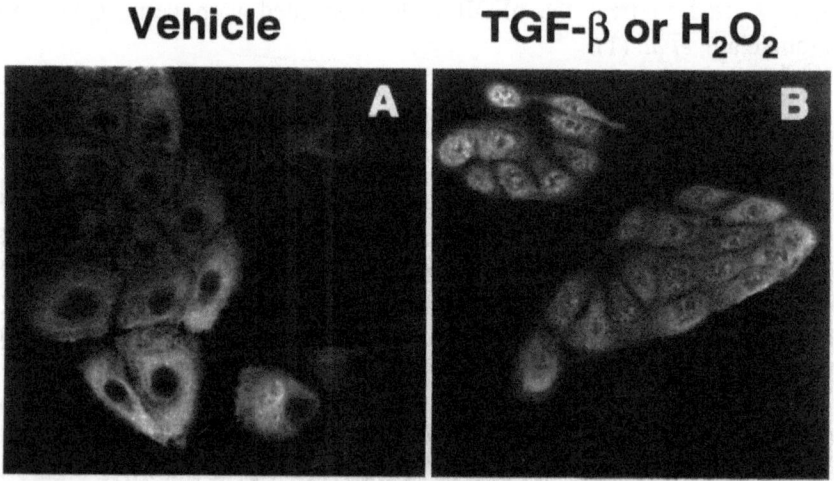

Figure 4. Confocal microscopy using polarized fluorescent excitation light of fluorescent tagged anti-TIEG protein antibodies. Panel A = TIEG protein in untreated keratinocytes and Panel B = TIEG protein in TGFβ or H$_2$O$_2$ treated cells. Reprinted with permission from Subramaniam, *et al.* (2).

Overexpression of TIEG in Cells Inhibits Cell Proliferation and Induces Apoptosis in Human Osteoblasts and Pancreatic Epithelial Cells

Figure 5 shows that the hFOB cells, stably transfected with a TIEG expression vector, display increase TIEG mRNA and protein levels and markedly reduced DNA synthesis/cell proliferation, compared to nontransfected or vector control transfected cells (2, 3). These results support that TIEG is an early responding regulatory gene for E_2 in human osteoblast cells, which inhibits DNA synthesis. In addition, the overexpression of TIEG in the TGF-β-sensitive epithelial cell line, PANC1, is sufficient to reduce cell proliferation and to induce apoptosis (4). Together, these results support a role for TIEG in linking E_2 and TGF-β-mediated signaling cascades to the regulation of cell proliferation. Since TIEG overexpression inhibits cell proliferation, as does the treatment of cells with E_2 or TGF-β, it is speculated that TIEG may play a role in the signaling pathway for TGF-β or E_2 that inhibit cell proliferation. More recent studies with human osteosarcoma cells not only show that the overexpression of TIEG inhibits cell proliferation in transformed cells, but mimics the patterns of TGF-β regulation of late gene expression (Hefferan, *et al.,* in preparation).

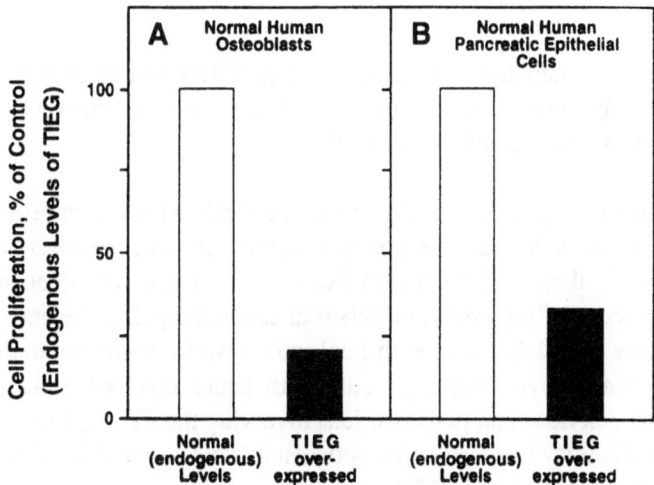

Figure 5. Rate of cell proliferation in (Panel A) stably transfected normal human osteoblasts (hFOB) or (Panel B) transiently transfected pancreatic carcinoma cells with the TIEG expression constructs.

TIEG as a Potential Marker for Certain Human Malignancies

Immunohistochemical studies have demonstrated that TIEG protein is expressed in epithelial cells of the placenta, breast, and pancreas, as well as in osteoblast cells of bone and selected other cells of the bone marrow and cerebellum. Some cells show a cytoplasmic localization while others show a nuclear localization (3). All cells of the kidney display a negative staining for this protein. Interestingly, a stage specific expression of TIEG protein is found in a dozen (BC) biopsies using immunohistochemistry. As shown in Figure 6, the cells in normal breast epithelium displays a high expression of TIEG protein, while those in the *in-situ* carcinoma (stage II/III) display less than half the levels, and those in the invasive carcinoma (stage IV) show a complete absence of the TIEG protein.

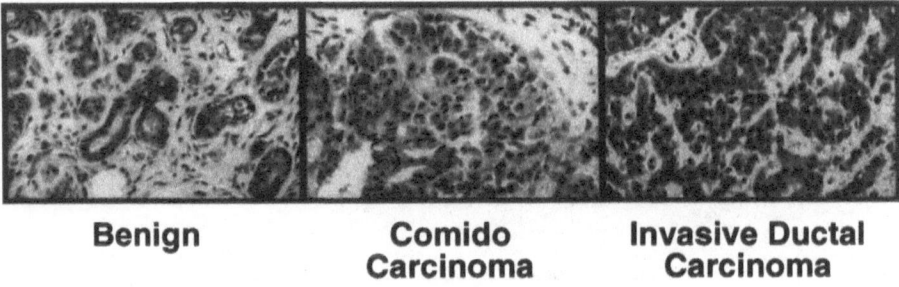

Benign   **Comido   Invasive Ductal
                    Carcinoma   Carcinoma**

Figure 6. Immunohistochemical detection of TIEG protein in normal (Panel A), stage II carcinoma (Panel B), and stage IV carcinoma (Panel C). Taken with permission from Subramaniam *et al.* 1998.

As shown in Figure 7, the TIEG gene was localized to chromosome 8q22.2 locus, the same locus as the genes involved in osteopetrosis and acute myelogenous leukemia. This region lies close to the c-*myc* gene locus and represents a locus of high polymorphism in cancer biopsies. Recent studies by this laboratory in collaboration with Jalal and co-workers (in preparation), have found that lymphocytes from patients with acute myeloid leukemia show chromosome deletions and translocations involving the TIEG gene. Studies are underway to identify the correlation between this disease and the chromosomal abnormalities involving the TIEG gene.

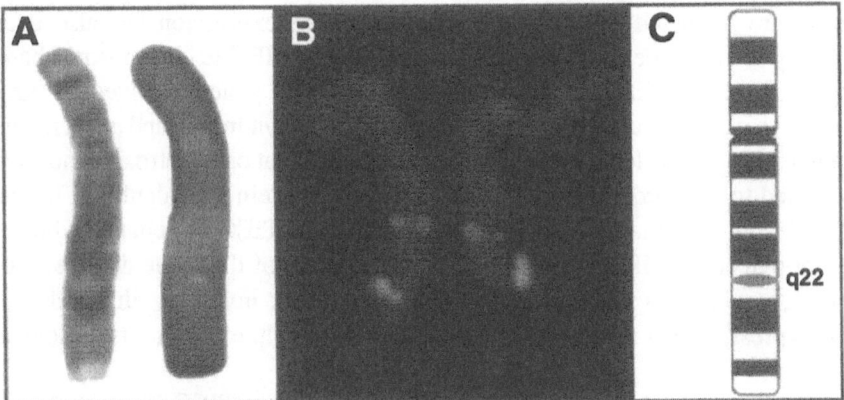

Figure 7. Localization of the putative tumor suppressor gene, TIEG, by *in-situ* hybridization to 8q22.2. Panel A: Sequential staining of GTL-banded chromosome 8 by TIEG genomic DNA probe labeled with biotin-UTP. Panel B: A pair of chromosome 8 where TIEG is labeled with digoxigennin (solid arrows), and a control probe for c-myc at 8q24.2 is labeled at broken arrows. Panel C: An ideogram of chromosome 8 at 400 band stage indicating the band q22.2.

Summary and Overview

BC, pancreatic carcinoma, and other cancer cells produce TGF-ß and their growth is inhibited by this growth factor (12). More recently, TGF-ß has been implicated in the antiestrogen-induced apoptosis of BC cells (13). Thus, if TIEG is a key participant in the TGF-ß action on breast or pancreatic carcinoma cells, it might be involved in the primary pathway of TGF-ß inhibition of cell proliferation. Support that TIEG may be involved in the cell cycle with properties of a tumor suppressor arises from recent studies in pancreatic carcinoma cells, TGF-ß induces TIEG expression and inhibits cell proliferation. Interestingly, TIEG overexpression in these cells was shown to induce apoptotic mediated growth inhibition (4). In studies presented here, reduced TIEG protein levels were found in the *in-situ* breast carcinomas and an absence of TIEG protein was found in invasive carcinomas. Although these preliminary observations certainly require more study with a significant number of samples, a pattern is evolving wherein TGF-ß induces TIEG protein levels which in turn inhibits proliferation. The TGF-ß does inhibit cell proliferation in pancreatic carcinoma cells.

It is interesting to note that the tumor suppressor gene, p53 (14), and the BRCA-1 gene (15), which are important in BC metastasis and in apoptosis/cell death, are regulated by E_2 in BC cells, the TIEG expression has also been recently shown to be E_2 regulated. The mapping of TIEG to chromosome band 8q22.2 is also of interest since this locus contains genes involved in bone disease, e.g., the renal tubular acidosis osteopetrosis syndrome, and cancer, e.g., acute myelogenous leukemia. It is well established that osteopetrosis syndrome is related to a disorder in osteoclasts. The TIEG protein was identified in and cloned from osteoblasts. The biological functions of TIEG protein and whether or not defects in TIEG are involved in the etiology of this bone disease or of cancer, remains to be determined. Further studies involving the under or overexpression and mutations of this gene should help elucidate its biological function.

In any event, the data presented here, support that TIEG is a novel gene implicated in cell cycle and tumor suppressor-like activities of bone and pancreatic carcinoma cells. Also, it might serve as primary target of TGF-ß to inhibit apoptosis and gene expression in human osteoblasts and other cells.

As outlined in Table 1, the correlation between the levels of TIEG protein, cell proliferation, and the stage of BC, its prime location in human chromosome 8q22.2, and its high frequency deletion in acute leukemia, suggest that TIEG may play a role in tumor suppressor gene activities, apoptosis, or some other regulatory function of cell cycle regulation.

Table 1. TIEG as a novel candidate tumor suppressor gene.

1.	Upregulated by inhibitors of cell proliferation
2.	Overexpression mimics TGF-β action
3.	Overexpression inhibits cell proliferation
4.	Underexpression with cell transformation
5.	Levels correlate with stage of cancer

The model in Figure 8 outlines the putative role for TIEG as a candidate for early transcription factor in the TGF-β (or E_2) pathway to regulate late gene expression and cell processes such as cell proliferation. The endogenous TIEG protein in the cytoplasmic (perinuclear) regions of the cell are rapidly triggered by E_2 or TGF-β to translocate to the nucleus. The TIEG protein triggers the transcription of additional TIEG, and other immediate early genes to produce more TIEG and other late genes involved in cell division, etc.

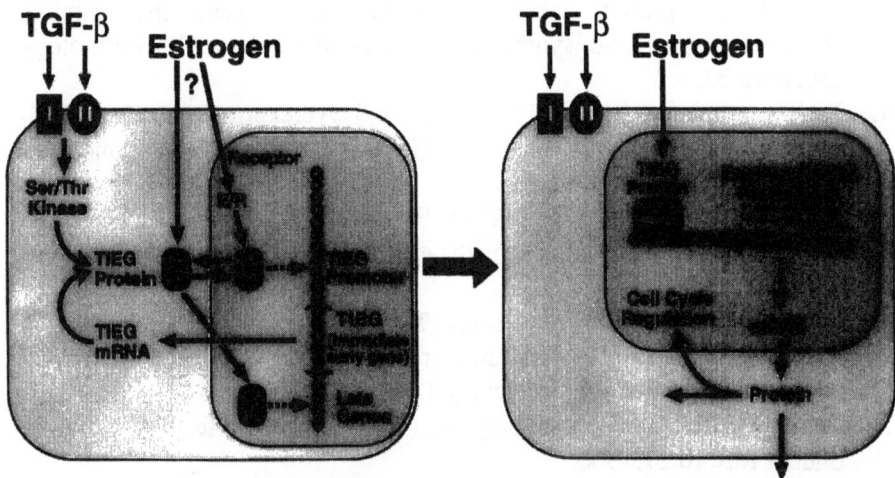

Figure 8. Putative role(s) of TIEG in the TGF-β or estrogen pathways. Model of the mechanism of action of TIEG in human cells. On the left, TGF-β and E₂-induce TIEG and other immediate early gene transcription via modifying TIEG to undergo nuclear translocation and serve as an active transcription factor. On the right, TIEG protein is shown to bind to the promoters to regulate the transcription of late genes, including cell proliferation.

Acknowledgments

The authors would like to thank Ms. Jacquelyn House for her excellent clerical assistance and Ms. Kay Rasmussen for her excellent technical help. This work was supported, in part, by NIH training grants CA90441 (M.S., K.T.), DK07352 (T.E.H.), HD07108 (G.R.) and NIH grants AR43627, AG04875, and the Mayo Foundation.

References

1. Subramaniam M, Harris SA, Oursler MJ et al (1995) Identification of a novel TGF-β-regulated gene encoding a putative zinc finger protein in human osteoblasts. Nucleic Acids Res 23:4907-12.
2. Subramaniam M, Hefferan TE, Tau KR et al (1998) Tissue, cell type, and breast cancer stage-specific expression of a TGF-β inducible early transcription factor gene. J Cell Biochem 68:226-36.

3. Tau KR, Hefferan TE, Waters KM et al (1998) Estrogen regulation of a transforming growth factor-β inducible early gene that inhibits deoxyribonucleic acid synthesis in human osteoblasts. Endocrinology 139:1346-53.

4. Tachibana I, Imoto M, Adjei PN et al (1997) Overexpression of the TGFβ-regulated zinc finger-encoding gene, TIEG, induces apoptosis in pancreatic epithelial cells. J Clin Invest 99:2365-74.

5. Roberts AB, Sporn MB (1993) Physiological actions and clinical applications of transforming growth factor-beta (TGF-beta). Growth Factors 8:1-9.

6. Oursler MJ, Riggs BL, Spelsberg TC (1993) Glucocorticoid induced activation of latent transforming growth factor -ß by normal human osteoblast-like cells. Endocrinology 133:2187-96.

7. Turner RT, Riggs BL, Spelsberg TC (1994) Skeletal effects of estrogen. Endocr Rev 16:275-300.

8. Ericksen EF, Colvard DS, Berg NJ et al (1980) Evidence of estrogen receptors in normal human osteoblast-like cells. Science 241:84-6.

9. Komm BS, Terpening CM, Benz DJ et al (1988) Estrogen binding receptor mRNA and biologic response in osteoblast-like osteosarcoma cells. Science 241:81-3.

10. Harris SA, Tau KR, Turner RT et al (1996) Estrogens and Progestins. In: Bilezikian JP, Raisz LG, Rodan GA, editors. Principles of Bone Biology. San Diego, Academic Press 507-20.

11. Robinson JA, Harris SA, Riggs BL et al (1997) Estrogen regulation of human osteoblastic cell proliferation and differentiation. Endocrinology 138:2919-27.

12. Valverius EM, Walker-Jones D, Bates SE et al (1989) Production of and responsiveness to transforming growth factor-ß in normal and oncogene-transformed human mammary epithelial cells. Cancer Res 49:6269-74.

13. Chen H, Tritton TR, Kenny N et al (1996) Tamoxifen induces TGF-ß1 activity and apoptosis of human MCF-7 breast cancer cells *in vitro*. J Cell Biochem 61:9-17.

14. Hurd C, Khattree N, Alban P et al (1995) Hormonal regulation of the p53 tumor suppressor protein in T47D human breast carcinoma cell line. J Biol Chem 270:28507-10.

15. Gudas J, Nguyen H, Li T et al (1995) Hormone-dependent regulation of BRCA1 in human breast cancer cells. Cancer Res 55:4561-65.

PART 7. AROMATASE: IMPLICATIONS FOR BREAST CANCER

Introduction

Aromatase:
Implications for Breast Cancer

Gregory A. Reed

Estrogens have been established clearly as causative agents for mammary cancer in animal models and as facilitating factors in human breast cancer (BC) (1). Proposed roles for 17β-estradiol (E_2) and other estrogens (E) in mammary carcinogenesis include control of the proliferation and differentiation of normal mammary epithelial cells, initiation of the carcinogenic process by Es or their metabolites, the promotion of initiated pre-malignant cells, and the Es requirement the maintenance and continued proliferation of hormone-dependent tumor cells. Excessive or inappropriate exposure to Es could enhance any stage of tumor development, thus the source of Es and the control of this source become key targets for study in the investigation of experimental carcinogenesis and for possible clinical intervention in human BC.

Endocrine modulation of tumor development and progression has become a fertile area for both experimental models and clinical applications (2). The earliest demonstration of the importance of Es in BC was derived from the effects of oophorectomy on the progression of BC in humans. Removal of the ovaries, the major site for the production of Es in pre-menopausal women, had a pronounced protective effect. As Es were known to be promoters of the development and maintenance of normal breast epithelium, it was surmised that they also played a similar role for mammary epithelial-derived tumor cells. Subsequent applications of endocrine modulation for the treatment of BC involved the use of androgens as opposing endocrine factors, and of adrenalectomy, which removes the source of steroid precursors for both androgens and Es. More recent interventions have targeted Es and their effects more directly, first, by the use of estrogen receptor (ER) antagonists (antiestrogens), and secondly, by specific inhibition of the biosynthesis of Es. The latter centers on inhibition of aromatase.

Aromatase and Estrogen Supply

The biosynthetic pathway for Es requires the oxidative demethylation of C19 steroid precursors and subsequent aromatization of the A-ring (Figure 1) (3).

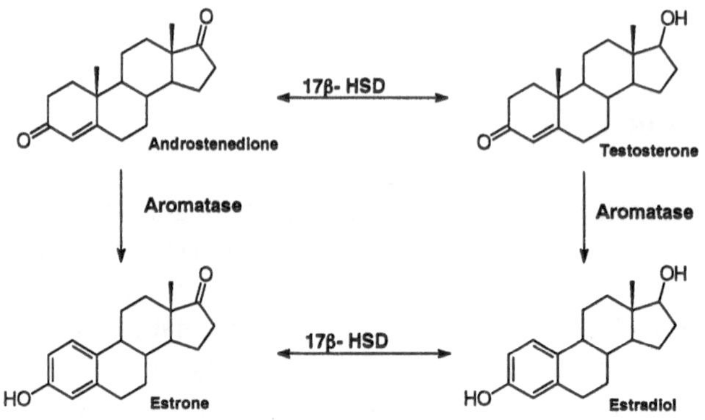

Figure 1. Conversion of androgens to estrogens by aromatase.

This aromatization, an irreversible reaction, represents the rate-limiting step in E production. The reaction is catalyzed by an enzyme with the trivial name aromatase. This is the only known aromatization reaction to occur in vertebrates. Aromatase will accept androstenedione or testosterone as its substrate, as shown in Figure 1, but also 16α-hydroxytestosterone and related androgens. Each is converted to the corresponding E. Androstenedione is converted to estrone, testosterone is converted to E_2, and 16α-hydroxytestosterone is converted to estriol by aromatase. The biosynthetic pathways which produce the presenting androgen precursor are tissue-specific, and determine the identity of the initial E produced in a given tissue. E_2 is the predominant product, particularly in the ovary, whereas estriol and estrone are produced by aromatase in placenta and in adipose tissue, respectively. Once the Es have been produced, they may be interconverted reversibly by the actions of 17α-hydroxysteroid dehydrogenase (17α-HSD), which catalyzes both the oxidation of the 17α-hydroxyl to the corresponding ketone and the reduction of the ketone to the 17α-hydroxyl. Further transformations by hydroxylation at various positions on the steroid nucleus are, like the aromatization, irreversible reactions.

Aromatase is a member of the cytochrome P450 superfamily of enzymes, and is coded for by the gene CYP19 (3). Although distantly related in sequence to other steroidogenic cytochrome P450s, aromatase is the sole member of its family. This protein catalyzes a series of reactions comprised of two successive hydroxylations of the C19 methyl group of androgen substrates, and a final oxidation to release formic acid and the resulting E. Like most P450s, this enzyme is localized primarily in the endoplasmic reticulum. The enzyme is found in all vertebrate species examined, with highest levels of expression in the gonads and the brain. Humans and higher primates exhibit a broader tissue distribution, with the placenta and adipose tissue as additional sites for aromatase expression and activity. The latter suggests the possibility of local E biosynthesis in the breast, and also serves to distinguish the human distribution of E biosynthesis from that of rodents and many other animal models.

Although differential expression of aromatase is observed in various cell types and tissues of an organism, only a single gene product is expressed (3). The differential expression results from the tissue-specific utilization of one of several defined promoters upstream of the coding region for the enzyme. Although well established for the tissue-specific expression of other proteins, this scheme of multiple promoters for site-specific regulation of the expression of aromatase appears to be unique among cytochrome P450s.

Hormonal therapy for BC and other responsive tumors provides a targeted approach for therapy with the potential for far less severe adverse effects than are observed with the majority of chemotherapeutic regimens. Although ER antagonists are currently the most widely used and most effective hormonal agents used against BC, aromatase inhibition remains a viable target for this type of chemotherapy. Indeed, the development of more effective aromatase inhibitors remains an important goal in drug development. Such drugs may be used as sole agents, or perhaps in combination with the receptor antagonists. Of equal importance is the investigation of the regulation of aromatase expression. The use of tissue-specific promoters raises the possibility that specific suppressors of aromatase expression may be found which could block local production of Es in breast, for example, while not affecting synthesis and actions of the hormone in other tissues.

Key Questions: Aromatase and Breast Cancer

Defining the true role of aromatase activity in the development and progression of BC will require answers to several key questions. Chief among them are what cell types express aromatase, and what level of aromatase activity is maintained in those cell types. These answers will define the potential for peripheral and local (i.e. in-situ) production of Es. Second will be the elucidation of factors which control the expression of aromatase in these different cells and tissues. Control of expression directly affects the actual level of activity present. Finally, more applied studies will determine the actual effects of aromatase inhibition on the causation, progression, and the treatment of BC in animal models and in humans. This inhibition might be at the level of suppression of expression or the more typical inhibition of catalytic activity of the enzyme. Given the variety of promoters used in different tissues for the activation of aromatase transcription, modulation of expression might be the most highly targeted means of decreasing aromatase activity and subsequent E production in the cells surrounding a tumor, while maintaining levels of Es systemically for other beneficial purposes. With a clear picture of when and where Es are produced in animals and humans, with the ability to specifically block the production of Es, and moreover with an understanding of the tissue-specific control of expression of the rate-limiting enzyme for E production, the tools will be at hand to tease out the contributions of local and systemic Es to the development of cancer. These insights may then be applied to the development of more effective and better tolerated therapies for this disease.

References

1. Li JJ, Li SA (1996) The effects of hormones on tumor induction. In: Arcos JC, Arcos MS, and Woo Y (eds) Chemical Induction of Cancer. Boston: Birkhauser Press, pp. 397-449.
2. Kaufmann K. A review of endocrine options for the treatment of advanced breast cancer. Oncology 1997; 54:2-5.
3. Simpson ER, Mahendroo MS, Means GD et al (1994) Aromatase cytochrome P450, the enzyme responsible for estrogen biosynthesis. Endocrine Rev 15:342-355.

20

Control of Estrogen Biosynthesis in Breast Cancer

Shiuan Chen, Dujin Zhou, Yeh-Chih Kao, Chun Yang, and Baiba Grube

Introduction

Estrogens (Es) play a crucial role in breast cancer (BC) development. Aromatase (CYP19), a cytochrome P450, is the enzyme that synthesizes Es. Using enzyme activity measurements (1-3), immunocytochemistry (4-7), and RT-PCR analysis (8, 9), aromatase is expressed at a higher level in human BC tissue than in normal breast tissue. Cell culture (10, 11), animal experiments using aromatase-transfected BC cells (12, 13), and transgenic mouse studies (14) have demonstrated that *in-situ* produced E plays a more important role than circulating Es in breast tumor promotion. In addition, tumor aromatase has been shown to stimulate BC growth in both an autocrine and a paracrine manner (15). RT-PCR and gene transcriptional studies have revealed that in normal tissue, the aromatase promoter switches from a glucocorticoid-stimulated promoter, I.4, to the cAMP-stimulated promoters, I.3 and II, in cancerous tissue (9, 16, 17). Suppression of *in-situ* E biosynthesis can be achieved by the prevention of aromatase expression, or by the inhibition of aromatase activity in breast tumors. Our laboratory has devoted significant effort to understand the regulatory mechanism of aromatase expression in BC tissue and to determine the structure-function relationship of aromatase. The information obtained from our studies will help in developing approaches to repress aromatase/E biosynthesis in BC tissue.

Gene Regulation Studies of Aromatase Expression in Breast Cancer

It is known that a complex mechanism is involved in the control of human aromatase expression. At least nine exon Is have been reported (18). It is thought that aromatase expression in these tissues is driven by the promoters situated upstream from these exon Is, providing tissue-specific controls of aromatase expression. In order to understand the regulatory mechanism of aromatase expression in breast tumors, we decided to first determine which promoters are used to drive aromatase expression in breast tumors. RT-PCR using exon 1-specific primers was performed to determine the exon I usage in aromatase mRNA in 70 breast tumor specimens (16). Exon PII was found to be present in aromatase mRNA in 73% of the specimens (49 samples) and to be the major exon I in 78% (38 of the 49 samples) of the specimens containing RNA messages with exon PII. Exon I.3 has been found to be present in aromatase mRNA in 78% of specimens (52 samples) and to be the major exon I in 60% (31 of the 52 samples) of the specimens containing messages with exon I.3. Exon I.4 was detected in a lesser number of breast tumor specimens (49%; 33 samples) and to be the major exon I in 33% (11 of the 33 samples) of the specimens containing RNA messages with exon I.4. These results have shown that exons PII and I.3 are the two major exons I present in aromatase mRNA isolated from breast tumors, suggesting that promoters II and I.3 are the major promoters driving aromatase expression in BC and surrounding adipose stromal cells. On the other hand, exon I.4 was found to be the major exon I in aromatase mRNA in normal adipose stromal tissue (19). Similar findings were reported by Bulun, *et al.* (17), and Harada (9). These results indicate that there is a switch of the regulatory mechanism of aromatase expression from normal breast tissue to cancerous tissue.

Promoters I.3 and II are 200-bp apart and promoter I.3 is up stream from promoter II. Promoter II has been determined to be a cAMP-driven promoter by Simpson, *et al.* (20). While we have performed functional analysis of the region containing promoter II (21), recent efforts from our laboratory are in the characterization of the genomic region containing promoter I.3. A TATA box containing promoter was identified 21 bp up stream from exon I.3 by DNA deletion and DNAse 1 footprinting analysis (22) (Figure 1). Two important features are associated with promoter I.3. First, the footprinted regions are different with nuclear extracts from BC MCF-7 cells and from adipose stromal cells. Using nuclear extracts from MCF-7 cells, a region of protection at -23bp/-9bp (5'-CTTATAATTTGGCAA-3Õ) was observed. This region contains a TATA box-like sequence and was termed RE1. The proteins in the nuclear extract from adipose stromal cells protected the adjacent sequences at -11bp/+5bp (5'-CAAGAAATTTG-GCTTT-3'). This region was termed RE2. There is a 3-bp overlap between RE1 and RE2.

Together, RE1 and RE2 were termed binding region 1 (B1) (5'-CTTATAATTTGGCAAGAAATTTGGCTTT-3', Figure 1).   Transient expression analyses with CAT constructs containing RE1, RE2 or B1 fragments in MCF-7 and adipose stromal cells showed that RE1 activated the transcription of the CAT gene, and this transcriptional activation activity appears to be orientation-dependent as well as copy-independent (22). These results and those obtained from DNA deletion analysis led us to conclude that there is a promoter present in RE1 region. The CAT activity of B1 containing MCF-7 cells showed a 2-fold increase over that of RE1 containing cells. Therefore in MCF-7 cells, the presence of RE2 enhanced the promoter function of RE1. Conversely, in adipose stromal cells, RE2 suppressed the promoter of RE1 by 9-fold, and therefore functioned as a negative regulatory element. The above experiments showed that the promoter activity of RE1 was affected by the presence of RE2.

Second, RE1 and RE2 both contain the sequence (5'-AATTTGGC-3') forming a direct repeat. A double-stranded oligonucleotide corresponding to the entire B1 but with a three-base pair deletion between the two repeats (5'-CTTATAATTTGGCAAATTTGGCTTT-3'), MuB1, was prepared, ligated to CAT gene and tested by transient expression analysis. No CAT activity was detected in the cell extract from both MCF-7 and adipose stromal cells transfected with this CAT construct (22). This result was interesting in that the deletion construct still contains the entire RE1 sequence which would have been expected to have promoter activity. Therefore, not only does RE2 have an effect on the promoter activity of RE1, but also its orientation with respect to RE1 is critical.

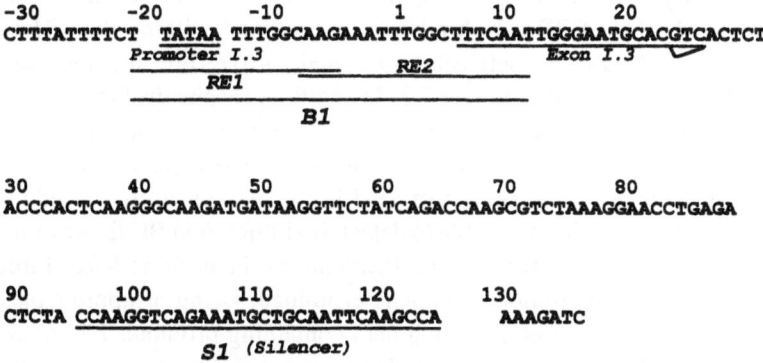

Figure 1. The nucleotide sequence of the genomic region containing B1, RE1, RE2, and S1.

Silencer and CREaro

In addition to the finding that the immediate region down stream (i.e., RE2) from promoter I.3 (i.e., RE1) can modulate the promoter activity, we characterized two additional regions that regulate the activity of promoter I.3. A negative regulatory silencer element (S1) was originally identified while we characterized promoter II (21). Recent DNA deletion and DNAse 1 footprinting analyses determined the position of the silencer, between +94 and +123bp(5'-GAGACTCTACCAA<u>GGT</u>CA<u>GAAA</u>TGCT<u>GCA</u>A<u>TTC</u>AAG<u>CC</u>A-3') (Figure 1) (23). Promoter functional analysis revealed that the silencer suppresses both promoters I.3 and II. UV cross-linking experiments with [^{32}P]-labeled, BrdU-substituted S1 as probe and nuclear extracts from MCF-7 cells and skin fibroblasts were also performed. S1 was found to be mainly cross-linked to four nuclear proteins, with molecular weights of approximately 150 kd, 45 kd, 30 kd, and 25 kd (23). All the protein-S1 interactions could be competed by unlabeled S1 but not by poly(dI-dC). Interestingly, two smaller proteins could also be competed by unlabeled B1 fragment which contains promoter I.3. The latter result may imply that the inhibitory effect of the silencer element toward promoter I.3 in the B1 region is probably accomplished through the interactions of the two smaller nuclear proteins with both silencer element and promoter I.3.

We have applied the yeast one-hybrid screening method to search for proteins binding to the silencer element. Most proteins identified belong to the nuclear receptor family. Fifty percent of the positive clones encode for ERRα-1, and other positive clones include EAR-2, EAR-3 (COUP-TF1), RARγ, and p120E4F. Since ERRα-1 was found to be the major protein interacting with the S1, we decided to characterize first the regulatory action of ERRα-1 on promoter I.3 of the human aromatase gene. ERRα-1 is a member of the orphan nuclear receptor family, with a molecular weight of 45 kd. DNase I footprinting analysis has revealed that ERRα-1 binds to a region within the S1, 5Õ-AAGGTCAGAAAT-3Õ, between +96 and +107 bp relative to the transcriptional start site of promoter 1.3. In addition, despite the fact that nuclear receptor SF-1 was previously shown to bind to the same site and to mediate a cAMP-dependent response in ovary (24), our yeast one-hybrid screening did not find any SF-1 clones. The absence of SF-1 in BC tissue was confirmed by our RT-PCR analysis which was unable to detect SF-1 mRNA in BC tissue or in SK-BR-3 cells. On the other hand, our RT-PCR analysis identified ERRα-1 mRNA in 28 out of 32 breast tumor specimens examined. Using a reporter plasmid including the aromatase genomic fragment containing promoter I.3 and S1, in BC SK-BR-3 cells, ERRα-1 was found to have a positive regulatory function. These results are interesting, but they are insufficient to explain the negative regulatory action of S1. Now, experiments are being performed to study the interaction of ERRα-1 with co-regulatory proteins, and the regulatory roles carried out by these protein complexes.

Recently, we have also found that promoter 1.3 is a cAMP-responsive promoter by the identification of a cAMP responsive element, CREaro, between -66 and -59 bp relative to the transcription start site of promoter 1.3. CREaro was identified by DNA deletion and mutation analyses together with CAT functional analysis (25). Since after forskolin treatment, the CAT activity in tumor fibroblasts transfected with a plasmid containing both CREaro and the silencer has been found to be similar to that in cells transfected with a plasmid containing only CREaro, this result suggests a functional interaction between the CREaro and the silencer elements. In the presence of cAMP, the positive regulatory CREaro can overcome the negative regulatory action of the silencer on the promoter function of promoter 1.3. We feel that this finding is very important in that it provides a molecular basis regarding the switching mechanism of aromatase promoter usage from normal to cancerous tissue. Our current hypothesis is that in normal breast stromal cells, aromatase expression is regulated by promoter 1.4 mediated through glucocorticoid, and the action of promoter 1.3 and II is suppressed by the silencer. However, in cancer tissue, cAMP production increases and aromatase promoters are switched to cAMP-dependent promoters, i.e., 1.3 and II.

Results from our and other laboratories reveal that cAMP plays a critical role in up regulating the expression of aromatase/increasing E biosynthesis in BC tissue. Several factors have been suggested to induce the level of cAMP in BC tissue. For example, Zhao, et al.(26), suggested that prostaglandin PGE2 synthesized in BC cells induces cAMP response. Furthermore, E is capable of increasing cAMP production in BC cells by stimulating adenylate cyclase (27). These observations suggest a paracrine loop between E production (by aromatase), and cAMP synthesis in BC tissue.

While we characterized CREaro, an additional negative regulatory region approximately 80 bp up stream from CREaro was observed. Initial studies suggest a cooperative interaction between the newly identified negative regulatory region and the silencer element S1. Although the region contains a nucleotide sequence resembling a TGF-β response element, extensive functional experiments have not clearly demonstrated the effect of TGF-β. We are investigating the effect of this negative regulatory region on the activity of promoter I.3.

Aromatase Inhibitor Studies

As indicated in the introduction, an abnormal expression of aromatase has been detected in a significant number of breast tumors, as well as cancerous and surrounding adipose stromal cells. In view of this, the inhibition of the enzyme has been considered as a potential therapy for BC. Aromatase-inhibitor therapy is considered as a second-line therapy in patients who fail antiestrogen treatment. Twenty to thirty percent of the patients who fail antiestrogen treatment respond to aromatase-inhibitor therapy. Throughout the years, a number of very potent and highly selective aromatase inhibitors have been synthesized and tested as drugs for the treatment of BC. Aromatase inhibitors can be categorized as steroidal and nonsteroidal. In general, steroidal aromatase inhibitors are analogues of androgen substrates, and nonsteroidal inhibitors perturb the catalytic properties of the heme prosthetic group of aromatase. While a number of the inhibitors have been shown to be very potent and specific inhibitors of aromatase, the exact nature of their interactions with aromatase are not known. This is especially true for nonsteroidal inhibitors since these compounds have very diverse structures. Although the structures of these compounds are different, it is thought that they bind to the active site of aromatase, as indicated by competitive inhibition studies of the enzyme.

One of the major purposes of our structure-function relationship of human aromatase was to determine the binding characteristics of the substrate and inhibitors. During the last several years, we have made attempts to identify functionally critical amino acids and the active site region, initially, by an alignment of the amino acid sequences of aromatase from five species with those of cytochrome P450cam and P450bm3, and later, by examining three-dimensional models of the enzyme that were generated by computer modeling based on the x-ray structures of cytochrome P450cam and P450bm3. Using a mammalian cell-expression system, site-directed mutagenesis experiments were performed to evaluate the importance of the selected amino acid residues and the proposed model of the active site of the enzyme (28-31). The kinetic properties and the reaction intermediate profiles of the mutants were determined. Furthermore, the inhibition profiles of a number of aromatase inhibitors on different mutants were determined.

Through the inhibition profile studies, we determined the relative potency of seven known aromatase inhibitors, according to their IC_{50} values for the inhibition of the wild-type aromatase, CGS 20267 (Letrozole) (IC_{50} = 1.3 nM) > vorozole (IC_{50}=2.5 nM) > MDL 101,003 (IC_{50}=12 nM) > ICI D1033 (Arimidex) (IC_{50}=25 nM) > 4-hydroxyandrostenedione (Lentaron) (IC_{50}=60 nM) > 7aAPTADD (IC_{50}=165 nM) > aminoglutetimide (IC_{50}=6 μM). The molecular basis of the interaction of these inhibitors with aromatase has been determined (32).

With the active site model generated from studies with known inhibitors, the binding characteristics and the structure requirement for flavone and isoflavone phytoestrogens to inhibit human aromatase were also obtained (33). The data indicated that these compounds bind to the active site of aromatase in an orientation in which their rings A and C, mimic rings D and C of the androgen substrate, respectively. The data also provided a molecular basis as to why isoflavones are significantly poorer inhibitors of aromatase than flavones. The potential usage of phytoestrogens in suppressing aromatase activity and BC development was demonstrated in a recent study involving grape juice (34). Inhibition kinetic analysis indicated that grape juice contains phytochemicals which inhibit aromatase by competing for the binding of the substrate androstenedione. Results from cell culture experiments suggest that chemicals in grape juice can act as weak agonists/antagonists of the estrogen receptor (ER), and as aromatase inhibitors. Finally, the BC-protective action of grape juice was demonstrated in a nude mouse model using MCF-7aro, an aromatase-transfected MCF-7 cell line (15). The data showed that, in mice fed (by gavage) 0.5 ml of grape juice/day/5 weeks, the tumor size was reduced 70% compared to the tumor size of mice not fed grape juice. These findings suggest that grape juice may be useful in BC prevention by inhibiting *in-situ* aromatase/E biosynthesis.

Summary

Suppression of *in-situ* E biosynthesis can be achieved by the prevention of aromatase expression in breast tumors, or by the inhibition of aromatase activity. It is our hope that through an understanding of the regulatory mechanism of aromatase expression in BC tissue, a therapy based on suppressing aromatase expression can be developed. We have identified several transcriptional factors that bind to these regulatory elements. We anticipate that we will learn a great deal more about the regulatory mechanism of aromatase expression in BC tissue by studying the interaction between transcriptional factors and cis-regulatory elements in the genomic region containing promoters I.3 and II.

Aromatase inhibitors are used in thre treatment of BC. Complete or partial tumor regression has been reported in postmenopausal patients treated with aromatase inhibitors, such as aminoglutethimide or 4-hydroxyandrostenedione (2, 35). Aromatase-inhibitor therapy is a second-line treatment for those who fail antiestrogen therapy. Furthermore, aromatase inhibitors may be useful as a chemopreventive agent against BC by suppressing aromatase activity. Using a N-methyl-N-nitrosourea (NMU)-induced rat mammary cancer model, vorozole, an aromatase inhibitor, has been shown to be a more effective chemopreventive agent against mammary cancer than 9-cis-retinoic acid, N-(4-hydroxyphenyl)-retinamide (4-HPR), and dehydroepiandosterone (DHEA) (36, 37). Vorozole at 0.08 mg/kg body weight/day (by gavage) reduced the number of mammary tumors/rat by 73%. NMU-induced tumor incidence is E dependent (38), and vorozole is thought to act as a chemopreventive agent by suppressing aromatase activity in the animal. Our recent experiments on grape juice demonstrate that grape juice contains chemicals which may also prevent BC development by suppressing *in-situ* aromatase/E biosynthesis.

Acknowledgments

This study was supported in part by NIH grants CA44735 and ES08258. Baiba Grube is a surgical oncology fellow supported by the Department of Surgery, City of Hope National Medical Center.

References

1.   James VHT, McNeill JM, Lai LC et al (1987) Aromatase activity in normal breast and breast tumor tissues: *in vivo* and *in vitro* studies. Steroids 50: 269-279.
2.   Miller WR, O'Neill J (1987) The importance of local synthesis of estrogen within the breast. Steroids 50: 537-548.
3.   Miller WR, Mullen P, Sourdaine P et al (1997) Regulation of aromatase activity within the breast. J Steroid Biochem Molec Biol 61:193-202.
4.   Esteban JM, Warsi Z, Haniu M et al (1992) Detection of intratumoral aromatase in breast carcinomas, an immunohistochemical study with clinico-pathologic correlation. J Amer Pathol 140:337-343.
5.   Sasano H, Nagura H, Harada N et al (1994) Immunolocalization of aromatase and other steroidogenic enzymes in human breast disorders. Hum Pathol 25:530-535.
6.   Santen RJ, Martel J, Hoagland M et al (1994) Stromal spindle cells contain aromatase in human breast tumors. J. Clin Endocrinol Metab 79: 627-632.
7.   Lu Q, Nakamura J, Savinov A et al (1996) Expression of aromatase protein and messenger ribonucleic acid in tumor epithelial cells and evidence of functional significance of locally produced estrogen in human breast cancers. Endocrinology 137:3061-3077.
8.   Bulum SE, Price TM, Mahendroo MS et al (1993) A link between breast cancer and local estrogen biosynthesis suggested by quantification of breast adipose tissue aromatase cytochrome P450 transcripts using competitive polymerase chain reaction after reverse transcription. J Clin Endocrinol Metab 77:1622-1628.
9.   Harada N (1997) Aberrant expression of aromatase in breast cancer tissues. J Steroid Biochem Molec Biol 61:175-184.
10.   Santner SJ, Chen S, Zhou D et al (1993) Effect of androstenedione on growth of untransfected and aromatase-transfected MCF-7 cells in culture. J Steroid Biochem Molec Biol 44:611-616.
11.   Macaulay VM, Nicholls JE, Gledhill J et al (1994) Biological effects of stable overexpression of aromatase in human hormone-dependent breast cancer cells. Br J Cancer 69:77-83.
12.   Yue W, Zhou D, Chen S et al (1994) A new nude mouse model for postmenopausal breast cancer using MCF-7 cells transfected with the human aromatase gene. Cancer Res 54:5092-5095.
13.   Dowsett M, Lee K, Macaulay M et al (1996) The control and biological importance of intratumoural aromatase in breast cancer. J Steroid Biochem Molec Biol 56:145-150.
14.   Tekmal RR, Ramachandra N, Gubba S et al (1996) Overexpression of int-5/aromatase in mammary glands of transgenic mice results in the induction of hyperplasia and nuclear abnormalities. Cancer Res 56: 3180-3185.

15. Sun XZ, Zhou D, Chen S (1997) Autocrine and paracrine actions of breast tumor aromatase. A three-dimensional cell culture study involving aromatase transfected MCF-7 and T-47D cells. J Steroid Biochem Molec Biol 63:29-36.
16. Zhou C, Zhou D, Esteban J et al (1996) Aromatase gene expression and its exon I usage in human breast tumors. Detection of aromatase messenger RNA by reverse transcription-polymerase chain reaction (RT-PCR). J Steroid Biochem Molec Biol 59:163-171.
17. Bulun SE, Noble LS, Takayama K et al (1997) Endocrine disorders associated with inappropriately high aromatase expression. J Steroid Biochem Molec Biol 61: 133-139.
18. Shozu M, Zhao Y, Bulun SE et al (1998) Multiple splicing events involved in regulation of human aromatase expression by a novel promoter I.6. Endocrinology 139: 1610-1617.
19. Mahendroo MS, Mendelson CR, Simpson ER (1993) Tissue-specific and hormonally controlled alternative promoters regulate aromatase cytochrome P450 gene expression in human adipose tissue. J Biol Chem 268:19463-19470.
20. Means GD, Kilgore MW, Mahendroo MS et al (1991) Tissue-specific promoters regulate aromatase cytochrome P450 gene expression in human ovary and fetal tissues. Molecular Endocrinol 5:2005-2013.
21. Wang J, Chen S (1992) Identification of a promoter and a silencer at the 3Õ-end of the first intron of the human aromatase gene. Molecular Endocrinol 6:1479-1488.
22. Zhou D, Clarke P, Wang J et al (1996) Identification of a promoter that controls aromatase expression in human breast cancer and adipose stromal cells. J Biol Chem 271:15194-15202.
23. Zhou D, Chen S (1998) Characterizaiton of a sliencer element in the human aromatase gene. Arch Biochem Biophys 353:213-220.
24. Michael MD, Kilgore MW, Morohashi KI et al (1994) Ad4BP/SF-1 regulates cyclic AMP-induced transcription from the proximal promoter (PII) of the human aromatase P450 (CYP19) gene in the ovary. J Biol Chem 270:13561-13466.
25. Zhou D, Chen S (1998) Identification and characterization of a cAMP-responsive element in the region upstream from promoter 1.3 of the human aromatase gene. Molecular Endocrinol submitted.
26. Zhao Y, Agarwal VR, Mendelson CR et al (1997) Transcriptional regulation of CYP19 gene (aromatase) expression in adipose stromal cells in primary culture. J Steroid Biochem Molec Biol 61:203-210.
27. Aronica SM, Kraus WL, Katzenellenbogen BS (1994) Estrogen action via the cAMP signaling pathway: Stimulation of adenylate cyclase and cAMP-regulated gene transcription. Proc Natl Acad Sci USA 91:8517-8521.

28. Zhou D, Pompon D, Chen S (1991) Structure-function studies of human aromatase by site-directed mutagenesis: Kinetic properties of mutants Pro308 - Phe, Tyr361 - Phe, Tyr361 - Leu, and Phe406 - Arg. Proc Natl Acad Sci USA 88:410-414.

29. Zhou D, Korzekwa KR, Poulos T et al (1992) A site-directed mutagenesis study of human placental aromatase. J Biol Chem 267: 762-768.

30. Chen S, Zhou D (1992) Functional domains of aromatase cytochrome P450 inferred from comparative analyses of amino acid sequences and substantiated by site-directed mutagenesis experiments. J Biol Chem 267: 22587-22594.

31. Zhou D, Cam LL, Laughton CA et al (1994) A mutagenesis study at a postulated hydrophobic region near the active site of aromatase cytochrome P450. J Biol Chem 269:19501-19508.

32. Kao YC, Cam LL, Laughton CA et al (1996) Binding characteristics of seven inhibitors of human aromatase. A site-directed mutagenesis study. Cancer Res 56:451-460.

33. Kao YC, Zhou C, Sherman M et al (1998) Molecular basis of the inhibition of human aromatase (estrogen synthetase) by flavone and isoflavone phytoestrogens: A site-directed mutagenesis study. Environmental Health Perspectives 106:85-92.

34. Chen S, Sun XZ, Kao YC et al (1998) Suppression of breast cancer cell growth with grape juice. Pharmaceutical Biol, in press.

35. Coombes RC, Goss PE, Dowsett M et al (1987) 4-Hydroxyandrostenedione treatment for postmenopausal patients with advanced breast cancer. Steroids 50:245-252.

36. Steele V, Lubet R, Eto I et al (1997) Effect of animal age on the chemopreventive effects of selected agents using a MNU-induced rat mammary cancer model. Proceedings of the 88th Annual Meeting of American Association for Cancer Research, 12-16 April 1997, San Diego, CA; Abst. 2438.

37. Lubet RA, Bowden C, DeCoster R et al (1997) Vorozole: Effects on MNU-induced rat mammary tumors. Proceedings of the 88th Annual Meeting of American Association for Cancer Research, 12-16 April 1997, San Diego, CA; Abst. 2491.

38. Kumar R, Sukumar S, Barbacid M (1990) Activation of ras oncogenes preceding the onset of neoplasia. Science 248:1101-1104.

21

Regulation of Aromatase in Normal and Malignant Breast Tissues: The Role of the Immune System

A. Singh, A. Purohit, M.W. Ghilchik and M.J. Reed

Introduction

The crucial role that the aromatase enzyme complex has in regulating the synthesis of estrogens (E) in breast tumors has stimulated research to identify factors that regulate its activity. Es are the main hormones that support the growth of breast tumors and a number of potent aromatase inhibitors are currently being evaluated in clinical trials (1-3). Some years ago, it was discovered that concentrations of estrone and estradiol were much higher in normal and malignant breast tissues than in blood (4-6). Surprisingly, while blood E concentrations decrease at the menopause, breast tissue E concentrations are similar in pre- and postmenopausal women (7).

The finding of elevated E concentrations in breast tumors led to investigations to examine whether they originated by uptake from the circulation or *in-situ* synthesis. A double isotopic infusion technique was developed for use in postmenopausal women with breast cancer (BC) to differentiate uptake from *in-situ* synthesis (8). Convincing evidence was obtained that in a proportion of breast tumors, *in-situ* synthesis of estrone from androstenedione made a major contribution to the elevated E levels in breast tumors. Support for this finding was recently obtained in an animal model showing that under physiological conditions, reflecting those in postmenopausal women, *in-situ* aromatase in mammary tumors makes a significant contribution to tissue E levels (9).

While *in-situ* aromatase activity is now considered to be an important regulator of tissue Es, there was initially some difficulty in reconciling such high tissue E concentrations with the level of aromatase activity in breast tumors (10). Aromatase activity, when assayed in peripheral tissues, such as adipose or breast tissues, is relatively low. It was originally thought that insufficient E could be synthesized *in-situ* via the aromatase pathway to activate the estrogen receptor (ER) (10). During the last few years, however, it has become apparent that there are a number of important mechanisms by which aromatase activity can be markedly increased. Furthermore, it is now evident that the location of a tumor

277

within the breast can influence aromatase activity in adipose tissue proximal to the tumor. Aromatase activity or expression has now been shown to be consistently elevated in the adipose tissue in the tumor-bearing quadrant of the breast (11-13).

Identification of Aromatase Regulating Factors

The finding of an association between breast tumor location and aromatase activity in proximal tissue suggested that breast tumors might produce factors that could stimulate aromatase activity. Alternatively, it is also possible that the increased aromatase activity in a breast quadrant resulted in a favorable estrogenic environment in which tumor growth could occur.

A number of investigations have been undertaken in an attempt to identify aromatase regulating factors in normal and malignant breast tissues. Stromal fibroblasts from normal and malignant breast tissues were cultured in conditioned medium (CM), and analyzed for the presence of growth factors, cytokines and other potential regulating factors. Cytosols from normal and malignant breast tissues were prepared, fractionated, and tested for their ability to stimulate aromatase activity in cultured fibroblasts. Fluid collected from women with gross cystic breast disease (breast cyst fluid, BCF) was also found to stimulate aromatase activity in cultured fibroblasts. BCF was also examined for growth factors and cytokines, and subjected to a number of purification procedures in an attempt to identify the nature of the aromatase stimulatory factors in this fluid.

Results from this research led to the identification of several factors that have now been confirmed as having important roles in regulating aromatase activity. The cytokines interleukin 1 (IL-1) and IL-6 were identified in BCF and the ability of this fluid to stimulate aromatase activity correlated with its IL-6 concentration (14). In BCF, the concentrations of IL-6 was considerably higher than that of IL-1, suggesting that IL-6 is the main cytokine in BCF, and that is responsible for its aromatase stimulatory properties. High concentrations of IL-6 were also detected in CM collected from cultured breast-tumor derived fibroblasts (15). Other cytokines, such as IL-11 and oncostatin M have also been shown to stimulate aromatase activity (16).

Therefore, the cytokine IL-6 has emerged as having an important role in regulating aromatase activity (17). Plasma IL-6 concentrations increase with ageing (18, 19), and this finding offers a likely explanation for the increase in peripheral aromatase activity that occurs in older subjects (20). Two mechanisms have also been identified by which the ability of IL-6 to stimulate aromatase activity may be potentiated. Another cytokine, tumor necrosis factor α (TNF-α) can also stimulate aromatase activity (21). TNF-α, however, can act synergistically with IL-6 to markedly increase aromatase activity (22). Cytokines act by binding to membrane-spanning receptors. The IL-6 receptor (IL-6R) complex consists of an 80 kDa (gp80) ligand-binding sub-unit, and a 130 kDa (gp130) signal transducing protein. TNF-α increases expression of the gp130 component of the IL-6 signalling pathway (23). Such a mechanism may account for the synergistic stimulation of aromatase activity by IL-6 and TNF-α (17). It has been known for many years that peripheral aromatase activity is correlated with body weight (24). Increased production of TNF-α by adipocytes from obese, as compared to lean subjects (25, 26), offers a possible explanation for the association between peripheral aromatase activity and body weight.

In addition to the IL-6 receptor (IL-6R), a soluble form of the receptor (IL-6sR) also exists (27). Unlike all other known soluble cytokine receptors that antagonise the effects of their respective cytokines, IL-6sR enhances the response of IL-6 in some biological systems. The combination of IL-6 plus IL-6sR resulted in a 21-fold greater stimulation of aromatase activity than that achieved by IL-6 alone (28). As IL-6sR is present in CM from breast tumor, but not normal fibroblasts and is also detectable in breast tumor cytosol, regulation of *in-vivo* aromatase by IL-6 plus IL-6sR represents another important mechanism by which breast tumor aromatase activity may be markedly increased.

The Role of the Immune System in Regulating Aromatase Activity

Having identified cytokines as important regulators of aromatase activity, attention turned to locating the major source of cytokines available to stimulate breast tumor aromatase activity. An important clue as to their likely origin was provided by a study in which aromatase activity was measured in breast tissue obtained from a women who had previously undergone breast augmentation with an injection of silicone (13). Aromatase activity in this tissue was considerably higher than ever previously measured. Histological examination of this tissue revealed the presence of numerous tumor-associated macrophages and tumor-infiltrating lymphocytes. This finding suggested the possibility that these immune cells may be an important source of the cytokines that stimulate aromatase activity. Evidence to support this concept was obtained by the demonstration that CM collected from lipopolysacchoride stimulated peripheral monocytes and lymphocytes markedly stimulated fibroblast aromatase activity (13). Further support for the immune system having a role in regulating breast tumor aromatase activity was obtained from a similar study that employed monocytes and lymphocytes from a kidney transplant recipient (29). The incidence of BC in immunosuppressed transplant recipients is about 25% lower than the expected rate (30). The ability of CM collected from cells of an immunosuppressed subject to stimulate aromatase activity was considerably lower than similar CM collected from a woman with BC.

The investigations with CM collected from the immunosuppressed subject has recently been extended to examine its effect in aromatase activity in co-cultured malignant epithelial cells and fibroblasts. As shown in Figure 1, a preparation of cultured breast tissue cells was obtained that had approximately equal number of spindle-shaped fibroblasts and more rounded epithelial cells. Using these cells it was found, as previously reported, that stripped fetal calf serum (SFCS) in the absence of dexamethasone, resulted in the detection of minimal aromatase activity (Figure 2). However, the addition of dexamethasone to the SFCS resulted in maximal stimulation of aromatase activity in these cells with CM from monocytes or lymphocytes having no further stimulatory effect. These data were in marked contrast to the results obtained using only breast tumor-derived fibroblasts where CM from monocytes and lymphocytes of a woman with BC was required to maximally stimulate aromatase activity (30). The finding from the experiment employing co-cultured cells suggests that in addition to the cytokines that are known to stimulate aromatase activity other, as yet unidentified factors, produced by tumor epithelial cells may also be involved in regulating tumor aromatase activity.

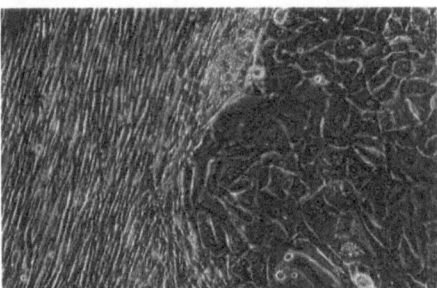

Figure 1. A mixed cell population cultured from a breast tumor. Cells consist of the spindle-shaped fibroblasts and more rounded epithelial cells.

Regulation of Cytokine Production by Immune Cells

Macrophages and lymphocytes are now considered to be an important source of tumor cytokines, and regulation of cytokine production by lymphocytes is currently under investigation. T-helper (Th) lymphocytes can develop a Th-1 or Th-2 phenotype, each of which secretes a characteristic profile of cytokines (31). IL-6 is, as previously discussed, an important regulator of aromatase activity, and is produced by Th-2 lymphocytes.

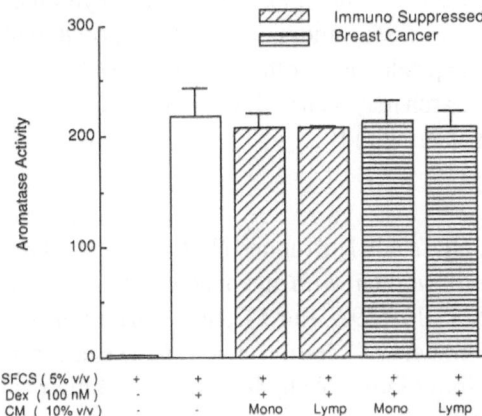

Figure 2. Effect of dexamethasone (Dex) or conditioned medium (CM) from peripheral monocytes (Mono) or lymphocytes (Lymp) from a woman with BC or an immunosuppressed subject in the presence of stripped fetal calf serum (SFCS) on aromatase activity in a mixed cell population of tumor-derived fibroblasts and epithelial cells.

There is now good evidence that whether Th cells progress to a Th-1 or Th-2 phenotype is regulated by the balance of the adrenal androgen, dehydroepiandrosterone (DHEA) to that of glucocorticoid (32, 33). In the presence of DHEA and glucocorticoid, a Th-1 phenotype predominates whereas if DHEA levels are low, a Th-2 response occurs. Stress, which has been implicated in the development of BC (34), results in an increase in glucocorticoid production and a Th-2 response. This in turn would give rise to an increase in production of IL-6 and thus enhanced aromatase activity. Although this is an attractive hypothesis to explain how stress might influence the development of BC, further studies are required to confirm its validity.

Recently, it has been found that alternative promoters may be involved in the control of breast tumor aromatase to that in normal breast tissue (35, 36) and that the prostaglandin PGE_2 may be involved in the regulation of breast tumor aromatase (37). However, PGE_2 is also produced by macrophages and there is evidence that PGE_2 in fact regulates IL-6 production by fibroblasts and macrophages (38, 39).

Summary

It is now evident that factors produced by cells of the immune system, such as IL-6 and TNF-α, have an important role in regulating breast tumor aromatase activity. If T-helper cells are an important source of cytokines that can stimulate aromatase activity in breast tumors, it should be possible to develop drugs to block Th-2 cytokine production or the interaction of Th-2 cytokines with their receptors. Such research may lead to the development of important therapies for the treatment of women with BC.

References

1. Svenstrup B, Herrstedt J, Brunner N et al (1994) Sex hormone levels in postmenopausal women with advanced breast metastatic breast cancer treated with CGS 169 49A. Eur J Cancer 30A:1259-1258.
2. Dowsett M, Smithers D, Moore J et al (1994) Endocrine changes with the aromatase inhibitor fadrozole hydrochloride in breast cancer. Eur J Cancer 30A:1453-1458.
3. Johnston SRD, Smith IE, Doody D et al (1994) Clinical and endocrine effects with oral aromatase inhibitor vovozole in postmenopausal patients with advanced breast cancer. Cancer Res 54:5875-5881.
4. Bonney RC, Reed MJ, Davidson K et al (1983) The relationship between 17β-hydroxysteroid dehydrogenase activity and oestrogen concentrations in human breast tumours and in normal breast tissue. Clin Endocrinol 19:727-739.
5. Van Landeghem AJJ, Poortman J, Nabuurs M et al (1985) Endogenous concentrations and subcellular distribution of estrogens in normal and malignant human breast tissue. Cancer Res 45:2900-2906.
6. Vermeulen A, Deslypere JP, Paridaens R et al (1986) Aromatase, 17β-hydroxysteroid dehydrogenase and intratissular sex hormone concentrations in cancerous and normal glandular breast tissue in postmenopausal women. Eur J Cancer 22:515-525.
7. Thijssen JHH, Blankenstein MA (1989) Endogenous oestrogens and androgens in normal and malignant endometrial and mammary tissues. Eur J Cancer Clin Oncol 25:1953-1959.
8. Reed MJ, Owen AM, Lai LC et al (1989) In situ oestrone synthesis in normal breast and breast tumour tissue: effect of treatment with 4-hydroxyandrostenedione. Int J Cancer 44:233-237.
9. Yue W, Wang J-P, Hamilton CJ et al (1998) *In situ* aromatization enhances breast tumor estradiol levels and cellular proliferation. Cancer Res 58:927-932.
10. Bradlow HL (1982) A reassessment of the role of breast tumor aromatase. Cancer Res 42 (Suppl):3382s-3386s.
11. O'Neill JS, Elton RA, Miller WR (1988) Aromatase activity in adipose tissue from breast quadrants: a link with tumour site. Br J Med 296:741-743.

12. Bulun SE, Price TM, Aitken J et al (1993) A link between breast cancer and local estrogen biosynthesis suggested by quantification of breast adipose tissue aromatase cytochrome P450 transcripts using competitive polymerase chain reaction after reverse transcription. J Clin Endocrinol Metab 77:1622-1628.

13. Purohit A, Ghilchik MW, Duncan L et al (1995) Aromatase activity in interleukin-6 production by normal and malignant breast tissues. J Clin Endocrinol Metab 80:3052-3058.

14. Reed MJ, Coldham NG, Patel SR et al (1992) Interleukin-1 and interleukin-6 in breast cyst fluid: their role in regulating aromatase activity in breast cancer cells. J Endocrinol 132:R5-R8.

15. Reed MJ, Topping L, Coldham NG et al (1993) Control of aromatase activity in breast cancer cells: the role of cytokines and growth factors. J Steroid Biochem Molec Biol 44:1033-1039.

16. Zhao Y, Nichols JE, Bulun SE et al (1995) Aromatase P-450 gene expression in human adipose tissue: a role of Jak/STAT pathway in regulation of the adipose-specific promoter. J Biol Chem 270:16449-16457.

17. Reed MJ, Purohit A (1997) Breast cancer and the role of cytokines in regulating estrogen synthesis: an emerging hypothesis. Endocrine Rev 18:701-715.

18. Wei J, Xu H, Davies JL et al (1992) Increase of plasma IL-6 concentrations with age in healthy subjects. Life Sci 51:1953-1956.

19. Daynes RA, Araneo BA, Ershler WB et al (1993) Altered regulation of IL-6 production with normal aging. J Immunol 150:5219-5230.

20. Hemsell DL, Grodin JM, Brenner PF et al (1974) Plasma precursors of estrogens. II. Correlation of the extent of conversion of plasma androstenedione to estrone with age. J Clin Endocrinol Metab 34:476-479.

21. Macdiarmid F, Wang D, Duncan LJ et al (1994) Stimulation of aromatase activity in breast fibroblasts by tumour necrosis factor α. Mol Cell Endocrinol 106:17-21.

22. Purohit A, Duncan LJ, Wang DY et al (1997) Paracrine control of oestrogen production in breast cancer. Endocr Rel Cancer 4:323-330.

23. Sayers L, Content J (1992) Enhancement of IL-6 receptor β chain (gp130) expression by IL-6, IL-1 and TNFα in human epithelial cells. Biochem Biophys Res Commun 185:902-908.

24. Grodin JM, Siiteri PK, MacDonald PC (1973) Source of estrogen production in postmenopausal women. J Clin Endocrinol Metab 36:207-214.

25. Hotamisligil GS, Shargill NS, Spiegleman BM (1993) Adipose expression of tumor necrosis factor α: a direct role in obesity linked insulin resistance. Science 259:87-91.

26. Hotamisligil GS, Arner P, Caro JF et al (1995) Increased adipose tissue expression of tumor necrosis factor α in human obesity and insulin resistance. J Clin Invest 95:2409-2415.

27. Rose-John S, Heinrich PC (1994) Soluble receptors for cytokines and growth factors: generation and biological function. Biochem J 300:281-290.

28. Singh A, Purohit A, Wang DY et al (1995) IL-6sR: release fromMFC-7 breast cancer cells and role in regulating peripheral oestrogen synthesis. J Endocrinol 147:R9-R12.

29. Singh A, Purohit A, Duncan LJ et al (1998) Control of aromatase activity in breast tumours: the role of the immune system. J Steroid Biochem Molec Biol, in press.

30. Stewart T, Tsai S-CJ, Grayson H et al (1995) Incidence of de-novo breast cancer in women chronically immunosuppressed after organ transplantation. Lancet 346:796-798.

31. Romagnani S (1992) Human Th1 and Th2 subsets: doubt no more. Immunol Today 12:256-257.

32. Daynes RA, Araneo BA, Dowell TA et al (1990) Regulation of murine lymphokine production *in vivo*. J Exp Med 171:979-996.

33. Rook GAW, Hernandex-Pando R, Lightman S (1994) Hormones, peripherally activated prohormones and regulation of Th1/Th2 balance. Immunol Today 15:301-303.

34. Chen CC, David AS, Nunnerly H et al (1995) Adverse life events and breast cancer: case-controlled study. Br Med J 311:1527-1530.

35. Mahendroo MS, Mendelson CR, Simpson ER (1993) Tissue-specific and hormonally-controlled alternative promoters regulate aromatase cytochrome P450 gene expression in human adipose tissue. J Biol Chem 268:19463-19470.

36. Utsumi T, Harada N, Maruta M et al (1996) Presence of alternatively spliced transcripts of aromatase gene in human breast cancer. J Clin Endocrinol Metab 81:2344-2349.

37. Zhao Y, Agarwal VR, Mendelson CR (1996) Estrogen biosynthesis proximal to a breast tumor is stimulated by PGE2 via cyclic AMP, leading to activation of promoter II of the CYP 19 (aromatase) gene. Endocrinology 137:5739-5742.

38. Hinson RM, Williams JA, Shacter E (1996) Elevated interleukin 6 is induced by prostaglandin E_2 in a murine model of inflammation: possible role of cyclooxygenase-2. Proc Natl Acad Sci USA 93:4885-4890.

39. Zhang Y, Lin J-X, Vilcek J (1988) Synthesis of interleukin 6 (interferon-β2/B cell stimulatory factor 2) in human fibroblasts is triggered by an increase in intracellular cyclic AMP. J Biol Chem 263:6177-6182.

22

Regulation of Aromatase in Breast Cancer and Correlation of Aromatase and Cyclooxygenase Gene Expression

Robert W. Brueggemeier, Anne L. Quinn, Yasuro Sugimoto, Young C. Lin, Michelle L. Parrett, Farahnaz S. Joarder, Randall E. Harris, and Fredika M. Robertson

Introduction

Approximately two-thirds of newly diagnosed breast cancers (BC) in the USA are hormone-dependent BC, requiring estrogen (E) for tumor growth. E is important for the local stimulation of growing malignancies in the breast. 17β-Estradiol (E_2), the most potent endogenous E, is biosynthesized from androgens by the cytochrome P450 enzyme complex called aromatase (1-3). The highest levels of aromatase enzymatic activity are present in the ovaries of premenopausal women, in the placenta of pregnant women, and in the peripheral adipose tissues of postmenopausal women and of men. Aromatase activity has also been demonstrated to be present in breast tissue *in vitro* (4-7). Furthermore, expression of aromatase is highest in or near breast tumor sites (5, 8). The gene expressing cytochrome P450$_{arom}$ protein is referred to as *CYP19* and is part of the cytochrome P450 superfamily. The cDNA for aromatase encodes a 55 kDa protein containing 503 amino acids (1, 9). The regulation of aromatase expression varies due to the different promotors in each tissue (10, 11); thus, aromatase biosynthesis is tissue-specific and tightly regulated (1). The increased expression of aromatase cytochrome P450$_{arom}$ observed in BC tissues was recently associated with a switch in the major promoter region utilized in gene expression, resulting in promoter II as the predominant promoter used in BC tissues (12, 13). As a result of the use of the alternate promoter, the regulation of E biosynthesis switches from one, controlled primarily by glucocorticoids and cytokines, to another regulated through cAMP-mediated pathways (12). The prostaglandin PGE$_2$ increases intracellular cAMP levels and stimulates E biosynthesis (12), whereas other autocrine factors such as IL-1β do not appear to act via PGE$_2$ (14).

Cellular processes such as growth and differentiation are mediated through complex regulation of key genes that are expressed in a well-controlled temporal and tissue specific pattern (15). Paracrine interactions, including cell-cell mediated communication, are an important physiological process by which surrounding cells can modulate other cells' activity and maintain proper tissue integrity. An additional level of organization is provided by the surrounding extracellular matrix which provides the three-dimensional framework upon which the tissue is structured. These extracellular matrix proteins interact via specific receptor mediated events and alter transcriptional activity of the cell (16). The extracellular matrix (ECM) generally consists of at least 50 different proteins, which provide a framework of tissue throughout the body (17). In the breast, the basement membrane, which is a specialized form of the ECM, surrounds epithelial cells and other cell types and is primarily composed of laminin, type IV collagen, and proteoglycans. The interstitial tissue matrix is made up of structural ECM proteins (primarily collagen I and fibronectin), stromal fibroblasts, and adipocytes (18). Expression of specific genes is highly dependent on receiving coordinated extracellular signals. These signals represent a cooperation of ECM signals with other regulatory molecules such as hormones and growth factors (19).

The exact paracrine interactions between normal epithelial and stromal cells remain to be fully understood, and the importance of ECM in these interactions in BC is obscure. Studies reported herein focus upon the role of the ECM protein, collagen I, on aromatase activity in breast stromal cells in culture, and evaluates the direct paracrine interactions of soluble factors produced by the stroma that can support tumor growth.

Aromatase Activity of Primary Breast Stromal Fibroblasts

Primary normal stromal fibroblasts cells obtained from breast tissue samples from twelve female patients of varying age (16-80 years) were evaluated for aromatase activity, when grown under different culturing conditions. The effect of the ECM protein, collagen I, on aromatase activity was studied. Collagen I is the major ECM protein in the breast stroma. Although several studies have examined fibroblasts aromatase activity, no study has used an appropriate substratum which mimics in-vivo conditions.

The results of this twelve-patient study are presented in Figure 1. Constitutive aromatase activity was determined by measuring the release of $[^3H]$-H_2O from $[1\beta\text{-}^3H]$-androst-4-ene-3,17-dione, and the ability of these cells to respond to dexamethasone (DEX) with increased aromatase activity. Normal fibroblasts utilize promoter I.4 which has a glucocorticoid responsive element located upstream of the untranslated exon I.4, making them responsive to treatment with 100 nM DEX. Constitutive aromatase activity was lower when cells were grown on a collagen gel for 4-7 days (6.0-fold lower) using

DMEM/F12 media containing 10% dextran coated charcoal stripped serum. Fibroblasts grown on collagen I also appeared to be significantly more responsive to stimulation by 100 nM DEX (plastic:7.0-fold induction, collagen: 33.2-fold induction) when pretreated with DEX for 12 h prior to measurement of aromatase activity. This data show that growing primary fibroblasts on a collagen I matrix results in a decrease in constitutive aromatase activity. This decrease corresponds to a 6.0-fold reduction in activity. These values were corrected to the number of cells so this reduction is not a reflection of differences in the number of cells.

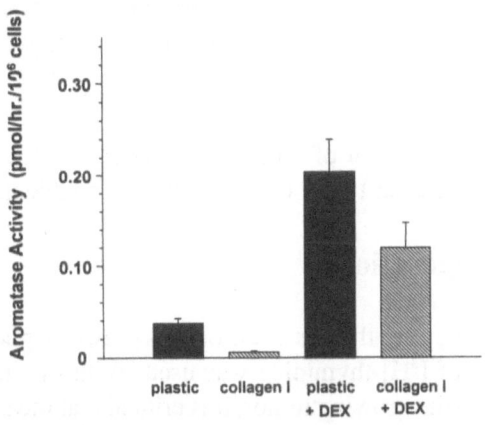

Figure 1. Aromatase activity in breast stromal cells cultured on plastic or collagen I gels ± 100 nM DEX, (n = 12 patients).

Aromatase in Primary Breast Epithelial Cells

Aromatase activity is much lower in cultures of primary breast epithelial cells. To evaluate the effect of the ECM on aromatase in breast epithelial cell cultures, the relative levels of aromatase mRNA expression in cells cultured on different supports were assessed. Breast epithelial cells were isolated by culturing with media containing low [Ca^{++}] levels, on either plastic, collagen I, or Matrigel supports for 2 days, and the levels of steady state mRNA were determined using competitive RT-PCR. Aromatase expression in epithelial cells grown on collagen I support was about 2.8 times greater than the expression in cells grown on plastic. Moreover, cells grown on Matrigel exhibited approximately 4.0 times greater expression of aromatase mRNA than cells grown on plastic (Figure 2). No differences were observed in the expression of two other enzymes involved in steroid biotransformations, steroid sulfatase and 3β-hydroxysteroid dehydrogenase.

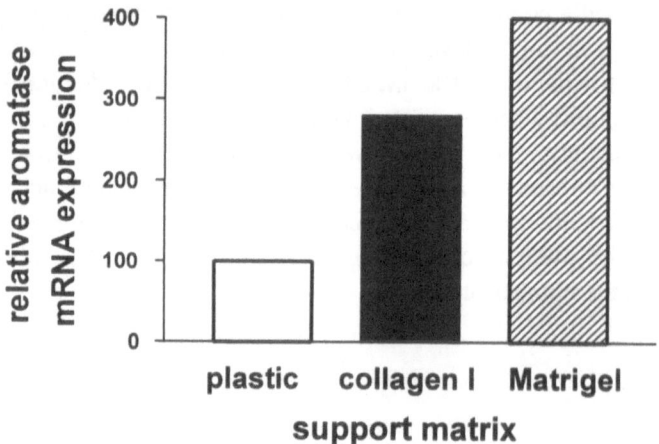

Figure 2. Relative expression of aromatase mRNA in breast epithelial cells cultured on plastic, collagen I gels, or Matrigel, (n = 5 patients).

Thymidine Incorporation

To evaluate the relative growth rates of fibroblasts grown on plastic and collagen I, the incorporation of [³H]-thymidine was used. With the importance of the stromal fibroblasts to the growing tumor, it is critical that measurement of gene expression and enzyme function be carried out under circumstances seen in the normal breast. Since growth and differentiation are two mutually exclusive cellular functions, a cell culture system that offers maintenance of cells rather than supporting maximal proliferation is more representative of *in-vivo* conditions. Therefore, the rationale of growing cells on a collagen I substratum was because this medium is more relevant to the normal breast.

Fibroblasts were grown on plastic or collagen I for 1 to 7 days. [³H]-Thymidine was added to separate plates every day. The incorporation of thymidine can be related to the growth rates of these cells (Figure 3). The fibroblasts which were grown on collagen I showed a significant reduction in the incorporation of thymidine from day 1 to day 5. The cells that were grown on plastic had a faster growth rate and reached confluence at around day 5. At this time, these cells became contacted inhibited, which resulted in the drastic decrease seen after 5 days for the cells grown on plastic. During the time frame that the aromatase activity measurements were taken (day 4), the difference in thymidine incorporation was substantial.

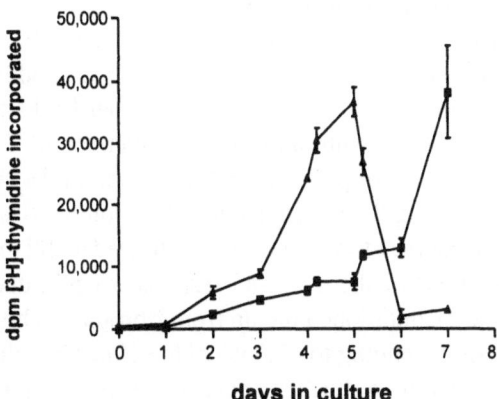

Figure 3. Thymidine incorporation in breast stromal cells cultured on plastic
(♦), or collagen I gels (■), (n = 6 wells).

Conditioned Media Experiments for Paracrine Interactions

To further characterize stromal interactions with the epithelial cells, conditioned
media experiments were used to indirectly measure aromatase activity.
Fibroblasts were cultured under a variety of conditions and, subsequently, the
media was used to treat MCF-7 cells. The soluble factors produced by the
fibroblasts would be able to interact with the epithelial MCF-7 cells.
Additionally, if provided to the fibroblasts, turnover of androgen precursors
would elicit an E-mediated response in the epithelial cells if E levels were of
sufficient magnitude.

MCF-7 cells are known to express a small trefoil protein, pS2. This small
84 residue protein, containing at its amino terminus a signal peptide
characteristic of secreted proteins, was isolated from a human breast carcinoma
cell line. Transcriptional activation of the pS2 gene is a primary response to Es
in the MCF-7 cell line (20, 21). The proximal 5 flanking region of the pS2 gene
contains a transcriptional enhancer E responsive element, a 13 base pair
imperfect palindromic sequence. Cells which are E deprived for 48 h show a
low level of this message and is markedly stimulated by the addition of E_2. The
increase in pS2 message is rapid, with an increase in gene expression after 12 h
of E_2 treatment, reaching a maximum after 48 h.

If the fibroblasts were producing Es, then the E responsive MCF-7 cells
would respond by an increase in pS2 gene expression. This was determined by
Northern analysis and was an indirect measure of the level of fibroblast-derived
E. If the cultured fibroblasts produce sufficient E_2 in the media, an increase in
pS2 expression in the epithelial cells would be seen.

Conditioned media from fibroblasts supplemented with either 100 nM testosterone (T), or vehicle alone (ethanol) was given to MCF-7 cells which had been E deprived for 48 h. Other flasks were given DEX in addition to T which is known to increase aromatase activity. Finally, other flasks were dosed with T and 7α-APTADD, a potent inhibitor of the conversion of T to E_2. Figure 4 depicts a Northern analysis for pS2 and 36B4, and shows the combined results of these experiments using T as a substrate. The control flasks, which were deprived of E for the course of the experiment, showed a pS2 expression which was 21.52% (SEM 4.41) of the maximal response of pS2 upon E_2 treatment (normalized to 100%). Conditioned media from fibroblasts showed an increase in pS2 expression corresponding to 67.36% of the 10nM E_2 value. The addition of 100 nM T resulted in a further increase in pS2 expression over the conditioned media alone, equaling 87.46% (SEM 16.86). It was anticipated that the addition of DEX and T would result in a further enhancement of the pS2 expression. DEX is known to increase aromatase activity in fibroblasts. To maximize the amount of E formed, the DEX was added at the beginning of the 3 day treatment. Figure 4 shows that, in all cases, this resulted in a reduction of pS2 expression, 50.4% (SEM 4.45) over that seen for 100 nM T alone. A report evaluating the result of longer term DEX treatment determined that long term treatment >36 h alters aromatase activity and decreases glucocorticoid receptor (GR) levels (22). There is no statistical difference in the pS2 expression between conditioned media alone and the T and DEX treatment. This supports the hypothesis that long term treatment of DEX reduces aromatase activity in addition to decreasing GR levels (22). The addition of 7α-APTADD, results in a further reduction in pS2 expression, as would be expected (23).

Correlation of Aromatase and Cyclooxygenase Gene Expression in Human Breast Cancer Specimens

The prostaglandin PGE_2 increases intracellular cAMP levels and stimulates E biosynthesis (12), whereas other autocrine factors such as IL-1β do not appear to act via PGE_2 (14). Therefore, local production of PGE_2 via the cyclooxgenase isozymes may influence E biosynthesis and E-dependent BC growth. Prostaglandin G/H endoperoxide synthase, also called cyclooxygenase (COX), is the key rate limiting enzyme which catalyzes the conversion of arachidonic acid to prostaglandins. Two isoforms of this enzyme have been identified, COX-1 and COX-2 (24-26). Both isoforms of the COX gene have been shown to be constitutively co-expressed at low but detectable levels in most human tissues (25).

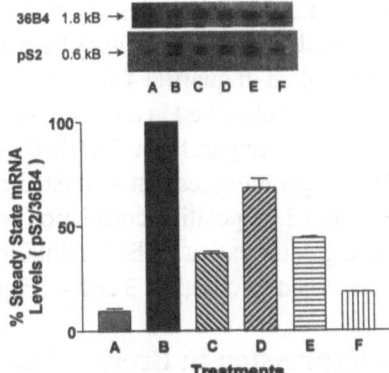

Figure 4. Northern analysis of the effect of fibroblast-derived conditioned media on pS2 mRNA expression in MCF-7 cells. (A) Control media. (B) Media containing 10 nM E_2. (C) Conditioned media from untreated breast stromal cells. Conditional media from breast stromal cells treated with: (D) 100 nM T, (E) 100 nM T + 100 nM DEX, (F) 100 nM T + 100 nM of 7α-APTADD.

COX-1 is believed to be responsible for synthesis of prostaglandins during homeostasis, whereas COX-2 gene expression is an immediate-early response gene that is inducible following stimulation by serum, tumor promoters, mitogens. endotoxin, cytokines, and hormones (27, 28). The induction of COX-2 and the prostanoids subsequently produced have been associated with the inflammatory response (29, 30), and with the process of tumor promotion (31-33). COX inhibition is believed to be one of the mechanisms by which these compounds inhibit the growth of colon and mammary tumors in rodent models of chemical carcinogenesis (34-39). Recent epidemiological studies found a significant inverse association between the intake of non-steroid anti-inflammatory drugs (NSAIDs) and the risk of BC (40-42), which provides support for the role of eicosanoids and COX gene isoforms in growth and invasive potential of human breast tumors. RT-PCR techniques were used to analyze both CYP19 and COX gene expression in 23 human breast tumors and normal breast tissue samples.

CYP19 Expression in Breast Tissue Specimens

Tissue specimens were ranked into one of five quartiles based on assessment of extent of inflammatory infiltrate, presence of necrosis, and evidence of invasion (Table 1) (43). Normal breast tissue with no tumor cells were ranked in quartile 0 (n = 3), tissue specimens with a tumor cell density of ~1-25% were ranked in quartile 1 (n = 4), those with a tumor cell density of ~26-50% were ranked in quartile 2 (n = 4), those with a tumor cell density of 51-75% were ranked in quartile 3 (n = 8), and those with a tumor cell density between 76-100% and with evidence of invasion were ranked in quartile 4 (n = 4).

CYP19 gene expression was observed in all tissue samples analyzed (Table 1), and the levels of expression ranged from CYP19/36B4 ratios of 0.144 to 0.949. The levels of CYP19 gene expression remained relatively constant in breast tissue in quartiles 1 and 2. A positive correlation was observed between CYP19 expression and the greater extent of BC cellularity, i.e., an increase in CYP19 expression was observed in quartiles 3 and 4 (Figure 5).

COX-1 and COX-2 Expression in Breast Tissue Specimens

COX-1 and COX-2 gene expression was also measured in the same normal human breast tissue samples and human breast tumors. COX-1 was present in 1/3 normal human breast tissues and 18/21 human breast tumors (Table 1). In contrast, COX-2 was not present in normal breast tissue specimens, and was detectable and heterogeneous in each of the 21 breast tumor tissue samples examined, with a significant linear association between tumor cell density and COX-2 gene expression (p<0.0001) (Figure 6). The greatest COX-2 expression was found in human breast tumors, ranked within quartile 4, which had high tumor cellularity and 75% of the samples had evidence of invasion across the basement membrane. The relationship between the levels of COX-2 gene expression and high tumor cell density was statistically significant after adjusting for the presence/absence of inflammation and the level of COX-1 gene expression.

Correlation of CYP19, COX-1, and COX-2 Expression in Breast Tissue Specimens

Linear regression analysis using a bivariate model was performed for correlation of the levels of CYP19 gene expression with COX-1 and COX-2 gene expression. This bivariate analysis shows a strong linear association (R=0.80, p<0.0001) between both COX-1 and COX-2 expression and CYP19 expression (Figure 7). These data suggest a strong relationship between the expression of CYP19 aromatase in breast tissue specimens and the COX isoforms (both COX-1 and -2) which produce prostaglandins locally in the breast tissue. This implies that the expression of both COX-1 and COX-2 together serve as better predictors of aromatase expression in BC patients. Higher levels of COX-1 and COX-2 expression would produce higher levels of PGE_2, resulting in elevated CYP19 expression through increases in intracellular cAMP levels and activation of promoter II.

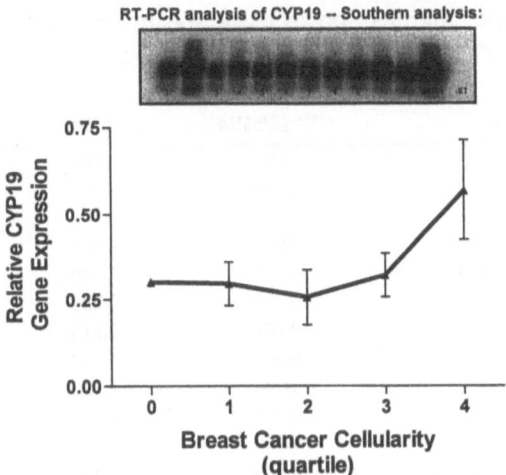

Figure 5. Relationship of CYP19 gene expression in human breast tissue specimens and BC cellularity. Southern analysis of the cDNA amplification products derived from RT-PCR amplification was performed using CYP19 primers. The lane numbers refer individual patient samples, with aromatase cRNA used as a positive control, and the reaction without reverse transcriptase as a negative control. The ratio of CYP19/36B4 is plotted versus the quartile score for BC cellularity in the human breast tissue specimens. Each data point represents the mean for the samples in each quartile from Table 1.

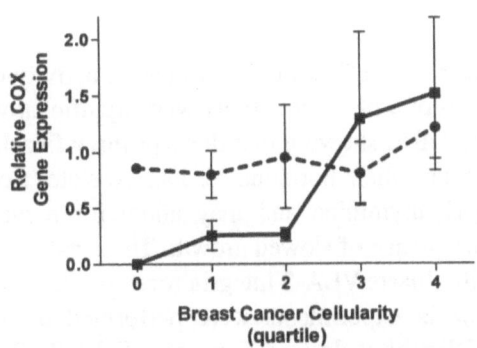

Figure 6. Relationship of COX-1 and COX-2 gene expression in human breast tissue specimens to BC cellularity. The ratios of COX-1/HPRT (●) and of COX-2/HPRT (■) were plotted versus the quartile score for BC cellularity in the human breast tissue specimens. Each data point represents the mean for the samples in each quartile from Table 1.

Table 1. Quartile ranking of breast tissue specimens based on tissue cellularity and levels of CYP19, COX-1, and COX-2 expression.

Quartile	CYP19/36B4	COX-1/hprt	COX-2/hprt
0	N/A	0.892	0
0	0.300	0	0
0	N/A	0	0
1	N/A	0.968	0.587
1 (well differentiated CA)	0.443	1.240	0.190
1	0.251	0.480	0.055
1	0.208	0.518	0.175
2	0.391	1.770	0.165
2	N/A	1.420	0.295
2	0.237	0.624	0.385
2	0.144	0	0.197
3 (50% inflammation)	0.359	1.130	1.130
3	0.599	1.900	2.390
3	0.603	1.030	0.860
3	0.288	0.875	0.268
3	0.160	0	0.523
3 (50% inflammation)	0.208	0.148	1.880
3 (inflammation)	0.196	0	2.160
3 (50% inflammation)	0.164	1.070	1.110
4 (invasive CA)	0.498	1.430	1.080
4 (invasive CA)	0.949	2.450	3.240
4 (invasive CA)	0.602	1.470	1.060
4	0.257	0.500	0.667

N/A = not analyzed, insufficient sample available

Discussion

A collagen I matrix has an affect on the aromatase activity of primary breast fibroblasts. The levels of aromatase activity were significantly increased by the presence of 100 nM DEX, showing that these primary fibroblasts grown on a collagen I matrix retain their hormone responsive state. Collagen I reduced incorporation of [^{3}H]-thymidine and may allow for a more differentiated phenotype as a consequence of slowed growth. These data support the specific interaction of the fibroblasts VLA-2 integrin receptor with a collagen I.

Conditioned media experiments were performed in order to examine paracrine effects of fibroblast-derived-E on epithelial cells. T administration to fibroblasts resulted in the production of E_2 into the media in sufficient concentrations to elicit an increase in pS2 expression when the conditioned media was administered to MCF-7 cells. Co-incubation of MCF-7 cells with conditioned media supplemented with T + DEX produced a decrease in pS2 expression over a 3 day treatment. Addition of an aromatase inhibitor resulted in suppression of fibroblast-derived-E and showed no increase in pS2 expression.

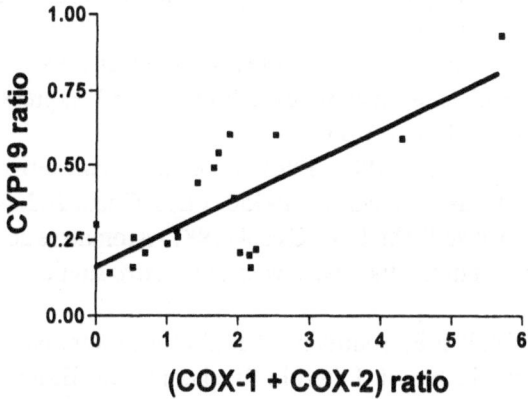

Figure 7. Correlation of CYP19 gene expression with COX-1 and COX-2 gene expression in human breast tissue specimens. A bivariate linear regression analysis shows a strong linear association (R=0.80, p<0.0001) between both COX-1 and COX-2 expression and CYP19 expression.

The potential for high aromatase activity in breast stromal cells may more critically depend upon tumor-derived factors. One group of potential tumor-derived factors may be prostaglandins biosynthesized by the COX isozymes. A linear regression analysis using a bivariate model shows a strong linear association between both COX-1 and -2 expression and CYP19 expression. This implies that the expression of both COX-1 and -2 together serve as better predictors of aromatase expression in BC patients. Higher levels of COX-1 and -2 expression would produce higher levels of PGE_2, resulting in elevated CYP19 expression through increases in intracellular cAMP levels and activation of promoter II. Moreover, a strong relationship between the aromatase and COX enzyme systems suggests that autocrine and paracrine mechanisms may be involved in hormone-dependent BC development via growth stimulation from local E biosynthesis and invasive potential from prostaglandins and related prostanoids.

Acknowledgments

This work was supported in part by grants R01 CA73698, T32 CA09498, R21 CA66193, and P30 CA16058 from the NCI/NIH, the Charlotte Geyer Foundation, and the Wendy Will Case Cancer Foundation.

References

1. Simpson ER, Mahendroo M S, Means GD et al (1994) Aromatase cytochrome P450, the enzyme responsible for estrogen biosynthesis. Endocr Rev 15:342-355.
2. Simpson ER, Mahendroo M S, Means GD et al (1993) Tissue-specific promoters regulate aromatase cytochrome P450 expression. J Steroid Biochem Mol Biol 44:321-330.
3. Kellis JT, Vickery LE (1987) Purification and characterization of human placental aromatase cytochrome P-450. J Biol Chem 262:4413-4420.
4. James VHT, McNeill JM, Lai LC et al (1987) Aromatase activity in normal breast and breast tumor tissues: *in vivo* and *in vitro* studies. Steroids 50:269-279.
5. Miller WR, Mullen P, Sourdaine P et al (1997) Regulation of aromatase activity within the breast. J Steroid Biochem Molec Biol 61:193-202.
6. Reed MJ, Topping L, Coldham NG et al (1993) Interleukin-I and interleukin-6 in breast cyst fluid: their role in regulating aromatase activity in breast cancer cells. J Steroid Biochem Molec Biol 44:589-596.
7. Reed MJ (1994) The role of aromatase in breast tumors. Breast Canc Res Treat 30:7-17.
8. Bulum SE, Price TM, Mahendroo MS (1993) A link between breast cancer and local estrogen biosynthesis suggested by quantification of breast adipose tissue aromatase cytochrome P450 transcripts using competitive polymerase chain reaction after reverse transcriptase. J Clin Endocrinol Metab 77:1622-1628.
9. Sanghera M K, Simpson ER, McPhaul MJ et al (1991) Immunocytochemical distribution of aromatase cytochrome P450 in the rat brain using peptide-generated polyclonal antibodies. Endocrinology 129:2834-2844.
10. Means GD, Kilgore MW, Mahendroo MS et al (1991) Tissue-specific promoters regulate aromatase cytochrome P450 gene expression in human ovary and fetal tissues. Mol Endocrinol 5:2005-2013.
11. McPhaul MJ, Herbst MA, Matsumine H et al (1993) Diverse mechanisms of control of aromatase gene expression. J Steroid Biochem Mol Biol 44:341-346.
12. Zhao Y, Agarwal V, Mendelson C et al (1996) Estrogen biosynthesis proximal to a breast tumor is stimulated by PGE_2 via cyclic AMP, leading to activation of promoter II of the CYP19 (aromatase) gene. Endocrinol 137:5739-5742.
13. Zhou C, Zhou D, Esteban J et al (1996) Aromatase gene expression and its exon I usage in human breast tumors. J Steroid Biochem Molec Biol 59:163-171.

14. Hughes R, Timmermans P, Schrey MP (1996) Regulation of arachidonic acid metabolism, aromatase activity, and growth in human breast cancer cells by interleukin-1β and phorbol ester. Int J Cancer 67:684-689.
15. Sekeris CE (1991) Hormonal steroids act as tumor promoters by modulating oncogene expression. J Cancer Res Clin Oncol 117:96-101.
16. Lin CQ, Bissell MJ (1993) Multi-faceted regulation of cell differentiation by extracellular matrix. FASEB J 7:737-743.
17. Lochter A, Bissell MJ (1995) Involvement of extracellular matrix constituents in breast cancer. Semin Cancer Biol 6:165-173.
18. Jones PL, Schmidhauser C, Bissell MJ (1993) Regulation of gene expression and cell function by extracellular matrix. Crit Rev Eukaryotic Gene Expr 3:137-154.
19. Howlett AR, Bissell MJ (1993) The influence of tissue microenvironment (stroma and extracellular matrix) on the development and function of mammary epithelium. Epithelial Cell Biol 2:79-89.
20. Rio M-C, Chambon P (1990) The pS2 gene, mRNA and Protein: A potential marker for human breast cancer. Cancer Cells: A Monthly Review. 2:269-274.
21. Rio MC, Bellocq JP, Gairard B et al (1987) Specific Expression of pS2 gene in a subclass of breast cancers in comparison with expression of the estrogen and progesterone receptors and ERBB2. Proc Natl Acad Sci 84:9243-9247.
22. Berkovitz GD, Chen S, Migeon CJ et al (1992) Induction and superinduction of messenger ribonucleic acid specific for aromatase cytochrome P-450 in cultured human skin fibroblasts. J Clin Endocrinol Metab 74:629-634.
23. Snider CE, Brueggemeier RW (1987) Potent enzyme-activated inhibition of aromatase by a 7?-substituted C_{19} steroid. J Biol Chem 262:8685-8689.
24. Smith WL, Garavito RM, DeWitt DL (1996) Prostaglandin endoperoxide H synthases (cyclooxygenase)-1 and –2. J Biol Chem 271:33157-33160.
25. Williams CS, DuBois RN (1996) Prostglandin endoperoxide syjthase: Why two isoforms? Am J Physiol 270:G393-400.
26. Herschman HR (1994) Regulation of prostaglandin synthase-1 and prostaglandin synthase-2. Cancer Metastasis Rev 13:241-256.
27. Hershman HR (1996) Prostaglandin synthase 2. Biochem Biophys Acta 1299:125-140.
28. Wu KK (1996) Cyclooxygenase 2 induction: molecular mechanism and pathophysiologic roles. J Lab Clin Med 128:242-245.
29. Seibert K, Zhang Y, Leahy K et al (1994) Pharmacological and biochemical demonstration of the role of cyclooxygenase 2 in inflammation and pain. Proc Natl Acad Sci USA 91:12013-12017.

30. Vane JR, Mitchell JA, Appleton I et al (1994) Inducible isoforms of cyclooxygenase and nitric-oxide synthase in inflammation. Proc Natl Acad Sci USA 91:2046-2050.
31. Furstenberger G, Gross M, Marks F (1989) Eicosanoids and multi-stage carcinogenesis in NMRI mouse skin: role of prostaglandin El and F in conversion (first stage of tumor promotion) and promotion (second stage of tumor promotion). Carcinogenesis 10:91-96.
32. Maldve RE, Fischer SM (1996) Multifactor regulation of prostaglandin H synthase-2 in murine keratinocytes. Molec Carcinogen 17:207-216.
33. Muller-Decker K, Scholz K, Marks F et al (1995) Differential expression of prostaglandin H synthase isozymes during multistage carcinogenesis in mouse epidermis. Molec Carcinogen 12:31-41.
34. Giardello FM, Offerhaus OJA, Dubois RN (1995) The role of nonsteroidal anti-inflammatory drugs in colorectal cancer prevention. Eur J Cancer 31A:1071-1076.
35. Rao CV, Rivenson A, Simi B, Zang E, Kelloff G, Steele VE, Reddy BS. Chemoprevention of colon carcinogenesis by sulindac, a nonsteroidal anti-inflammatory agent. Cancer Res 1995 55:1464-1472.
36. McCormick DL, Moon RC (1983) Inhibition of mammary carcinogenesis by flurbiprofen, a nonsteroidal anti-inflammatory agent. Br J Cancer 48:859-861.
37. Fulton AM (1984) In vivo effects of indomethacin on the growth of murine mammary tumors. Cancer Res 44:2416-2420.
38. Carter CA, Ip MM, Ip CA (1989) Comparison of the effects of the prostaglandin synthesis inhibitors indomethacin and carprofen in 7,12-dimethylbenz(a)anthracene-induced mammary tumorigenesis in rats fed different amounts of essential fatty acids. Carcinogenesis 10:1369-1374.
39. Lee PP, Ip MM (1992) Regulation of proliferation of rat mammary tumor cells by inhibitors of cyclooxygenase and lipoxygenase. Prostagland Leukotrien Essen Fat Acid 45:21-31.
40. Harris RE, Namboodiri KK, Steilman SD et al (1995) Breast cancer and NSAID use: heterogeneity of effect in a case-control study. Preven Med 24:119-120.
41. Harris RE, Namboodiri KK, Farrar WB (1996) Nonsteroidal anti-inflammatory drugs and breast cancer. Epidemiology 7:203-205.
42. Harris RE, Namboodiri KK, Farrar WB (1995) Epidemiological study of nonsteroidal anti-inflammatory drugs and breast cancer. Oncology Reports 2:591-592.
43. Parrett ML, Harris RE, Joarder FS (1997) Cycooxygenase-2 gene expression in human breast cancer. Inter J Oncology 10:503-507.

PART 8. ORGAN SITE: PROSTATE/OVARY

Introduction

Androgen Receptor and its Role in the Development and Control of Androgen-independent Prostate Cancer

Shutsung Liao, John M. Kokontis, and Richard A. Hiipakka

Prostate cancer (PC) is the most commonly diagnosed malignancy and the second leading cause of cancer death among American men. Generally, prostate tumors are initially dependent on androgen for growth even after metastasis and, therefore, can be treated effectively by androgen deprivation as Charles Huggins showed in 1941 (1). Unfortunately, after 1 to 3 years of endocrine therapy, prostate tumors usually reappear as androgen-independent tumors and androgen deprivation or antiandrogen therapies are no longer effective. Presently, no effective therapy is available for recurrent advanced PCs that are androgen-independent for their survival or growth.

The emergence of an androgen-independent prostate tumor can be due to selective out-growth of androgen-independent cancer cells after androgen-dependent cancer cells are suppressed by androgen deprivation, assuming that these two forms of cancer cells co-metastasize from the primary tumor (2). Much evidence exists, however, for the ability of androgen-dependent PC cells to adapt to a low-androgen environment and progress to androgen-independent forms. Loss of androgen-dependency can be due to a defect or a loss in androgen receptor (AR) gene expression (3) but, in most instances, continued AR expression and function have been observed in hormone-independent tumors (4, 5). These androgen-independent cells may utilize growth factors (6) or recruit alternative pathways (such as protein kinase) for AR activation in the absence of androgen (7). Androgen-independent cells may also utilize an alternative growth regulatory pathway that does not require AR-dependent signaling (8, 9).

Progression of Androgen-dependent Prostate Cancer Cells to Androgen-independent Prostate Cancer Cells

In our study, we subjected an androgen-dependent clone of the LNCaP cell line, called 104-S, to long-term (several years) androgen deprivation during culture *in vitro* (5). During culture, the 104-S cells progressed through an intermediate form, 104-R1 cells, and, subsequently, transformed to a faster-growing stage of cells, 104-R2 cells, which could grow in the absence of androgen and in the presence of the antiandrogen bicalutamide (Casodex) (9). The proliferation of 104-R1 or -R2 cells is repressed by androgen (17β-hydroxy-17-methyl-estra-4,9,11-trien-3-one or R1881) at a concentration (0.1 nM) that is optimal for 104-S cell growth. Paradoxically, the transition of androgen-dependent 104-S cells to androgen-independent 104-R1 or -R2 cells, was accompanied by an increase in the cellular level of AR mRNA by ~2.0-3.0-fold, and the AR protein level by ~10.0-20.0-fold (5). During this progression from androgen-dependent to androgen-independent cells, AR transcriptional activity, measured by androgen induction of prostate-specific antigen (PSA) mRNA and an androgen-dependent chloramphenicol acetyltransferase (CAT) reporter gene in transfected cells, increased up to 20-fold (5). Therefore, AR in the androgen-independent 104-R cells is functional, but is dissociated from the pathways that in 104-S cells can lead to cell proliferation. It is also possible that the androgen-induced repression of 104-R cell proliferation is related to the high level of AR in these cancer cells. Excessive AR may, for example, sequester factors and/or disrupt an orderly sequence of events that are required for cell growth and proliferation.

Androgen-dependent Induction of Cell Cycle Arrest in Androgen-independent Prostate Cancer Cells

Androgen repression of 104-R cells is apparently due to a G1 arrest during cell cycling. Therefore, we studied (10) the mechanism of androgen-dependent repression by examining the role of regulatory factors that are involved in the control of cell cycle progression (Figure 1). In both, 104-R1 and -R2 cells, R1881, at concentrations (0.1-1 nM) that repressed cell growth, induced the cyclin-dependent kinase (cdk) inhibitor, p27^{kip1}. In contrast, in androgen-dependent 104-S cells, the same concentrations of R1881 that promote cell proliferation reduced the cellular level of p27^{kip1}.

The effect of androgen on c-*myc* gene expression correlated well with the proliferative activity of both, the androgen-dependent and the androgen-independent cancer cells (5). At 0.1 nM, R1881 induced c-*myc* mRNA level over 2.0-fold in 104-S cells, but reduced the mRNA level to less than 20% of the control value in 104-R cells. At higher concentrations (~20 nM), R1881 inhibited both cell proliferation and c-*myc* expression in both types of cells. The androgen repression of cell proliferation of these cells could be blocked by retroviral overexpression of c-*myc*. (Table 1).

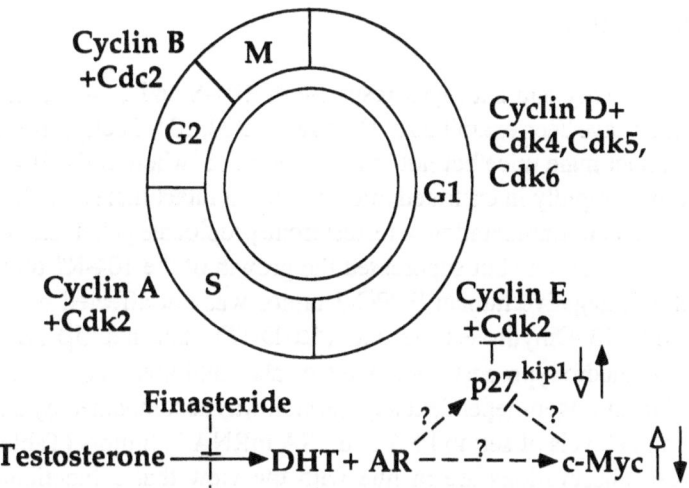

Figure 1. The role of androgen and AR during LNCaP cell cycle progression. In androgen-dependent LNCaP 104-S cells, testosterone (T) is converted to 5α-DHT that binds to AR. The 5α-DHT-AR complex promotes cell cycling by upregulation of c-*myc* expression and downregulation of the synthesis of p27^{kip1} (open arrows), that otherwise can inhibit the activity of the cyclin E-cdk2 complex. In androgen-independent but androgen-repressed LNCaP 104-R cells that were originally derived from LNCaP 104-S cells through a long period of culture in an androgen deprived medium, 5α-DHT-AR complex induces G1 arrest by downregulation of c-*myc* and upregulation of p27^{kip1} (black arrows). Finasteride, a 5α-reductase inhibitor, can stimulate cell cycle and growth of LNCaP 104-S tumors but can induce cell cycle arrest and suppress the growth of LNCaP 104-R tumors. The mechanism involved in the progression of androgen-dependent LNCaP 104-S cells to androgen-independent LNCaP-104-R cells is not known but this process is reversible (10, 11).

Table 1. AR and androgen dependent responses in PC cells.

Cancer cells	AR level	Response to androgen[a]			
		Tumor growth PSA		p27^{kip1}	c-*myc*
PC-3	−	No effect	nr	nr	nr
104-S	+	Stimulation	+	−	+
104-R1>10	+	Suppression	+	+	−
104-R1Ad[b]	+	Stimulation	+	−	+

[a] Cellular level   nr, no response   +, upregulation   −, downregulation

[b] Cells that were reverted from 105-R1 back to androgen-dependent state

Androgen Receptor-dependent Suppression of Prostate Tumors in Mice

The tumorigenicity and androgen response of 104-S and 104-R cells in male athymic mice have been examined (11). As expected, 104-S cells formed tumors readily in intact male mice but not in castrated mice, whereas the 104-R2 cells formed tumors rapidly in castrated mice but not in intact males. With castrated mice, subcutaneous implantation of testosterone propionate pellets stimulated the growth of 104-S tumors but suppressed the growth of the 104-R2 tumors. The growth of AR-negative human PCPC-3 tumor was not affected by androgen implantation. 5α-Dihydrotestosterone (5α-DHT), but not 5β-DHT, 17β-estradiol, or medroxyprogesterone acetate, also inhibited the 104-R2 tumor growth. This androgen-dependent suppression was accompanied by a transient increase in the levels of serum PSA and PSA mRNA in tumors (Table 1).

These observations are in line with the view that a functional AR is possibly required for tumor suppression. Similarly, we have observed that antiandrogens, such as bicalutamide, can antagonize AR function and tumor suppression, and stimulate the growth of the 104-R2 tumor in androgen-treated castrated or intact adult mice. Suppression of the 104-R2 tumor growth by T was apparently dependent on the conversion of T to 5α-DHT; administration of a 5α-reductase inhibitor, such as finasteride (Proscar), to the T-treated mice inhibited T-dependent tumor suppression and stimulated the growth of the 104-R2 tumors in mice. These findings indicated that the use of a 5α-reductase inhibitor or antiandrogens, in the general treatment of metastatic PC may require careful assessment.

Reversion of Androgen-independent Prostate Tumors Back to Androgen-dependent Tumors

Using a cell culture system, we have observed that over time 104-R1 cells can adapt to high concentrations of androgen, and become androgen-dependent again (10). During this adaptation, the AR content in these cells (104-R1Ad) was reduced to a level comparable with that in the original androgen-dependent 104-S cells. Androgen failed to induce the cdk inhibitor p27^{kip1} in these adapted cells. This reversion from androgen-independent cancer cells to androgen-dependent cancer cells has also been observed in athymic mice (11). When 104-R2 cells were implanted in normal mice, tumor growth was not seen for about 5 weeks, but from the 7th-week, new tumors gradually appeared and they behaved like 104-S tumors in their response to androgen (unpublished observation).

Intermittent Androgen Replacement Therapy (IART) and Androgen Suppression/Reversion Therapy (ASRT)

Based on the assumption that androgen-dependent and androgen-independent tumors coexist in PC patients and that suppression of androgen-dependent tumors can accelerate the growth of independent tumors, a trial of Intermittent Androgen Replacement Therapy (IART) (12) is ongoing. In this trial (Southwest Oncology Group Study), the intermittent supply of androgen is expected to stimulate and maintain a low level of growth of androgen-dependent tumors which restricts the growth of the androgen-independent tumors (Figure 2). Our findings that androgens can suppress certain AR positive, androgen-independent tumors suggests another clinical trial of Androgen Suppression/Reversion Therapy (ASRT). In such a trial, androgens would potentially suppress the growth of androgen-independent tumors and revert some tumors to androgen-dependent state. Such suppressed and reverted tumors could be retreated by androgen-withdrawal or by administration of antiandrogen (Figure 2).

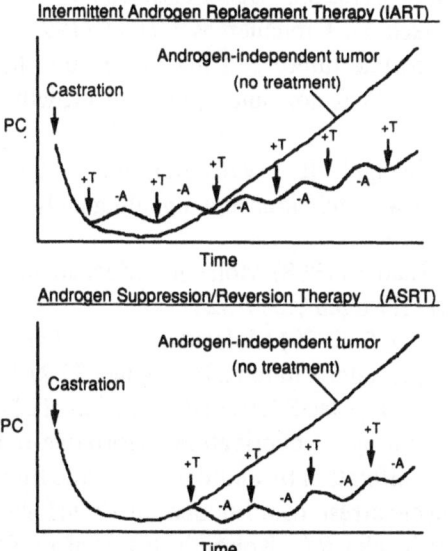

Figure 2. Hypothetical consequences of Intermittent Androgen Replacement Therapy (IART) (upper figure) and Androgen Suppression/Reversion Therapy (ASRT). Castration can be replaced by 'chemical castration' using antiandrogens or drugs that limit testicular androgen production. If this method is used, re-supply of androgen (+T) can be achieved by stopping administration of these antiandrogens or other drugs. Re-administration of these drugs can stop androgen action (-A). Ordinate, Severity of PC as measured by a method such as bone scan. Abscissa, period of treatment.

References

1.   Huggins C, Stevens RE, Hodges CV (1941) Studies on prostatic cancer. II. The effects of castration on advanced carcinoma of the prostate gland. Arch of Surg 43:209-223.
2.   Isaacs JT, Coffey DS (1981) Adaptation versus selection as the mechanism responsible for the relapse of prostate cancer to androgen ablation therapy as studied in the Dunning R-3327-H adenocarcinoma. Cancer Res 41:5070-5075.
3.   Bruchovsky N, Rennie PS, Coldman AJ et al (1990) Effects of androgen withdrawal in the stem cell composition of the Shionogi carcinoma. Cancer Res 50:2275-2282.
4.   Hobisch A, Culig Z, Radmeyer C et al (1995) Distant metastasies from prostatic carcinoma express androgen receptorprotein. Cancer Res 55:3068-3072.
5.   Kokontis J, Takakura K, Hay N et al (1994) Increased androgen receptor activity and altered c-myc expression in prostate cancer cells after long-term androgen deprivation. Cancer Research 54:1566-1573.
6.   Culig Z, Hobisch A, Cronauer MV et al (1994) Androgen receptor activation in prostate tumor cell lines by insulin-like growth factor-1, keratinocyte growth factor, and epidermal growth factor. Cancer Res 54:5474-5478.
7.   Nazareth LV, Weigel NL (1996) Activation of the human androgen receptor through a protein kinase A signaling pathway. J Biol Chem 271: 19900-19907.
8.   Hiipakka RA, Liao S (1998) Molecular Mechanism of androgen action. Trend Endocrinol Metab 9:317-324.
9.   Kokontis JM, Liao S (1999) Molecular action of androgen in the normal and neoplastic prostate. Vitamins Hormones 55:219-307.
10.   Kokontis JM, Hay N, Liao S (1998) Progression of LNCaP prostate tumor cells during androgen deprivation: Hormone-independent growth, repression of proliferation by androgen, and role for p27^{kip1} in androgen-induced cell cycle arrest. Mol Endocrinol 12:941-953.
11.   Umekita Y, Hiipakka RA, Kokontis JM et al (1996) Human prostate tumor growth in athymic mice: Inhibition by androgens and stimulation by finasteride. Proc Natl Acad Sci USA 93:11802-11807.
12.   Akakura K, Bruchovsky N, Goldenberg SL et al (1993) Effects of intermittent androgen suppression on androgen-dependent tumors. Apoptosis and serum prostate-specific antigen. Cancer 71:2782-2790.

23

Etiologic Mechanisms in Epithelial Ovarian Cancer

Harvey A. Risch

Introduction and Background

Ovarian cancer (OC) is a moderately common neoplasm of older women that is both difficult to diagnose and treat. Almost 2% of women are affected over the lifetime. It is the fourth most frequent cause of cancer death among women, after lung, breast, and colorectal cancer. The established risk factors (low parity, non-use of oral-contraceptives, germline BRCA1/2 mutation) account for a portion of disease occurrence, but mechanisms by which these factors affect risk of developing OC are not fully understood. The purpose of this chapter is to consider evidence for and against the two main etiologic hypotheses, concerning incessant ovulation and excessive gonadotropins. We use the term "ovarian cancer " to denote the borderline (low malignant potential) and invasive tumors of the surface epithelium of the ovary that constitute the more than 90% of all nonbenign ovarian neoplasms of adult women. Germ-cell, stromal, and other primary tumors also occur but are not the main focus here. Some etiologic heterogeneity may also exist among the epithelial subtypes, this is discussed by the author in detail elsewhere (1).

In 1971, Fathalla (2) suggested that long-term, repeated ovulation without pregnancy-related pauses may provoke neoplasia of the ovarian epithelium. He noted that the ovarian surface epithelium rapidly proliferates during the 24 h postovulation, and that invaginations of the epithelium to form clefts and inclusion cysts within the ovarian stroma are most pronounced just after ovulation. Casagrande et al. (3) extended this, to decreased risk associated with anovulation resulting from oral-contraceptive use. Those authors suggested that exposure to estrogen (E) -rich follicular fluid following ovulation was the cause of the proliferation and/or malignant transformation. In 1983, Cramer and Welch (4) combined these ideas: Given lifelong repeated invaginations of the ovarian epithelium to form clefts and inclusion cysts, under excessive gonadotropin (FSH or LH) stimulation of the ovarian stroma, and the resulting E stimulation, then the epithelium may undergo malignant transformation. They thus concluded that factors affecting systemic E regulation would influence gonadotropin stimulation and, indirectly, the paracrine E milieu of the epithelium. The gonadotropin model is consistent with the known protective effects of parity and oral contraceptive use, inverse associations seen in the great majority of OC studies (5, 6). Both pregnancy and oral contraceptives suppress ovulation, and may lower basal as well as peak gonadotropin stimulation. In the postmenopausal years, the Cramer-Welch model relates systemic Es, exogenous or through obesity or perhaps diet, to estrogenic stimulation of the ovarian epithelium. The main point of Cramer and Welch was that it is excessive gonadotropins, leading ultimately to increased estrogenic exposure of the epithelial cells, which is responsible for the elevated risk of malignancy. In the following discussion, we evaluate current evidence related to these two hypotheses, on incessant ovulation and gonadotropin stimulation.

Incessant Ovulation

The proliferative behavior of the ovarian epithelium following ovulation supports a potential role for ovulation in the etiology of OC . Hyperovulatory poultry hens under chronic photostimulation are extremely likely to develop ovarian or tubal adenocarcinomas (7), and repeatedly recultured rat ovary epithelial cells, forced to proliferate, spontaneously acquire malignant features, and produce serous cystadenocarcinomas when injected into nude athymic mice (8). After each ovulation, in addition to the repair of the ovulatory wound, the epithelium has a tendency to form clefts extending into the cortical stroma (2). These clefts frequently close off, becoming inclusion cysts. Increased prevalence of inclusion cysts in contralateral ovaries of women with unilateral OC suggests that germinal inclusion cysts may be related to cancer development (9). However, greater density of inclusion cysts among cancer cases was not seen in another, larger study (10). The latter study found that both germinal inclusion cysts and unilateral OC occur more frequently in the right ovary than the left, and other groups have also reported a higher frequency of right-sided OC (11), though this finding was not confirmed in the large SEER cancer-incidence database (12). Ovulation has also been reported to occur somewhat more often in the right ovary than in the left (13), but this finding too has not been confirmed (14).

p53 and Ovulation

Inactivation and/or somatic mutation of the p53 cell-cycle checkpoint regulator gene has been implicated in neoplasia in a variety of organs. p53 mutations appear to be involved early in the neoplastic process of glioblastoma, esophageal cancer, and hepatocellular carcinoma (15), but late in the development of colon cancer (16). Dysfunction in p53 is observed in about 46% of invasive ovarian tumors (17), but in only 8% of borderline (low malignant potential) ones (18, 19), and not at all in benign tumors or normal ovarian epithelium (18, 19). Thus, p53 inactivation is likely to be a late event in OC, though given a high degree of concordance between primary tumors and metastases (20), it may occur prior to metastatic spread. Nevertheless, the types of mutations seen in OCs suggest that many p53 mutations are caused by generalized genomic instability, rather than being the cause of the instability (21).

A recent paper by Schildkraut, et al. (22), asserted that exposure to a high lifetime number of ovulatory cycles was associated with increased risk of p53-overexpressing OC, but not of p53-negative OC. Based on the claimed specificity of the association for p53-positive tumors only, it was concluded that both repetitive ovulation and p53 inactivation were involved in the etiology of OC. However, the given analysis showed that two of the three principal factors determining calculated lifetime number of ovulatory cycles, attained parity and duration of oral contraceptive use, were equally associated with p53-positive and p53-negative cancers (23). Only age at diagnosis differed between p53-positive and p53-negative subjects. Similarly, borderline ovarian tumors are known to have the same risk-factor associations with low parity and with non-use of oral contraceptives as invasive tumors (1), yet the borderline tumors rarely show p53 mutations. The Schildkraut results (22) also showed p53-positive OC s to be more associated with distant rather than local/regional stage at diagnosis; even more importantly, p53 positivity was strongly associated with tumor grade $(P<10^{-5})$ (22), and this relationship has been seen by a number of others (17). Thus, we are left with the view that p53-overexpressing OCs are likely to be those diagnosed later in the disease process, after the accumulation of more genetic errors, and not with evidence for a role of ovulation in causing p53 damage leading to neoplasia.

Breastfeeding, Menstrual Variability, and Ovulation

Breastfeeding can suppress ovulation, especially if the breastfed infant is not supplemented with bottle feeding. Total duration of breastfeeding, or average amount of breastfeeding per pregnancy, have been observed to be associated with reduced risk of OC in a number of studies (6, 24). Also, certain features of the menstrual cycle reflect the probability of anovulation. Cycles <25 or >35 days in length, or with more than eight days of flow, are appreciably more likely to be anovulatory (25). Moderate physical activity and/or significant weight loss can induce menstrual changes. Few epidemiologic studies of OC have considered menstrual cycle factors. In one large case-control study, Parazzini, et al. (26) observed significantly lower risk (adjusted OR 0.45, 95% CI 0.31-0.65) among women with cycles <25 or >35 days long. No case-control difference in menstrual cycle length was seen in some older studies, though the particular studies apparently did not allow for the fact that overly long cycles might have the same effect on risk as excessively short ones. However, an OC case-control study by the author (24) found that menstrual cycles on average <25 days long, ≥35 days long, generally irregular, or with >8 days of flow, all were associated with odds ratios below one (OR 0.67, 0.77, 0.75, and 0.40, respectively).

Magnitude of Effect of Ovulatory Events

While we have not completely ruled out a role for ovulation, it is apparent that, by itself, ovulation is insufficient to account for the pathogenesis of OC. Ovulations occur over at least 20 years (25). Each full-term pregnancy suppresses ovulation for about a year, at most 5% of the total number of ovulations. Epidemiologic studies show that the reduction in risk among parous women for each subsequent pregnancy after the first one is about 14-16% (6, 24), and this is statistically inconsistent with the 5% ($P<10^{-5}$) reported previously reported (6). Each year of oral contraceptive use, also suppresses ovulation for a year, but the lowered risk for an additional year of use among ever-users is only about 9%, and that too is not consistent with the lowered risk with each pregnancy (P=0.001) reported (6).

Hormonal Factors in General

Even if ovulation is etiologically involved in OC, additional mechanisms must also operate. These mechanisms are probably hormonal. Salazar, et al. (27) found significantly greater frequencies of hyperplastic or metaplastic changes in the ovarian epithelium, and excessive stromal activity, in women with family histories of ovarian or breast cancer. Resta, et al. (28), observed metaplastic or hyperplastic changes in the surface epithelium or in inclusion cysts in 92% of ovaries of women with epithelial tumors of the contralateral ovary (benign and malignant), in 76% of ovaries of women with endometrial adenocarcinoma, in 68% of women with polycystic ovary syndrome, but in only 22% of control women with incidental oophorectomy during surgery for various nonneoplastic gynecologic conditions. Since excessive ovulation does not occur in polycystic ovary syndrome, some other factor may be responsible for the increased proliferation. Resta, et al. (28), also saw a loss of surface epithelium more often in the ovaries of the control women than among those of the other three groups. The greater presence of epithelium on the ovarian surface in the three case groups seems not to be attributable to ovulation but to some other factor.

In addition, OCs seem to arise most frequently in the cortical stroma, in epithelial inclusion cysts, compared to the same cells of the ovarian surface epithelium (29), and even less often in the related pelvic peritoneal mesothelium which has a much greater surface area. In the Resta study (28), hyperplastic or metaplastic changes were observed more often in inclusion cysts than in surface epithelium in all four subject groups. Inclusion cysts are not affected by the trauma and repair processes of ovulation. Within the ovarian cortex, the epithelial cells of the inclusion cysts are in closer proximity to the vasculature and to the steroid hormone-producing cells and activity (29). In summary, the evidence to date thus appears to suggest hormonal influences on the behavior of the ovarian epithelial cells.

Gonadotropins

The gonadotropin hypothesis initially arose from observations that ovarian tumors occurred in rodents following bilateral oophorectomy and subcapsular splenic transplantation (30). Intact ovarian function suppressed tumor formation, apparently by reducing gonadotropin hypersecretion. Aside from long-term photostimulation of poultry hens, ovarian tumors can be produced in animals by treatment with chemical carcinogens, X-irradiation, or neonatal thymectomy, the three methods causing destruction of follicles and ovarian failure. Ovarian tumors also occur spontaneously in certain strains of animals that are congenitally deficient in or that rapidly lose oocytes. These animals experience excessive gonadotropin stimulation, and tumor occurrence is reduced or blocked by treatment with depot gonadotropin releasing-hormone agonists, which suppress the gonadotropins. The neoplasms seen in animals are tubular adenomas, benign epithelial tumors which grow within and replace the ovarian stroma, but which do not invade in the uncontrolled fashion typical of malignant cancers, and which do not metastasize. Non-epithelial tumors, particularly of granulosa-cell type, also occur. Thus, the generalization of the various animal models to human OC is unclear. Nevertheless, Cramer has suggested that, under the same physiologic stimuli, the presence of epithelial inclusion cysts within human ovarian stroma could lead to a different spectrum of tumor types than occurs in rodents (31).

In the USA, the average age of occurrence of OC (total borderline and invasive) is about 57-59 years (24), while childbirth and oral contraceptive usage are frequent at ages 25-35, suggesting a latency of some 25-30 years. Follow-up of the atomic bomb survivors cohort, also shows a consistent estimate of 25 years latency among the most heavily exposed women, especially those younger than 40 at the time of the bombing (32). Serum FSH and LH climb to maximal values around and immediately after the menopause, paralleling the depletion of oocytes (33), and remain elevated thereafter. Age-specific OC incidence peaks in the mid- to late-70's, the same 25 years latency after the menopause. This suggests that a relationship may exist between the rise in gonadotropins and the later peak in incidence rates. However, given the average age of OC occurrence in the late-50's, the peri- and postmenopausal exposure to elevated gonadotropins would relate to incidence mostly after age 70, after some three-quarters of cases have occurred.

Ovarian epithelial cells near the time of ovulation are receptive to human chorionic gonadotropin (hCG) stimulation, in that they progress with lysosome secretion and ovulation. About 25% of benign ovarian tumors have been observed to bind hCG (and by implication, LH, which is very similar in protein sequence) (34). However, the epithelial binding seen was quite weak, in all cases <5 fmol/mg protein homogenate, values usually considered negative in studies of receptor binding. Also, in *in-vitro* cell culture, high concentration of hCG has been seen to stimulate the proliferation of rabbit ovarian epithelial cells, but FSH + LH applied together did not result in growth stimulation (35). The applicability of this finding to human epithelial cells *in vivo* is uncertain however.

Work over the last decade has suggested that insulin and insulin-like growth factors (IGFs) may modulate the effects of the gonadotropins (36). IGFs are found at relatively high serum concentrations, and are produced in the ovaries, as well as in the liver and elsewhere. *In vitro*, both insulin and IGF-I stimulate granulosa-cell and granulosa-lutein cell aromatase to increase conversion of androgens to E (36, 37). *In vivo*, however, the hormonal relationships are less clear. Insulin-dependent diabetes mellitus is characterized by hypoinsulinemia and normal insulin sensitivity of target tissues. Among insulin-treated postmenopausal diabetic women, increased serum total estrone (E_1) and 17β-estradiol (E_2) levels are seen, but because sex-hormone binding globulin (SHBG) also appears to be significantly elevated, the free fractions of these hormones remain normal. Non-obese women with non-insulin-dependent diabetes mellitus (NIDDM) tend to have slight insulin resistance, with inadequate insulin production as their main abnormality, whereas obese women with NIDDM have severe insulin resistance and hyperinsulinemia (38). Thus, it is unclear whether (or which forms of) diabetes mellitus, as opposed to obesity, might be related to the ovarian hormonal climate. A number of epidemiologic studies have shown significant positive associations between "history of diabetes mellitus" and risk of endometrial cancer (39), a disease considered to be related to unopposed E stimulation. However, the same and other studies have failed to show positive associations between history of diabetes and risk of OC. Whether an association exists, and what the implications for the gonadotropin hypothesis would be, remains to be seen; stratification by or adjustment for obesity is likely to be important. Obesity itself, if anything, may increase the risk of OC.

Finally, a recent prospective study gives direct evidence relating to the effects of the gonadotropins. Among participants to a specimen bank who were followed for more than 15 years after giving blood samples, 31 cases of OC occurred (40). These cases were compared to 62 matched non-cancer cohort controls on prediagnosis serum hormone levels. Cases were found to have significantly lower FSH levels than controls (P=0.04), but were without significant differences in serum LH levels. Thus, the evidence in total seems to suggest that the gonadotropins, while participating in the feedback regulation of ovarian steroid hormones, may not in themselves be responsible for alterations in OC risk, but could reflect certain hormonal circumstances that may be related to risk.

Estrogens

As we have seen, the evidence in support of hormonal mechanisms is largely indirect. The ovarian surface epithelium is avascular, suggesting a paracrine rather than endocrine influence of hormonal factors. Concerning Es, the ovarian epithelium is not itself normally (i.e., in the non-neoplastic state) very steroidogenically active (41). Most of ovarian steroidogenesis occurs under the control of FSH and LH in the granulosa and theca interna cells of developing and mature follicles, and under LH stimulation within secondary interstitial stromal cells which are derived from the theca cells following follicular atresia (33). E biosynthesis peaks sharply in the granulosa cells prior to ovulation (33), again somewhat in the midluteal phase, and falls after cycle day 22 (42). At ovulation, the epithelium is bathed in follicular fluid which may contain E_2 at levels about 10,000 times higher than circulating concentrations (42). Immediately after, the epithelial cells proliferate at the edges of the ovulatory wound, migrate over it, and contribute to wound repair. As a whole, during menstrual cycles the epithelium proliferates at times when estrogenic influences are relatively stronger, and the increased mitotic activity may enhance the risk of mutations occurring, which could then propagate clonally with additional epithelial cell division in further cycles.

Additional epidemiologic evidence bears on the role of Es in the etiology of OC. Breastfeeding, which appears protective (6, 24), is associated with lower serum E_2 (and also LH, but higher levels of FSH). Menopausal exogenous E therapy raises serum E_2 and E_1 levels and lowers gonadotropin levels. Increased risk of OC following menopausal E use was not generally seen in older studies, but a number of recent large studies do suggest increased risk with usage (43), and one older study found significantly increased risk with use of Premarin, and especially following use of diethylstilbestrol (44).

However, certain other observations imply that Es may not be the most relevant etiologic factor. Pregnancy increases serum Es about 100-fold, but is protective, thus some other hormone must be involved. If ovarian epithelial cells were responsive to estrogenic stimulation, then estrogen receptors (ER) should be found in them. Early studies did suggest that ERs are detectable in cytosols of normal human ovaries (45). However, more recent studies using monoclonal antibodies directed against E and other receptors have shown no ERs in surface epithelial cells or in inclusion cysts, but almost all of the sections of surface epithelium and all of the epithelial inclusion cysts expressed PRs (46), a fact relevant for the progesterone discussion, below. Finally, the recent cohort study of Helzlsouer, et al. (40). observed at baseline slightly lower E_2 levels for the cases compared to the matched controls.

Progesterone

Given our discussion above, it is likely that other hormonal factors are involved in the etiology of OC. One possibility is progesterone. Evidence for a protective role of progesterone begins with consideration of the increased sex hormone activity during pregnancy. Over the first mo. of pregnancy, maternal LH and FSH decline strongly with the increase in trophoblast hCG. The hCG also stimulates the corpus luteum to continue making progesterone and prevents its regression. By weeks 7-8, luteal-placental shift occurs, in which the massive placental production of progesterone starts. During pregnancy, the placental synthesis thus causes a 10.0-fold increase in maternal circulating progesterone levels. Thus, the protective aspect of pregnancy, not mediated through suppression of ovulation, might be the 8-9 mo. of elevated progesterone. After all, it seems unlikely to be due to the pregnancy Es, since most of the evidence relating Es to risk of OC points either to no effect or to increase in risk.

With respect to oral contraceptive usage, the synthetic progestogens in these agents could directly convey the reduced risk consistently seen according to duration of use. Alternatively, the magnitude of risk decrease could be consistent with protection due to ovulation suppression. During use of oral contraceptives, endogenous progesterone synthesis appears to be as low as it is during the early follicular phase of the menstrual cycle, without follicle maturation or corpus luteum functioning. However, given that the progestational potency of the synthetic 19-nortestosterone progestins is more than 100 times that of progesterone (47), and that serum levels of progestins absorbed from oral contraceptives are comparable to luteal-phase progesterone levels, e.g., 5 ng/ml (48), the total progestational exposure of the ovary is probably quite high (49). Thus, the decreased risk of OC with oral contraceptive use could also be due to the cyclic progestational climate.

Another piece of evidence implies that combined oral contraceptives offer OC protection beyond that potentially from suppressing ovulation. A recent case-control study identified a sufficiently large number of subjects who had used progestin-only types of oral contraceptives (50). These progestin-only formulations do not totally suppress ovulation and some ovulatory cycles generally occur (49); up to 40% of women using these agents have regular ovarian function, with normal E and luteal-phase progesterone synthesis (51). In the case-control study, relative to never use of progestin-only contraceptives, the risks were 0.39 for total use less than 3 years, and 0.21 for more than 3 years of use, with trend P=0.009. These lower risks are comparable to those associated with use of combined oral contraceptives, or perhaps even a little more protective (50). Thus, the progestin-only contraceptives create a progestational hormonal environment with a lowered risk that cannot be totally attributed to suppression of ovulation. Given that combined oral contraceptives convey a similar degree of protection but with less ovulation, it seems apparent that OC risk reduction associated with ovulation suppression cannot comprise the total protection given by the combined preparations, and that the net benefit is likely to be due to the progestogen.

A similar degree of protection may exist with usage of depot medroxyprogesterone acetate (DMPA). DMPA is a long-acting 17-acetoxy progesterone which suppresses endogenous progesterone synthesis and ovulation. E_2 levels also stay low, in the early to midfollicular phase range, <100 pg/ml (52). Serum levels of DMPA remain about 1 ng/ml for three mo. after injection; these levels inhibit the midcycle peak in gonadotropins but do not seem to change basal LH and FSH levels (52). Only one adequate study has examined usage of DMPA and risk of OC. This was the large WHO international case-control study, which found for nonmucinous OC a significantly reduced risk of 0.42 (95% CI 0.15-0.96) with ever usage (53). DMPA use may thus protect against the development of OC, though further studies would help to confirm this fact.

The effects of physical exercise may also bear on a possible relationship between progesterone activity and OC. In a prospective study of 31,000 Iowa women followed for seven years (54), a significant increasing trend in risk of OC was seen according to increasing value of an index of usual physical activity. Other reports have also suggested greater risk with employment in jobs categorized as having moderate (compared to low) physical activity levels: manual workers, physical education teachers, and jobs with little sitting time. Increased physical activity is associated with a shortened luteal phase, resulting in lower luteal progesterone levels. This finding applies to female nonathletes as well as athletes. Even moderate recreational physical activity without amenorrhea or other menstrual disturbances may be associated with decreased progesterone levels (55). However, if ovulation is indeed involved in the pathogenesis of OC, then women whose regular physical activity is intense or frequent enough to cause amenorrhea may be at decreased risk due to the ovulation suppression.

Summary

Overall, it appears that incessant ovulation could play a part in the pathogenesis of OC, but that an additional factor, probably hormonal, must also be involved. Independent evidence for the gonadotropins as that factor is not obvious at present. Some evidence supports E, although perhaps stronger evidence implicates a protective role of progesterone in the etiology.

Acknowledgment

Supported by grants 1R01 CA63682 and 1R01 CA74850 from NIH.

References

1. Risch HA, Marrett LD, Jain M et al (1996) Differences in risk factors for epithelial ovarian cancer by histologic type: results of a case-control study. Am J Epidemiol 144:363-372.
2. Fathalla MF (1971) Incessant ovulation -a factor in ovarian neoplasia? Lancet 2:163.
3. Casagrande JT, Pike MC, Ross RK et al (1979) "Incessant ovulation" and ovarian cancer. Lancet 2:170-173.
4. Cramer DW, Welch WR (1983) Determinants of ovarian cancer risk. II. Inferences regarding pathogenesis. J Natl Cancer Inst 71:717-721.
5. Franceschi S, Parazzini F, Negri E et al (1991) Pooled analysis of 3 European case-control studies of epithelial ovarian cancer: III. Oral contraceptive use. Int J Cancer 49:61-65.
6. Whittemore AS, Harris R, Itnyre J et al (1992) Characteristics relating to ovarian cancer risk: collaborative analysis of 12 US case-control studies. II. Invasive epithelial ovarian cancers in white women. Am J Epidemiol 136:1184-1203.
7. Wilson JE (1958) Adeno-carcinomata in hens kept in a constant environment. Poultry Sci 37:1253.
8. Godwin AK, Testa JR, Handel LM et al (1992) Spontaneous transformation of rat ovarian surface epithelial cells: Association with cytogenetic changes and implications of repeated ovulation in the etiology of ovarian cancer. J Natl Cancer Inst 84:592-601.

9. Mittal KR, Zeleniuch-Jacquotte A, Cooper JL et al (1993) Contralateral ovary in unilateral ovarian carcinoma: A search for preneoplastic lesions. Int J Gynecol Pathol12:59-63.

10. Westhoff C, Murphy P, Heller D et al (1993) Is ovarian cancer associated with an increased frequency of germinal inclusion cysts? Am J Epidemiol 138:90-93.

11. Cruickshank DJ (1990) Aetiological importance of ovulation in epithelial ovarian cancer: a population based study. Br Med J 301:524-525.

12. Hartge P, Devesa S (1995) Ovarian cancer, ovulation and side of origin. Br J Cancer 71:642-643.

13. Potashnik G, Insler V, Meizner I et al (1987) Frequency, sequence, and side of ovulation in women menstruating normally. Br Med J 294:219.

14. Balasch J, Penarrubia J, Marquez M et al (1994) Ovulation side and ovarian cancer. Gynecol Endocrinol 8:51-54.

15. Montesano R, Hainaut P, Wild CP (1997) Hepatocellular carcinoma: from gene to public health. J Natl Cancer Inst 89:1844-1851.

16. Fearon ER, Vogelstein B (1990) A genetic model for colorectal tumorigenesis. Cell 61:759-767.

17. Eltabbakh GH, Belinson JL, Kennedy AW et al (1997) p53 overexpression is not an independent prognostic factor for patients with primary ovarian epithelial cancer. Cancer 80:892-898.

18. Berchuck A, Kohler MF, Hopkins MP et al (1994) Overexpression of p53 is not a feature of benign and early-stage borderline epithelial ovarian tumors. Gynecol Oncol 52:232-236.

19. Eltabbakh GH, Belinson JL, Kennedy AW et al (1997) p53 and HER-2/neu overexpression in ovarian borderline tumors. Gynecol Oncol 65:218-224.

20. Mazars R, Pujol P, Maudelonde T et al (1991) p53 mutations in ovarian cancer: a late event? Oncogene 6:1685-1690.

21. Sood AK, Skilling JS, Buller RE (1997) Ovarian cancer genomic instability correlates with p53 frameshift mutations. Cancer Res 57:1047-1049.

22. Schildkraut JM, Bastos E, Berchuck A (1997) Relationship between lifetime ovulatory cycles and overexpression of mutant p53 in epithelial ovarian cancer. J Natl Cancer Inst 89:932-938.

23. Risch HA (1997) Re: Relationship between lifetime ovulatory cycles and overexpression of mutant p53 in epithelial ovarian cancer. J Natl Cancer Inst 89:1726-1727.

24. Risch HA, Marrett LD, Howe GR (1994) Parity, contraception, infertility, and the risk of epithelial ovarian cancer. Am J Epidemiol 140:585-597.

25. Harlow SD, Ephross SA (1995) Epidemiology of menstruation and its relevance to women's health. Epidemiol Rev 17:265-286.

26. Parazzini F, La Vecchia C, Negri E et al (1989) Menstrual factors and the risk of epithelial ovarian cancer. J Clin Epidemiol 42:443-448.

27. Salazar H, Godwin AK, Daly MB et al (1996) Microscopic benign and invasive malignant neoplasms and a cancer-prone phenotype in prophylactic oophorectomies. J Natl Cancer Inst 88:1810-1820.

28. Resta L, Russo S, Colucci GA et al (1993) Morphologic precursors of ovarian epithelial tumors. Obstet Gynecol 82:181-186.

29. Godwin AK, Perez RP, Johnson SW et al (1992) Growth regulation of ovarian cancer. Hematol Oncol Clin North Am 6:829-841.

30. Biskind MS, Biskind GR (1944) Development of tumors in the rat ovary after transplantation into the spleen. Proc Soc Exp Biol Med 55:176-179.

31. Cramer DW (1990) Epidemiologic aspects of early menopause and ovarian cancer. Ann N Y Acad Sci 592:363-375.

32. Tokuoka S, Kawai K, Shimizu Y et al (1987) Malignant and benign ovarian neoplasms among atomic bomb survivors, Hiroshima and Nagasaki, 1950-1980. J Natl Cancer Inst 79:47-57.

33. Carr BR (1993) The ovary. In: Carr BR, Blackwell RE (eds) Textbook of reproductive medicine. Appleton and Lange, Norwalk, CT, pp. 183-207.

34. Rajaniemi H, Kauppila A, Ronnberg L et al (1981) LH(hCG) receptor in benign and malignant tumors of human ovary. Acta Obstet Gynecol Scand Suppl 101:83-86.

35. Osterholzer HO, Streibel EJ, Nicosia SV (1985) Growth effects of protein hormones on cultured rabbit ovarian surface epithelial cells. Biol Reprod 33:247-258.

36. Yong EL, Baird DT, Yates R et al (1992) Hormonal regulation of the growth and steroidogenic function of human granulosa cells. J Clin Endocrinol Metab 74:842-849.

37. Erickson GF, Garzo VG, Magoffin DA (1989) Insulin-like growth factor-I regulates aromatase activity in human granulosa and granulosa luteal cells. J Clin Endocrinol Metab 69:716-724.

38. Henry RR (1996) Glucose control and insulin resistance in non-insulin-dependent diabetes mellitus. Ann Intern Med 124:97-103.

39. La Vecchia C, Negri E, Franceschi S et al (1994) A case-control study of diabetes mellitus and cancer risk. Br J Cancer 70:950-953.

40. Helzlsouer KJ, Alberg AJ, Gordon GB et al (1995) Serum gonadotropins and steroid hormones and the development of ovarian cancer. J Am Med Ass 274:1926-1930.

41. Guraya SS (1980) Histochemistry of the ovary. In: Motta PM, Hafez ESE (eds) Biology of the ovary. Martinus Nijhoff Publishers, New York, pp.33-51.

42. Clement PB (1987) Histology of the ovary. Am J Surgical Pathol 11:277-303.

43. Risch HA (1996) Estrogen replacement therapy and risk of epithelial ovarian cancer. Gynecol Oncol 63:254-257.

44. Hoover R, Gray LA Sr, Fraumeni JF Jr (1977) Stilboestrol (diethylstilbestrol) and the risk of ovarian cancer. Lancet 2:533-534.
45. Toppila M, Tyler JPP, Fay R et al (1986) Steroid receptors in human ovarian malignancy: a review of four years tissue collection. Br J Obstet Gynaecol 93:986-992.
46. Zeimet AG, Müller-Holzner E, Marth C et al (1994) Immunocytochemical versus biochemical receptor determination in normal and tumorous tissues of the female reproductive tract and the breast. J Steroid Biochem Molec Biol 49:365-372.
47. Ryder TA, Mobberley MA, Whitehead MI (1995) The endometrial nucleolar channel system as an indicator of progestin potency in HRT. Maturitas 22:31-36.
48. Brenner PF, Mishell DR Jr, Stanczyk FZ et al (1977) Serum levels of d-norgestrel, luteinizing hormone, follicle-stimulating hormone, estradiol, and progesterone in women during and following ingestion of combination oral contraceptives containing dl-norgestrel. Am J Obstet Gynecol 129:133-140.
49. King RJB (1991) Biology of female sex hormone action in relation to contraceptive agents and neoplasia. Contraception 43:527-542.
50. Rosenberg L, Palmer JR, Zauber AG et al (1994) A case-control study of oral contraceptive use and invasive epithelial ovarian cancer. Am J Epidemiol 139:654-661.
51. Stubblefield PG (1993) Contraception. In: Copeland LJ, Jarrell JF, McGregor JA (eds) Textbook of gynecology. WB Saunders Co., Philadelphia, pp.156-188.
52. Mishell DR Jr (1996) Pharmacodynamics of depot medroxyprogesterone acetate contraception. J Reprod Med 41:381-390.
53. Stanford JL, Thomas DB (1991) Depot-medroxyprogesterone acetate (DMPA) and risk of epithelial ovarian cancer. The WHO Collaborative Study of Neoplasia and Steroid Contraceptives. Int J Cancer 49:191-195.
54. Mink PJ, Folsom AR, Sellers TA et al (1996) Physical activity, waist-to-hip ratio, and other risk factors for ovarian cancer: a follow-up study of older women. Epidemiology 7:38-45.
55. Ellison PT, Lager C (1986) Moderate recreational running is associated with lowered salivary progesterone profiles in women. Am J Obstet Gynecol 154:1000-1003.

24

Stromal Influences in Prostatic Carcinogenesis

Gerald R. Cunha, Simon W. Hayward, Thea Tlsty, and Gary D. Grossfeld

Introduction

It has been estimated that 184,500 new cases of prostate cancer (PRCA) will be diagnosed in the USA during 1998 and that 39,200 deaths will result from this disease. Thus, PRCA is the most commonly diagnosed malignancy, and the second leading cause of cancer-related death amongst American men. Our laboratory has investigated some of the unique biological characteristics of PRCA with the ultimate goal of formulating new, less invasive therapeutic strategies. We have recently hypothesized that epigenetic influences from adjacent stromal cells may be crucial in determining whether a particular prostate tumor remains dormant or becomes invasive (1). This hypothesis (Figure 1) suggests that subsequent to initial genetic damage to prostatic epithelium (PRE), signaling from epithelium to the surrounding stroma/mesenchyme (SM) cells becomes abnormal, resulting in dedifferentiation of SM towards a fibroblastic phenotype. One of the predicted consequences of such a change in differentiation state of SM is that the local microenvironment of the epithelium becomes altered, and thus the influence of stroma on epithelium changes from homeostatic to mitogenic. These changes subsequently lead to increased epithelial proliferation, migration and ultimately, to an increase in invasive potential of genetically altered prostatic epithelial cells.

Genetic Changes in Cancer

Carcinogenesis has been described as a complex multi-step process in which a series of genetic alterations involving oncogenes and tumor suppressor genes may be required during progression. This has been illustrated in colorectal cancer where both early and late events have been identified and in which roles of specific "gatekeeper" gene products (specific proteins protective against neoplastic progression) have been described (2). For example, adenomatous polyposis coli gene (APC) has been shown to be the gatekeeper for colon cancer. Other gatekeeper genes have also been identified, such as Rb in retinoblastoma and VHL gene in renal cell carcinoma. However, for PRCA and the vast majority of human malignancies gatekeeper genes have not yet been identified.

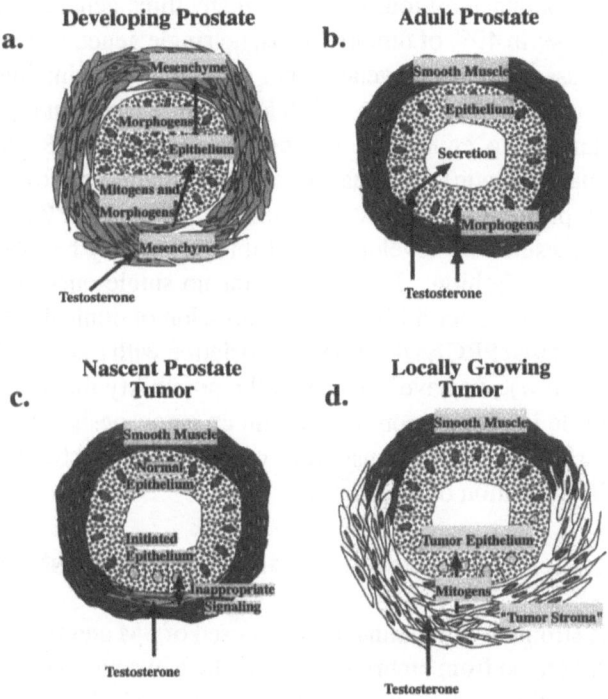

Figure 1. Interactions between epithelial and SM of prostate during development and adulthood. During prostatic development, (a) low levels of androgens, acting through mesenchymal androgen receptor (AR), stimulate proliferation and differentiation of PRE. Concurrently, epithelium induces differentiation of mesenchyme into SM. In the normal adult, (b) high levels of circulating androgens, acting through AR located in SM, maintain morphology of growth-quiescent adult epithelium. Secretory function is elicited by direct androgenic stimulation of AR in differentiated columnar epithelium. Epithelial and SM differentiation is maintained by paracrine acting morphogenic factors. In early tumors we have hypothesized that following genetic insult to epithelium (c) signaling between epithelium and adjacent SM becomes abnormal, leading to (d) formation of a fibroblastic "tumor stroma" which can respond to androgenic stimulation by producing paracrine acting mitogens, fueling a cycle of tumor proliferation and stromal and epithelial dedifferentiation.

Even though for certain carcinomas there appears to be a preferred sequence of genetic alterations, it should be noted that specific genetic changes do not necessarily lead consistently to the same type of lesion. For example, Vogelstein examined four genetic abnormalities and proposed that these occurred in a specific order during colorectal tumor formation (3). However, only 10% of tumors actually contained all four lesions, and any three genetic changes were only found together in 40% of tumors. Thus, no single genetic alteration could be cited as necessary for carcinogenesis, nor could any combination of genetic lesions be characterized as common, much less required for tumor progression.

Genetic damage to epithelium is clearly a feature of PRCA. Genetic analysis of human prostatic tumors has consistently found genetic abnormalities in PRE in both primary and metastatic tumors. Studies on PRCA in certain families has suggested that development of this tumor may be inherited in an autosomal dominant fashion. However, so far no single oncogene has been conclusively linked to either initiation or progression of clinical PRCA.

Given the fact that PRCAs develop in association with a stroma that is itself abnormal (see below), we have considered the possibility that stroma may be playing a key role in progression of prostatic carcinogenesis. This possibility stems from earlier studies demonstrating central roles of stroma in normal growth and differentiation of the prostate.

Stromal-Epithelial Interactions in the Normal Prostate

Adult prostatic stroma is predominantly composed of SM and fibroblastic cells which are both derived from embryonic urogenital sinus mesenchyme (UGM). Adult PRE are intimate associated with a mixture of SM cells and a few interspersed fibroblasts. Differentiation of prostatic SM from UGM occurs via reciprocal androgen-dependent mesenchymal-epithelial interactions (4). During development UGM induces and specifies patterns of epithelial morphogenesis, regulates epithelial proliferation, promotes epithelial cytodifferentiation, and induces and specifies epithelial functional or biochemical activity (4). In reciprocal fashion, as the induced PRE differentiates, it in turn signals UGM to differentiate into SM (5). Both epithelial and prostatic SM differentiation require androgens (6). As AR-positive UGM differentiates into prostatic SM, these SM cells continue to express AR. In regard to prostatic epithelial development, analysis of tissue recombinations composed of AR-positive wild-type (wt) UGM plus AR-deficient testicular feminized (Tfm) epithelium has demonstrated that androgen-induced epithelial ductal morphogenesis, epithelial mitogenesis, and certain aspects of epithelial differentiation are elicited via AR in stroma/mesenchyme (4). Epithelial AR are only required for expression of androgen-dependent secretory proteins (7, 8).

In adulthood, androgenic stimulation is required to maintain both PRE and SM in a fully differentiated, growth-quiescent state. Epithelial AR, required for expression of epithelial secretory activity, are not required to maintain the basic simple columnar morphology of PRE (4). In contrast, experiments using so-called Tfm/wt tissue recombination model strongly suggests that in adulthood maintenance of prostatic homeostasis by androgens is primarily due to action of androgens on AR-positive SM cells that in turn signal to maintain epithelial cytodifferentiation and growth-quiescence.

Androgens have several effects on prostate: (a) induction of prostatic morphogenesis, (b) stimulation of epithelial proliferation, (c) prevention of epithelial cell death, (d) maintenance of adult prostatic epithelial structure and function, and (e) maintenance of prostatic SM differentiation (9). Androgens stimulate normal prostatic epithelial proliferation only during fetal, neonatal, and pubertal growth periods. In adulthood, androgens stimulate epithelial proliferation if the prostate has been previously subjected to a period of androgen-deprivation. All periods when prostatic epithelial growth occurs have in common an elevated stromal/epithelial ratio and presence of mesenchymal/fibroblastic cells in the stroma (9). Thus, prostatic epithelial proliferation *in vivo* is induced by androgens action on a mesenchymal/fibroblastic stroma. Conversely, if stromal cells associated with PRE are fully differentiated SM cells, androgens do not elicit epithelial proliferation, but instead maintain a growth-quiescent secretory epithelium. This idea is supported by studies in adult rodent prostate suggesting that presence of fibroblastic cells in association with prostatic ductal tips is important in mediating epithelial proliferation that occurs specifically at tips of prostatic ducts (10). Epithelial proliferation is exceedingly low in proximal ducts where thick SM sheaths surround the ducts. Thus, status of prostatic stroma, whether it be predominantly SM or fibroblastic/mesenchymal, appears be a critical determinant in regulating epithelial differentiation and proliferation.

In summary, in developing prostate, low levels of androgens act upon mesenchyme to induce prostatic ductal morphogenesis, epithelial proliferation and differentiation, while in adulthood, high levels of androgens act upon prostatic SM to maintain a growth-quiescent, functional secretory epithelium. Epithelial proliferation is mediated *in vivo* via stromal AR. In contrast, functional epithelial AR is required for expression of prostatic secretory proteins (8). In castrated males, administration of exogenous androgens initially promotes prostatic epithelial proliferation and differentiation via partially dedifferentiated SM cells expressing fibroblastic markers. As a result of androgen replacement, fully differentiated prostatic SM cells reappear and maintain a fully differentiated functional growth-quiescent PRE through cell-cell interactions. Thus, local control of prostatic epithelial proliferation and differentiation is a result of androgenic stimulation of prostatic stroma. The type of response (proliferation versus differentiation) is determined by the nature of the stromal cells. Apparently, prostatic SM responds to androgens by inhibiting epithelial proliferation and maintaining epithelial functional differentiation (perhaps through activity of TGFβs), while AR expressing prostatic mesenchymal cells/fibroblasts (such as those of fetal prostate or androgen-deprived adult prostate) elicit epithelial proliferative activity.

Tumor Associated Stromal Cells

Considerable evidence supports the concept of "tumor stroma", which is defined as connective tissue cells and extracellular matrix in immediate association with carcinoma cells. Such an abnormal stroma has been documented in a variety of carcinomas. For example, stromas surrounding invasive carcinomas of the breast, cervix, colon, ovary, and skin cancer is composed of "activated" or abnormal myofibroblastic cells (11). Such myofibroblastic cells are not found in normal stroma. In addition, stromal cells associated with breast and other types of carcinomas abnormally over-express certain matrix metalloproteinases (MMP) or inhibitors of metalloproteinases (12). MMPs are thought to contribute in a paracrine manner to epithelial cell malignancy (13). Phenotypic changes associated with carcinoma-associated fibroblasts (CAF) include changes in migratory behavior of these fibroblasts in vitro as well as increased agglutinability by concanavalin-A (14). Composition of intra- and peritumoral extracellular matrix is also altered (11), which may augment invasive potential of malignant epithelial cells. Given the many abnormal features of tumor stroma, it has been suggested that without tumor stroma there would be no tumors (15).

By altering the local micro-environment of carcinoma cells, the "tumor stroma" may modulate malignant phenotype and behavior. For example, when MCF-7 breast carcinoma cells are co-cultured with various types of fibroblasts, their phenotype, including expression of estrogen receptor, progesterone receptor, pS2, and cathepsin-D, was found to be influenced by the type of fibroblasts with which they were co-cultured (16).

With respect to prostatic carcinogenesis, we have hypothesized that following genetic alteration of PRE, a sequential disruption occurs in reciprocal homeostatic interactions between the prostatic SM and the associated epithelium. This results in de-differentiation of both emerging PRCA cells and surrounding SM (1). Thus, genetic insult to PRE may lead to inappropriate or abnormal signaling from initiated epithelium to surrounding SM. This elicits conversion of a predominantly SM stroma into a predominantly fibroblastic stroma either through dedifferentiation or apoptosis of SM. As cellular composition of stroma changes, signaling from prostatic stroma to PRE becomes aberrant resulting in progressive change in epithelial differentiation and proliferation. During progression of prostatic carcinogenesis a vicious cycle is initiated in which de-differentiation occurs in both PRE and SM, a concomitant increase in both epithelial and stromal proliferation.

This hypothesis predicts a change in cellular composition of PRCAs as compared to normal human prostate. Indeed, using immunohistochemistry, we have demonstrated that whereas stroma of normal human prostate is predominantly composed of SM cells, stroma of human prostatic adenocarcinomas is predominantly composed of fibroblastic cells (Figure 2). Another prediction of our hypothesis is that CAF should profoundly affect phenotypic expression of adjacent epithelial cells through promotion of carcinogenesis and tumorigenesis. This has been verified recently both *in vivo* and *in vitro*.

We have developed an *in-vivo* model which involves analysis of tissue recombinants composed of an immortal but non-tumorigenic clonally derived human prostatic epithelial cell line plus CAF derived from human prostatic adenocarcinomas. In this model, the initiated epithelial cell population is represented by the human prostatic cell line BPH-1, which was immortalized using SV40T antigen (17). While BPH-1 cells clearly have acquired genetic abnormalities, these human prostatic epithelial cells are non-tumorigenic when grown alone either subcutaneously or beneath the renal capsule of athymic hosts for up to one year (17, and unpublished results). Primary human prostatic CAF were obtained from human prostate tumors. BPH-1 cells and CAF, grown individually as grafts for 20 to 85 days in nude mice, survived at the graft site but exhibited minimal growth with a median wet weight of 10 mg or less. Histologic examination demonstrated that grafts of BPH-1 cells alone formed keratinized pearls demonstrating their well-differentiated phenotype, while grafts of CAF alone demonstrated a benign appearing fibroblastic stroma (18). Experimental tissue recombinants contained 1×10^5 BPH-1 cells and 2.5×10^5 human prostatic CAF in 50 µl of type I rat tail collagen. These resultant gels were grafted beneath renal capsules of male athymic rodents.

Tissue recombinants composed of CAF + BPH-1 cells exhibited striking growth reaching wet weights of over 5 grams in 41 days (from an initial weight of 10 mg). The large size of many tumors and local destruction of the renal graft site compromised health of the nude mouse hosts. Composition of individual tumors was approximately 80% epithelial, as judged by morphometric analysis. Histopathologic appearance of tumors was consistent with poorly-differentiated prostatic adenocarcinoma. Tumors contained poorly differentiated, irregular epithelial cords of varying sizes, small nests of aberrant glands and single epithelial cells intermingled within a fibrous stroma (Figure 3).

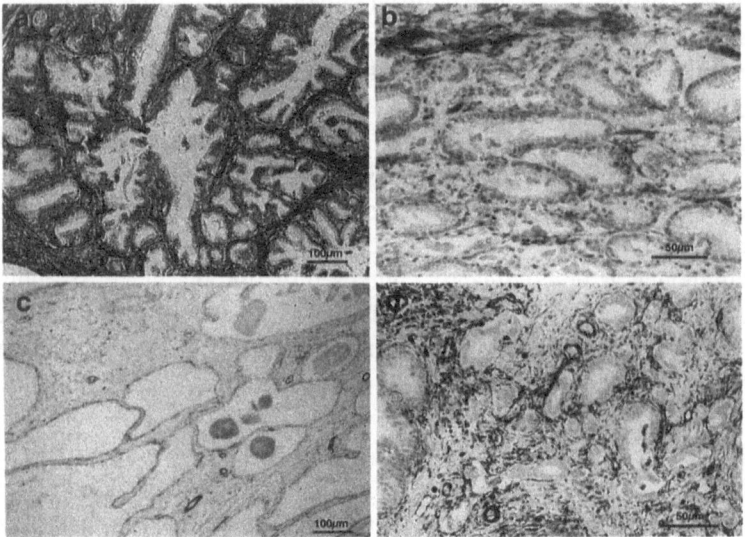

Figure 2. Expression of SM α-actin (a and b) and vimentin (c and d) in normal prostate (a and c) and in prostatic tumors (b and d). Stroma of normal prostate in the region of glandular epithelium is predominantly SM with vimentin expression localized to blood vessels (arrows). In prostatic tumors, α-actin expression is much less prominent while the fibroblast marker vimentin is much more widely distributed.

Epithelial nature of the tumor cells was confirmed by immunostaining and the BPH-1 origin of tumor cells was confirmed by nuclear staining with an antibody to SV40T antigen. Intermixed with these poorly differentiated epithelial cells were areas of a more highly differentiated stratified squamous cornified epithelium. Stromal cells were intermingled between epithelial cell islands throughout the tumor making tissue boundaries difficult to discern. In contrast to the malignant histologic appearance of CAF + BPH-1 recombinants, growth was minimal when BPH-1 cells were grown in association with stromal cells derived from non-malignant human prostates (NHPF). By histological analysis NHPF + BPH-1 recombinants appeared benign. Epithelial cells in NHPF + BPH-1 tissue recombinants formed small solid cords that could only be found by serial section of consistently small grafts. Even more striking were UGM + BPH-1 recombinants, in which BPH-1 cells formed highly differentiated branched ductal structures resembling developing prostatic tissue. UGM + BPH-1 recombinants were notable for highly ordered tissue architecture, which was in stark contrast to chaotic tissue architecture seen in CAF + BPH-1 recombinants. These studies demonstrated that stromal cells derived from normal versus neoplastic prostates exerted differential effects on non-tumorigenic human PRE *in vivo*. Normal stromal cells induced BPH-1 cells to form branched prostatic ductal structures. In contrast, tumor-derived stromal cells induced chaotic tissue organization, rapid epithelial proliferation (Figure 3), and tumor formation. Thus, these data suggest that both genetic and epigenetic mechanisms are important in human prostatic carcinogenesis.

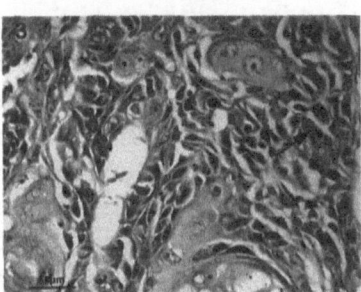

Figure 3. A tissue recombinant composed of human prostate tumor derived fibroblasts and the non-tumorigenic epithelial cell line BPH-1 grown as a subrenal capsule graft for 42 days in an adult male athymic rat host. Note glandular epithelial morphology characteristic of adenocarcinoma.

As an *in-vitro* counterpart of the *in-vivo* model described above, a system was developed in which BPH-1 cells are plated onto a confluent lawn of fibroblastic cells derived from either malignant CAF or NHPF. For this purpose, stromal cells were grown to confluence on microscope slides after which BPH-1 cells were plated at low density onto the confluent stromal layer and grown for 48 h. Control cultures of stromal cells only or BPH-1 cells only were also grown on microscope slides for 48 h. BPH-1 cells cultured for 48 h on a confluent monolayer of "normal" human prostatic fibroblasts grew as discreet coherent colonies with few single cells between epithelial colonies (Figure 4). BPH-1 cells of these multi-cellular colonies expressed E-cadherin along adjacent cell membranes. Individual epithelial colonies had smooth regular borders and were round or oval shaped. In contrast, BPH-1 cells cultured for 48 h on a confluent monolayer of CAF grew as single cells or small colonies with ragged edges. Many cells overlapped each other suggesting a loss of contact inhibition. E-cadherin expression was markedly decreased, and in many cases undetectable in BPH-1 cells co-cultured with CAF. Mean colony size of BPH-1 cells cultured on CAF was significantly lower than that of BPH-1 cells cultured on normal fibroblasts. Thus, the nature of stromal micro-environment can influence phenotypic expression of human prostatic epithelial cells both *in vitro* and *in vivo*.

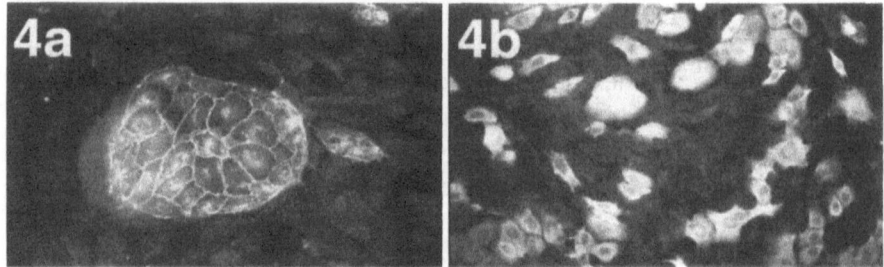

Figure 4. Expression of E-cadherin (a) in a BPH-1 epithelial colony growing on a confluent layer of stromal cells derived from normal prostate. Note the even smooth-edged colony morphology, and expression of E-cadherin along cell margins. BPH-1 cells grown on fibroblasts derived from a prostate tumor (b) have a very different morphology. Many single scattered cells are seen, and the edges of the few epithelial colonies have a ragged appearance.

The concept that stroma plays a role in prostatic carcinogenesis is supported by studies of Thompson, *et al.* (19), who demonstrated a regulatory role of stroma during prostatic carcinogenesis. A novel *in-vivo* mouse prostatic reconstitution system was developed by these workers who infected either urogenital sinus or its individual mesenchymal (UGM) or epithelial (UGE) components with a virus containing the *myc* and *ras* oncogenes. Prostatic reconstitutions composed of uninfected UGM + infected UGE gave rise to epithelial hyperplasias. Stromal desmoplasias developed when prostatic reconstitutions were made with infected UGM + uninfected UGE. Carcinomas developed only in prostatic reconstitutions in which both UGM and UGE were infected (19). Thus, aberrant expression of *ras* and in both UGM and UGE were required to achieve epithelial malignancy, and carcinomas only developed when stromal change accompanied epithelial alteration, suggesting that an abnormal stroma may be a requirement or a facilitator of the carcinogenic process.

Several studies examining the role of stromal cells in prostatic tumorigenesis have originated from the laboratory of Leland Chung. Coinoculation of tumorigenic NbF-1 (sarcomatous) fibroblasts with human PC-3 prostatic carcinoma cells accelerated tumor growth and shortened tumor latency (20). Similar studies have been performed on the human LnCaP prostatic carcinoma cell line (21, 22). These studies further demonstrated that fibroblasts differed in their ability to enhance prostatic carcinogenesis (21). Fibroblasts derived from rat UGM and human bone, but not other sources, accelerated tumorigenesis of human LnCaP cells *in vivo*. It should be noted that the above studies by Chung, et al. (20-22), have utilized anaplastic, highly tumorigenic PRCA cell lines growing in association with either tumorigenic or benign fibroblasts. In contrast, our CAF + BPH-1 recombinants have utilized non-tumorigenic fibroblasts and non-tumorigenic, but immortalized, PRE. Thus, Chung's studies deal with enhancement of tumorigenesis in established carcinoma cells, whereas our CAF + BPH-1 recombinant studies deal with progression of benign prostatic epithelial cells to form carcinomas.

Chung's initial studies attempted to examine the ability of prostatic stromal cells to promote carcinogenic progression of benign prostatic epithelial cells. These experiments involved coinoculating tumorigenic NbF-1 fibroblasts with a non-tumorigenic prostatic epithelial cell line (NbE-1 cells). The tumorigenic rat NbF-1 prostatic fibroblasts formed sarcomas when grown alone (23). Coinoculation of NbF-1 fibroblasts with benign NbE-1 prostatic epithelial cells formed large "carcinosarcomas" as early as 9 days. The epithelium comprised only 2-5% of tumor mass. Histopathologic changes, that may have occurred in epithelium as a result of coinoculation with the tumorigenic NbF-1 cells, were not specified.

Benign Stroma as an Inhibitor of Prostatic Tumorigenesis

The concept that interactions between epithelium and stroma can inhibit tumorigenesis has been examined using rat Dunning prostatic adenocarcinoma R3327 (DT). The interface between epithelium and stroma in this tumor is highly abnormal as the basement membrane separating epithelial and stromal cells is frequently discontinuous or excessively reduplicated. Moreover, stromal cells within Dunning tumor are abnormal, being comprised almost exclusively of fibroblastic cells with an absence of SM cells. Thus, stromal-epithelial interactions in Dunning tumor are clearly abnormal, which suggested the possibility that Dunning carcinoma cells might be "normalized" through interaction with normal stroma. To test this hypothesis, small fragments of DT, or epithelial DT epithelial cell suspensions were grown for one mo. in male athymic rodent hosts either alone or in association with "normal" stroma derived for embryonic UGM or neonatal seminal vesicle mesenchyme (SVM). Grafts of DT alone maintained a characteristic histopathology of the DT, forming large tumors containing small ducts lined by one or more layers of undifferentiated squamous or cuboidal epithelial cells. In grafts of UGM or SVM + DT, the DT epithelial cells differentiated into tall columnar secretory cells organized into large cystic ducts (24). Mesenchyme-induced phenotypic changes in DT epithelial histodifferentiation were associated with striking changes in growth (25). DT cells induced to differentiate by SVM or UGM were shown to have an 8.0-fold reduction in growth rate and marked reduction of tumorigenic abilities when compared to parental Dunning tumor cells (25). For example, ducts from primary SVM + DT recombinants were subsequently grafted directly to new

330 G.R. Cunha, et al.

male hosts or were recombined with fresh SVM to form secondary SVM + DT recombinants. Both types of grafts exhibited minimal growth during a 3.0-mo. period in nude mouse hosts, and maintained a highly differentiated state. Control grafts of primary DT alone formed large tumor masses weighting 5 to 7 grams during the same time period. It was interesting and significant to note that in SVM + DT recombinants SM cells (apparently derived from the SVM) were found in close apposition to highly differentiated DT epithelium. This supports the idea that prostatic SM plays a role in maintaining (or inducing) epithelial differentiation and epithelial growth-quiescence.

Conclusions - The Importance of both Genetic and Epigenetic Effects

The studies described above suggest that both genetic and epigenetic events are important in promotion of PRCA, and suggest the following concepts. (A) Carcinoma-associated fibroblasts can promote carcinogenesis in a genetically altered human PRE but not in genetically normal human PRE. (B) Normal stroma does not promote tumorigenesis in genetically altered human PRE, but may in some cases cause certain carcinoma cells to differentiate with a concomitant abrogation in tumorigenesis. (C) Carcinoma-associated stromal cells do not form tumors when grown in absence of epithelium. These concepts apply particularly to emerging carcinoma in-situ as stromal microenvironment may play a determining role in the slow in-vivo progression from a normal PRE to an invasive carcinoma. These concepts probably do not apply to highly anaplastic tumorigenic cell lines such as LnCaP, DU-145 and PC-3, which are adapted for cell culture.

Implications of "tumor stroma" as a determinant of tumor growth are potentially important from both a diagnostic and therapeutic perspective. For example, the ability to identify tumor stromal populations that promote down-regulation of E-cadherin in the carcinoma cells would be immensely important in identifying patients at risk for malignant progression of their prostatic adenocarcinoma. Traditional therapy for all epithelial malignancies, including PRCA, has been targeted at carcinoma cells. These cells, however, represent a "moving target" due to their genetic instability. Although carcinoma-associated stromal cells are abnormal, preliminary studies using comparative genomic hybridization have shown that these cells are genetically normal. Therefore, "tumor stroma" may represent a more stable target at which to direct treatment. For example, therapy targeted at carcinoma-associated stroma to up-regulate epithelial E-cadherin could be used to maintain prostatic tumors in a highly differentiated, non-invasive phenotype.

References

1. Hayward SW, Rosen MA, Cunha GR (1997) Stromal-epithelial interactions in normal and neoplastic prostate. Br J Urology 79 (Suppl. 2):18-26.
2. Kinzler KW, Vogelstein B (1996) Lessons from hereditary colorectal cancer. Cell 87:159-170.
3. Vogelstein B, Fearon ER, Hamilton SR et al (1988) Genetic alterations during colorectal-tumor development. N Engl J Med 319:525-532.
4. Cunha GR, Donjacour AA, Cooke PS et al (1987) The endocrinology and developmental biology of the prostate. Endocrine Rev 8:338-362.
5. Cunha GR, Battle E, Young P et al (1992) Role of epithelial-mesenchymal interactions in the differentiation and spatial organization of visceral smooth muscle. Epithelial Cell Biol 1:76-83.
6. Hayward SW, Cunha GR, Dahiya R (1996) Normal development and carcinogenesis of the prostate: A unifying hypothesis. Ann N Y Acad Sci 784:50-62.
7. Cunha GR, Young P (1991) Inability of Tfm (testicular feminization) epithelial cells to express androgen-dependent seminal vesicle secretory proteins in chimeric tissue recombinants. Endocrinology 128:3293-3298.
8. Donjacour AA, Cunha GR (1993) Assessment of prostatic protein secretion in tissue recombinants made of urogenital sinus mesenchyme and urothelium from normal or androgen-insensitive mice. Endocrinology 131:2342-2350.
9. Hayward SW, Baskin LS, Haughney PC et al (1996) Stromal development in the ventral prostate, anterior prostate and seminal vesicle of the rat. Acta Anatomica 155:94-103.
10. Nemeth JA, Lee C (1996) Prostatic ductal system in rats: Regional variation in stromal organization. Prostate 28:124-128.
11. Ronnov-Jessen L, Peterson O, Bissell M (1996) Cellular changes involved in conversion of normal to malignant breast: Importance of the stromal reaction. Physiological Rev 76:69-125.
12. Basset P, Wolf C, Chambon P (1993) Expression of the stromelysin-3 gene in fibroblastic cells of invasive carcinomas of the breast and other human tissues: a review. Breast Cancer Res Treat 24:185-193.
13. Masson R, Lefebvre O, Noel A et al (1998) In vivo evidence that the stromelysin-3 metalloproteinase contributes in a paracrine manner to epithelial cell malignancy. J Cell Biol 140:1535-1541.
14. Oishi K, Romijn JC, Schroeder FH (1981) The surface character of separated prostatic cells and cultured fibroblasts of prostatic tissue as determined by concanavalin-a hemadsorption. Prostate 2:11-21.
15. Bosman FT, de Bruine A, Flohil C et al (1993) Epithelial-stromal interactions in colon cancer. Int J Dev Biol 37:203-211.

16. Adam L, Crepin M, Lelong JC et al (1994) Selective interactions between mammary epithelial cells and fibroblasts in co-culture. Int J Cancer 59:262-268.

17. Hayward SW, Dahiya R, Cunha GR et al (1995) Establishment and characterization of an immortalized but non-tumorigenic human prostate epithelial cell Line: BPH-1. In Vitro 31A:14-24.

18. Olumi AF, Grossfeld GD, Hayward SW et al (1997) Human prostatic carcinoma-associated fibroblasts promote tumorigenesis, enhance proliferation and inhibit death of prostatic epithelial cells. Nature Medicine Submitted.

19. Thompson TC, Timme TL, Kadmon D et al (1993) Genetic predisposition and mesenchymal-epithelial interactions in ras+myc-induced carcinogenesis in reconstituted mouse prostate. Molec Carcinogenesis 7:165-179.

20. Camps JL, Chang S-M, Hsu TC et al (1990) Fibroblast-mediated acceleration of human epithelial tumor growth in vivo. Proc Natl Acad Sci USA 87:75-79.

21. Gleave ME, Hsieh JT, von Eschenbach AC et al (1992) Prostate and bone fibroblasts induce human prostate cancer growth in vivo: implications for bidirectional tumor-stromal cell interaction in prostate carcinoma growth and metastasis. J Urol 147:1151-1159.

22. Wu HC, Hsieh JT, Gleave ME et al (1994) Derivation of androgen-independent human LNCaP prostatic cancer cell sublines: role of bone stromal cells. Int J Cancer 57:406-412.

23. Chung LWK, Chang S, Bell C et al (1989) Co-inoculation of tumorigenetic rat prostate mesenchymal cells with non-tumorigenic epithelial cells results in the development of carcinosarcoma in syngeneic and athymic animals. Int J Cancer 43:1179-1187.

24. Hayashi N, Tsuji M, Sugimura Y et al (1996) Change in the morphological and functional cytodifferentiation induced by seminal vesicle mesenchyme in cell suspensions of rat Dunning prostatic adenocarcinoma cells. Int J Cancer 68:788-794.

25. Hayashi N, Cunha GR (1991) Mesenchyme-induced changes in neoplastic characteristics of the Dunning prostatic adenocarcinoma. Cancer Res 51:4924-4930.

25

Androgen Receptor Structure and Function in Prostate Cancer

Grant Buchanan and Wayne D. Tilley

Introduction

Androgens have diverse biological functions, playing a critical role during sexual development and in subsequent life to develop and maintain male secondary sex tissues. Like the normal prostate, prostate cancers (PRCA) are initially dependent on androgens for their growth, and androgen ablation or hormonal therapy remains the major form of systemic treatment for patients with metastatic disease. Although an initial response rate of 70-80% is observed following initiation of androgen ablation therapy, progression almost invariably occurs rapidly, with less than 20% of patients surviving 5 years (1). Nevertheless, the precise mechanisms involved in escape from androgenic control are poorly characterized. Alterations in one or more of the following determinants of androgen activity in the prostate could contribute to the development of unresponsiveness to conventional hormonal therapies: (a) the cellular bioavailability of the more potent metabolite of testosterone, 5α-dihydrotestosterone (5α-DHT), (b) the level and structure of the androgen receptor (AR), and (c) the expression profile of receptor specific cofactor molecules (Figure 1). This paper focuses on AR function in PRCA, with particular emphasis on the contribution of structural alterations in the AR to the failure of conventional hormonal therapies.

Mechanism of Prostate Cancer Progression

Alterations in the expression of the AR and/or receptor cofactors, amplification of the AR gene, ligand independent activation of the AR by alternative growth factor pathways, and structural changes in the AR, have all been proposed as mechanisms contributing to the development of hormone refractory prostate tumors (2, 3). Several early studies showed that AR expression is downregulated in androgen-independent Dunning rat tumor sublines, in parallel with tumor progression. Similarly, AR is not detectable in the androgen- independent human PRCA cell lines, DU145 and PC-3, leading to the proposal that loss of AR expression is a general mechanism by which prostate tumors acquire androgen independence. More recently, immunoreactive AR has been consistently demonstrated in the majority of hormone-sensitive and -refractory human prostate tumors (2), suggesting that loss of AR expression does not play a key role in the development of hormone refractory disease.

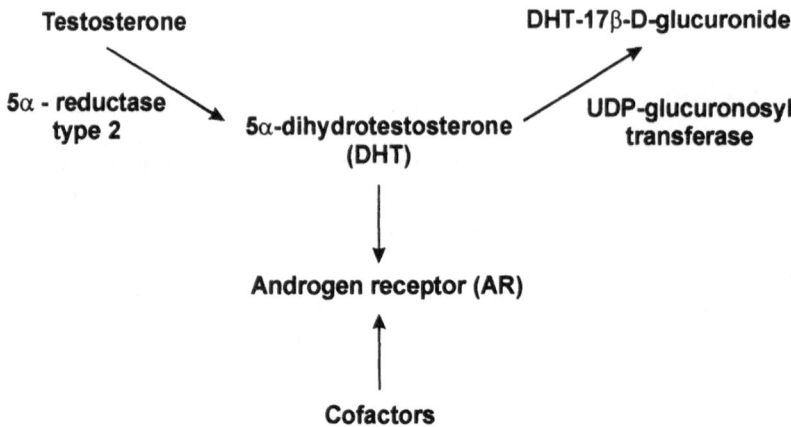

Figure 1. Determinants of androgen action in target tissues.

AR gene amplification has been identified in 30% of locally recurrent PRCA following orchidectomy (4), and in a tumor from a single patient treated with an AR antagonist, bicalutamide (5), but not in matched primary samples taken prior to therapy. Gene amplification was associated with a significant increase in the level of AR mRNA, and may reflect clonal selection of prostate cells with AR amplification in an environment of low circulating levels of androgens. However, it remains to be demonstrated whether amplification of the AR gene results in increased levels of AR protein in tumors that relapse following orchidectomy.

An increasing number of nuclear cofactors that modulate the activity of steroid receptors in the presence and absence of ligand are being identified (6). The cell specific profile of these coactivators and corepressors appears to be a major determinant of receptor activity (6). A recent study demonstrated that overexpression of an AR specific coactivator, ARA70, resulted in a 30.0-fold increase in activation of the AR in response to 17β-estradiol (E$_2$), but only a 6.0-fold increase in 5α-DHT-mediated activity (7). These findings suggest that the cellular level of specific cofactors may influence the response of nuclear receptors to alternative ligands. Amplification of a nuclear receptor coactivator, AIB1, was recently observed in four of five estrogen receptor (ER) positive breast cancer cell lines, and 10% of primary breast tumors. In addition, 64% of these tumors showed high levels of AIB1 expression relative to normal mammary epithelium (8). Taken together, these results suggest that amplification or overexpression of AR cofactors could contribute to the failure of hormonal effects by (i) inducing receptor activation in a low androgen environment (as exists following initiation of androgen ablation therapy) or (ii) facilitating the use of alternative ligands.

Recent studies have demonstrated ligand-independent activation of the AR by polypeptide growth factors and activators of protein kinase A (PKA) (3). In addition, synergistic activation of the AR by luteinizing hormone releasing hormone (LHRH) analogues, and low levels of androgens results in hypersensitization of the AR, and activation of AR growth regulatory pathways (3). Collectively, these studies suggest that alterations in paracrine signaling pathways in prostate tumors could facilitate activation of the AR independent of the ligand. This hypothesis is in agreement with observations in our laboratory of nuclear AR immunoreactivity in prostate tumor cells, following androgen deprivation (data not shown), as transformation of cytoplasmic AR to the active form is a requirement of nuclear localization.

The first indication that, structural alterations in the AR in PRCA could be an important mechanism in the failure of conventional therapies, came from studies of the androgen-responsive human PRCA cell line, LNCaP (2, 9). A single base substitution in the ligand binding domain of the AR gene in LNCaP cells results in a AR variant that, in addition to maintaining wild-type activity with 5α-DHT, is activated by estrogen, progesterone, and even the AR antagonists hydroxyflutamide (OHF) and cyproterone acetate (9). These observations provided a mechanism to explain that, although PRCAs remain initially responsive to androgens, androgen ablation provides a selective advantage for a sub-population of tumor cells containing AR variants that can be activated by alternative ligands, leading to the development of androgen-independent growth. In our laboratory, evidence for structural alterations in the AR gene in PRCA initially came from immunohistochemical studies of a cohort of patients with advanced disease. AR immunoreactivity was evaluated using video image analysis (VIA) of the staining for each tumor sample using antibodies directed against both the amino- and carboxy-termini of the AR. Despite heterogeneity of nuclear staining, there was concordance between the cellular concentration of immunoreactive AR, in tumors detected using both antibodies. In contrast, there was a distinct lack of concordance between the percentage of AR positive cells measured using each antibody (10). This result was suggestive of structural alterations in the AR protein in a subset of tumor cells resulting in the detection of the AR by only one or the other of the two antibodies. In this cohort of advanced prostate cancer patients, subsequent analysis of AR gene structure identified AR gene mutations in 44% of tumor samples (11).

AR gene mutations have been identified in PRCA at frequencies of <5% in early stage primary tumors to as high as 50% in metastatic lesions within bone (2). The majority of these mutations have arisen somatically within the tumor where they presumably conferred a significant growth advantage facilitating detection by current screening technologies. The variation in the frequency of mutations detected in individual studies may merely reflect differences between cohorts of PRCA patients examined. In addition, primary tumors can be sampled by core biopsy, radical prostatectomy and transurethral resection (TUR) which, due to the genetically heterogeneous nature of prostate tumors, may significantly contribute to the apparent discrepancy in the frequency of AR gene mutations. Similarly, racial and demographic differences in the populations studied, tumor stage at biopsy, micro-dissection of samples, the method of screening, and the extent of the AR analyzed (e.g., entire coding region versus the ligand binding domain) may influence detection. However, despite differences in detection frequency, six codons of the AR gene have been reported to contain a mutation by two or more independent studies of prostate tumors (12).

Our studies have identified an association between the presence of AR gene mutations in advanced prostate tumor samples taken prior to initiation of hormonal therapy, and subsequent disease progression (11). This is in agreement with *in-vitro* studies demonstrating that mutant AR present in prostate tumors retains functional activity in the presence of 5α-DHT, but has decreased specificity for ligand binding and transactivation (2, 3) (Figure 2). Mutant AR can be activated by adrenal androgens, non-testicular steroids such as progesterone or E_2, and by the AR antagonists, OHF and bicalutamide.

Two AR gene mutations identified in our studies (11) which result in missense amino acid substitutions [AR-Thr670 (ie Ile-Thr670) and AR-Asn780 (ie Ser-Asn780)], occur in distinct regions of the ligand binding domain (LBD) of the receptor from those identified in other studies (Figure 2), and exhibit different ligand mediated activities. Functional characterization of these two variant ARs using a prostate and androgen responsive reporter gene assay, revealed that each had a 2.0-3.0-fold increase in 5α-DHT (0.01-10.0 nM) induced transactivation activity compared to wild type AR. In addition, the adrenal androgens androstenedione and DHEA, the non-androgenic ligands, E_2 and progesterone, and the AR antagonists hydroxyflutanmide and bicalutamide (Casodex) collectively induced 2.0-10.0 fold greater activity of both AR-Thr670 and AR-Asn780 compared to wild type AR. These data are consistent with earlier studies suggesting that activation of variant AR, by low circulating levels of testicular or adrenal androgens, or aberrant activation by antiandrogens, may contribute to the maintenance of tumor growth in patients treated with androgen ablation therapies. Furthermore, increased activity in response to all ligands could explain a selective growth advantage of prostate tumor cell containing such mutations both prior to and during androgen ablation.

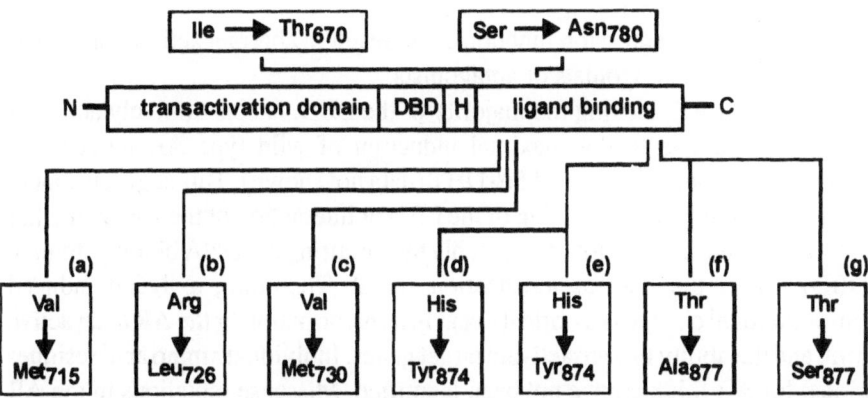

Figure 2. Position of missense mutations identified in the AR gene in human PRCA. (i) Functional analysis of AR variants identified in human prostate tumors, cell lines or xenografts in previous studies (2) (shown below the AR schematic) demonstrated broadening of specificity for ligand binding and/or transcriptional activation. a. Culig, *et al.* (13); b. Elo, *et al.* (14); c. Newmark, *et al.* (15); d. Taplin, *et al.* (16); e. Tan, *et al.* (18); f. Suzuki, *et al.* (17); g. Taplin, *et al.* (16). (ii) The positions of two missense mutations (ie AR-Thr670 and AR-Asn780) in the LBD of the AR gene identified in prostate tumors in our studies (11).

An increase in testosterone- and DHEA-induced activity was observed for a variant AR identified in the human PRCA xenograft, CWR22 (18). Our studies, however, are the first to identify a variant AR that exhibits increased activity compared to wild type AR in the presence of physiological concentration of the native ligand, 5α-DHT. There are several possible mechanisms that could explain an increased activity of the variant ARs in response to ligand. Alterations in the structure of the ligand binding domain may result in increased affinity for ligand, a slower dissociation rate or increased ligand induced stabilization of AR protein. However, ligand binding studies and western blot analysis of transfected AR-Thr670 and AR-Asn780 revealed no changes in binding affinity for 5α-DHT, and no differences in the level of AR protein in either the absence or presence of ligand (data not shown). In addition, the predicted structure of the LBD of the AR based on the recently delineated crystal structure of the progesterone receptor (PR) (19), suggests that residue 670 is unlikely to be directly involved in formation of the ligand binding pocket or in ligand binding. These results suggest that other mechanisms may be responsible for the observed increase in activity. Although the majority of the transactivation domains (TADs) are located in the amino terminal portion of the AR, a number of sub-domain structures of the LBD are essential for the full wild type activity of the AR. Mutations occurring in a region of the LBD containing a TAD or a domain that mediates transrepression function could result in aberrant activity of the AR in response to either agonists or antagonists.

Truncated AR, lacking the majority of the LBD, is constitutively active at a level comparable to the maximal induction of wild type AR induced by physiological concentrations of 5α-DHT (data not shown). This suggests that in the absence of ligand, the folding of the LBD or interaction of the AR with other factors inhibits transcription, presumably by obscuring the DNA binding domain (DBD) and/or the nuclear localization signal. Therefore, a ligand induced conformational change is a critical event in transformation of the AR to an active form, and the ability to transactivate target genes. Individual amino acid residues critical for AR folding have not been identified. Missense mutations in the AR gene could potentially alter the kinetics of receptor folding such that a lower concentration of 5α-DHT would result in receptor transformation, DNA binding and transcriptional activation.

It is now well documented that the level of individual coactivators and corepressors, in a particular cell type, can influence the level of transcriptional activity achieved by ligand bound and/or unbound nuclear receptors (6). Mutations in the AF-2 core in the LBD of the AR abolish receptor activity without altering ligand binding (12), indicating the potential importance of cofactors for activity of the AR. Although interaction of corepressors with the AR has not yet been demonstrated, it appears that for all related nuclear receptors examined, corepressors bind in the absence of ligand, or even constitutively. Limited trypsinization studies of the AR have demonstrated that, unlike 5α-DHT, binding of the AR antagonist OHF does not release protein factors bound to a region of the AR including residue 670 (20). In contrast, OHF was able to release these factors from an AR containing the LNCaP mutation (20). As LNCaP AR is activated by OHF, these results suggest that the antagonist ability of antiandrogens may be mediated by their inability to release corepressors from the AR. If mutations in the AR prevent or alter the binding of constitutive corepressors, or alter the ability of ligands to release corepressors, the basal level of transcriptional activity achieved for individual ligands, as observed for both AR-Thr670 and AR-Asn780 mutants, may be increased. Recently, it was reported that the AR specific coactivator ARA70 was able to enhance the agonist potential of several antiandrogens, including OHF and bicalutamide, in a dose dependent manner (21). In addition, mutations in the AF-2 core of the ER have been reported to enhance the agonist activity of several antiestrogens without altering ligand or DNA binding ability, presumably by altering the interaction of coactivators with the AF-2 domain (22). Therefore, AR gene mutations that enhance interactions with coactivators such as ARA70 could result in an increase in basal levels of AR activity and/or increased agonist activity of antiandrogens.

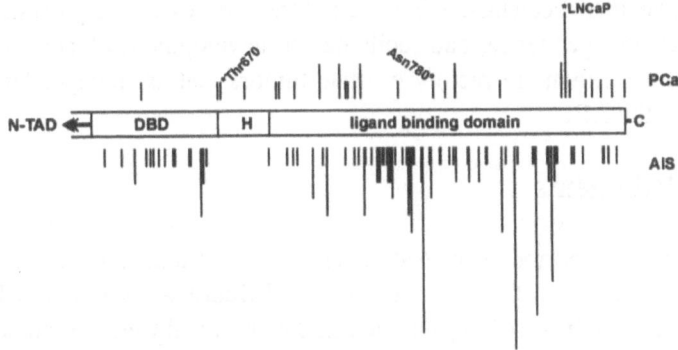

Figure 3. Location and frequency of AR gene mutations identified in PRCA and the inherited form of androgen insensitivity. Schematic diagram of the DNA binding (DBD), hinge (H) and ligand binding domains of the AR protein showing the position of missense mutations identified in (a) clinical PRCA (PCa) (above the diagram), and (b) patients with the inherited form of androgen insensitivity (AIS) (below the diagram) (12). The positions of two missense mutations, Ile-Thr670 and Ser-Asn780, identified in our studies (11) and discussed in the text are indicated (*). The position of the AR gene mutation first identified in the LNCaP prostate cancer cell line (9) and subsequently by several groups in human prostate tumors is also shown. The length of the line denoting each mutation is proportional to the number of individual reports of a mutation at that codon. At least two mutations in the same codon have been reported in human PRCA at 6 positions in the AR. However, none of the codons containing amino acid substitutions identified in PRCA have been reported as containing a mutation in AIS.

Summary

A distinct clustering of AR gene mutations identified in prostate tumors occurs in regions of the AR devoid of inactivating mutations identified in the inherited syndrome of androgen insensitivity (AIS) (Figure 3) (2, 12). Functional characterization of variant AR identified in PRCA consistently reveals a broadening of specificity for ligand binding and/or transactivation. Collectively, our studies and those of others, provide an explanation for the development of resistance to current hormonal therapies in a subset of advanced PRCA. Further investigation of the functional consequences of AR gene mutations identified in PRCA and the interactions of these AR variants with nuclear cofactors will facilitate identification of important subdomain structures within the AR protein necessary for optimal AR activity. Moreover, these studies will provide insight into the molecular mechanisms involved in the progression of prostate tumors to androgen independence, and facilitate the development of new treatment strategies for hormone refractory prostate tumors that are independent of the structure of the AR.

Acknowledgments

This work was supported by the National Health and Medical Research Council of Australia, the Anti-Cancer Foundation of South Australia, the Flinders University of South Australia, and the Flinders Medical Center Foundation.

References

1. Kozlowski JM, Ellis WJ, Grayhack JT (1991) Advanced prostatic carcinoma: early v's late endocrine therapy. In: Andriole GL and Catalona WJ (eds) The Urologic Clinics of North America. Philadelphia, WB Saunders Company, pp. 15-24.
2. Bentel JM, Tilley WD (1996) Androgen receptors in prostate cancer. J Endocrinol 151:1-11.
3. Culig Z, Hobisch A, Hittmair A et al (1998) Expression, structure, and function of androgen receptor in advanced prostatic carcinoma. Prostate 35:63-70.
4. Koivisto P, Kononen J, Palmberg C et al (1997) Androgen receptor gene amplification: a possible molecular mechanism for androgen deprivation therapy failure in prostate cancer. Cancer Res 57:314-319.
5. Palmberg C, Koivisto P, Hyytinen E et al (1997) Androgen receptor gene amplification in a recurrent prostate cancer after monotherapy with the nonsteroidal potent antiandrogen Casodex (bicalutamide) with a subsequent favorable response to maximal androgen blockade. Eur Urol 31:216-219.
6. Horwitz KB, Jackson TA, Bain DL et al (1996) Nuclear receptor coactivators and corepressors. Mol Endocrinol 10:1167-1177.
7. Yeh S, Miyamoto H, Shima H et al (1998) From estrogen to androgen receptor: A new pathway for sex hormones in prostate. Proc Natl Acad Sci USA 95:5527-5532.
8. Anzick SL, Kononen J, Walker RL et al (1997) AIB1, a steroid receptor coactivator amplified in breast and ovarian cancer. Science 277:965-968.
9. Veldscholte J, Ris-Stalpers C, Kuiper GG et al (1990) A mutation in the ligand binding domain of the androgen receptor of human LNCaP cells affects steroid binding characteristics and response to anti-androgens. Biochem Biophys Res Commun 173:534-540.

10. Tilley WD, Lim-Tio SS, Horsfall DJ et al (1994) Detection of discrete androgen receptor epitopes in prostate cancer by immunostaining: measurement by color video image analysis. Cancer Res 54:4096-4102.
11. Tilley WD, Buchanan G, Hickey TE et al (1996) Mutations in the androgen receptor gene are associated with progression of human prostate cancer to androgen independence. Clin Cancer Res 2:277-285.
12. Gottlieb B, Lehvaslaiho H, Beitel LK et al (1998) The AndrogenReceptor Gene Mutations Database. Nucleic Acids Res 26:236-240.
13. Culig Z, Hobisch, A, Cronauer, MV et al (1993) Mutant androgen receptor detected in an advanced-stage prostatic carcinoma is activated by adrenal androgens and progesterone. Mol Endocrinol 7:1541-1550.
14. Elo JP, Kvist L, Leinone K et al (1995) Mutated human androgen receptor gene detected in a prostatic cancer patient is also activated by estradiol. J Clin Endocrinol Metab 80:3494-3500.
15. Newmark JR, Hardy DO, Tonb DC et al (1992) Androgen receptor gene mutations in human prostate cancer. Proc Natl Acad Sci USA 89:6319-6323.
16. Taplin ME, Bubley GJ, Shuster TD et al (1995) Mutation of the androgen-receptor gene in metastatic androgen-independent prostate cancer. N Engl J Med 332:1393-1398.
17. Tan J, Sharief Y, Hamil KG et al (1997) Dehydroepiandrosterone activates mutant androgen receptors expressed in the androgen-dependent human prostate cancer xenograft CWR22 and LNCaP cells. Mol Endocrinol 11:450.
18. Suzuki H, Sato N, Watabe Y et al (1993) Androgen receptor gene mutations in human prostate cancer. J Steroid Biochem Mol Biol 46:759-765.
19. Tan J, Sharief Y, Hamil KG et al (1997) Dehydroepiandrosterone activates mutant androgen receptors expressed in the androgen-dependent human prostate cancer xenograft CWR22 and LNCaP cells. Mol Endocrinol 11:450-459.
20. Williams SP, Sigler PB (1998) Atomic structure of progesterone complexed with its receptor. Nature 393:392-396.
21. Kuil CW, Berrevoets CA, Mulder E (1995) Ligand-induced conformational alterations of the androgen receptor analyzed by limited trypsinization. Studies on the mechanism of antiandrogen action. J Biol Chem 270:27569-27576.
22. Miyamoto H, Yeh S, Wilding G et al (1998) Promotion of agonist activity of antiandrogens by the androgen receptor coactivator, ARA70, in human prostate cancer DU145 cells. Proc Natl Acad Sci USA 95:7379-7384.
23. Mahfoudi A, Roulet E, Dauvois S et al (1995) Specific mutations in the estrogen receptor change the properties of antiestrogens to full agonists. Proc Natl Acad Sci USA 92:4206-4210.

PART 9. OSTEOPOROSIS AND ESTROGEN

Introduction

Hormone Replacement Therapy: A Clinical Overview

James H. Pickar

The average life expectancy of women has been increasing (1) while the average age of onset of menopause has remained relatively stable (2, 3). Today women have an average life expectancy of about 80 years and the average age of menopause is approximately 51. Women spend more than one-third of their life after menopause. The substantial decrease in estrogen (E) associated with the menopause is accompanied by both short and long term effects. Perhaps the most common early effect is vasomotor instability experienced by approximately 85% of postmenopausal women (4). Additionally, effects include vaginal atrophy and osteoporosis.

In the USA, there are more than 250 thousand hip fractures/year occurring in women (5). Clinical trials have demonstrated that hormone replacement therapy (HRT) is effective in relieving vasomotor instability, treating and preventing vaginal atrophy, and maintaining or increasing bone mass, thus reducing the risk for fracture. Data from the PEPI trial demonstrated that over a three-year period bone mineral density in the lumbar spine decreased by 1.8% in the placebo group, while it increased by 3.5 to 5.0% in the E and E/progestin groups. At the hip, the placebo group lost 1.7% while the E and E/progestin groups gained 1.7% in bone mineral density (6). Data comparing the SERM raloxifene and E have demonstrated a significantly greater increase in bone mineral density with E (7).

Observational studies have suggested that HRT is also effective in significantly reducing the risk of coronary heart disease, the leading cause of death among postmenopausal women (8, 9). Additionally, areas of future investigation include the relationship between E use and possible reduction in the risk of Alzheimer's disease, and reduction in the risk for colon cancer. Results from a case control study demonstrated a 35% reduction in risk for Alzheimer's disease and related dementias among ever users of estrogen replacement therapy (ERT). The risk decreased significantly in association with increasing dosage and duration of use(10). As regards colon cancer, data from a recent study from the American Cancer Society suggested a 45% reduction in risk of fatal colon cancer in current users of ERT with a significant trend for decreasing risk with increasing years of use (11).

Observational studies have described an increase in risk associated with HRT for venous thromboembolism (12, 13), and pulmonary emboli, although the absolute increase in pulmonary emboli attributable to HRT is small, approximately 5 cases/100,000 person-years in women aged 50-59 years (14). Breast cancer and its possible association with HRT, at doses customarily used today, would likely remain an issue until data from extremely large clinical trials become available.

The concern over the relationship of unopposed E use and the development of endometrial hyperplasia and endometrial carcinoma has now largely been addressed by large clinical trials demonstrating a reduction in risk compared to E alone, with the addition of appropriate doses and duration of progestin use to hormone replacement therapy (15, 16).

References

1. Menopause and Postmenopausal Hormone Therapy (1994) In: Speroff L, Glass RH, Kase NG (eds) Clinical Gynecologic Endocrinology and Infertility, 5th Edition. Williams and Wilkins Publishing Group, Baltimore, Maryland, pp. 583-649.
2. Speroff L (1994) The Menopause. A signal for the Future. In: Lobo RA (ed) Treatment of the Postmenopausal Woman, Basic and Clinical Aspects. Raven Press, New York, pp. 1-7.
3. Rekers H (1991) Mastering the Menopause. In: Burger H, Boulet M (eds) A Portrait of the Menopause. The Parthenon Publishing Group Ltd., Parkridge, New Jersey, pp. 23-43.
4. Oldenhave A, Jaszmann LJB, Haspels AA et al (1993) Impact of climacteric on well-being. A survey based on 5213 women 39 to 60 years old. Am J Obstet Gynecol 168:772-780.
5. Lindsay R, Thorne JF (1987) Alterations in skeletal homeostasis with age and menopause. In: Mishell, Jr.,DR (ed) Menopause, Physiology and Pharmacology. Year book Medical Publishers Inc., Chicago, Illinois, pp. 77-90.
6. The Writing Group for the PEPI Trial (1996) Effects of hormone therapy on bone mineral density. Results from the Postmenopausal Estrogen/Progestin Interventions (PEPI) trial. J Am Med Ass 276: 1389-1396.
7. Evista Product Labeling (U.S.) Eli Lilly and Company, 12/11/97.
8. Grodstein F, Stampfer MJ, Manson JE et al (1996) Postmenopausal estrogen and progestin use and the risk of cardiovascular disease. N Engl J Med 335:435-461.
9. Sullivan JM, Vander Zwaag R, Lemp GF et al (1998) Postmenopausal estrogen use and coronary atherosclerosis. Arch Intern Med 108:3358-363.

10. Paganini-Hill A, Henderson VW (1996) Estrogen replacement therapy and risk of Alzheimer disease. Arch Internal Med 156:2213-2217.
11. Calle E, Miracle-McMahill HL, Kosinski AS et al (1995) Estrogen replacement therapy and risk of fatal colon cancer in aprospective cohort of postmenopausal women. J Natl Cancer Inst 87:517-523.
12. Jick H, Derby LE, Myers MW et al (1996) Risk of hospital admission for idiopathic venous thromboembolism among users of postmenopausal oestrogens. Lancet 348:981-983.
13. Daly E, Vessey MP, Hawkins MM et al (1996) Risk of venous thromboembolism in users of hormone replacement therapy. Lancet 348:977-980.
14. Grodstein F, Stampfer MJ, Goldhaber SZ et al (1996) Prospective study of exogenous hormones and risk of pulmonary embolism in women. Lancet 348:983-987.
15. Woodruff JD, Pickar JH, for the Menopause Study Group (1994) Incidence of endometrial hyperplasia in postmenopausal women taking Premarin with medroxyprogesterone acetate or Premarin alone. Am J Obstet Gynecol 170:1213-1223.
16. The Writing Group for the PEPI Trial (1996) Effects of hormone replacement therapy on endometrial histology in postmenopausal women. J Am Med Ass 275:370-375.

26

Role of Estrogen and Bone Morphogentic Protein Signaling in Osteoblast Differentiation

Stephen E. Harris

Introduction

The three major cell types involved in bone formation and remodeling are the osteocyte, osteoclast, and the osteoblast. The osteocyte, which is embedded in a lacunae of the bone matrix and extends dendritic processes through the bone matrix, is thought to be the key sensory cell for bone and detects mechanical stress generated by fluid flow, stress, and pressure changes. The osteoclast, derived from the hemopoetic precursor monocyte-macrophage lineage, is the key cell involved in bone resorption and remodeling. The osteoblast is the key cell that lays down new bone matrix, and is the precursor to the osteocyte. It has now been demonstrated, at least *in vitro* and in some cases *in vivo* that estrogen (E_2) is a direct target for all three bone cell components (1-10).

Osteocytes

Osteocytes are thought to be derived from some fraction of the mature osteoblast that becomes incorporated into the bone matrix. These osteocyte precursors must produce factors that suppress local mineralized matrix, creating extensive channels throughout the bone matrix. The osteocytes send dendrites through the matrix and form an osteocyte inter-connected network. This network responds to mechanical strain and sends signals to both osteoblast and osteoclast precursors. Recent data indicate that E_2 can block apoptosis of osteocytes by increasing the anti-apoptotic gene *bcl-2* (1). In the absence of E_2, osteocytes produce nitric oxide that is a known homing signal for osteoclasts that in turn may lead to local bone resorption (1). This is one hypothesis of how E_2 may regulate osteocyte-osteoclast communication and is being tested in new model systems.

Osteoclasts

Chick osteoclast and human osteoclastomas contain estrogen receptor (ER-α) (2). This suggests a direct role of E_2 on osteoclast (2). In the *in-vitro* systems,

E_2 has been shown to block apoptosis of osteoclast indirectly by stimulating TGF-β production from osteoblast or stromal cell precursors (3). E_2 can also block production of osteoclast differentiation factors, such as IL-1, IL-6, and TNF-like factors, from stromal cells (4). The partial E_2 agonist for bone, Tamoxifen (TAM), can also block production of these factors (4).

Osteoblasts

The presence of both ER-α and ER-β in osteoblasts suggests they are direct targets for E_2 action (5). E_2 alone has been shown to stimulate proliferation of rat long bone osteoblasts, similar to the level seen with dynamic 4 point bending strain (mechanical stress) (6). The strain plus E_2 are additive. TAM blocks both E_2 and strain induced osteoblast proliferation. This suggests that the strain effects on osteoblasts are in part mediated through the ER. EGF-like factors may be mediators of these responses (6).

Bone Morphogenetic Proteins and Estrogen on Osteoblast Differentiation

The bone morphogenetic proteins (BMPs) are a class of ligands involved in differentiation of a large variety of tissues, including bone and cartilage (11). They belong to the TGF-β super-family and can promote the growth and differentiation of osteoblasts to a mature mineralization state. There are over 15 members of this family (BMP2-16). Many of the BMPs can induce cartilage and bone when implanted in a muscle site. This demonstrates they can redirect muscle precursors to osteoblasts and chondroblasts (11). Recent data has shown that E_2 can directly stimulate BMP6 production in human osteoblasts transfected with ER-α (8). We have demonstrated that E_2 plus recombinant BMP2 can synergistically interact to increase the rate of bone formation *in vitro* (9). TAM has been shown to block proliferation of osteoblasts, but can accelerate terminal differentiation of osteoblast to a mineralized matrix (10). This effect is thought to be through the ERβ, which increases 10.0-fold during later phases of osteoblast differentiation (5).

2T3 Model for Osteoblast Differentiation

We have used a transgenic approach to develop an immortalized osteoblast model that can undergo the entire cascade of bone formation *in vitro*. The weak BMP2 promoter was linked to T-antigen and transgenic mice were developed (13). From the calvarae of these mice, a clonal osteoblast cell line was obtained that responds to BMP2 by producing an extensive mineralized matrix that is very similar to bone made *in vivo* (13). This model we refer to as 2T3. It is clonal and can be stably transfected with a variety of genes.

Figure 1 shows the BMP2 response of 2T3 cells overtime, as assayed by Von Kossa stain for mineralized structures (black). 2T3 cells form a small amount of mineral without BMP2. However, BMP2 greatly accelerated bone formation as can be seen in this figure.

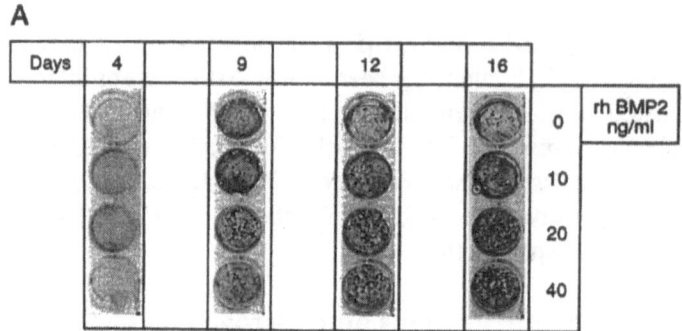

Figure 1. Clonal 2T3 preosteoblasts produce a mineralized matrix (bone nodules) during a 9-16 day period. BMP2 greatly increases the net amount of bone at 10-40 ng/ml. Media: αMEM + 7% FCS + 100 μg/ml Ascorbic Acid and 5 mm β-glycerolphosphate. Photograph of 2T3 cultures stained Von Kossa for mineral (black) and Van Giesen for matrix. BMP2 added at day 0 and media changed every 3 days.

BMP2 Signaling Requires the BMP Receptor 1B for Bone Formation in 2T3 Osteoblasts

BMP2 signaling requires a BMP receptor type II (BMPR II) and BMP receptor type I, that forms heteromers and signals to the Smad proteins (Smad, 1, 5, 8) by specific serine phosphorylation on the C-terminal end of these "signaling" Smads. The phosphorylated Smad 1, 5, or 8 forms heteromers with Smad 4 and are translocated to the nucleus to interact with other cell specific nuclear transcription factors. These interactions result in specific gene expression (11,12) mediated by BMP2, 4, or 7 ligands.

There are several BMP type I receptors. We have demonstrated, at least *in vitro*, the BMP receptor 1B (BMPR-1B) is required for BMP2 induced bone cell differentiation (12). When BMPR-1B signaling is blocked using a dominant negative BMPR-1B gene, osteoblasts cannot differentiate into mature mineralizing osteoblasts but are re-specified to differentiate into adipocytes in the appropriate media (12). We have also shown that 2T3 cells containing a constitutively active BMP receptor 1B can differentiate into bone structure without added BMP2 ligand. BMP2 added to these ca BMPR-1B 2T3 cells further increases bone formation (12).

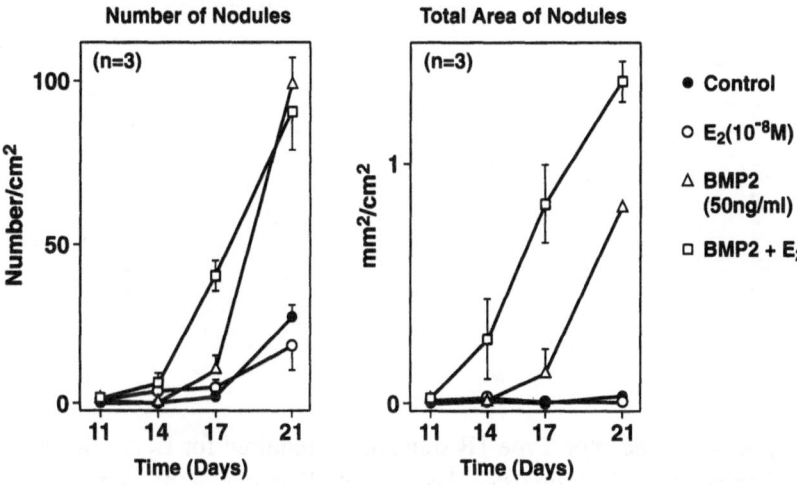

Figure 2. 17β-Estradiol (E₂) and BMP2 synergistically interact to stimulate the rate of bone nodule formation in wild-type 2T3 preosteoblasts. Cells were grown to confluence in αMEM + 7% charcoal-stripped (2x) FCS (day 0), as in Figure 1. The media was changed to αMEM + 7% charcoal-stripped (2x) FCS + 100 μg/ml Ascorbic acid, and 5 mm β-glycerol phosphate. Mineral formation (bone nodules) were monitored by Von Kossa stain and quantitated by image analysis (13). The total number of nodules is shown on the Left panel and total bone area/cm² is shown on the Right panel. ●, Control; ○, E₂ 10⁻⁸M; ✳, BMP2, 50 ng/ml; ☐, BMP2 + E₂.

Estrogen and BMP2 Synergize to Increase the Rate of Bone Formation

As shown in Figure 2, E₂ can interact with BMP signaling to increase the rate of bone formation in this 2T3 model. Both the number of mineralized nodules and total area of bone are accelerated when both E₂ and BMP2 are added together in E₂-depleted media.

Using the wild-type and mutant BMPR-1B 2T3 clones, we now can ask whether E₂ stimulates bone formation in the absence of BMPR-1B signaling, using the 2T3 cells with the dominant-negative kinase truncated receptor (trBMPR-1B 2T3) or the presence of a constitutively active BMPR-1B that does not require BMP2 ligand for bone formation (12).

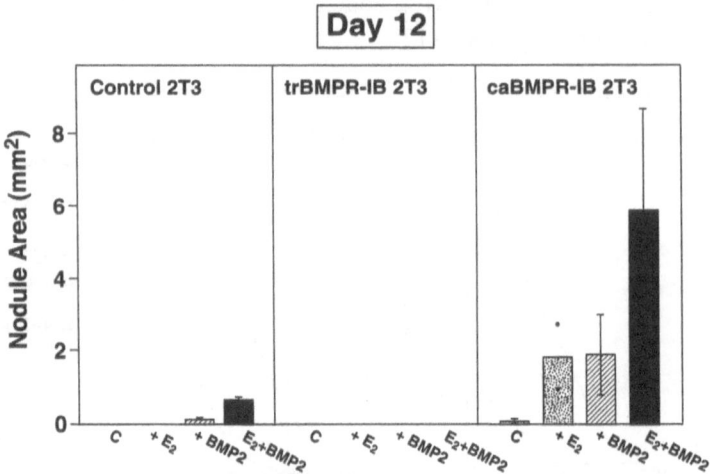

Figure 3. BMP receptor Type 1B signaling is required for E_2 acceleration of bone formation in 2T3 preosteoblasts. Left Panel: Control, empty vector containing 2T3 cells. Middle Panel: 2T3 cells stably transfected with dominant-negative truncated BMP receptor Type 1B (trBMPR-1B 2T3). Right Panel: 2T3 cells stably transfected with the constitutively active BMP receptor Type 1B (caBMPR-1B 2T3). All assays were done at 12 days post-confluence.

BMPR-1B Signaling Is Required for Estrogen-accelerated Bone Formation

In Figure 3, we measure the interaction of BMP2 and E_2 in wild-type (empty vector clones) control 2T3 cells, in 2T3 cells containing the dominant-negative BMPR-1B (trBMPR-1B 2T3), and in 2T3 cells containing the constitutively active BMPR-1B (caBMPR-1B 2T3). In the control cells, BMP2 stimulates mineralized nodules and E_2 + BMP2 gives a 4.0-fold increase in mineralized nodules over BMP2 alone. This was measured at 12 days of culture. By 21 days BMP2 + E_2 was approximately the same as BMP2 alone. Thus, E_2 + BMP2 does not effect the net amount of bone formed, but E_2 accelerates the rate of bone formation in the presence of BMP2.

When BMP2 signaling is blocked, as in the trBMPR-1B 2T3 cells, no bone formation was seen in the absence or presence of BMP2 and/or E_2, indicating BMPR-1B signaling is required for E_2 action on osteoblast differentiation. We suspect, without BMPR-1B signaling and subsequent differentiation, the ER-β is not induced.

As expected, bone formation occurs in caBMPR-1B 2T3 cells without BMP2 (Figure 3, Right panel). BMP2 can further increase the amount of mineralized nodules. However, E_2 alone can also stimulate bone formation in caBMPR-1B 2T3 osteoblast. This again demonstrates that BMPR-1B signaling is required for E_2 acceleration of bone formation. BMP2 and E_2 even gave a further 2.5-fold increase in mineralized nodules (Figure 2, Right panel). We presume that the endogenous wild-type BMPR-1B or other BMP receptor 1 types is contributing to this synergy. Thus, BMPR-1B signaling is playing a major role in the E_2/BMP2 synergy observed on the rate of bone formation in this model.

PPARγ-Ligand Induced Adipocyte Differentiation of 2T3 Osteoblasts

2T3 cells can be considered primarily a mesenchymal osteoblast precursor, capable of complete differentiation to bone in the presence of BMP2. However, in the presence of a PPARγ-ligand and the phosphodiesterase inhibitor, isobutyl-methyl-xanthine, a small fraction of the osteoblast re-specify and differentiate into oil-red positive adipocytes (12). In the 2T3 cells containing the dominant-negative BMPR-1B (trBMPR-1B), massive differentiation into adipocytes occurs in the presence of PPARγ-ligand and is further stimulated by BMP2 (12). These trBMPR-1B 2T3 cells have highly elevated PPARγ2 mRNA and adipsin mRNA that is further stimulated by BMP2 (12). We then tested the effect of E_2 on adipocyte differentiation in both wild-type and mutant trBMPR-1B 2T3 cells.

Estrogen Inhibits PPARγ-ligand Induced Adipogenesis of Wild-type 2T3 Cells

When wild-type 2T3 cells were treated with 10^{-7} M combination of the specific PPARγ-ligand, BRL49653 and RXR specific ligand, LG100346, approximately 5% of the 2T3 cells differentiate into oil-red positive adipocytes by 12 days of culture. BMP2 further increased the number of adipocytes 3-fold (Figure 4). No adipocytes wee seen without the PPARγ-Ligand mixture. As shown in Figure 4, E_2 at 10^{-8} M decreases PPARγ-induced adipocyte formation by over 60% in either the absence or presence of BMP2. These data suggest estrogens may play a key role in specifying bone-marrow precursors toward an osteoblast lineage, and suppressing these precursors from differentiating into adipocytes.

Estrogen Inhibits Adipogenesis of Mutant trBMPR-1B 2T3 Cells in the Absence of PPARγ-ligand

When trBMPR-1B 2T3 cells are grown in the absence of PPARγ-ligand mixture, they form 2-3% adipocytes that are increased 3.0-fold in the presence of BMP2. Again E_2 suppresses adipogenesis ~70% in either the presence or absence of BMP2. However, in the presence of PPARγ-ligand, trBMPR-1B 2T3 cells form massive amounts of adipocytes (Figure 5). Approximately 50% of the culture stains oil-red positive by 12 days. Again E_2 suppresses oil-red positive cells, but only 30-40% in these mutant trBMPR-1B 2T3 cells in the presence of the PPARγ-ligand. Thus, even with defective BMP receptor 1B signaling in the mutant 2T3 clones, E_2 can suppress terminal differentiation of mesenchymal to mature adipocytes.

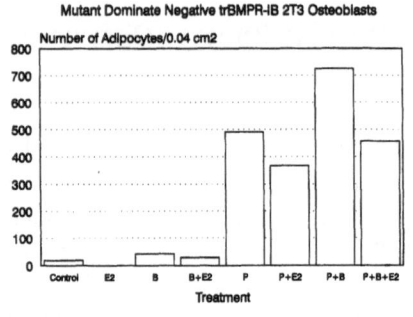

E_2 = estradiol 17βb 10-8M
B = BMP2 @ 40 ng/ml
P = PPARg-Ligand 10-7M

12 Day Culture
aMEM 7% Charcoal-stripped Fetal Calf Serum
Isobutyl-Methyl Xanthine

Figure 4. Estrogen suppresses adipogenesis of wild-type 2T3 or empty vector 2T3 osteoblasts cells in the presence of the PPARg-ligand mix, BRL49653 and LG100346. E_2 was at 10^{-8} M and BMP2 was at 40 ng/ml.

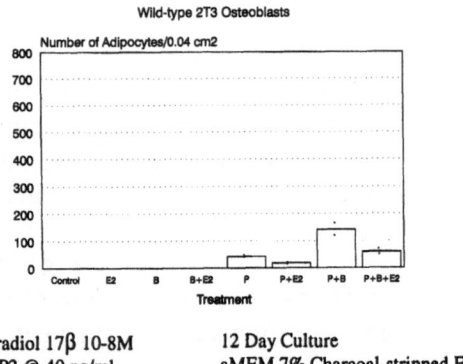

E_2 = estradiol 17β 10-8M
B = BMP2 @ 40 ng/ml
P = PPARg-Ligand 10-7M

12 Day Culture
aMEM 7% Charcoal-stripped Fetal Calf Serum
Isobutyl-Methyl Xanthine

Figure 5. Estrogen suppresses adipogenesis of mutant trBMPR-1B 2T3 cells in the absence or presence of PPARg-Ligand mix, BRL49653 and LG100346. E_2 was at 10^{-8} M and BMP2 was at 40 ng/ml.

Model for Role of Estrogen and BMP Receptor Signaling in Osteoblast and Adipocyte Differentiation

In summary, using the 2T3 model for osteoblast and adipocyte differentiation, we have shown that 1.) E_2 can synergize with BMP2 signaling through the BMP receptor type 1B to accelerate the rate of bone formation, but not the net amount of bone and 2.) E_2 can suppress the potential of these mesenchymal cells to differentiate to adipocytes. Our model is presented in Figure 6.

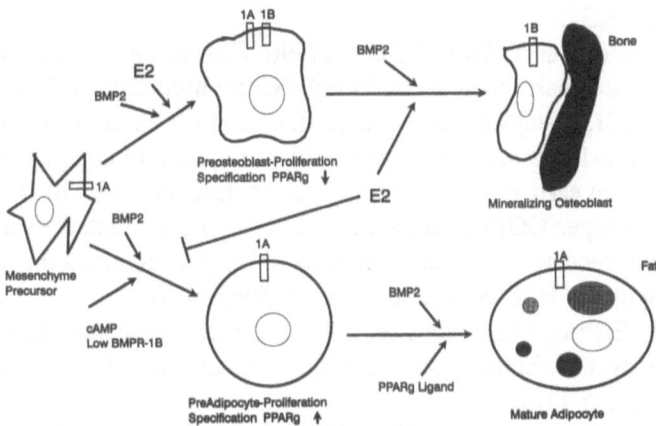

Figure 6. Model of how estrogens can interact with BMP2 to increase the rate of bone formation and suppress mesenchyml precursors from differentiating to adipocytes. High levels of BMP receptor type 1B and BMP ligands drive cells toward mineralizing matrix. High levels of BMP receptor 1A or absence of BMPR-1B allow mesenchyml precursors to respecify toward preadipocytes. In the presence of PPARg-Ligand they form mature fat cells.

Mesenchymal precursors cells predominately express the BMP receptor type 1A, also found on most fibroblastoid-like cells (12). BMP2 acting on the type 1A receptor increases growth and proliferation of preosteoblast and, eventually decreases BMP receptor type 1A expression, as cell slow growth and commit to mature osteoblast. There is a subsequent increase in BMP receptor type 1B. Recent data suggests that caBMPR-1A can in fact induce BMPR-1B levels. BMP2 and E_2 may decrease PPARγ expression, possibly through ER-β. E_2 interacts with the type 1B pathway to drive osteoblast to the mineralizing state. Mesenchymal precursors in the presence of high cAMP and PKA activity, and low BMPR-1B signaling preferentially differentiate towards proliferating preadipocytes with increased PPARγ levels. In the presence of BMP2 and PPARγ-ligand, these preadipocytes differentiate into mature fat cells. BMP2 can accelerate this process. The implication for this model are that post-menopausal women exposed to PPARγ-ligands, such as thiozolidinediones, may have bone cell precursors that preferentially differentiate to fat and not to bone.

References

1. Tomkenson A, Gevers EF, Wit JM et al (1998) The role of estrogen in the control of rat osteocyte apoptosis. J Bone Mineral Res 13:1243-1250.
2. Oursler MJ, Peterson L, Fitzpatrick L et al (1994) Human giant cell tumors of bone (osteoclastomas) are estrogen target cells. Proc Natl Acad Sci USA 91:5227-5231.
3. Hughes DE, Dai A, Tiffee JC et al (1996) Estrogen promotes apoptosis of murine osteoclast mediated by TGFβ. Nature Med. 2:1132-1136.
4. Kimble RB, Matayshi AB, Vannice JL et al (1995) Simultaneous block of interleukin-1 and tumor necrosis factor is required to completely prevent bone loss in early post ovariectomy period. Endocrin 136:3054-3061.
5. Arts J, Kuiper GGJM, Janssen J et al (1997) Differential expression of estrogen receptors α and β mRNA during differentiation of human osteoblast SV-HFO cells. Endocrin 138:5067-5070.
6. Damien E, Price JS, Lanyon LE (1998) The estrogen receptor's involvement in osteoblasts adaptive response to mechanical strain. J Bone and Mineral Res 13:1275-1282.
7. Paech K, Webb P, Kuiper GGJM, Nilsson S et al (1997) Differential ligand activities of estrogen receptors ERα and ERβ at AP1 sites. Science. 277:1508-1510.
8. Richard DJ, Hoffbauer LC, Bonde SK et al (1998) Bone morphogenetic protein-6 production in human osteoblastic cell lines. Selective regulation by estrogen. J Clin Invest 101: 413-422.
9. Harris SE Unpublished.
10. Takeuchi M, Tokin M, Nagata K (1995) Tamoxifen directly stimulates the mineralization of human osteoblast-like cells through a pathway independent of estrogen response element. Biochem Biophys Res Comm 210:295-301.
11. Hogan BLM (1996) Bone morphogenetic proteins: multifunctional regulators of vertebrate development. Genes Dev 10:1580-1594.
12. Chen D, Ji X, Harris MA et al (1998) Differential roles for bone morphogenetic protein (BMP) receptor Type 1B and 1A in differentiation and specification of mesenchymal precursor cells to osteoblast and adipocyte lineages. J Cell Biol 142 (1):295-305.
13. Ghosh-Choudhury N, Windle JJ, Koop BA et al (1996) Immortalized murine osteoblasts derived from BMP2-T-antigen expressing transgenic mice. Endocrin 137:331-339.

27

Estrogen and the Skeleton

Michael Kleerekoper

Introduction

The crucial role of estrogen (E) in the normal growth and development of the skeleton in girls has been known for decades. Recent studies in a man with estrogen receptor (ER) deficiency has underscored an equally important role for E in boys. Similarly the role of declining ovarian E production in bone loss in women has been well documented since the initial hypothesis of Albright in the 1940's (1). Important studies in the last several years have provided insight into possible mechanisms underlying these clinical observations, particularly the role of E in modulating local cytokine production in skeletal tissues. The finding of ER-β as the dominant ER in bone (2) answers many questions regarding the previously documented low ER density in this clearly E-dependent tissue.

Estrogen and Skeletal Growth

There are no significant differences in bone mineral density (BMD) between girls and boys at ages 8 through 11 (3), even though there are already significant BMD differences between non-Hispanic whites and African-American children at this age. This ethnic difference continues throughout life accelerating at puberty (4, 5), while the lack of gender difference begins to disappear at puberty (6). The earlier puberty in girls is accompanied by an earlier growth spurt than in boys including an earlier increase in BMD. Clear relationships between stages of puberty and BMD increases have been well documented in girls (7). Girls with delayed or absent puberty do not have this normal pubertal increase in BMD (8).

A recent report of a 28 year-old male with ER deficiency (9) highlights the importance of E on skeletal growth and development in males. This patient had delayed epiphyseal closure with marked skeletal under-mineralization in the presence of normal circulating testosterone levels and elevated E levels.

Estrogen Deficiency and Bone Loss

In all experimental animal models, bilateral oophorectomy (BO) is associated with a decrease in bone mass, a disruption of the microarchitecture of the skeleton, and a decrease in bone strength (10). E deficiency induced in this manner stimulates osteoclast-mediated bone resorption. Several lines of evidence point to an increase in local cytokine production, particularly IL-1 and IL-6, as the stimulus for increased osteoclastic activity (11, 12). There is both an increase in osteoclast number and increase in activity of each osteoclast. Antibodies to IL-6 block the rise in bone resorption induced by BO. BO followed by E administration prevents the increase in IL-1 and IL-6 and prevents the increase in osteoclastic activity. Repression of the IL-6 promoter by E appears to be mediated via NF-kappa B and C/EBP beta (13).

Surgical menopause (BO) (14) and natural menopause (15) in women have also been shown to be associated with acceleration of bone loss due to stimulation of osteoclast-mediated bone resorption. Studies implicate increased IL-1 and IL-6 production in this event in women, as it does in experimental animals. Diseases and therapies associated with a significant reduction in ovarian E production, are also associated with increased bone resorption and increased bone loss. This includes premature ovarian failure, and declining ovarian function due to disease of the hypothalamus (athletic amenorrhea, anorexia, bulimia), or pituitary (prolactinoma). Intermittent therapy with gonadotropin releasing hormone (GnRH) agonists lowers pituitary gonadotrophin synthesis and release with the resultant decrease in ovarian E production. This too is associated with bone loss that can be prevented by concomitant administration of E.

Osteoclast-mediated bone resorption occurs on skeletal surfaces, cancellous, endocortical, and to a lesser extent periosteal. Per unit of bone mass, or bone volume, there is substantially greater cancellous bone surface than endocortical or periosteal surface. At menopause, only 20% of total skeletal mass is cancellous bone, but 80% of total skeletal surface is cancellous bone. As a direct result of this, the major affects of E deficiency-induced increases in bone resorption are seen in cancellous bone, with cortical thinning due to endocortical bone resorption occurring later (16). In the bone remodeling cycle, osteoclast-mediated bone resorption is tightly coupled to osteoblast-mediated bone formation (17). However, the increase in bone formation resulting from E deficiency, is not sufficient to overcome the E deficiency-induced increase in bone resorption. Nonetheless, this coupling of resorption and formation, to a great extent, controls the rate of bone loss. This is in contrast to other circumstances, such as the effects of glucocorticosteroids on the skeleton which increase bone resorption, but also inhibit bone formation. Glucocorticosteroid-induced bone loss is substantially more rapid than the bone loss associated with E deficiency. While low levels of E persist throughout life following BO or the naturally occurring menopause, the rate of bone loss appears to slow down within 10 years after menopause. The mechanism for the slowing down of postmenopausal bone loss is unclear. One possibility is that this is simply a reflection of the reduced amount of skeletal surface, particularly cancellous bone surface, induced by the more rapid early postmenopausal bone loss. Throughout the postmenopausal period, the rate of bone loss remains higher than in the E replete premenopausal woman.

Several recent studies indicate just how precisely E levels modulate bone metabolism. In women in their 70's and older, where measurable E levels in the circulation are quite low, there is nonetheless a relationship between the variability even in these low E levels and bone density, as well as hip fracture rates (18).

The comments made about E deficiency and bone loss in women, apply equally well to testosterone deficiency and bone loss in men. Bilateral orchiectomy in men is associated with accelerated bone loss (19) just as is BO in women, and both primary and secondary diseases of the testes, with the declining testosterone production, are associated with accelerated bone loss. Surprisingly, in the older male, cross-sectional studies have shown a closer relationship between circulating E levels and bone mass than between circulating testosterone levels and bone mass (20).

Estrogen Replacement and the Prevention of Bone Loss

As previously mentioned, in experimental animals, BO induces accelerated bone loss and this can be prevented by administration of E. The same is true following a surgical menopause in women (14). The situation is a little different following natural menopause in women because the decline in ovarian E production is more gradual and begins up to four years prior to the last menstrual period. There is probably a threshold level of E, or a threshold for the rate of decline in E that triggers the increase in osteoclastic bone resorption (21). These theoretical thresholds are almost certainly reached, at least in some women, prior to the last menstrual period. This means that many women at the time of their last menstrual period have a substantial increase in the surface extent of resorption cavities. When E is given, the birth rate of new resorption cavities is substantially curtailed, but the coupled bone formation process continues to fill in existing resorption cavities. This phenomenon is known as closure of the remodeling space. This will be seen as a transient increase in bone mass reaching a plateau as the remodeling space is completely closed. This has been amply demonstrated in the recent NIH-sponsored postmenopausal E-progestin intervention studies (PEPI) (22). There is substantial variability in the size of the remodeling space at the time of the last menstrual period. There is substantial matching variability in the measured apparent increase in bone mass when E is replaced. Some of the bone loss induced by E deficiency is irreversible. The longer the E deficiency is allowed to proceed uncorrected, the greater the amount of irreversible bone loss (14). However, as noted above, E deficiency is associated with ongoing bone loss throughout life. Whenever E is provided to an E deficient woman, no matter how long she has been E deficient, there will be inhibition of bone resorption and a dramatic slow-down in the rate of loss. Again, if there is a large remodeling space at the time E is given, there will be a seeming increase in bone mass; if there is a very small remodeling space, because the rate of bone loss is very small, there will be little measurable increase in bone mass (23). These observations, however, suggest that it is possible to consider E replacement at any time in the life of a postmenopausal E deficient woman. The earlier the E is administered, the less irreversible bone loss will occur. If E replacement is discontinued or interrupted, then rates of bone loss increase seemingly to the rate that was operative at the time E was administered. The effects of E deficiency on bone resorption are most evident at the time of BO, with the most rapid decline in ovarian E production. If adequate E is given at the time of BO, bone loss will be prevented, and will be prevented as long as E is administered. However, as soon as E is discontinued, the rate of loss will approach that which would have operated at the time of the BO; similarly for rates of loss following natural menopause (15).

Estrogen and the Prevention of Osteoporotic Fractures

The major determinants of risk of a fragility fracture complicating osteoporosis are bone mass, bone microarchitecture, and propensity to fall. From the preceding discussion, it is apparent that E deficiency affects both bone mass and bone microarchitecture such that osteoporotic fragility fractures are increasingly prevalent in older postmenopausal women (24). It is equally apparent that E replacement will preserve skeletal mass and microarchitecture that is present at the time E replacement is begun. Finally, the beneficial effects of E will be apparent only as long as E is continued. Cross-sectional epidemiologic studies have demonstrated that E use for a minimum of ten years postmenopause is associated with a significant reduction in the occurrence of osteoporotic hip fracture (25). Some studies have suggested that five years of E therapy may be sufficient, but not as effective as ten years. By age 75, a time when most women who have begun postmenopausal E therapy have long since discontinued that therapy, a history of ever-use of E is no more protective against hip fracture than a history of never-use of E (26). Importantly, current use of E, even at age 75, remains protective against hip fracture. The most logical conclusion from all of this is that maximum benefit from E replacement therapy for the prevention of osteoporotic fragility fractures will be derived in the woman who starts E as early as possible after the E and continues with that E therapy for as long as possible, preferably throughout the remainder of her life.

References

1. Albright F, Smith, PH, Richardson AM (1941) Postmenopausal osteoporosis. J Am Med Ass 116:2465-2473.
2. Grandien K, Berkenstam A, Gustafsson JA (1997) The estrogen receptorgene: promoter organization and expression. Int J Biochem & Cell Biol 29:1343-1369.
3. Nelson DA, Simpson PM, Johnson CC et al (1997) The accumulation of whole body skeletal mass in third- and fourth-grade children: effects of age, gender, ethnicity, and body composition. Bone 20:73-78.
4. Gilsanz V, Roe TF, Mora S et al (1991) Changes in vertebral bone density in black girls and white girls during childhood and puberty. N Engl J Med 325:1597-1600.
5. Gilsanz V, Skaggs DL, Kovanlikaya A et al (1998) Differential effects of race on the axial and appendicular skeletons of children. J Clin Endocrinol Metab 83:1420-1427.
6. Takahashi Y, Minamitani K, Kobayashi Y et al (1996) Spinal and femoral bone mass accumulation during normal adolescence: comparison with female patients with sexual precocity ad hypogonadism. J Clin Endocrinol Metab 81:1248-1253.
7. Theintz G, Buchs B, Rizzoli R et al (1992) Longitudinal monitoring of bone mass accumulation in healthy adolescents: evidence for a marked reduction after 16 years of age at the levels of lumber spine and femoral neck in female subjects. J Clin Endocrinol Metab 79:1060-1065.
8. Holmes SJ, Shalet SM (1996) Role of growth hormone and sex steroids in achieving and maintaining normal bone mass. Hormone Res 45:86-93.
9. Smith EP, Boyd J, Frank GR et al. (1994) Estrogen resistance caused by a mutation in the estrogen-receptor gene in a man. N Engl J Med 331:1056-1061.
10. Schot LP, Schuurs AH (1990) Pathophysiology of bone loss in castrated animals. J Steroid Biochem & Mol Biol 37:461-465.
11. Ershler WB, Harman SM, Keller ET (1997) Immunologic aspects of osteoporosis. Develop & Comp Immunol 21:487-499.
12. Pacifici R (1998) Cytokines, estrogen, and postmenopausal osteoporosis - the second decade. Endocrinol 130:2659-2661.
13. Stein B, Yang MX (1995) Repression of the interleukin-6 promoter by estrogen receptor is mediated by NF-kappa B and C/EBP beta. Mol & Cell Biol 15:4971-4979.
14. Lindsay R, Hart DM, Forrest C et al (1980) Prevention of spinal osteoporosis in oophorectomized women. Lancet 2:1151-1154.
15. Slemenda C, Longcope C, Peacock M et al (1996) Sex steroids, bone mass, and bone loss: A prospective study of pre-, peri-, and postmenopausal women. J Clin Invest 97:14-21.

16. Riggs BL, Melton LJ (1986) Medical progress series: Involutional osteoporosis. N Engl J Med 314:1676-1686.
17. Han ZH, Palnitkar S, Rao DS et al (1997) Effects of ethnicity and age or menopause on the remodeling and turnover of iliac bone: implications for mechanisms of bone loss. J Bone Miner Res 12:498-508.
18. Cummings SR, Browner WS, Bauer D et al. (1998) Endogenous hormones and the risk of hip and vertebral fractures among older women. N Engl J Med 339:733-738.
19. Stepan JJ, Lachman M, Zverina J et al (1989) Castrated men exhibit bone loss. Effect of calcitonin treatment on biochemical indices of bone remodeling. J Clin Endocrinol Metab 69:523-527.
20. Riggs BL, Khosla H, Melton LJ (1998) A unitary model for involutional osteoporosis: Estrogen deficiency causes both type I and type II osteoporosis in postmenopausal women and contributes to bone loss in aging men. J Bone Miner Res 13:763-773.
21. Falch JA, Oftebro H, Haug E (1987) Early postmenopausal bone loss is not associated with a decrease in circulating levels of 25-hydroxyvitamin D, 1,25-dihydroxyvitamin D or vitamin D binding protein. J Clin Endocrinol Metab 64:836-841.
22. Anonymous (1996) Effects of hormone therapy on bone mineral density: results of the postmenopausal estrogen/progestin interventions (PEPI) trial. The writing group for PEPI. J Am Med Ass 276:1389-1396.
23. Rosen CJ, Chesnut CH, Mallinak NJ (1997) The predictive value of biochemical markers of bone turnover for bone mineral density in early postmenopausal women treated with hormone replacement or calcium supplementation. J Clin Endocrinol Metab 82:1904-1910.
24. Looker AC, Orwoll ES, Johnston CC Jr et al (1997) Prevalence of low femoral bone density in older U.S. adults from NHANES III. J Bone Miner Res 12:1761-1768.
25. Michaelsson K, Baron JA, Farahmand BY et al (1998) Hormone replacement therapy and risk of hip fracture: population based case-control study. The Swedish hip fracture study group. Brit Med J 316:1858-1863.
26. Felson DT, Zhang Y, Hannan MT et al (1993) The effect of postmenopausal estrogen therapy on bone density in elderly women. N Engl J Med 329:1141-1146.

PART 10. CARDIOVASCULAR DISEASE AND ESTROGEN/PROGESTINS

28

Mechanisms of Estrogen Action on the Cardiovascular System

John C. Stevenson

Population studies have repeatedly shown a beneficial effect of postmenopausal estrogen (E) use on coronary heart disease (CHD) (1), with an overall reduction of around 50% in the incidence. Prospective randomized controlled clinical trials are now under way to confirm these epidemiological findings (2). However, it is clearly important to understand the biological basis of these actions of E on the cardiovascular (CV) system in order to optimize current hormone replacement therapies (HRT) and develop new HRT with maximum CV impact for the future.

E has both metabolic effects and direct effects on the vasculature, both of which may improve arterial function and reduce or reverse atheroma formation. The metabolic effects include changes in lipids and lipoproteins, glucose and insulin metabolism, and coagulation and fibrinolysis. The direct arterial effects include changes in endothelium-dependent processes, ion channels, renin-angiotensin system, and remodeling processes.

Estrogen and Lipids

Lipids and lipoproteins are important in the development of atheroma. Elevated low density lipoprotein (LDL) concentrations are associated with increased CHD risk because their by hepatic receptors operates at near saturation and is slow. Thus, the LDL will have a relatively long half-life in the circulation, making them more susceptible to modification or damage, and hence more likely to be retained intramurally in the arteries giving rise to atheromatous plaque. Small dense LDL particles are particularly atherogenic because they are more readily cleared through scavenger mechanisms rather than by the apoB100 receptors, and also because they may be more susceptible to oxidative damage. Postprandial lipoprotein remnants are also atherogenic and thus the efficiency of the clearance of such remnants is also important. Lipoprotein (a) is atherogenic largely because of its propensity for intramural retention in arteries, particularly in the presence of elevated LDL concentrations. In contrast, high density lipoproteins (HDL) are inversely associated with CHD risk. HDL may participate in reverse cholesterol transport whereby they remove cholesterol from tissues, such as arterial walls, and return it to the liver for excretion or resecretion. Triglycerides are associated with increased CHD risk (3), and high concentrations may be of considerable significance in women.

The effects of E on lipids and lipoproteins depend on the type and dose of E used, and its route of administration. It should be noted that these estrogenic effects may be modified by progestogen addition.

It is well established that natural E lowers total cholesterol, irrespective of the type or route of administration, and this effect is maintained with long term treatment (4). This lowering of cholesterol results primarily from a decrease in LDL cholesterol concentrations due to an up-regulation of apoB100 receptors, and oral E administration appears to be slightly more effective than transdermal E in this respect. E may also reduce the levels of lipoprotein (a), although this effect appears rather small.

E appears to increase the proportion of small dense LDL particles (5), but this is not disadvantageous as it also increases their clearance rate (6). Other actions of E are to protect against lipoprotein oxidation (7, 8), and to improve the postprandial clearance of potentially atherogenic lipoprotein remnants (9).

E inhibits hepatic lipase activity and increases the hepatic synthesis of apolipoprotein AI. Thus, oral E increases HDL cholesterol, particularly the HDL2 subfraction which is thought to confer a protective effect against atherosclerosis development, whereas transdermal estradiol appears to have a less marked effect on HDL cholesterol (10), but it may cause a small increase in HDL2.

E effects on triglycerides are determined by the type and route of administration. Conjugated equine Es cause a significant increase in triglycerides (10), an effect which is pharmacological resulting from the hepatic first-pass effect of this steroid. Oral 17β-estradiol (E_2) may also raise triglycerides (11), but transdermal E_2 causes a reduction in triglycerides (10), which is probably the physiological effect of E_2.

Estrogen and Insulin

Decreased tissue sensitivity to insulin action, insulin resistance, is a pivotal metabolic disturbance linked with adverse changes in many CHD risk factors. It is accompanied by hyperinsulinaemia which itself may increase CHD risk by directly promoting atherogenesis (12).

Experimental studies both *in vitro* and *in vivo* have demonstrated increased pancreatic insulin secretion in response to E administration. In clinical studies, E_2 administered to postmenopausal women brings about an improvement in insulin resistance (13, 14). However, conjugated equine Es at high doses and alkylated Es, such as ethinylestradiol or mestranol, impair glucose tolerance and increase insulin concentrations (15).

In one study of healthy postmenopausal women (16), we found that transdermal therapy with E_2 and cyclic norethisterone had no significant effect on glucose tolerance or insulin concentrations. In contrast, oral therapy with conjugated equine Es and cyclic norgestrel caused a reduction in the initial plasma insulin response to intravenous glucose, which in turn resulted in a reduction in glucose elimination rate at the outset of the test, and an overall elevation in glucose concentrations. These changes increased the stimulation of pancreatic insulin secretion and hence the overall insulin response during the test. In another study (11), we found that oral E_2 given with cyclic dydrogesterone reduced insulin concentrations without any change in glucose tolerance, suggesting a reduction in insulin resistance. It should be noted that the addition of certain other progestogens, such as medroxyprogesterone acetate, may produce adverse effects on glucose and insulin metabolism.

Estrogen and Hemostatic Factors

The effects of HRT on homeostasis are somewhat complex (17), but overall are associated with a reduced incidence of arterial thromboembolism (18). Oral HRT causes reductions in fibrinogen and possibly factor VII, but these effects are perhaps counterbalanced by reductions in antithrombin III (19). Thus, an increase in prothrombotic activity, as evidenced by increased concentrations of prothrombin fragments 1 + 2, is observed (19). However, oral E is associated with a reduction in plasminogen activator inhibitor-1 (8) and tissue plasminogen activator, with increased fibrinolytic activity (19). Transdermal E_2 has little or no effect on hemostatic parameters (8, 19, 20).

Estrogen and Direct Arterial Effects

Estradiol receptors (ER) are found throughout the human arterial tree, suggesting that Es have direct effects on arteries, and there is mounting evidence from *in vitro* and *in vivo* studies to confirm this. E_2 has an inotropic effect in animals, causing systemic vasodilation and increased cardiac output (21). In humans, a decrease in carotid arterial waveform pulsatility index, a change reflecting increased arterial compliance, is observed with the administration of E_2 to postmenopausal women (22), an effect not abolished by progestogen administration (23). The acute administration of E_2 causes a reduction in myocardial ischemia, as shown by an increase in time to 1 mm ST segment depression, and in overall exercise time during the ECG exercise test, in postmenopausal women with established CHD (24).

The action of E on the arteries is mediated through both endothelium-dependent and endothelium-independent mechanisms. E_2 at physiological levels causes relaxation of coronary arteries (25), and stimulates nitric oxide (NO) synthase production by vascular endothelial cells (26). Studies both in animals (27) and in women (28, 29) have shown that the endothelium-dependent vasodilator response to acetylcholine is improved by E_2 administration. E_2 also inhibits the release of the powerful vasoconstrictor, endothelin-1, by vascular endothelial cells (26).

E_2 may also act through Ca^{++}-dependent mechanisms. In studies of isolated arterial rings, an increase in the Ca^{++} concentration of the medium resulted in contraction of the arterial rings, but this effect was inhibited in a dose-dependent manner by the addition of E_2 (30). E_2 also inhibits inward Ca^{++} currents and reduces intracellular free Ca^{++} in isolated cardiac myocytes (30). In addition, E_2 activates K^+ channels to cause coronary artery relaxation (31).

Es may also affect arterial function through changes in the renin-angiotensin system. Enhanced angiotensin-1 conversion is found in patients with the deletion allele of the angiotensin-1 converting enzyme (ACE) gene polymorphism, and such patients show impaired NO release from vascular endothelium (32). An association of the ACE gene deletion allele and CHD has been shown, particularly in women (33). We have shown that HRT with continuous E and progestogen given to postmenopausal women reduces circulating ACE activity (34).

Regulation of vascular remodeling is important for vascular health, and dysfunctional regulation may be associated with CV disease. Remodeling of vascular extracellular matrix occurs at all stages of atheroma progression, and restoration of the regulation of these processes may inhibit atherogenesis. A key group of enzymes involved in these processes are the matrix metalloproteinases (MMPs), which degrade collagen and have been implicated in the development of CV disease (35). We have recently demonstrated that MMP release by vascular smooth muscle cells is increased by E_2 in a dose-dependent manner (36). Thus, the effect of modest increases in MMPs induced by low dose E_2 in HRT may be to counteract increased vascular collagen deposition in postmenopausal women, thereby contributing to improved arterial health.

References

1. Stampfer MJ, Grodstein F (1994) Role of hormone replacement in cardiovascular disease. In: Lobo RA (ed) Treatment of the Postmenopausal Woman: Basic and Clinical Aspects. Raven Press Ltd, New York, pp. 223-233.
2. Spencer CP, Cooper AJ, Stevenson JC (1996) Clinical trials in progress with hormone replacement therapy. Exp Opin Invest Drugs 5:739-749.

3. Bengtsson C, Björkelund C, Lapidus L et al (1993) Associations of serum lipid concentrations and obesity with mortality in women: 20 year follow up of participants in prospective population study in Gothenburg, Sweden. Br Med J 307:1385-1388.

4. Whitcroft SI, Crook D, Marsh MS et al (1994) Long-term effects of oral and transdermal hormone replacement therapies on serum lipid and lipoprotein concentrations. Obstet Gynecol 84:222-226.

5. van der Mooren MJ, de Graaf J, Demacker PN et al (1994) Changes in the low-density lipoprotein profile during 17 beta-oestradiol-dydrogesterone therapy in postmenopausal women. Metabolism 43:799-802.

6. Campos H, Walsh BW, Judge H et al (1997) Effect of estrogen on very low density lipoprotein and low density lipoprotein subclass metabolism in postmenopausal women. J Clin Endocrinol Metab 82:3955-3963.

7. Sack MN, Rader DJ, Cannon RO (1994) Oestrogen and inhibition of oxidation of low-density lipoproteins in postmenopausal women. Lancet 343:269-270.

8. Koh KK, Mincemoyer R, Bui MN et al (1997) Effects of hormone replacement therapy on fibrinolysis in postmenopausal women. N Engl J Med 336:683-690.

9. Westerveld HT, Kock LAW, van Rijn JM et al (1995) 17β-estradiol improves postprandial lipid metabolism in postmenopausal women. J Clin Endocrinol Metab 80:249-253.

10. Crook D, Cust MP, Gangar KF et al (1992) Comparison of transdermal and oral estrogen/progestin hormone replacement therapy: effects on serum lipids and lipoproteins. Am J Obstet Gynecol 166:950-955.

11. Crook D, Godsland IF, Hull J et al (1997) Hormone replacement therapy with dydrogesterone and 17β-oestradiol: effects on serum lipoproteins and glucose tolerance during 24 month follow up. Br J Obstet Gynaecol 104:298-304.

12. Stout R (1990) Insulin and atheroma: 20-yr perspective. Diabetes Care 13: 631-654.

13. Notelovitz M, Johnston M, Smith S et al (1987) Metabolic and hormonal effects of 25mg and 50mg 17β estradiol implants in surgically menopausal women. Obstet Gynecol 70:749-754.

14. Cagnacci A, Soldani R, Carriero P et al (1992) Effects of low doses of transdermal 17β-estradiol on carbohydrate metabolism in postmenopausal women. J Clin Endocrinol Metab 74:1396-1400.

15. Spellacy WN, Buhi WC, Birk SA (1972) The effects of estrogens on carbohydrate metabolism: glucose, insulin and growth hormone studies on one hundred and seventy one women ingesting Premarin, mestranol and ethinyl estradiol for six months. Am J Obstet Gynecol 114:378-392.

16. Godsland IF, Gangar KF, Walton C et al (1993) Insulin resistance, secretion, and elimination in postmenopausal women receiving oral or transdermal hormone replacement therapy. Metabolism 42:846-853.

17. Winkler UH (1992) Menopause, hormone replacement therapy and cardiovascular disease: a review of haemostaseological findings. Fibrinolysis 6 suppl 3:5-10.

18. Paganini-Hill A, Ross RK, Henderson BE (1988) Postmenopausal oestrogen treatment and stroke: a prospective study. Br Med J 297:519-522.

19. Scarabin P-Y, Alhenc-Gelas M, Plu-Bureau G (1997) Effects of oral and transdermal estrogen/progesterone regimens on blood coagulation and fibrinolysis in postmenopausal women. Arterioscler Thromb Vasc Biol 17: 3071-3078.

20. Fox J, George AJ, Newton JR et al (1993) Effect of transdermal oestradiol on the haemostatic balance of menopausal women. Maturitas 18:55-64.

21. Magness RR, Rosenfeld CR (1989) Local and systemic estradiol-17 beta: effects on uterine and systemic vasodilation. Am J Physiol 256:E536-E542.

22. Gangar KF, Vyas S, Whitehead M et al (1991) Pulsatility index in internal carotid artery in relation to transdermal oestradiol and time since menopause. Lancet 338:839-842.

23. Hillard TC, Bourne TH, Whitehead MI et al (1992) Differential effects of transdermal estradiol and sequential progestogens on impedance to flow within the uterine arteries of postmenopausal women. Fertility and Sterility 58:959-963.

24. Rosano GMC, Sarrel PM, Poole-Wilson P et al (1993) Beneficial effect of oestrogen on exercise-induced myocardial ischemia in women with coronary artery disease. Lancet 342:133-136.

25. Collins P, Shay J, Jiang C et al (1994) Nitric oxide accounts for dose-dependent estrogen-mediated coronary relaxation after acute estrogen withdrawal. Circulation 90:1964-1968.

26. Wingrove CS, Stevenson JC (1997) 17β-oestradiol inhibits stimulated endothelin release in human vascular endothelial cells. Eur J Endocrinol 137: 205-208.

27. Williams JK, Adams MR, Klopfenstein HS (1990) Estrogen modulates responses of atherosclerotic coronary arteries. Circulation Res 81:1680-1687.

28. Gilligan DM, Badar DM, Panza JA (1994) Acute vascular effects of estrogen in postmenopausal women. Circulation 90:786-791.

29. Collins P, Rosano GMC, Sarrel PM et al (1995) 17β-estradiol attenuates acetylcholine-induced coronary arterial constriction in women but not men with coronary heart disease. Circulation 92:24-30.

30. Jiang C, Poole-Wilson P, Sarrel P et al (1992) Effects of 17β-oestradiol on contraction, Ca2+ current and intracellular free Ca2+ in guinea-pig isolated cardiac myocytes. Br J Pharmacol 106:739-745.

31. White RE, Darkow DJ, Falvo Lang JL (1995) Estrogen relaxes coronary arteries by opening BKCa channels through a cGMP-dependent mechanism. Circ Res 77:936-942.

32. Buikema H, Pinto YM, Rooks G et al (1996) The deletion polymorphism of the anfiotensin-converting enzyme gene is related to phenotypic differences in human arteries. Eur Heart J 17:787-794.

33. Schuster H, Wienker TF, Stremmler U et al (1995) An angiotensin-converting enzyme gene variant is associated with acute myocardial infarction in women but not in men. Am J Cardiol 76:601-603.

34. Proudler AJ, Ahmed AIH, Crook D et al (1995) Hormone replacement therapy and serum angiotensin-converting-enzyme activity in postmenopausal women. Lancet 346:89-90.

35. Dollery CM, McEwan JR, Henney AM (1995) Matrix metalloproteinases and cardiovascular disease. Circ Res 77:863-868.

36. Wingrove CS, Garr E, Godsland IF et al (1998) 17β-oestradiol enhances release of matrix metalloproteinase-2 from human vascular smooth muscle cells. Biochim Biophys Acta 1406:169-174.

29

Atherosclerosis and Hormone Replacement Therapy: The Role of Estrogen in Secondary Prevention of Cardiovascular Events

Jay M. Sullivan

Introduction

For over sixty years, it has been appreciated that young and middle aged women have far fewer heart attacks than men of comparable age. It has also been noted that the myocardial infarction (MI) rate increases as women age after menopause (1). More than thirty five observational studies have examined the effect of estrogen replacement therapy (ERT) on survival and have found that current users of estrogen (E) have a reduction in the rate of cardiovascular (CV) events of 42% (RR 0.58, 95% CI -0.42-0.64) (2). Recent studies have indicated that the addition of progestins does not reduce this apparent benefit (3).

There has been serious concern about recommending hormone replacement therapy (HRT) for women with known CV diseases. This concern rose from the adverse effects of E therapy for men in the Coronary Drug Project and from the increased risk of MI in older women who smoked cigarettes and used early preparations of oral contraceptive agents. A British study found that 45% of general practitioners and gynecologists considered ischemic heart disease to be a relative contraindication to hormone replacement and a Finnish study found that 24% of generalists thought that HRT increased the risk of developing CV disease.

This review will examine the experience of women with CV disease who receive E or HRT.

Estrogen Therapy After an Acute Coronary Event

There are few studies of E use after MI. The first was the Coronary Drug Project, which randomized male survivors of acute MI into several therapeutic arms, two of which involved conjugated equine Es in daily doses of 2.5 or 5.0 mg. The men receiving 5 mg per day suffered more CV events than the control group. Definite MI occurred in 6.2% of E-treated men, but in only 3.2% of those receiving placebo. There was a statistically significant increase in incidence of definite pulmonary embolism or thrombophlebitis in the E-treated men, 3.5%, compared to 1.3% in the control group. Although the men receiving 2.5 mg/day of Es did not have a statistically significant increase in heart attacks, this part of the study was stopped when malignancy was found more often in the E-supplemented men than in those receiving placebo.

Women enrolled in The Group Health Cooperative of Puget Sound in the state of Washington were the subject of a retrospective cohort study involving 726 individuals. All were discharged from the hospital after surviving an acute MI between 1980 and 1991. Pharmacy records disclosed that 122 women received ERT. One hundred eighty three women died and 135 suffered a second MI. After adjustment for age and time since infarction, the relative risk for reinfarction among current users of ERT was 0.64 (95% CI, 0.32-1.30). For women who had used E in the past, the relative risk was 0.90 (95% CI, 0.62-1.31). The reduction of total mortality in current users was greater, RR 0.50 (95% CI, 0.25-1.00), than for past users 0.79 (95% CI, 0.56-1.09). Adjustment for congestive heart failure, diabetes mellitus, and other CV risk factors altered the relative risk calculation very little. Although this study did not show that E use significantly reduced the recurrence of MI, it did provide evidence that E use is safe for women with a history of MI and suggests that E use may be beneficial.

Estrogen Replacement in Women With a History of Cardiovascular Disease

Two large observational studies included women known to have CV disease at the time that the study began. Both found that ERT was associated with a greater survival benefit in the group with pre-existing disease, than in women who lacked historical or clinical evidence of CV disease. The Lipid Research Clinics Program (4) included a cohort of 2,270 women who were followed for an average of 8.5 years. In women free of CV disease, the mortality rate was 12.8/10,000 in E users and 30.2/10,000 in non-users, a decline of 58%. In women with CV disease, the CV death rate was 13.8/10,000 in E users, and 66.3/10,000 in non-users, a greater decrease of 79%.

The Leisure World Study included 8,881 postmenopausal women who were followed for 7.5 years. In women with no history of angina or MI, all-cause mortality was 21.8/1,000 in E users, and 26.7/1,000 in non-users. A decrease of 18%. In women with a positive history, all-cause mortality was 27.5/1,000 in E users and 41.7/1,000 in non-users, 34% less.

Estrogen Replacement in Women with Positive Coronary Angiography

The effect of E on survival in patients with angiographically-demonstrated coronary artery disease was studied in 2,268 women who underwent catheterization (5). Actuarial methods were used to analyze survival over 10 years. Patients free of coronary artery disease at baseline had 10-year survival rates greater than 90% regardless of E use. In patients with mild to moderate coronary lesions at baseline, 10-year survival was significantly better among E users than in non-users. Among those who never took E, 85% were still alive, compared with 96% in those who used E ($p=0.027$). The difference in survival was most marked in patients with severe stenotic lesions. Sixty percent of those who never used Es were alive at 10 years, compared with 98% of those who had ever taken E ($p=0.007$).

A Cox stepwise proportional hazards analysis was used to determine which factors had a statistically significant independent effect on total mortality. The most powerful determinants were the number of coronary arteries involved, the severity of cardiac functional impairment, age, and stenosis of the left main coronary artery. The only significant factor predicting improved survival was E use. Relative risk equaled 0.16 with 95% confidence intervals of 0.04-0.66.

Estrogen Replacement after Coronary Revascularization

The relationship between postmenopausal E use and survival has also been studied in women who underwent coronary artery bypass surgery. Life-tables analysis was used to compare postsurgical survival in women who received ERT with those who did not. The 10.0-year survival was 81.4% in the E users and 65.1% in the non-users ($p=0.0001$). A Cox proportional hazards model selected the number of vessels diseased, E use, left main coronary stenosis, and diabetes mellitus as significant independent predictors of survival.

Two studies have examined the effect of E on outcome after percutaneous transluminal coronary arterioplasty. One study involved 293 women of whom 100 received E replacement. The MI rate during follow-up was 6% and their 7.0-year survival rate was 95%. In contrast, in the group of 193 women who did not receive E, the MI rate was 12% and 7.0-year survival was 78% ($p=0.001$). A second study, involving 23 E users and 84 non-users, found no differences in the rate of restenosis by angiographic criteria at 6 mo., 48% versus 50%. The same study observed a 57% restenosis rate after coronary atherectomy in 79 women who did not use E, and a significantly lower rate of 27% in 18 E users ($p=0.038$).

Estrogen Replacement in Women with Cardiovascular Risk Factors

The Nurses' Health Study also supports the concept that those women who are at the greatest risk of CV disease benefit most from ERT (6). The major CV risk factors examined were current cigarette smoking, high cholesterol, high blood pressure, diabetes mellitus, parentenal history of premature MI, and body mass index greater than 29. In women with one or more major CV risk factors, the relative risk of survival was 0.51 (0.45-0.57) while in those without CV risk factors, the relative risk was 0.83 (0.62-1.28).

Adverse Cardiovascular Effects of Estrogen

Recent data indicate that ERT increases the risk of deep vein thrombosis and pulmonary embolism. A British study of 103 cases of idiopathic venous thromboembolism and 178 women controls found that users had an odds ratio of 3.5 (95% CI, 1.8-7.0) compared to those who did not use HRT. Another case control study, the Group Health Cooperative of Puget Sound observed a relative risk of thromboembolism of 3.2 (95% CI, 1.5-6.8) comparing current users with non-users. The Nurses' Health Study observed a 2.0-fold increase in the risk of a more definite endpoint, confirmed pulmonary embolism, among current E users. Although the three studies found that E use was associated with an increase in the relative risk of venous thromboembolism, the absolute risk was low as venous thrombosis occurred infrequently. When weighed against a 42% reduction in CV disease, a highly prevalent disorder, the increased risk of venous thromboembolism does not contraindicate ERT, but does point out the need for attention to a prior history of unprovoked thrombosis.

Mechanisms of Cardioprotection (Table 1)

Observational and animal studies suggest that the effect of ERT on lipids accounts for about 25% to 50% of its cardioprotective effect. Prior to menopause, women have higher HDL levels than men. After menopause, low density lipoprotein (LDL) levels increases while HDL levels decline. ERT decreases LDL and total cholesterol levels, and increase levels of HDL cholesterol and triglycerides (7).

Table 1. Estrogen: mechanisms of cardioprotection.

I. LIPID EFFECTS
Increased hepatic clearance of LDL
Increased synthesis of apolipoprotein A_1 and A_2
Decreased clearance of HDL
Increased synthesis of VLDL and triglycerides*
II. ENDOTHELIAL EFFECTS
Increased release of nitric oxide
Increased expression of genes that encode for nitric
Oxide synthase (Controversial)
Decreased release of endothelin I
Decreased response to endothelin I
Increase release of PGI_2
Decreased formation of thromboxane A_2
Increased endothelial proliferation
Increased endothelial cell migration
Increased capillary tube formation
Decreased endothelial cell apoptosis
III. OXIDATIVE EFFECTS
Antioxidant
Decreased formation of Oxygen-derived free radicals
IV. CLOTTING EFFECTS
Decreased plasma fibrinogen
Decreased plasminogen activator inhibitor
Antiplatelet effect
Increased fibrinolysis
Decreased antithrombin III*
Decreased protein C*
V. CARBOHYDRATE EFFECTS
Increased insulin sensitivity
Decreased blood glucose
Decreased blood insulin
VI. ION CHANNEL EFFECTS
Ca^{++} channel blockade
K^+ channel opening
VII. ARTERIAL WALL EFFECTS
Vasodilation (decreased vasospasm)
Decreased myointimal proliferation
Decreased uptake of LDL
*Potentially adverse effect

To reduce the risk of endometrial carcinoma, ERT is usually given along with a progestin. There are relatively few studies focusing on the cardioprotective effects of combined HRT. The PEPI Trial (8) observed that conjugated Es, with or without progestins, lowered LDL by 14.5-17.2 mg/dl. E alone raised HDL by 5.6 mg/dl. The addition of a progestin attenuated the HDL rise to 1.2 to 1.5 mg/dl, while micronized progesterone raised HDL by 4.2 mg/dl.

In a study of surgically menopausal non-human primates, both E and E with progesterone reduced the extent of aortic atherosclerosis, even though combination therapy reduced HDL levels (9). Combination therapy also reduced LDL cholesterol uptake by arterial walls to the same extent as E. Recent studies have shown that the addition of medroxyprogesterone acetate (MPA) reduces the antiatherosclerotic effect of E.

In long-term human cohort studies, HDL levels did not differ significantly between women taking ERT or HRT (10). The Uppsala Study (11) showed that both ERT or HRT reduced the risk of first MI or stroke about equally. Nachtigall, *et al* (12), in the only completed randomized trial of HRT, showed a reduction in the rate of MI in 84 pairs of hospitalized women that was not statistically significant.

The Puget Sound Area Health Group study provided additional evidence that HRT reduced CV risk to the same degree as E alone. The relative risk of first MI was 0.69 (95% CI 0.54 to 1.25) in ERT, and 0.53 (0.30 to 0.87) in HRT (13).

The sixteen year follow-up of the Nurses' Health Study provides important information about combined HRT (14). In this study of 59,337 women, the relative risk of coronary heart disease in women who took HRT was 0.39 (0.19 to 0.78) compared to women who did not take it The relative risk in women who took ERT was 0.60 (0.43 to 0.83).

The Effects of Estrogen on Endothelium

Es have an effect on vascular reactivity. The endothelium plays an important role in the regulation of blood vessel tone. Furchgott, *et al*. (15), demonstrated that when endothelium was removed the response of arterial strips to acetylcholine changed. Intact strips relaxed. After removal, acetylcholine caused constriction. Acetylcholine stimulates the release of endothelial-derived relaxing factor, which causes vasodilatation. Relaxing factor has been identified as nitric oxide, formed from l-arginine. Release of nitric oxide activates guanylate cyclase. This triggers synthesis of cyclic GMP, which in turn alters Ca^{++} movement.

Impaired endothelial function has been described in the elderly, in patients with hypertension, hypercholesterolemia or diabetes, in cigarette smokers and in menopausal women. Studies in animals (16) and humans (17) show that E improves endothelium-dependent vasodilatation and increases release of nitric oxide. Certain evidence suggests that E induces nitric oxide synthase, but the data are contradictory. Oxygen-derived free radicals inactivate nitric oxide. E has recently been shown to reduce the generation of oxygen-derived free radicals, thus increasing the effect of nitric oxide (18). E also modifies the release and effect of endothelin I, a potent vasoconstrictor released by the endothelium (19).

The expression of adhesion molecules by injured endothelial cells is one of the first events in the formation of an atherosclerotic plaque. Molecules such as E-selectin, VCAM, and ICAM cause monocytes to adhere to endothelium and to migrate into the subendothelial space and become macrophages. E_2 has been shown to inhibit the expression of adhesion molecules (20).

E_2 has also been found to stimulate endothelial cell proliferation, to increase the ability of the endothelium to spread and cover wounds, and to form vascular tubes (21). E_2 inhibits apoptosis, or programmed cell death, in endothelial cells exposed to tumor necrosis factor α (22).

Infusion of acethycholine into normal human coronary arteries causes vasodilatation, but infusion into arteries with atherosclerotic lesions produces vasoconstriction of the stenotic and adjacent areas. This suggests that atherosclerotic involvement of the vessel wall impairs endothelial function. Williams, et al. (16), demonstrated that acetylcholine causes constriction when infused into coronary vessels of ovariectomized monkeys fed a high fat diet, suggesting loss of endothelial function. When the monkeys received ERT, acetylcholine produced a more normal response. Four human studies have made similar observations.

Other evidence that ERT alters blood vessel function includes; demonstration of ERs in endothelial and vascular smooth muscle cells, the Ca^{++} channel blocking and K^+ channel opening properties of E, stimulation of the production of prostacyclin, and reduction of the production of thromboxane A_2 (23).

In addition to being actively involved in regulating vascular tone through the regulation of vasorelaxing and vasoconstricting factors, the endothelium also regulates the growth of vascular smooth muscle, an important component in the growth of atherosclerotic plaques; limits the passage of LDL cholesterol into the blood vessel wall, which in turn retards the growth of the atherosclerotic plaque; and increases the metabolism of triglycerides through the action of cell membrane lipoprotein lipase.

The Importance of Correcting Other Coronary Risk Factors in Women

A National Center for Health Statistics survey found that 29% of adult American women smoke cigarettes. Eighty-four percent of women under age 50 with a history of acute MI are cigarette smokers. In the USA, 30% of white women and 50% of black women weigh 20% more than their ideal body weight. Twenty-three percent of American women are hypertensive. With aging, the prevalence of hypertension rises to 35% in white women and 55% in black women.

Table 2. Cardiovascular risk factors for women.

GENETIC	LIFESTYLE
Diabetes mellitus	Cigarette smoking
Hypertension	High fat, High
Elevated LDL cholesterol	Cholesterol disease
Low HDL cholesterol	Sedentary lifestyle
Small, dense LDL Stress (?)	
Elevated Lp(a)	
Elevated homocysteine	
Elevated fibrinogen	
Elevated PAI	
Estrogen deficiency	
Obesity	

A meta analysis of randomized antihypertensive drug treatment trials, in which 47% of participants were women, showed a 42% decrease in stroke and a 14% decline in coronary disease. Based on these trials, women with systolic blood pressure over 160 mm Hg and diastolic pressure over 90 mm Hg should change lifestyle to reduce weight, lower sodium and alcohol intake, and increase exercise.

The Lipid Research Clinics Follow-Up Study followed 2,270 women and found no association between total or LDL cholesterol and CV death. Triglycerides were found to be a significant risk factor for CV death in women and that HDL cholesterol was protective. The Framingham Study reported that total and LDL cholesterol are definite risk factors for coronary disease in women in their fifth, sixth, and seventh decades of life.

Two randomized trials of the effects of dietary and drug interventions on atherosclerosis involved cohorts containing 52% women. These studies showed that lowering LDL and increasing HDL slowed the progression of atherosclerosis in both men and women. However, data were insufficient to show reduction of coronary events. The results of one primary prevention trial and six secondary prevention trials suggested that women and men both benefit from lipid lowering. Based on the available data, it is reasonable to propose that lowering cholesterol is beneficial for women.

Evidence that diabetes mellitus is a very powerful predictor of CV risk for women is strong. In premenopausal women, diabetes mellitus increases CV risk to that of comparably aged men.

Also, the U.S. Nurses' Health Study found that women who took 1-6 aspirin tablets a week had 32% fewer first episodes of MI; and women who took the most vitamin E for over 2 years had a 44% lower rate of coronary artery disease compared with others.

Addendum

The Heart and Estrogen/Progestin Replacement Study (HERS) (26) was the first randomized, placebo-controlled, double-blind study to test the hypothesis that HRT therapy reduced recurrent coronary events in women with coronary heart disease. The trial was unique in that it used conjugated equine E 0.625 mg daily plus combined, continuous MPA in a daily dose of 2.5 mg. No prior observational study has examined this regimen.

The trial involved 2,763 women who were followed an average of 4.1 years. Their average age was 67 years. Most were white, overweight and on aspirin therapy.

Over the 4.1 years of follow-up, there were no difference in the primary endpoints of coronary deaths or non-fatal MIs between the two groups (RR 0.99, 95% CI, 0.8-1.22). Examination of the time course of these results showed that there was an early increase in the risk of a cardiac event during the first year (RR 1.52, 95% CI, 1.01-2.29) while a significantly lower event rate was found in years 4 and 5 (RR 0.67, 95% CI, 0.43-1.04). Most of the coronary events occurred during the first 4.0-mo. period. There was also a significant increase in the risk of venous thromboembolism during the same period. There was no difference in the occurrence of breast cancer, endometrial cancer, or hip fracture.

The explanation for this result is not clear. It is possible that MPA interferes with the anti-atherosclerotic effects of E or that HRT therapy or ERT causes thrombotic events in the coronary and venous circulations of susceptible individuals. The authors of the study concluded that this regimen of HRT could not be recommended for the secondary prevention of heart disease, however women who are already on this or other forms of ERT or HRT should continue therapy because of the favorable long-term trends.

Acknowledgment

This chapter was reproduced with permission from Menopausal Medicine, Sullivan, JM. The role of E in secondary prevention of CV events. Menopausal Medicine 1998;6. Copyright American Society for Reproductive Medicine, 1998.

References

1. Kannel WB, Hjortland MC, McNamara PM et al (1976) Menopause and the risk of cardiovascular disease. The Framingham Study. Ann Intern Med 85:447-452.
2. Stampfer MJ, Colditz GC (1991) Estrogen replacement therapy and coronary heart disease: A quantitative assessment of the epidemiologic evidence. Preventive Medicine 20:47-63.
3. Grodstein F, Stampfer MJ, Manson JE et al (1996) Postmenopausal estrogen and progestin use and the risk of cardiovascular disease. N Engl J Med 335:453-461.
4. Bush TL, Barrett-Connor E, Cowan LD et al (1987) Cardiovascular mortality and noncontraceptive use of estrogen in women: results from the Lipid Research Clinics Program Follow-up Study. Circulation 75:1102-1109.
5. Sullivan JM, Vander Zwaag R, Hughes JP et al (1990) Estrogen replacement and coronary artery disease: effect on survival in postmenopausal women. Arch Intern Med 150:2557-2562.
6. Grodstein F, Stampfer MJ, Colditz GA et al (1997) Postmenopausal hormone therapy and mortality. N Engl J Med 336:1769-1775.
7. Walsh BW, Schiff I et al (1991) Effects of postmenopausal estrogen replacement on the concentrations and metabolism of plasma lipoproteins. N Engl J Med 325:1196-1204.
8. The Writing Group for the PEPI Trial (1995) Effects of estrogen or estrogen/progestin regimens on heart disease risk factors in postmenopausal women. The Postmenopausal Estrogen/Progestin Interventions (PEPI) Trial. J Am Med Ass 273:199-208.
9. Clarkson TB, Shively CA, Morgan T et al (1990) Oral contraceptives and coronary artery atherosclerosis of cynomolgus monkeys. Obstet Gynecol 75:217-222.
10. Nabulsi AA, Folsom AR, White A et al (1993) Association of hormone-replacement therapy with various cardiovascular risk factors in postmenopausal women. N Engl J Med 328:1069-1075.
11. Falkeborn M, Persson I, Adami HO et al (1992) The risk of acute myocardial infarction after oestrogen and oestrogen-progestogen replacement. Br J Obstet Gynaecol 99:821-8928.
12. Nachtigall LE, Nachtigall RH, Nachtigall RD et al (1979) Estrogen replacement therapy II: a prospective study in the relationship to carcinoma and cardiovascular and metabolic problems. Obstet Gynecol 54:74-79.
13. Psaty BM, Heckbert SR, Atkins D et al (1994) The risk of myocardial infarction associated with the combined use of estrogens and progestins in postmenopausal women. Arch Intern Med 154:1333-1339.

14. Grodstein F, Stampfer MJ, Manson JE et al (1996) Postmenopausal estrogen and progestin use and the risk of cardiovascular disease. N Engl J Med 335:453-461.

15. Furchgott RF, Zawadzk JV (1980) The obligatory role of endothelial cells in the relaxation of arterial smooth muscle by acetylcholine. Nature 288:373-376.

16. Williams JK, Adams MR, Klopfenstein HS (1990) Estrogen modulates responses of atherosclerotic coronary arteries. Circulation 81:1680-1687.

17. Reis SE, Gloth ST, Blumenthal RS et al (1994) Ethinyl estradiol acutely attenuates abnormal coronary vasomotor responses to acetylcholine in postmenopausal women. Circulation 89:52-60.

18. Arnal JF, Clamens S, Pechet C et al (1996) Ethinylestradiol does not enhance the expression of nitric oxide synthase in bovine endothelial cells but increases the release of bioactive nitric oxide by inhibiting superoxide anion production. Proc Natl Acad Sci 93:4108-4113.

19. Jiang C, Sarrel PM, Poole-Wilson PA et al (1992) Acute effect of 17B-estradiol on rabbit coronary artery contractile responses to endothelin-1. Am J Physiol 263:H271-H275.

20. Caulin-Glaser T, Watson CA, Pardi R et al (1996) Effects of 17 beta-estradiol on cytokine-induced endothelial cell adhesion molecule expression. J Clin Invest 98(1):36-42.

21. Morales DE, McGowan KA, Grant DS et al (1995) Estrogen promotes angiogenic activity in human umbilical vein endothelial cells in vitro and in a murine model. Circulation 91:755-763.

22. Spyridopoulos I, Sullivan AB, Kearney M et al (1997) Estrogen-receptor-mediated inhibition of human endothelial cell apotosis. Estradiol as a survival factor. Circulation 95:1505-1514.

23. Fogelberg M, Vesterquist O, Dicfalusy U et al (1990) Experimental atherosclerosis: effects of estrogen and atherosclerosis on thromboxane and prostacyclin formation. Europ J Clin Invest 20:105-110.

24. Sullivan JM (1998) Estrogen replacement after coronary artery thrombosis. In: Studd JWW (ed) Chapter 6 in the Management of the Menopause, Annual Review 1998. Parthenon Publishin,g Carnforth, UK.

25. Rich-Edwards JW, Manson JE, Hennekens CH et al (1995) The primary prevention of coronary heart disease in women. N Engl J Med 332:1758-1766.

26. Hulley S, Grady D, Bush T et al (1998) E for the Heart and Estrogen/progestin Replacement Study (HERS) Research Group. Randomized trial of estrogen plus progestin for secondary prevention of coronary heart disease in postmenopausal women. J Am Med Ass 280:605-613.

VIEWPOINT

30

Long-term Hormone Replacement Therapy: A Contrary Point of View

Jacques E. Rossouw

Known Benefits and Risks

Benefits of short term hormone replacement therapy (HRT) include the relief of symptoms of peri-menopausal vasomotor instability and vaginal atrophy. Improvement in cognitive functioning has been reasonably well established (1). Controlled clinical trials have demonstrated that estrogen (E) halts loss of bone mass at menopause and thereafter, yet there is no clinical trial evidence that HRT prevents fractures (2).

Known risks of HRT include gallbladder disease, pancreatitis, and venous thromboembolism (3-7). These risks are present soon after the onset of therapy, and may continue for some years thereafter. E unopposed by a progestin increases the risk of endometrial cancer (8-9). Addition of a progestin prevents the emergence of endometrial cancer for up to 3 years, but some studies suggest the re-emergence of increased risk after a longer duration of therapy (8-9).

Unknown Benefits and Risks

However, fifty years after the introduction of HRT, little in known about the benefits and risks of long-term treatment. Despite widespread assumptions to the contrary, there is no incontrovertible evidence that HRT will prevent coronary heart disease (CHD) (10-11). A reduction in risk of CHD, and lack of a substantial increase in risk of breast cancer, is critically important to the calculation of overall benefit and risk (see below). Effects on strokes are not clear, with observational studies reporting no effect, decreases, or increases in risk of stroke (12). At least one study has reported an increase in thrombotic stroke in E users, and a dose-response relationship for all strokes (5). Despite promising effects on cognitive function, it is not known whether HRT will prevent or ameliorate dementia (1). The evidence that HRT will prevent colorectal cancer is limited (13).

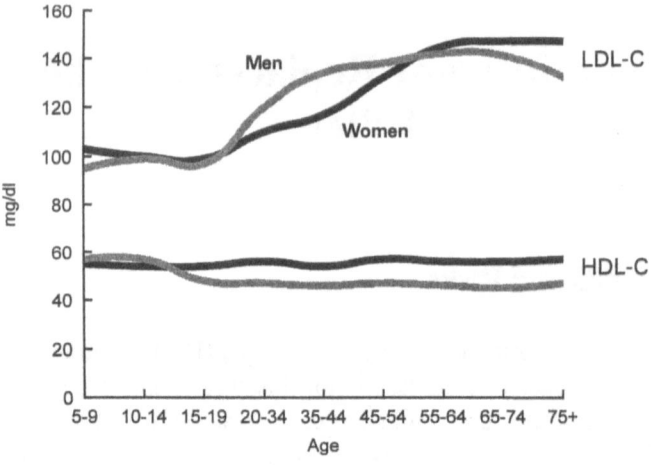

Figure 1. Levels of LDL- and HDL-cholesterol in men and women by age (15).

Coronary Heart Disease

Endogenous Sex Hormones, Blood Lipids, and CHD. The mediator of the putative protective effect of E is generally thought to be the higher levels of high density lipoprotein cholesterol (HDL-C) in women (14). In adults, HDL-C levels are some 10 mg/dl higher in women than in men, and a difference of that magnitude could explain much of the sex difference in CHD (15). However, it is unclear whether the sex difference in HDL-C over the lifespan is due to endogenous E raising HDL-C, or to androgens lowering it. Interestingly, the sex difference manifests itself at puberty, when the HDL-C levels of boys drop (16). Prior to puberty, HDL-C levels in boys and girls are identical (Figure 1). By contrast, the HDL-C levels in women remain fairly constant throughout life, including during the childhood years, with only a minor drop during the menopause. This pattern of HDL-C levels by age is compatible with an androgen effect in men, rather than an E effect in women. The low density lipoprotein (LDL-C) levels in young adult men is higher than that of young adult women; after the age of about 55 years this pattern reverses as the LDL-C levels in men flatten out and decline while the levels in women continue to rise. Though there are other potential explanations, the changes in LDL-C levels in men are compatible with androgens raising LDL-C in younger men, with a waning effect in later years as androgen levels decline. In women, E may help keep LDL-C levels relatively lower up to middle age, thereafter, the increases in LDL-C may be associated with declining E levels. The rate of increase of CHD by age and gender is instructive in that there is no increase around the age of menopause in women, as might be expected if decreasing E levels were important, while there is a flattening of the rate in men, consistent with waning androgen levels (16).

Exogenous Estrogen and Potential Metabolic Mechanisms for Reduction in Risk of CHD. The data on the effects of exogenous Es are quite consistent for lipids: Given orally, E decreases LDL-C, and Lp(a), and increases HDL-C and triglycerides. Oral progestins do not modify the E effects on LDL-C and Lp(a), but do blunt the increases in HDL-C and triglycerides (1, 17-19). The data on coagulation factors are not easy to interpret, but generally, exogenous E appears to be is pro-coagulant but at the same time pro-fibrinolytic (20-21). Some of the estrogenic effects on coagulation are partially countered by progestins (17-18). The observational and clinical trial data on venous thromboembolism indicate that the overall estrogenic effect is to promote clot formation in the veins (3-7). The balance between unfavorable changes in coagulation factors and favorable lipid changes may determine the outcome for CHD, stroke, and venous thromboembolism (7, 22). E administered though a skin patch, which does not undergo first-pass circulation through the liver, has much less effect on both lipids (23-24) and coagulation factors (20, 25). However, this does not mean that skin patches are preferable to oral Es if the purpose is to prevent CHD, since it may well be that the metabolic changes in lipid levels are the mediators of any benefit. On the other hand, if the mediators of benefit are direct effects on the arterial wall, then the skin patch may have an advantage. However, there is no epidemiologic data supporting either the use of the skin patch to prevent CHD or for oral E use.

Direct Effects on the Arterial Wall. Evidence is accumulating from animal and human studies that E has direct effects on the arterial wall (26). In a model of diet-induced atherosclerosis in ovariectomized monkeys, oral E reduced atherosclerosis through direct effects on LDL turnover and oxidation in the vessel wall (27). These effects were not correlated with plasma lipoprotein levels, including levels of HDL-C (which do not change), but are countered by oral progestins. Similarly, in monkeys with coronary atherosclerosis, E improved endothelium-mediated coronary vasodilation, and this effect was countered by progestin (28). However, E with or without progestin did not augment regression of established coronary atherosclerosis in monkeys (29). In postmenopausal women, E, at physiological doses, increased endothelium dependent coronary vasodilation, and this response was dampened or abolished by progestins (30-33).

Observational Studies. The observational studies form the most important body of evidence supporting the view that HRT in postmenopausal women may prevent CHD. Observational studies comparing the CHD rates in women who choose to take HRT to those who do not have generally suggested a risk reduction of about 40-50% in current HRT users compared to never-users (5, 34, 35, 37). However, observational studies are likely to be confounded by various biases, which will lead to an overestimation of the benefits and an underestimation of risks (10-11). For example, women who choose HRT were healthier than those who do not, and would have lower rates of CHD, and many other diseases, by virtue of their better prior health status (38). Women who continue HRT for many years fit the definition of good compliers, and good compliance to any medication is associated with lower risk. For example, CHD patients in a trial of β-blocking agents who took more that 75% of their study medications had a 68% reduction in mortality compared to those who took less than 75% of study medications (39). One interpretation could be that the drug works, and the more drug is taken, the better it works; however, the participants who took 75% of placebo also had 60% fewer deaths. Clearly, there is something about the good compliers that makes them less likely to die. This compliance bias is substantial and is very difficult to correct for in observational studies.

Another source of bias is occasioned by the fact that women who are prescribed HRT are likely to be under more regular medical care, leading to earlier diagnosis and treatment of risk factors and early disease. This surveillance bias leads to a reduced risk for death from a variety of diseases, and may explain why the mortalities from CHD and stroke in HRT users appear to be reduced to a greater extent than the incidence of these diseases (5, 37). The final likely source of bias is survivor bias, meaning that women who discontinue HRT often do so because they are ill, and in subsequent years they have a very high mortality (40). In turn, those who remain on HRT are much healthier and have a lower mortality, but of course the HRT may not the reason they are healthier. Yet, since even the best observational studies cannot correct for all these biases, the apparent benefit will be erroneously attributed to HRT use.

Breast Cancer

It seems increasingly likely that E plays some role in encouraging the growth of breast cancer (BC). Most of the identified risk factors for BC have a link with increased exposure to E, early menarche, late menopause, timing and number of pregnancies, obesity, alcohol consumption. After the menopause, the rate of increase of BC mortality drops off, consistent with a loss of E effect. Most tellingly, selective estrogen receptor modulators (SERMs) with anti-estrogenic effects on the breast, e.g. Tamoxifen (TAM) and Raloxifene, reduce the risk for

BC (41- 42). TAM is well established as a first-line treatment to prevent recurrence of BC. Despite the likely link between E and BC, however, the observational studies have not been very compelling in demonstrating increased risk in HRT users. Individual studies have provided inconsistent results, while the meta-analyses have suggested little increased risk for ever-use of HRT, or for less than 5 years' use (34, 43-45). The meta-analyses have been more consistent in suggesting an increased risk in long-term users. The best quantitative estimate comes from a collaborative study combining the worldwide data of 52,705 women with BC and 108,411 controls (46). This analysis confirmed the association of current HRT use with an increased risk for BC. The risk increased by approximately 2.3% for every year of use, similar to the increased risk of 2.8% for every year that the menopause is delayed. For the subset of women who used E alone for 5 years or more (average duration of use 11 years), the increased risk was 35% (the increased risk was 53% for those who also used a progestin).

As indicated earlier, observational studies tend to bias findings towards underestimating adverse outcomes, which may be part of the explanation for the unconvincing nature of the studies in regard to HRT and BC. In fact, in the Nurses' Health Study and the Breast Cancer Detection Demonstration Project (BCDDP), current users of HRT had a lower mortality from BC than never-users (37, 40). However, in the BCDDP study, women who used HRT for more than 10 years, and women who discontinued HRT had a higher mortality from BC. The lower initial mortality is consistent with selection bias for commencing HRT (e.g. women with a BC family history might not commence HRT), compliance and surveillance bias during HRT use, and survivor bias. The higher mortality with prolonged use is consistent with a real effect of E increasing the risk for BC to the extent that the biases are overwhelmed.

Endometrial Cancer

Recognition of the increased risk of endometrial cancer in users of unopposed E led to a dramatic decrease in the prescriptions for E, until it was discovered that adding progestins could counteract the stimulatory effect of E on the endometrium. This combination is now standard practice when prescribing HRT for women with an intact uterus, particularly after the PEPI study showed that even with careful monitoring, unopposed E use led to the development of adenomatous hyperplasia in a substantial proportion of women, but not in the women also receiving progestin (48). It is less certain that progestin will prevent endometrial cancer. Observational studies suggest that longer term use for more than 5 years may still be associated with increased risk, particularly if the progestin is given for less than 10 days of the cycle (8-9). Small short term (up to 3 years) clinical trials show no excess endometrial cancer, but longer and larger trials are needed (48). The combined data from the current long-term clinical trials should have sufficient power to examine this issue.

Overall Benefit and Risk

An estimate of the degree of residual bias for CHD can be made by comparing the reduction in CHD in current users with the reduction in all cancers (49). Since all cancers should not decrease in HRT users (in fact increases in endometrial cancer and BC can be expected), a reduction in all cancers can be used as an index of the degree of residual bias (Figure 2).

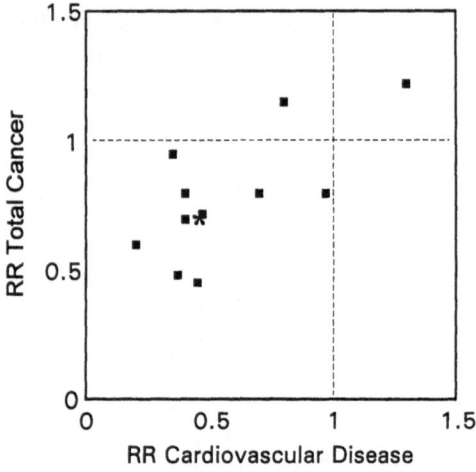

Figure 2. Plot of the relative risks for cancer against the relative risks for cardiovascular disease in observational studies comparing hormone users with non-users. Adapted from Postuma (49), with the addition of the mortality data from the Nurses' Health Study (37) marked with a * symbol.

On average, the observational studies show about a 20% reduction in all cancers, and a 40% reduction in CHD; thus, if the residual bias is 20%, then the real effect on CHD may be a more modest reduction of 20%. A 20% reduction in CHD may barely suffice to ensure overall benefit, even after accounting for a large reduction in deaths from complications of hip fracture (Table 1, Figure 3). A benefit of this degree might readily be countered by a combination of the anticipated increases of venous thromboembolism, and possible increases of endometrial and BC and thrombotic strokes (50). If there is severe bias in the observational studies, to the extent that no reduction in risk of CHD can be expected from HRT use, then the widespread adoption of HRT will result in substantial numbers of excess deaths from these HRT-related causes. At the other extreme, if there is no bias in the observational studies, then substantial benefit will accrue from the widespread use of HRT. The actual benefits and risks await the data from randomized controlled clinical trials.

Table 1. Estimated number of deaths from HRT-related causes, and estimates of the effect of level of bias on the relative risk if all USA women age 55 and older were to commence HRT (50).

		Relative Risk/Bias		
	No. of Deaths	None	Moderate	Severe
Coronary Heart	229,628	0.60	0.80	1.00
Stroke	88,768	1.00	1.15	1.30
Pulmonary Embolism	4,607	2.00	3.00	4.00
Breast Cancer	33,532	1.35	1.50	1.65
Endometrial Cancer	5,678	1.00	1.10	1.20
Hip Fracture	17,120	0.60	0.75	0.90

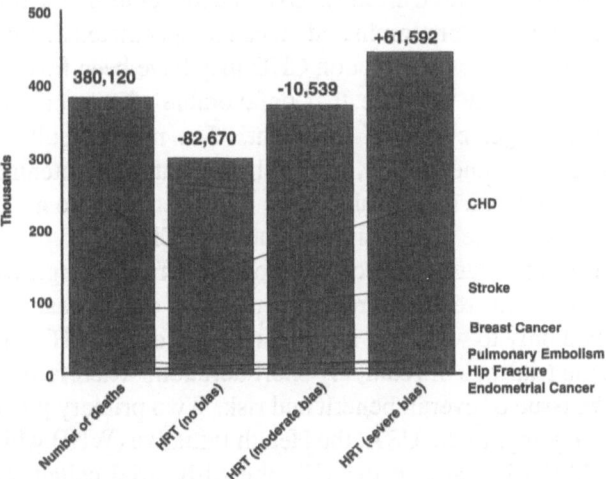

Figure 3. Potential effect of the level of bias in observational studies on the number of HRT-related deaths expected if all USA women age 55 and older were to commence HRT (50).

Randomized Controlled Clinical Trials

The clinical outcome trials now being done will provide unbiased estimates of the benefits and risks of HRT. The Heart and Estrogen/Progestin Study (HERS) was a secondary prevention trial which published its results in 1998 (7). HERS randomized 2,763 postmenopausal women with established CHD and an intact uterus to either conjugated equine Es (Premarin) 0.625 mg plus medroxyprogesterone 2.5 mg daily, and followed the participants for an average of 4.1 years. The lipid effects were in the expected direction, with a 10% reduction in LDL-C and a 11% increase in HDL-C in the HRT group compared to placebo. However, there was no overall effect on the primary outcome of CHD incidence, a significant 3.0-fold increase of venous thromboembolism, and a significant increase of gallbladder disease (Table 2). There were no significant effects on any other outcome, including BC; however, the trial was too small and too short in duration to have adequate statistical power to examine effects on these less common outcomes. For CHD, there was an interesting trend in that the results were in an adverse direction in the first year, followed by a reversal to apparent benefit after two years. This trend was statistically significant, but since it was not hypothesized before starting the trial, the finding should be viewed with some caution. Nevertheless, this trend overt time may suggest something about the mechanisms at play. The early adverse trend could be explained by pro-coagulant effects predominating early on, and causing an increased rate of CHD in women with diseased arteries. Over the longer term, the favorable lipid effects of HRT may have predominated. It can be speculated that if the trial had continued longer, the overall effect on CHD may have been favorable. On the other hand, it is equally possible that unfavorable effects on BC may have emerged after a longer period of treatment. The major result of no overall benefit for CHD was unexpected, and well illustrate the potential pitfalls of taking observational data a face value. The HERS findings do not lend support to the use of HRT for the secondary prevention of CHD.

Clearly, more information than could be obtained from a single trial is needed before evidence-based treatment recommendations can be made. The HERS findings applied only to women with existing heart disease, HERS did not test E alone, and the trial was of relatively short duration. Therefore, HERS could not address the issue of overall benefit and risk. Two primary prevention trials are currently ongoing: In the USA, the Health Initiative (WHI) which will have results after 2005 (51), and in the UK, the MRC trial called the Women's Intervention Study of Long Duration Oestrogen after the Menopause (WISDOM) which will have results a few years later (Madge Vickers, Ph.D., oral communication, March, 1998). These trials are large, with 27,500 women in WHI and 34,000 in WISDOM, and have long average follow-up period of 9 years. Each of these trials will randomize participants to E alone, E plus progestin, and placebo, and will study the effects of HRT on a wide spectrum of clinical outcomes. Thus, the combined results of WHI and WISDOM should provide a clear answer to the important question: *Should most postmenopausal women consider HRT?*

Table 2. Selected results of the heart and E/P replacement study (7).

Outcomes	Treatment Group		Relative Hazard (95%CI)	P value
	E/P (n=1380)	Placebo (n=1383)		
CHD events	172	176	0.99 (0.80-1.22)	.91
CHD death	71	58	1.24 (0.87-1.75)	.23
Nonfatal MI	116	129	0.91 (0.71-1.17)	.46
C artery bypass surgery	88	101	0.87 (0.66-1.16)	.36
Percutaneous C revascularization	164	175	0.95 (0.77-1.17)	.62
Stroke/transient ischemic attack	108	96	1.13 (0.85-1.48)	.40
Venous thromboembolic event	34	12	2.89 (1.50-5.58)	.002
Cancer	96	87	1.12 (0.84-1.50)	.44
Breast cancer	32	25	1.30 (0.77-2.19)	.33
Endometrial cancer	2	4	0.49 (0.09-2.69)	.41
Fracture	130	138	0.95 (0.75-1.21)	.70
Hip fracture	12	11	1.10 (0.49-2.50)	.82
Other fractures	119	129	0.93 (0.73-1.20)	.50
Gallbladder disease	84	62	1.38 (1.00-1.92)	.05
Deaths	131	123	1.08 (0.84-1.38)	.56

Summary

Very little is known with any degree of certainty about the long-term effects of HRT on the cardiovascular system (except for increases in VTE), the breast, and the brain. More is known about the bones and the endometrium, nonetheless, better estimates of the effects of HRT on fractures and endometrial cancer are needed. The lack of certainty stems directly from the fact that randomized controlled clinical trials that provide unbiased estimates of the effects of HRT on clinical outcomes have only recently been initiated. The observational data are extensive, especially for CHD and BC, but are so potentially confounded by various sources of bias that they cannot be used with any degree of confidence to provide an accurate prediction of the real effects of HRT. The observational data may systematically overestimate benefit and underestimate harm, and a computation of overall risk and benefit which does not take this effect into account will project a larger benefit than might be realized. Sensitivity analyses suggest that an overall benefit will only be achieved under the somewhat optimistic assumption that the observational study data provide accurate estimates of risks. Benefit would depend heavily on the achievement of a substantial reduction in CHD risk. A CHD risk reduction of 20% or more may result in overall benefit, while reductions of less than 15% may result in overall harm due to increases in BC and cardiovascular conditions caused by thrombosis.

Recommendations

Because of the uncertain basis of the current estimates of HRT effects, it is difficult to provide recommendations for the long-term use of HRT that will stand rigorous scrutiny. Such recommendations run the risk of being invalidated when the trial results become available.

  If the observational data do indeed overestimate benefit and underestimate risk, the large scale adoption of HRT by postmenopausal women might at best result in no benefit to them, or at worst might be putting them at risk for an adverse outcome. A more prudent interim course would be to promote the use of better proven and safe alternatives for the prevention and treatment of the common disorders that contribute to the morbidity and mortality of postmenopausal women. When considering prevention of disease in healthy people safety is of paramount concern. For example, CHD prevention through diet, exercise, smoking cessation, treatment of high blood cholesterol, and high blood pressure is safe and likely to be effective. For secondary prevention of CHD, aspirin, β-blockers, and lowering cholesterol will work as well in women as in men. Although of unproven efficacy for cancer prevention, a low fat dietary pattern with increase uptake of fruits, vegetables, grains, and cereals is certainly safer and may have multiple health benefits. Even for the prevention of osteoporosis, the alternatives of exercise and Ca^{++} are more benign and better suited as a primary prevention strategy than HRT. For the treatment of osteoporosis, alendronate is at least as effective as E. Alendronate has been proven to prevent fractures (52-53), and has the advantage of not affecting other organ systems. In the future, one or more of the SERMs might become an acceptable alternative to E for the treatment of osteoporosis. However, currently marketed SERMs are less effective than E or alendronate for maintaining bone mineral density, and there are concerns about their long-term safety (54).

References

1. Yaffe K, Sawaya G, Lieberburg I et al (1998) Estrogen therapy in postmenopausal women: effects on cognitive function and dementia. J Am Med Ass 279:688-695.

2. The Writing Group for the PEPI Trial Investigators (1995) Effects of estrogen or estrogen/progestin regimens on heart disease risk factors in postmenopausal women: the Postmenopausal Estrogen/Progestin Interventions (PEPI) Trial. J Am Med Ass 273:199-208.

3. Daly E, Vessey MP, Painter R et al (1996) Case-control study of venous thromboembolism risk in users of hormone replacement therapy (Letter). Lancet 348:1027.

4. Daly E, Vessey MP, Hawkins MM et al (1996) Risk of venous thromboembolism in users of hormone replacement therapy. Lancet 348:977-980.

5. Grodstein F, Stampfer MJ, Goldhaber SZ et al (1996) Prospective study of exogenous hormones and risk of pulmonary embolism in women. Lancet 348:983-986.

6. Jick H, Derby LE, Myers MW et al (1996) Risk of hospital admission for idiopathic venous thromboembolism among users of postmenopausal oestrogens. Lancet 348:981-983.

7. Hulley S, Grady D, Bush T et al for the Heart and Estrogen/Progestin Replacement Study (HERS) Research Group (1998) Randomized Trial of Estrogen Plus Progestin for Secondary Prevention of Coronary Heart Disease in Postmenopausal Women. J Am Med Ass 280:605-613.

8. Grady D, Gebretsadik T, Kerlikowski K et al (1995) Hormone replacement therapy and endometrial cancer risk: a meta-analysis. Obstet Gynecol 85:304-313.

9. Beresford SAA, Weiss NS, Voigt LF et al (1997) Risk of endometrial cancer in relation to use of oestrogen combined with cyclic progestagen therapy in postmenopausal women. Lancet 349:458-461.

10. Rossouw JE (1996) Estrogens for prevention of coronary heart disease: putting the brakes on the bandwagon (Editorial). Circulation 94:2982-2985.

11. Sotelo MM, Johnson SR (1997) The effects of hormone replacement therapy on coronary heart disease. Endocrinol Metab Clinics of North America 26:313-328.

12. Paganini-Hill A (1995) Estrogen replacement therapy and stroke. Prog Cardiovasc Dis 38:223-242.

13. Grodstein F, Martinez E, Platz EA et al (1998) Postmenopausal hormone use and risk for colorectal cancer and adenoma. Ann Internal Med 128:705-712.

14. Bush TL, Barrett-Connor E, Cowan LD et al (1987) Cardiovascular mortality and noncontraceptive use of estrogen in women: results from the lipid research clinics program follow-up study. Circulation 75:1102-1109.
15. National Heart, Lung, and Blood Institute (1980) The lipid research clinics population studies data book: Volume I: The prevalence study. U.S. Department of Health and Human Service, National Institutes of Health, NIH Pub. No. 80.
16. Godsland IF, Wynn V, Crook D et al (1987) Sex, plasma lipoproteins, and atherosclerosis: prevailing assumptions and outstanding questions. Am Heart J 114:1467-1503.
17. Lobo RA, Pickar JH, Wild RA et al (1994) Metabolic impact of adding medroxyprogesterone acetate to conjugated estrogen therapy in postmenopausal women. Obstet Gynecol 84:987-995.
18. Medical Research Council's General Practice Framework (1996) Randomized comparison of estrogen versus estrogen plus progestogen hormone replacement therapy in women with a hysterectomy. BMJ 312:473-478.
19. Darling GM, Johns JA, McCloud PI et al (1997) Estrogen and progestin compared with simvastatin for hypercholesterolemia in postmenopausal women. New Engl J Med 337:595-601.
20. Kroon UB, Silfverstolpe G, Tenghorn L (1994) The effects of transdermal estradiol and oral conjugated estrogens on hemostasis variables. Thromb Haemost 71:420-423
21. Scarabin P, Alhenc-Gelas M, Plu-Bureau G et al (1997) Effects of oral and transdermal estrogen/progesterone regimens on blood coagulation and fibrinolysis in postmenopausal women: a randomized controlled trial. Arterioscler Thomb Vasc Biol 17:3071-3078.
22. Psaty BM, Heckbert SR, Atkins D et al (1993) A review of the association of estrogens and progestins with cardiovascular disease in psotmenopausal women. Arch Intern Med 153:1421-1427.
23. Lemay A, Dodin S, Cedrin I, Lemay LT (1995) Phasic serum lipid excursion occur during cyclical oral conjugated oestrogens but not during transdermal oestradiol sequentially combined with oral medroxyprogesterone acetate. Clin Endocrinol Oxf 42:431-451.
24. Hanggi W, Lippuner K, Riesen W et al (1997) Long-term influence of different postmenopausal hormone replacement regimens on serum lipids and lipoprotein (a): a randomized study. Br J Obstet Gynaeco l104:708-717.
25. Koh KK, Mincemoyer R, Bui MN et al (1997) Effects of hormone-replacement therapy on fibrinolysis in postmenopausal women. N Engl J Med 336:683-690.

26. Guetta V, Cannon III RO (1996) Cardiovascular effects of estrogen and lipid-lowering therapies in postmenopausal women. Circulation 93:1928-1937.
27. Adams M, Register T, Golden D et al (1997) Medroxyprogesterone acetate antagonizes inhibitory effects of conjugated equine estrogens on coronary artery atherosclerosis. Ateriocler Thromb Vasc Biol 17:217-221.
28. Williams JK, Honore EK, Washburn SA et al (1994) Effects of hormone replacement therapy on reactivity of atherosclerotic coronary arteries in cynomolgus monkeys. J Am Coll Cardiol 24:1757-1761.
29. Williams JK, Anthony MS, Honore EK et al (1995) Regression of atherosclerosis in female monkeys. Ateriocler Thromb Vasc Bio 7:828-836.
30. Rosano GMC, Sarrel PM, Poole-Wilson PA et al (1993) Beneficial effect of estrogen on exercise-induced myocardial ischemia in women with coronary artery disease. Lancet 342:133-136.
31. Best PJM, Berger PB, Miller VM et al (1998) The effect of estrogen replacement therapy on plasma nitric oxide and endothelin-1 levels in postmenopausal women. Ann Internal Med 128:285-288.
32. Rosselli M, Imthurn B, Keller PJ et al (1995) Circulating nitric oxide (nitrite/nitrate) levels in postmenopausal women substituted with 17 beta-estradiol and noresthisteron acetate. Hypertension 25:848-853.
33. Sorensen KE, Dorup I, Hermann AP et al (1998) Combined hormone replacement therapy does not protect women against age-related decline in endothelium-dependent vasomotor function. Circulation 97:1234-1238.
34. Grady D, Rubin SM, Petitti D et al (1992) Hormone therapy to prevent disease and prolong life in postmenopausal women. Ann Internal Med 117:1016-1037.
35. Falkeborn M, Persson I, Adami H et al (1992) The risk of acute myocardial infarction after oestrogen and oestrogen-progestogen replacement. Brit J Obstet Gynecol 99:821-828.
36. Grodstein F, Stampfer MJ, Manson JE et al (1996) Postmenopausal estrogen and progestin use and the risk of cardiovascular disease. New Engl J Med 335:453-461.
37. Grodstein F, Stampfer MJ, Colditz GA et al (1997) Postmenopausal hormone therapy and mortality. New Engl J Med 336:1769-1775.
38. Matthews KA, Kuller LH, Wing RR et al (1996) Prior to use of estrogen replacement therapy, are users healthier than nonusers? Am J Epidemiol 143:971-978.
39. Horwitz RI, Viscoli CM, Berkman L et al (1990) Treatment adherence and risk of death after a myocardial infarction. Lancet 336:542-545.

40. Sturgeon SR, Schairer C, Brinton LA et al (1995) Evidence of a health estrogen user survivor effect. Epidemiology 6(3):227-231.
41. NIH News Release. Breast Cancer Prevention Trial. April 6, 1998.
42. Cummings S, Norton L, Eckert S et al (1998) Raloxifene reduces the risk of breast cancer and may decrease the risk of endometrial cancer in postmenopausal women (abstract). Two-year findings from the Multiple Outcomes of Raloxifene Evaluation (MORE) Trial. Proceedings of ASCO 17, 2a.
43. Colditz GA, Egan KM, Stampfer MJ (1993) Hormone replacement therapy and risk of breast cancer: results from epidemiologic studies. Am J Obstet Gynecol 168:1473-1480.
44. Colditz GA, Hankinson SE, Hunter DJ et al (1995) The use of estrogens and progestins and the risk of breast cancer in postmenopausal women. New Engl J Med 332:1589-1593.
45. Stanford JL, Weiss NS, Voigt LF et al (1995) Combined estrogen and progestin hormone replacement therapy in relation to risk of breast cancer in middle-aged women. JAMA 274:137-142.
46. Collaborative Group on Hormonal Factors in Breast Cancer (1997) Breast cancer and hormone replacement therapy: collaborative reanalysis of data from 51 epidemiological studies of 52,705 women with breast cancer and 108,441 women without breast cancer. Lancet 350:1047-1059.
47. The Writing Group for the PEPI trial (1996) Effects of hormone therapy on bone mineral density: results from the postmenopausal estrogen/progestin interventions (PEPI) trial. JAMA 276:1389-1396.
48. The Writing Group for the PEPI trial (1996) Effects of hormone replacement therapy on endometrial histology in postmenopausal women. The Postmenopausal Estrogen/Progestin Interventions (PEPI) Trial. JAMA 275:1880-1881.
49. Postuma WFM, Westendorp RG, Vanderbrouke JP (1994) Cardioprotective effect of hormone replacement therapy in postmenopausal women: is the evidence biased? BMJ 308:1268-1269.
50. Rossouw JE (1998) What we still need to learn about hormone replacement therapy. Infert Reprod Endocrinol Clin North America (in press).
51. The Women's Health Initiative Study Group (1998) Design of the Women's Health Initiative clinical trial and observational study. Controlled Clin Trials 19:61-109.
52. Black DM, Cummings SR, Karpf DB et al (1996) Randomized trial of effect of alendronate on risk of fracture in women with existing vertebral fractures. Lancet 348:1535-1541.

53. Delmas PD, Bjarnason NH, Mitlak BH et al (1997) Effects of raloxifene on bone mineral density, serum cholesterol concentrations, and uterine endometrium in postmenopausal women. New Engl J Med 337:1641-1647.
54. Rifkind BM, Rossouw JE (1998) Of designer drugs, magic bullets, and gold standards (Editorial). JAMA 279:1483-1486.

EPILOGUE

31

A Unified General Mechanism for Hormonal Carcinogenesis Begins to Emerge

Jonathan J. Li and Sara Antonia Li

It had long been established that early surgical oophrectomy or castration leads to a precipitous drop in breast and prostate cancer incidence in women and men, respectively (1, 2). The concept that sex hormones, primarily estrogens (Es) and androgens, are major players in the etiology of these neoplasms is not new. For instance, Miller and Bulbrook (3) emphasized twenty years ago that Es are the prime agents in breast cancer development, particularly during the critical periods of menarche and menopause. Additionally, since virtually all of the known risk factors for breast cancer are hormone-related, it was therefore not totally unexpected that the recent Tamoxifen clinical trials resulted in nearly a 50% decline is breast cancer incidence compared to placebo control groups (4). Because breast and prostate cancers are by far the most prevalent neoplasms in developed countries and have similar high incidences worldwide (5), and since sex hormones have emerged as major culprits in the development of these diseases, it has become obviously important to address the role of sex hormones in neoplastic processes in susceptible target tissues. While it is evident that sporadic non-familial breast and prostate cancers comprise the vast majority (>85%) of all cases reported, conceptual progress concerning the cellular and molecular mechanisms involved in these sporadic cases has thus far resisted elucidation.

If one fully appreciates the findings that have been widely reported (6), that only very low levels of hormones are associated with neoplastic development at these and other organ sites, then one is compelled to invoke hormone-receptor mediated mechanisms for hormonal carcinogenic processes. Since E-mediated genomic destabilization or instability has been observed in early tumoral lesions and in frank tumors in one well-established experimental model (7, 8), this finding has now been extended to early focal mammary dysplastic lesions and mammary tumors of two distinct rat strains induced solely by Es (9) and in a Leydig cell tumor in which E is implicated by an overexpression of aromatase in this tissue (10).

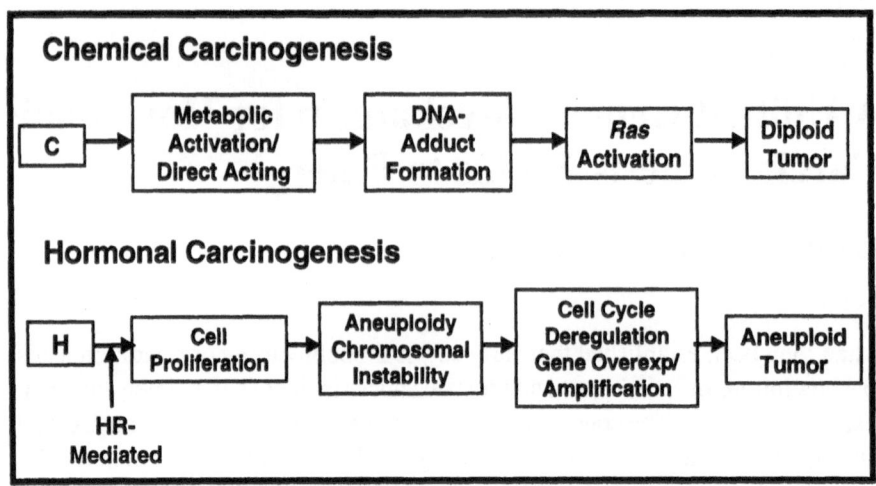

Figure 1. Mechanisms of chemical versus hormonal carcinogenesis.

To illustrate the significance of these findings, mammary tumors were induced in femage rats with either nitrosomethyl (NMU) or dimethylbenz[a]anthracene, either direct acting or metabolic-activating chemical carcinogens, respectively, exhibit a high diploid frequency (>85%). Therefore, the high frequency of aneuploidy now seen in four different solely E-induced neoplasms in three species strongly suggest that hormonally-induced neoplasms occur as a result of distinctly different oncogenic events from those induced by potent chemical carcinogens (Figure 1). The high frequency of genomic instability observed in early tumoral lesions of these E-induced neoplasms further suggest that this may be unique to hormonal carcinogenic processes. These results suggest that hormone-induced tumor models clearly resemble human breast and prostate cancers since both early lesions and primary tumors exhibit high frequencies of aneuploidy (11-13). Candidates which may either elicit or contribute to the genomic instability seen as a consequence of E treatment have been the subject of many of the studies presented in this volume (e.g., c-*myc*, cyclin E).

References

1. Lilienfeld AM (1956) The relationship of cancer of the female breast to artificial menopause and marital status. Cancer 9:927-934.
2. McMahon B, Cole P, Brown J (1973) Etiology of human breast cancer: A review. J Natl Cancer Inst 50:21-42.

3. Miller AB, Bulbrook RD (1980) The epidemiology and etiology of breast cancer. New Engl J Med 303:1246-1248.
4. Fisher B, Costantino JP, Wickerham DL, Redmond CK, Kavanah M, Cronin WM et al (1998) Tamoxifen for prevention of breast cancer: Report of the National Surgical Adjuvant Breast and Bowel Project P-1 Study. J Natl Cancer Inst 90:1371-1388.
5. Parkin DM, Pisani P, Ferlay J (1999) Global cancer statistics. CA Cancer J Clin 49:33-64.
6. Li JJ (2000) Preface. In: Li JJ, Daling J, Li SA (eds) Hormonal Carcinogenesis III. Springer-Verlag, New York, New York, pp. ix-xi.
7. Li JJ, Gonzalez, Banerjee SK, Li SA (1993) Estrogen carcinogenesis in the hamster kidney: Role of cytotoxicity and cell proliferation. Environ Health Perspect 101 (Suppl 5):259-264.
8. Li JJ, Hou X, Banerjee SK, Liao DZ, Maggouta F, Norris JS et al (1999) Overexpression and amplification of c-myc in the Syrian hamster kidney during estrogen carcinogenesis: A probable critical role in neoplastic transformation. Cancer Res 59:2340-2346.
9. Li JJ, Cansler M, Aldaz M, Weroha SJ, Ballenger J, Tawfik O et al (2000) Difference between hormone- and chemical-induced mammary tumors: Relation to human breast cancer. Proc Am Assoc Cancer Res 41:741.
10. Fowler KA, Gill K, Kirma ·N, Dillehay DL, Tekmal RR (2000) Overexpression of aromatase leads to development of testicular leydig cell tumors: An in vivo model for hormone-mediated testicular cancer. Am J Pathol 156: 347-353.
11. Makris A, Powles TJ, Dowsett M, Osborne CK, Trott PA, Fernando IN et al (1997) Prediction of response to neoadjuvant chemoendocrine therapy in primary breast carcinomas. Clin. Cancer Res 3:593-600.
12. Otteson GL, Chrisensen IJ, Larsem JK, Kerndrop GB, Hansen B, Anderson JA (1995) DNA aneuploidy in early breast cancer. Brit J Cancer 72:832-839.
13. Ross JS, Sheehan CE, Ambros RA, Nazeer T, Jennings TA, Kaufman RP Jr et al (1999) Needle biopsy DNA ploidy status predicts grade shifting in prostate cancer. Am J Surg Path 23(3):296-301.

COMMUNICATIONS

Session I. Epidemiology/Human Studies

The Risk of Post-menopausal Breast Cancer After Estrogen and Estrogen-Progestin Replacement

C. Magnusson, I.R. Persson, E. Weiderpass, and N. Correia

Summary

Hormone replacement therapy (HRT) in post-menopausal women is widely used for symptom relief and disease prevention. As sex hormones are involved in the etiology of breast cancer (BC), there is concern that hormone substitution after the menopause may increase BC risk. Accumulated epidemiological evidence shows that many years of recent or current HRT use leads to moderate excess risk of early stage BC, particularly in non-obese women. Results from our recently completed population-based study, including 3,345 cases of BC and 3,454 controls, aged 50-74 years, reveal clear and strong relationships between long-term intake of both estrogens (Es) and Es combined with progestins, seemingly confined to women with normal or lean body build. The results also suggest that the duration-dependent excess risk remains a long time after treatment cessation and that continuously/combined E-progestin treatment may be more adverse than those cyclically/combined. Our observations raise additional concern about the long-term safety of HRT and call for research efforts to define the safest possible HRT-regimens.

Introduction

HRT has become increasingly popular for alleviation of climacteric symptoms, as well as in selected women for prevention of osteoporosis and coronary heart disease. When assessing the overall benefit/risk balance, a possible adverse effect on BC risk is an important issue.

Established risk factors demonstrate the crucial role of sex hormones in the etiology of BC. Of particular relevance are the observations that premature oophorectomy and menopause, entailing a reduction of the level of endogenous ovarian hormones, are protective (1). Replacement of post-menopausal E deficiency with exogenous hormones could therefore, *a priori*, be suspected to increase the risk (2).

A reanalysis of most epidemiological evidence (3), show that several years of E intake confers, on average, about 50 % increased risk of BC, mostly for localised and early stage tumours. This risk increase was measurable for ongoing or recent exposure (use within 5 years after BC diagnosis), and seemingly confined to women of normal or lean body build. Effects of E-progestin combinations could not be evaluated. We undertook a large population-based, case-control study in Sweden to examine in detail the risk relationships between different treatment regimens and BC risk, taking into consideration the extensive use of mammography screening.

Material and Methods

During the period of October 1993 through March 1995, we ascertained in all of Sweden, 3,979 women with newly diagnosed BC and aged 50-74 years. These women were contacted after approval from their physicians. In all, 3,345 (84%) consented to participate. From the general Swedish population, an equal number of age frequency matched women, without BC, were randomly selected as controls; 3,454 out of 4,188 women (82%) were included (4).

Data were collected through a mailed questionnaire that covered details on HRT exposure, as well as on numerous reproductive and life-style factors, use of oral contraceptives, anthropomethric measures, previous diseases, family history, and number of previous mammography examinations. Among the control women, 15% agreed to be interviewed over the telephone only; in 50% of all subjects, missing data were supplemented through telephone calls.

We examined the associations between HRT and BC through logistic regression analyses, and adjusted for risk factors that could be confounders, including the number of mammography examinations.

Results

The distribution of established risk factors, e.g. nulliparity, late age at first full-time pregnancy, early menarche, etc., corresponded to what could be expected from the epidemiologic literature. Our detailed analyses of the effects of HRT revealed: The risk of BC increased monotonically with the duration of intake of regimens with medium potency Es (chiefly 17β-estradiol 2 mg and to a lesser extent conjugated Es). The risk estimates were 2.0-3.0-fold elevated after use for 10 years or longer.

These risk relationships seemed to be similar for women using Es alone or Es combined with a progestin, through any type of regimen (Figure 1).

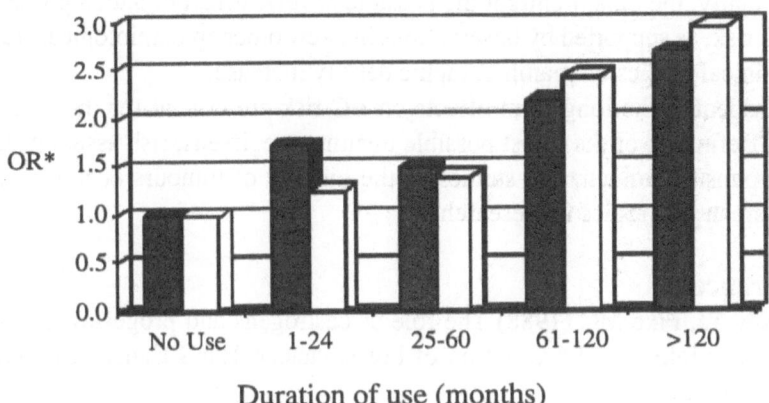

Figure 1. Risk for breast cancer in relation to use of E and E-progestin therapy. ■ E only. □ E-progestin. * Overall risk, OR (Adjusted for age, parity, ages at first birth and menopause, type of menopause, body mass index and height.)

The duration-dependent excess risk was observed in women who had ongoing treatment at or terminated within one year after diagnosis of the BC, and in those women who stopped their treatment more than 10 years ago. However, in the intermediate recency period, no clear association emerged.

The adverse effects of long-term HRT seemed to be confined to women with BMI-levels corresponding to a normal or lean body build. No significant risk increase was found in obese women.

When examining E-progestin combined use separately, continuously combined regimens (adding the progestin during all days of the E cycle) were associated with substantially higher estimates than those cyclically combined (usually 10 days of the progestin addition per cycle). There was no clear evidence of differential risks with the type of added progestins.

Conclusions

Our results, along with most previous epidemiological evidence, show that long-term HRT increases the incidence of post-menopausal BC. These new Swedish data also suggest that this adverse effect may carry on a long time after cessation of treatment, and that the excess risk may afflict mainly non-obese women. Importantly, the data highlight the possible adverse effect of added progestins on BC risk, as supported by observations in a few other epidemiological studies and clinical studies on mammographic density increase.

Evidently, the long-term effects on BC risk are crucial for the safety of HRT. Definition of the safest possible treatment regimens, risk assessments in sub-groups of women, and studies of the biology of tumours occurring after HRT are urgent topics for research.

References

1. Key TJ, Pike MC (1988) The role of oestrogens and progestagens in the epidemiology and prevention of breast cancer. Eur J Cancer Clin Oncol 24:29-43.
2. Pike MC, Spicer DV, Dahmoush L et al (1993) Estrogens, progestogens, normal breast cell proliferation, and breast cancer risk. Epidemiol Rev 15:17-35.
3. Collaborative Group on Hormonal Factors in Breast Cancer Breast cancer and hormone replacement therapy (1997) Collaborative reanalysis of data from 51 epidemiological studies of 52 705 women with breast cancer and 10 8411 women without breast cancer. Lancet 350:1047-1059.
4. Magnusson CM, Persson IR, Baron JA et al (1998) The role of reproductive factors and use of oral contraceptives in the aetiology of breast cancer in women aged 50-74 years. Int J Cancer 80:231-236.

No Significant Difference in Age at Menarche, Menstrual Cycle Length, Age at First Full-Term Pregnancy, and Nulliparity Among BRCA1 Mutation Carriers Compared with Their Unaffected Relatives

H. Jernström, O. Johannsson, Å. Borg, and H. Olsson

Summary

Early age at menarche, short menstrual cycle length, late age at first full-term pregnancy, and nulliparity are known risk factors for breast cancer (BC). These risk factors differ between BC patients with and without a family history of BC, and between BC patients and controls. Self-administered questionnaires were filled out by 95 women with a family history of known BRCA1 mutations; 39 were BRCA1 mutation carriers and 56 were not. Age at menarche did not significantly differ between BRCA1 mutation carriers and non-carriers, after adjustment for year of birth ($p = 0.40$). There were no significant differences between BRCA1 mutation carriers and non-carriers in: a) Menstrual cycle length (among women not using oral contraceptives) at age 30, or at the current age in younger women, after adjustment for year of birth and age at menarche ($p = 0.60$). b) Age at first full-term pregnancy, after adjustment for year of birth, age at menarche, and menstrual cycle length ($p = 0.69$). Nulliparity was not more common between BRCA1 mutation carriers compared with non-carriers, after adjustment for year of birth, age at menarche, and menstrual cycle length ($p = 0.81$). Our results suggest that reproductive risk factors for BC are not related to BRCA1 carrier status.

Introduction

Early age at menarche, short menstrual cycle length, and late age at first full-term pregnancy, or nulliparity are known risk factors for BC (1). In a study from our region, menstrual cycle length differs between BC patients with and without a family history of BC, and also between BC patients and controls (2). Previously, we reported that BRCA1 mutation carriers are small for gestational age compared to their unaffected relatives (3). Also, we reported that BRCA1 mutation carriers breast feed their children a shorter time than their unaffected relatives, which may be due to little or no milk production in several of the carriers (4). These findings may indicate that having only one intact BRCA1 allele affects the development *in-utero* and the differentiation of breast tissue in adulthood. However, if BRCA1 mutation carrier status affects reproductive risk factors for BC, it has not been investigated before.

Material and Methods

Genetic testing for BRCA1 germline mutations is offered through an Oncogenetic Clinic, in Lund if an individual has at least 3 first-degree relatives with BC and with 1 diagnosed before age 50, or 2 first-degree relatives with BC and with 1 diagnosed before age 40, or 1 first-degree relative with BC diagnosed before age 30. At the time of genetic testing, individuals are requested to fill out a detailed questionnaire. Questions asked include: Age at menarche, cycle length at age 30 or at present, oral contraceptive use, age at first full-term pregnancy, and number of pregnancies. Self-administered questionnaires were filled out by 95 women belonging to families with known BRCA1 mutations. Thirty nine women were BRCA1 mutation carriers and 56 women were non-carriers.

For the BRCA1 analyses, the entire coding region of the BRCA1 gene was screened for mutations using genomic DNA and the protein truncation test (PTT) or single stranded conformation polymorphism (SSCP) analysis, followed by direct sequence analysis in samples scored as positive in the PTT and SSCP analysis (5). For statistical analysis, the statistical program SPSS was used. Student's T-test was used to compare mean values between BRCA1 carriers and non-carriers. Pearson's correlation coefficient was used for correlation between carrier status and nulliparity. Comparisons between BRCA1 mutation carriers and non-carriers in multivariate models was carried out by logistic regression.

Results

No significant differences in means levels of age at menarche, menstrual cycle length, age at first-full term pregnancy, or nulliparity were found between BRCA1 carriers and non-carriers. However, the mean birth year among BRCA1 mutation carriers was significantly higher than in non-carriers (p=0.01).

Table 1. Mean levels of year of birth, age at menarche, menstrual cycle length at age 30 year or at current age in younger women, age at first full-term pregnancy, and % of nulliparous women in each group. Only birth year was significantly different between BRCA1 mutation carriers and non-carriers.

	BRCA1 positive n = 39 mean	BRCA1 negative n = 56 mean	p-value
Birth year	1953	1956	p=0.01
Age at menarche	13.1	12.8	N.S.
Menstrual cycle length (days)	28.1	27.8	N.S.
Age first full-term pregnancy (years)	24.5	23.0	N.S.
Nulliparous	25.6%	25.0%	N.S.

In a multivariate model, age at menarche did not differ significantly between BRCA1 mutation carriers and non-carriers after adjustment for year of birth (p = 0.40). There was no significant difference in menstrual cycle length (among women not using oral contraceptives) at age 30 or at the current age in younger women between BRCA1 mutation carriers and non-carriers, after adjustment for year of birth and age at menarche (p = 0.60). Neither there was a significant difference in age at first full-term pregnancy between BRCA1 mutation carriers and non-carriers, after adjustment for year of birth, age at menarche, and menstrual cycle length (p = 0.69). Nulliparity was not more common between BRCA1 mutation carriers compared with non-carriers, after adjustment for year of birth, age at menarche, and menstrual cycle length (p = 0.81).

Discussion

In this study, we found no significant difference between BRCA1 mutation carriers and non-carriers in age at menarche, menstrual cycle length, age at first full-term pregnancy, or nulliparity. In fact, non-carriers from these families tended to have a lower age at menarche and a shorter menstrual cycle length than mutation carriers. These findings are partly in contrast with Olsson *et al.* (2), who found a significantly shorter cycle length among women with familial BC, while there was no difference in the other reproductive factors between familial cases and controls. However, the majority of these familial cases did not have a true dominant inheritance viewed through the pedigree, which could indicate that less penetrant genes or multifactorial inheritance may be associated with some reproductive factors. Magnusson, *et al.* (6) found that there was no clear indication of a differential impact of hormonal risk factors such as age at menarche, parity, age at first birth, and age at menopause among post menopausal women with and without a positive family history among a population-based case-control group in all of Sweden, that included 3345 BC cases and 3454 controls. These findings are in agreement with ours. Narod, *et al.* (7) have found that reproductive factors modified susceptibility to cancer in women who were found by haplotype analysis to carry BRCA1 mutations. An increased risk for BC was associated with low parity and belonging to a recent birth cohort.

In the multivariate models, we adjusted for factors in a chronological order, starting with year of birth and age at menarche, adding menstrual cycle length, and then, age at first full-term pregnancy or nulliparity.

In conclusion, we found no evidence for changes in reproductive factors such as age at menarche, menstrual cycle length, age at first full-term pregnancy, and nulliparity in BRCA1 mutation carriers when compared with their relatives without mutations.

Acknowledgments

This study was supported by grants from the Swedish Cancer Society, Ingvar Kamprad's Foundation, Gunnar Nilsson's Foundation, The Medical Faculty at the University of Lund in Sweden, Knut and Alice Wallenberg's Foundation, and Tage Blücher's Foundation.

References

1. Kelsey JL, Gammon MD, John EM (1993) Reproductive factors and breast cancer. Epidemiol Rev 15:36–47.
2. Olsson H, Landin-Olsson M, Kristoffersson U et al (1985) Risk factors of breast cancer in relation to a family history of breast cancer in Southern Sweden. In: Müller HJ, Weber W (eds) Familial Cancer. Karger Publishing, Basel, Switzerland, pp. 34–35.
3. Jernström H, Johannsson O, Borg Å et al (1998) BRCA1-positive patients are small for gestational age compared with their unaffected relatives. Eur J Cancer 34:368–371.
4. Jernström H, Johannsson O, Borg Å et al (1998) Do BRCA1 mutations affect the ability to breast feed? Significantly shorter length of breast feeding among BRCA1 mutation carriers compared with their unaffected relatives. Breast (in press).
5. Håkansson S, Johannsson O, Johansson U et al (1997) Moderate frequency of BRCA1 and BRCA2 germline mutations in Scandinavian familial breast cancer. Am J Hum Genet 60:1068–1078.
6. Magnusson C, Colditz G, Rosner B et al (1998) Association of family history and other risk factors with breast cancer risk. Cancer Causes Control 9:259–267.
7. Narod SA, Goldgar D, Cannon-Albright L et al (1995) Risk modifiers in carriers of BRCA1 mutations. Int J Cancer 64:394–398.

Cell Proliferation and Apoptosis in the Normal Breast Epithelium of Pre, Peri, and Postmenopausal Women

Seema A. Khan and Scott Stickles

Summary

Estrogen exposure is widely believed to contribute to breast cancer (BC) risk through the induction of proliferation. We studied the rates of breast epithelial cell proliferation and apoptosis in pre, peri, and postmenopausal women. Archival paraffin embedded sections of normal epithelium were chosen from women undergoing breast surgery. Seventy-nine women were studied (46 pre, 6 peri, and 27 postmenopausal). Ki-67 index declined through menopause (2.33 for pre, 1.38 for postmenopausal women), as did the TUNEL index (0.20 in pre, 0.11 in postmenopausal women). Among premenopausal women, the expected late luteal peaks were seen in cell proliferation and apoptosis. Among postmenopausal women, there was a weak negative correlation between years from menopause and Ki-67 index (R =0.27, p=0.22), and a weaker positive correlation between years from menopause and TUNEL index (R=0.10, p=0.63). When comparing normal epithelium from women with and without BC, we found higher values for both indices in women with BC, regardless of menopausal status and menstrual cycle phase. No differences by cancer status were found in the ratio of Ki-67/TUNEL index. However, the product of Ki-67 and TUNEL index was significantly higher in premenopausal women with BC (3.18 vs 0.35, p = 0.004), and non-significantly higher in postmenopausal women with BC (0.26 vs 0.16). Finally, there was a significant association between higher TUNEL indices and the presence of BC (OR=3.7, 95% CI=1.2-11.0). For Ki-67 index, there was a weaker association with the presence of malignancy (OR 1.9, 95% CI 0.8-4.5). Thus, the high-risk breast appears to have increased cell turnover, with increased proliferation and apoptosis; the increase in apoptotic rate may reflect an increased burden of genetically damaged cells which need to be eliminated.

Introduction

Estrogen (E) stimulation of target tissue results in cell proliferation, and E withdrawal results in apoptosis. Normal premenopausal breast epithelium is exposed to cyclical E stimulation and withdrawal, and the total number of cycles of such exposure significantly influences the risk of developing BC. An imbalance in these events could lead to a change in the breast epithelial cell mass with a resulting increase in the cell population. We initiated a study of breast cell proliferation and apoptosis rates in the normal breast epithelium of women undergoing breast surgical procedures, to determine these rates in relation to BC and other epithelial lesions.

Methods

Subjects were recruited from the Breast Care Center at University Hospital, Syracuse. On the day of surgery, information regarding the date of their last menstrual period, oral contraceptive and exogenous hormone use was gathered. Blood samples were collected on the day of surgery to determine serum estradiol and progesterone levels. Paraffin sections from the surgical sample were screened for the presence of normal breast epithelium. Sections with a minimum of ten normal ducts/acini were chosen for analysis.

Ki-67 immunohistochemistry and the TUNEL assay were performed in 5 μ sections. Since the distribution of Ki-67 and TUNEL indices was found to be positively skewed, with relatively high standard deviations as seen in Figure 1, medians were used as summary values, and non-paraqmetric tests (Wilcoxon Rank Sum Test) were used to detect differences between groups. Logistic regression analysis was used to estimate odds ratios of a diagnosis of malignancy relative to Ki-67 and TUNEL indices. In order to obtain a more normal distribution of the labelling indices, log transformation of these indices was performed.

Results

A total of 79 women were studied, 21 being treated for BC, and 58 demonstrated benign changes on breast biopsy (Table 1). Perimenopausal women were considered premenopausal in the subsequent analyses because of their small numbers (rendering analysis as a separate subset meaningless) and high estradiol levels.

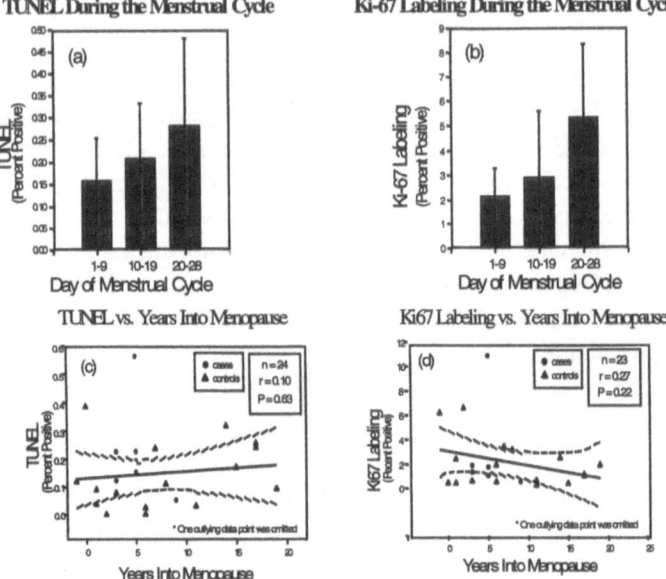

Figure 1. (a) Mean TUNEL and (b) Ki-67 (b) labeling indices during the cycle showing increased apoptosis and proliferation in late luteal phase versus early follicular phase. Error bars indicate that differences are not significant. (c) Patterns of TUNEL and Ki-67 labeling during menopause. Apoptosis appeared to increase slightly during menopause whereas (d) proliferation declined.

•, women with BC; ▲, women without BC.

Table 1. Population by menstrual and menopausal status (n = 79*)

	Premenopausal		Postmenopausal
	Follicular	Luteal	
With BC	3	9	7
Without BC	15	19	20
Total	18	28	27

*An additional 6 premenopausal women had irregular cycles, but were premenopausal by serum estradiol levels.

Median TUNEL labeling index (LI) was higher in both pre and postmenopausal women with BC, whereas Ki-67 LI was significantly higher in premenopausal women with BC, but was similar in postmenopausal women with and without BC (Table 2.2). Among premenopausal women, both TUNEL and Ki-67 LIs were higher in women with cancer, in follicular and luteal phases (Table 2.3).

Although the differences were not significant, the trends were consistent across all subsets. We calculated the ratio of Ki-67 to TUNEL index, since the ratio of mitotic to apoptotic index has been reported to be lower in the normal breast epithelium of women with cancer (1), but found no differences in this ratio in our study population (Table 2.4). However, the product of these indices was significantly higher in women with cancer, particularly in premenopausal women. Lastly, logistic regression was used to examine the association of increasing TUNEL and Ki-67 LI with the presence of cancer, using continuous values of both variables. We adjusted for menopausal status rather than age, since this was more significant in our data set (Table 3). Increasing TUNEL index was significantly associated with the presence of BC, whereas the association of Ki-67 LI with BC was less strong (see Table 3).

Table 2.1 Median TUNEL and Ki-67 LI.

All women	n	TUNEL	Ki-67 LI
Premenopausal	52	0.20	2.33
Postmenopausal	27	0.11	1.38

Table 2.2. Stratified by menopausal and cancer status.

	TUNEL		Ki-67	
	Cancer	No cancer	Cancer	No cancer
Premenopausal	0.22	0.14	6.38	2.16*
Postmenopausal	0.15	0.09	1.58	1.36

*Significantly lower than in premenopausal cases (p=.028).

Table 2.3. Premenopausal women stratified by menstrual cycle phase*.

	TUNEL		Ki-67 LI	
	Cancer	No cancer	Cancer	No cancer
Follicular	0.22	0.14	9.70	2.03
Luteal	0.26	0.20	6.38	4.70

* Differences not statistically significant.

Table 2.4. Median ratios[1] and products[2] of TUNEL and Ki-67 indices.

	Ratio		Product (Wilcoxon rank-sum p=0.0035)	
	Cancer	No cancer	Cancer	No cancer
Premenopausal	13.97	12.52	3.18	0.35
Postmenopausal	10.75	7.89	0.26	0.16

[1] Ratio=Ki-67/TUNEL   [2] Product=Ki67*TUNEL.

Discussion

Increased proliferation in response to E exposure is a key component of the current paradigm for the development of BC. The role of apoptosis in preserving the population balance of breast epithelium is beginning to attract attention, but has not been extensively studied so far. Initial results from the present study suggest that "at risk" breast epithelium from women with BC differs from normal epithelium of women with benign breast changes. These differences consist of a trend to greater proliferative activity and increased apoptosis. Thus the normal breast epithelium of women with BC appears to be in greater flux than that of women with benign breast changes, with increased cell turnover. This is reflected in the finding that the product of the Ki-67 and TUNEL labeling indices is significantly greater in premenopausal women with BC (see Table 2.4).

A recent study of apoptosis rates show that they were lowest for sclerosing adenosis, intermediate for duct hyperplasia, higher for *in-situ*, and highest for invasive BC (2). Our data are consistent with the idea that the normal breast epithelium of women who have demonstrated the ability to develop BC is perturbed, and shows some of the characteristics of more advanced lesions, such as increased proliferation and apoptosis.

The relative importance of increased apoptosis seems greater than that of increased proliferation, as seen in the logistic regression analysis presented in Table 3. The OR for BC is 3.66 for log transformed values of TUNEL, whereas the OR for Ki-67 is 1.93, and is not statistically significant. This lack of significant differences in measures of proliferation between cancer-containing breasts and those with benign changes is consistent with two previous studies which examined rates of proliferation and apoptosis in normal breast epithelium from women with and without BC (2, 3).

Table 3. Logistic regression model of Ki-67 and TUNEL indices in relation to breast cancer (n = 61)*.

	Odds Ratio	P>lzl	[95% Conf. Interval]
Log TUNEL	3.66	0.021	1.22 - 10.96
Log Ki-67	1.93	0.128	0.83 - 4.53
Menopausal status	4.46	0.072	0.88 - 22.69

*Logistic regression analysis was used to assess the relations between TUNEL and Ki-67 labeling and the presence of BC. Since the distribution of both indices was markedly skewed, with most patients having low values, log transformation was performed to normalize the distributions.

We did not find any differences in the ratio of proliferative index to TUNEL index as previously reported by Allan, *et al.* (2), and others (3). However, no information on menstrual cycle phase was available for the premenopausal women in these studies. This is of obvious importance in view of the well documented increase in apoptosis in late luteal phase..

Given our preliminary finding of increased cell turnover in the breasts of women with BC, we present an alternative hypothesis regarding the role of apoptosis in BC development, i.e. the high risk breast demonstrates increased cell turnover, which reflects both increased opportunities for the acquisition of genetic defects, as well as attempts to eliminate them. Thus, increased apoptosis may be a marker for a greater burden of cells with critical genetic defects, and therefore a marker of increased BC risk.

References

1. Allan DJ, Howell A, Roberts SA et al (1992) Reduction in apoptosis relative to mitosis in histologically normal epithelium accompanies fibrocystic change and carcinoma of the premenopausal human breast. J Pathol 167:25-32.
2. Mustonen M, Raunio H, Paakko P et al (1997) The extent of apoptosis is inversely associated with bcl-2 expression in premalignant and malignant breast lesions. Histopathology 31:347-354.
3. Hassan HI, Walker RA (1998) Decreased apoptosis in non-involved tissue from cancer-containing breasts. J Pathol 184:258-264.
4. Mundle SD, Gao XZ, Khan S (1995) Two in situ techniques reveal different patterns of DNA fragmentation during spontaneous apoptosis in vivo and induced apoptosis in vitro. Anticancer Research 15:1895-1904.

Expression and Estrogen Inducible Promoter Activity of Human Estrogen-responsive Finger Protein Gene in Breast and Ovarian Cancer Cells

Kazuhiro Ikeda, Satoshi Inoue, Akira Orimo, Hisahiko Hiroi, Fujiko Tsuchiya, ItsuoGorai, Yasuhiro Higashi, and Masami Muramatsu

Summary

In female reproductive organs, estrogen-responsive finger protein (efp), a member of RING finger family, which includes genes involved in carcinogenesis, is co-expressed with estrogen receptor (ER) α mRNA. RNase protection assay has shown that efp mRNA is expressed in both breast and ovarian cancer specimens and adjacent nontumoral tissues. It is also detected in breast and ovarian cancer cell lines (MCF-7, OVISE, OVKATE, OVMANA, OVSAHO, OVSAYO and OVTOKO cells). The concentration of efp mRNA varies among specimens and cell lines. In MCF-7 cells, estrogen treatment induces the efp mRNA expression. Furthermore, CAT assay showed that the activity of the efp promoter was enhanced by estrogen administration through the estrogen responsive element (ERE) in 3'-untranslated region (3'-UTR). These findings suggest that efp responds to estrogen, and mediates estrogen actions in cancer cells.

Introduction

Estrogen has important roles in cell proliferation and differentiation of female reproductive organs including uterus, mammary gland, and ovary. It is known that prolonged estrogen treatment causes increased cancer risk of these organs (1, 2). However, little is known about the mechanisms of these phenomena. Estrogen actions are assumed to be mediated by estrogen receptor (ER) and its target genes. Estrogen-responsive finger protein (efp) isolated by genomic-binding site cloning using an ER recombinant protein is a member of the RING finger family (3). The efp mRNA is predominantly expressed in female reproductive organs including uterus, ovary, and mammary gland (4). The efp gene has an estrogen responsive element (ERE) in the 3'-untranslated region (UTR) and estrogen-induced gene expression was found in the uterus, brain and mammary gland cells (3, 4). We have proposed that efp mediates estrogen actions in such estrogen target organs. In the present study, we investigated the expression of efp in human breast and ovarian cancer samples, and analyzed the expression and the estrogen responsiveness of the efp gene in breast and ovarian cell lines.

Materials and Methods

Breast and ovary tissue samples were collected from patients. Tumor and adjacent nontumoral tissues were obtained from the same resection specimen. MCF-7 cells were maintained in DMEM + 10% fetal calf serum (FCS), while other cell lines in RPMI 1640 + 10% FCS. To investigate estrogen responsiveness of efp mRNA, MCF-7 cells were maintained in phenol red-free DMEM + 10% dextran coated charcoal treated FCS for 24 h, and subsequently changed to medium with 10^{-8} M 17β-estradiol (E_2).

RNA Extraction and RNase Protection Assay (RPA)

Total RNAs were isolated using ISOGEN (NIPPONGENE). RNase protection assays were performed using RPA II (Ambion) according to the manufacturer's protocol, respectively. Efp and GAPDH RNA probes were generated as described elsewhere (5).

Results and Discussion

To investigate the expression of efp mRNA in breast and ovarian cancers, RNase protection assay was performed using total RNAs isolated from breast and ovarian cancer samples and adjacent nontumoral tissues. Tables 1 and 2 show that the intensity of efp signals normalized with GAPDH in breast and ovarian cancers, respectively. Efp was expressed in all breast cancer samples tested, however the amount of mRNA in a tumor, relative to adjacent non tumorous tissue varied among the specimens. Efp mRNA was also expressed in ovarian cancer samples tested. In these samples, the expression of efp was reduced in tumors. The expression of the efp mRNA was also detected in MCF-7 cells, and in all six ovarian cancer cell lines, OVISE, OVKATE, OVMANA, OVSAHO, OVSAYO and OVTOKO cells (6, 7) using RNase protection assay (data not shown). These results suggest that the efp might mediate estrogen actions in breast and ovarian cancers, and its expression may be regulated in a complex manner in these tumors.

Table 1. Expression of efp mRNA in breast cancer. Signals of efp were quantitated and normalized with GAPDH.

No. Sample	N^a	T^b
1	0.048	0.105
2	0.038	0.040
3	0.047	0.061
4	0.127	0.057
5	0.131	0.152
6	0.011	0.117
7	0.054	0.048
8	0.119	0.113
9	0.054	0.082
10	0.120	0.165
11	0.212	0.142
12	0.076	0.090
13	0.131	0.101
14	0.140	0.118
15	0.107	0.144
Mean ± SD	0.094 ± 0.053	0.102 ± 0.039

[a] Adjacent non tumorous tissue.
[b] Tumor tissue.

Table 2. Expression of efp mRNA in ovarian cancer. Signals of efp were quantitated and normalized with GAPDH.

No. Sample	N^a	T^b
1	0.276	0.049
2	0.122	0.051
3	0.129	0.095
4	0.135	0.081
Mean ± SD	0.166 ± 0.064	0.069 ± 0.020

[a] Adjacent non tumorous tissue.
[b] Tumor tissue.

Estrogen-induced Expression and Promoter Activity of the efp Gene

The estrogen-induction of efp mRNA in MCF-7 breast cancer cells is shown in Figure 1. RNase protection assay revealed that the efp mRNA was elevated after 10^{-8} M E_2 treatment for 4 h. The E_2 treatment also enhanced the activity of the efp promoter via ERE located in 3'-UTR by about 4.0-fold (data not shown). These observations suggest that the efp responds to estrogen and may mediate estrogen actions in cancer cells.

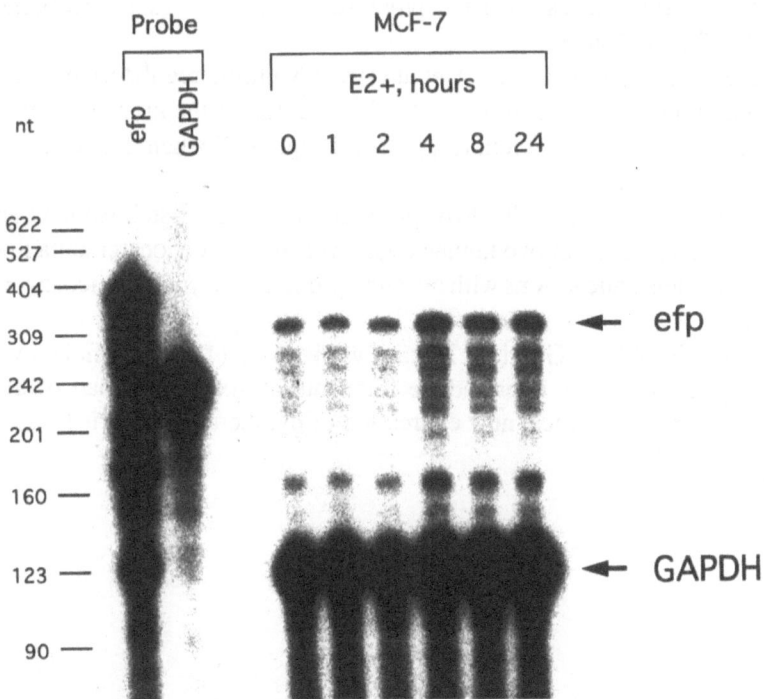

Figure 1. Effect of E_2 treatment on the expression of efp mRNA in MCF-7 cells. Total RNAs were isolated from MCF-7 cells untreated (0 h) or treated with 10^{-8} M E_2 for 1, 2, 4, 8, and 24 h. Aliquots, 20 μg of total RNA, were examined by RNase protection assay using efp and GAPDH probes. Full-length protected fragments for each probe are indicated.

Acknowledgment

K.I. is supported by The Asahi Glass Foundation and Sankyo Foundation of Life Science.

References

1. Brinton LA, Hoover R, Fraumeni JF, Jr (1986) Menopausal estrogen and breast cancer risk. An expanded case-control study. Brit J Cancer 54:825-832.
2. Weiss NS, Szekely DR, English DR et al (1979) Endometrial cancer in relation to patterns of menopausal estrogen use. J Am Med Ass 242:261-264.
3. Inoue S, Orimo A, Hosoi T et al (1993) Genomic binding-site cloning reveals an estrogen-responsive gene that encodes a RING finger protein. Proc Natl Acad Sci U S A 90:11117-11121.
4. Orimo A, Inoue S, Ikeda K et al (1995) Molecular cloning, structure, and expression of mouse estrogen- responsive finger protein Efp. Co-localization with estrogen receptor mRNA in target organs. J Biol Chem 270:24406-24413.
5. Ikeda K, Inoue S, Orimo A et al (1997) Multiple regulatory elements and binding proteins of the 5'-flanking region of the human estrogen-responsive finger protein (efp) gene. Biophys Biochem Res Commun 236:765-771.
6. Gorai I, Nakazawa T, Miyagi E et al (1995) Establishment and characterization of two human ovarian clear cell adenocarcinoma lines from metastatic lesions with different properties. Gynecol Oncol 57:33-46.
7. Yanagibashi T, Gorai I, Nakazawa T et al (1997) Complexity of expression of the intermediate filaments of six new human ovarian carcinoma cell lines: new expression of cytokeratin 20. Brit J Cancer 76:829-835.

Novel Small Molecule IL-6 Inhibitors as Anti-Cancer Drugs

Bernd Stein, May Sutherland, Stephanie Lipps, Joseph Lewcock, Helen Brady, and Lynn Ransone

Summary

Interleukin-6 (IL-6) has been demonstrated to play a key role in the pathophysiology of several important diseases including certain cancers such as multiple myeloma, renal cell, prostate, cervical and breast carcinomas. In vitro cancer proliferation models for autocrine IL-6 dependent proliferation were established. The production of IL-6 by these cancer cell lines was measured. Further, the autocrine and paracrine effects of IL-6 on cell proliferation were analyzed with a neutralizing IL-6 antibody.

IL-6 gene expression is inhibited by estrogen through a novel non-classical, estrogen receptor (ER) pathway (7). The expression of ER-α and ER-β in cancer cell lines was measured by RNase protection analysis. Surprisingly, the so-called ER-negative breast cancer cell line MDA-MB-231 expressed the novel ER-β. The other cancer cell lines investigated expressed various levels of ER-α and ER-β-mRNA.

High throughput screening identified a series of novel small molecules that blocked IL-6 gene expression through ER. These third generations Selective Estrogen Receptor Modulators (SERMs) strongly block proliferation of breast and prostate cancer cells. In summary, this study shows that ER-dependent small molecule IL-6 inhibitors that work through different molecular mechanisms than traditional estrogenic drugs will permit the discovery and development of new classes of anti-cancer drugs.

Introduction

The cytokine interleukin-6 (IL-6) has been shown to play a growth stimulatory role for various tumors, including prostate cancer, multiple myeloma and renal cell carcinoma. In addition, clinical and animal studies have shown that treatment of these tumors with neutralizing IL-6 antibodies inhibited tumor growth. In particular, IL-6 has been demonstrated to be an autocrine/paracrine growth factor for prostate cancer (1, 2). Neutralizing IL-6 antibodies reduced prostate cancer cell proliferation   (3, 4). Therefore, small molecule IL-6 inhibitors may represent a novel way for the treatment of certain cancers such as prostate tumors.

  Breast cancer cells such as MCF-7 and certain breast tumors have been shown to strictly depend on estrogen for proliferation. Therefore, the anti-estrogen tamoxifen (Nolvadex™) is being used in the clinic for prevention and treatment of breast cancer. However, tamoxifen also increases the risk of endometrial cancer 2-3 fold and has various other side effects. Therefore, there is a need for novel SERMs with a better safety/side-effect profile.

Material and Methods

Cell Culture. Cell lines (MCF-7, MDA-MB231, and DU-145) were obtained from American Type Culture Collection (ATCC, Manassas, Virgina) and cultured according to their recommendations.

Proliferation Assay. Cells were plated in phenol-red free culture media containing dextran-treated, charcoal-stripped sera and maintained in culture for 5 days (DU-145, MDA-MB 231) or 9 days (MCF-7). Cells were treated with vehicle or compounds (see figure legends for detail). Media with compounds or vehicle were replaced every 48-hours. Cell proliferation was assessed using the Cytoquant fluorescence-based dye assay (Molecular Probes, Eugene, OR).

Interleukin-6 Assay. IL-6 in culture media was assessed using a commercially available ELISA assay (Endogen, Cambridge, MA).

RNase Protection Analysis (RPA) for ER-α and ER-β. Total RNA from MCF-7, MDA-MB231 and DU-145 cells was prepared using the TRIZOL reagent (GIBCO Life Technologies, Grand Island, NY). Antisense RNA probes were synthesized against the coding sequences of the ER-α (positions 1018 to 1308), ER-β (180 bp of 3' coding and 3' untranslated region) and GAPDH genes using the In Vitro Transcription Kit (Pharmingen, San Diego, CA). The antisense probes were hybridized to the total RNA from the cancer cells using the RiboQuant RPA kit (Pharmingen) followed by electrophoresis on 6 % polyacrylamide-urea gels.

Results

IL-6 and estrogen have been demonstrated to play key roles in the proliferation of certain tumors *in vivo*. Therefore, we selected the estrogen-responsive MCF-7 and the non-responsive MDA-MB-231 cells as representative cell lines for breast cancer. Estrogen antagonists such as tamoxifen are effective in reducing MCF-7 cell proliferation but have no effect on MDA-MB-231 cells (5, 6). Further, we selected the IL-6 dependent DU-145 cell line as representative for prostate cancer.

In vitro cancer cell proliferation models were established. As expected MCF-7 cells demonstrated an estrogen-dependent increase in cell number (Figure 1A) but MDA-MB-231 did not (Figure 1B). The DU-145 prostate cancer cells secreted about 40 pg/ml of IL-6 into the media (data not shown) and a neutralizing antibody to IL-6 effectively blocked proliferation (Figure 1C). The MCF-7 and DU-145 *in vitro* cell proliferation models have similar growth characteristics as do *in vivo* tumors and are suitable for evaluation of drug effects on tumor proliferation.

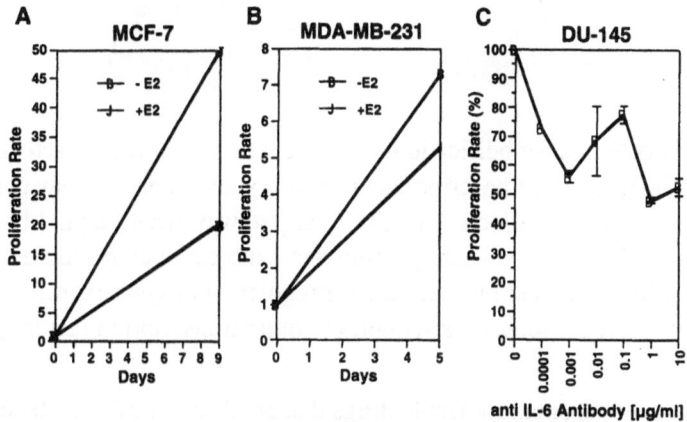

Figure 1. Proliferation of MCF-7 (**A**) and MDA-MB-231 (**B**) breast cancer cells *in vitro* in the presence of vehicle (-E2; 0.2 % EtOH) or 10 nM 17β-Estradiol in 0.2% EtOH (E2). (**C**) Proliferation of DU-145 prostate cancer cells *in vitro* in the presence of increasing amounts of IL-6 antibody. Cell number after 5 days in the absence of antibody was set to 100%.

ER-α and the recently cloned ER-β belong to a family of intracellular ligand-dependent transcription factors. The classical mechanism of estrogen-modulated transcription involves estrogen binding to the receptor, which then binds to a specific short DNA sequence, the estrogen response element (ERE), in the promoters of genes controlled by that specific hormone (Figure 2, Pathway A). We and others have demonstrated evidence for additional "non-classical" ERE pathways (7). This mechanism involves binding of ER to transcription factors such as NF-κB or AP-1 (Figure 2, Pathway B). This pathway explains estrogenic effects on genes without a classical ERE such as IL-6, which is regulated by NF-κB and C/EBP.

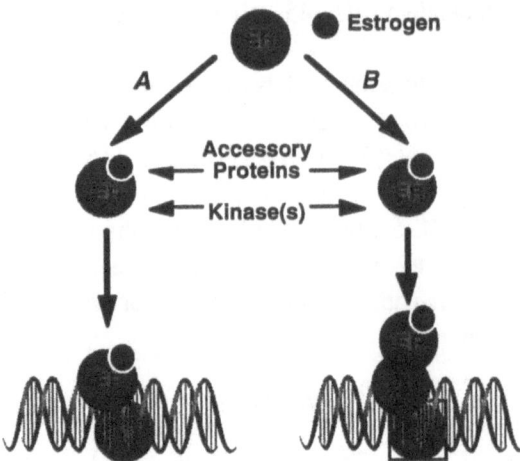

Figure 2. Biochemical modification of ER and interaction with co-activators/co-repressors influence its transcriptional regulatory activities and may contribute to cell/tissue-selective effects. **(A)** Classical pathway where ligand-bound ER modulates gene regulation through promoters with estrogen response elements (ERE); **(B)** Non-classical mechanisms for regulation of gene expression where ligand-bound ER complex cross-couples to other transcription factors (TF).

Therefore, novel small molecule drugs that act through ER may be useful as tissue selective estrogen antagonists for treatment of ER carrying as well as IL-6 dependent cancers. We first determined ER-α and ER-β mRNA levels in cancer cells by RNase protection. MCF-7 cells expressed very high levels of ER-α mRNA but hardly any ER-β mRNA (Figure 3). Surprisingly, the ER-negative breast cancer cell line MDA-MB-231 expressed ER-β mRNA (Figure 3). Prostate tissue and cancer cells have been shown to express ER-β (8). As expected, the DU-145 cell line expressed ER-β mRNA (Figure 3).

High throughput screening identified a series of small molecules that blocked IL-6 production through the estrogen receptor. Compounds 1 and 2 are lead compounds that bound with high affinity to ER-α and ER-β (data not shown).

However, in a human osteosarcoma cell line expressing ER-α compound 1 but not compound 2 blocked the production of IL-6 (data not shown). Conversely, in the corresponding cell line expressing ER-β, compound 2 was the most potent inhibitor. This differential functional ER selectivity of compound 1 versus compound 2 is also evident from cancer proliferation studies (Figure 4). Compound 1 blocked MCF-7 (ER-α expressing) but not significantly DU-145 (ER-β expressing) cell proliferation. In contrast, compound 2 strongly blocked DU-145 but not MCF-7 proliferation.

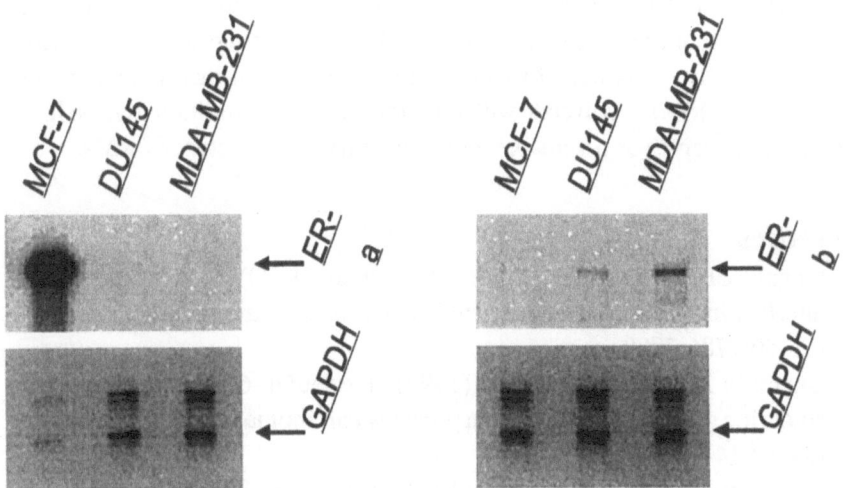

Figure 3. RNase protection analysis of RNA prepared from MCF-7, MDA-MB-231 and DU-145. The positions of ER-α, ER-β and GAPDH are marked.

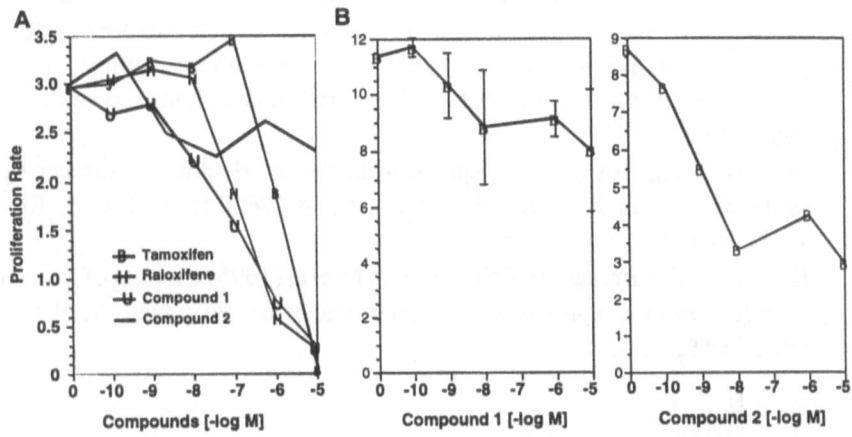

Figure 4. (A) Proliferation of MCF-7 breast cancer cells, (B) proliferation of DU-145 prostate cancer cells. Cells were treated with the indicated amounts of compounds and proliferation compared to vehicle control.

Conclusion

In summary, our data suggest that our ER-dependent small molecule IL-6 inhibitors represent a new generation of SERMs with *in vitro* properties superior to drugs currently being used for cancer treatment. We further show that ER binding affinity does not correlate with functional activity. Additionally, the IL-6 reporter screen serves as a valuable tool to identify ER-selective SERMs.

References

1. Siegall CB, Schwab G, Nordan RP, et al (1990) Expression of the interleukin 6 receptor and interleukin 6 in prostate carcinoma cells. Cancer Res 50:7786-7788.
2. Okamoto M, Lee C, Oyasu R (1997) Interleukin-6 as a paracrine and autocrine growth factor in human prostatic carcinoma cells in vitro. Cancer Res 57:141-146.
3. Okamoto M, Lee C, Oyasu R (1997) Autocrine effect of androgen on proliferation of an androgen responsive prostatic carcinoma cell line, LNCAP: role of interleukin-6. Endocrinology138:5071-5074.
4. Borsellino N, Belldegrun A, Bonavida B (1995) Endogenous interleukin 6 is a resistance factor for cis- diamminedichloroplatinum and etoposide-mediated cytotoxicity of human prostate carcinoma cell lines. Cancer Res 55:4633-4639.
5. Price JE, Polyzos A, Zhang RD et al (1990) Tumorigenicity and metastasis of human breast carcinoma cell lines in nude mice. Cancer Res 50:717-721.
6. Cailleau R, Olive M, Cruciger QVJ (1978) Long-term human breast carcinoma cell lines of metastatic origin: preliminary characterization. In Vitro 14:911-915.
7. Stein B, Yang MX (1995) Repression of the interleukin-6 promoter by estrogen receptor is mediated by NF-κB and C/EBPβ. Mol. Cell. Biol 15:4971-4979.
8. Kuiper GGJM, Enmark E, Pelto-Huikko M et al (1996) Cloning of a novel estrogen receptor expressed in rat prostate and ovary. Proc. Natl. Acad. Sci. USA 93:5925-30.

COMMUNICATIONS

Session II. Metabolism Studies/Cellular & Molecular Biology

Cellular Transforming Activity and Genotoxic Effects of 17β-Estradiol and its Eight Metabolites in Syrian Hamster Embryo Cells

Takeki Tsutsui, Yukiko Tamura, and J. C. Barrett

Summary

The abilities of 17β-estradiol (E_2) and its eight metabolites to induce cellular transformation and genetic effects were studied simultaneously using the Syrian hamster embryo (SHE) cell model. Treatment for 1-3 days with E_2, estrone (E_1), 2-hydroxyestrone (2-OHE_1), 4-hydroxyestrone (4-OHE_1), 2-methoxyestrone (2-$MeOE_1$), 16α-hydroxyestrone (16α-OHE_1), 2-hydroxyestradiol (2-OHE_2), 4-hydroxyestradiol (4-OHE_2), or estriol (E_3) inhibited SHE cell growth in a dose-dependent manner. Morphological transformation in SHE cells were induced by exposure for 48 hr to each estrogen (E), except for E_3. Somatic mutations in SHE cells at the Na^+/K^+ATPase and /or *hprt* loci were induced following treatment of cells with 4-OHE_1, 2-$MeOE_1$ or 4-OHE_2 for 48 hr. Chromosome aberrations were elicited only in cells treated with 4-OHE_1, 2-OHE_1, 4-OHE_2, 2-OHE_2 or E_1 for 24 hr. Aneuploidy induction in the near diploid range was observed in SHE cells treated with each E, except for 4-OHE_1 and E_3. The results indicate that the transforming activities of all Es tested correspond to at least one of genotoxic effects by each E, i.e., chromosome aberrations, aneuploidy or gene mutations, suggesting the involvement of genotoxicity in the initiation of E-induced carcinogenesis.

Introduction

Es are carcinogenic in humans and rodents (1), but the mechanisms by which these hormones induce cancer are not fully elucidated. There is strong evidence that Es are epigenetic carcinogens, acting via a promoting effect related to cellular proliferation, mediated through the estrogen receptor (ER) (2). However, it has been shown that estrogenic activity is not sufficient to explain the carcinogenic activity *in vivo* and *in vitro* under certain experimental conditions, because some Es are not carcinogenic. Another mechanism, related to mutagenic changes, has been suggested in studies of E-induced carcinogenesis (3, 4). We used Syrian hamster embryo (SHE) fibroblast cell cultures as a model system to study the ability of Es to directly transform cells (5-11). SHE cells do not express measurable levels of ER and E treatment is not mitogenic to the cells (12). Thus, estrogenic activity of the compounds can be excluded in this *in vitro* assay. The cells do, however, have the ability to metabolize Es (13, 14).

In the present study, we investigated the abilities of 17β-estradiol (E$_2$) and its eight metabolites to induce cellular transformation and genetic effects in SHE cells to examine a direct involvement of genotoxic effects of Es in the initiation of carcinogenesis. The results obtained indicate that the transforming activities of all Es tested correspond to at least one of genotoxic effects by each E, i.e., chromosome aberrations, aneuploidy or gene mutations, suggesting the involvement of genotoxicity in the initiation of E-induced carcinogenesis.

Materials and Methods

SHE cell cultures were established from 13-day gestation hamster fetuses and grown as previously described (6). E$_2$, estrone (E$_1$), 2-hydroxyestrone (2-OHE$_1$), 4-hydroxyestrone (4-OHE$_1$), 2-methoxyestrone (2-MeOE$_1$), 16α-hydroxyestrone (16α-OHE$_1$), 2-hydroxyestradiol (2-OHE$_2$), 4-hydroxyestradiol (4-OHE$_2$) and estriol (E$_3$) were purchased from Sigma (St. Louis, MO) and dissolved with DMSO at 3 mg/ml. DMSO was added to control cultures at a final concentration of 0.33%. 6-Thioguanine (TG) (Sigma), ouabain (Oua) (Sigma) and benzo[α]pyrene (B[α]P) (Aldrich Chemical Co., Milwaukee, WI) were obtained from the indicated sources.

Cells (3 x 10^4) in logarithmic growth phase were plated in triplicate on 35-mm dishes (Falcon, Oxnard, CA). After overnight incubation, the cells were treated with test Es at various concentrations for 1 to 3 days. The number of cells per 35-mm dish was determined after trypsinization.

For the cellular transformation and somatic mutation assays, cells (2.5 x 10^5) were plated into 75-cm^2 flasks (Falcon), incubated overnight and treated with test eatrogens for 48 hr. After trypsinization, a part of the cell suspension was assayed for morphological transformation, and the remaining cells were subcultured at the density of 4.0 x 10^5 cells per 75-cm^2 flask for mutation experiments. For morphological transformation, 2,000 cells were replated on 100-mm dishes (20 dishes for each group) and incubated for 7 days to form colonies. The cells were fixed with absolute methanol and stained with a 10% aqueous Giemsa solution. The number of surviving colonies with $\rangle$ 50 cells and morphologically transformed colonies were scored by previously established criteria (6).

For mutation experiments, the cells were grown for an expression time of 4 days, and then 10^5 cells were plated on 100-mm dishes (10 dishes for each group) with medium containing 18 μM TG or 1.1 mM Oua, and incubated 7 days for colony formation (15). The mutation frequency was calculated as described previously (15).

For scoring chromosome aberrations and chromosome number, SHE cells were plated into 75-cm^2 flasks at 1.3 x 10^5 cells/flask for the 72-hr group, 2.5 x 10^5 cells/flask for the 48-hr treatment group and 5.0 x 10^5 cells/flask for the 24-hr treatment group. After overnight incubation, the cells were treated with test Es for 24-72 hr. Three hours before the end of the treatment time, Colcemid (GIBCO, Grand Island, NY) was administered at 0.2 μg/ml, and metaphase chromosomes were prepared as described previously (6). After trypsinization, cells were treated with 0.9% sodium citrate at room temperature for 13 min, fixed in Carnoy's solution (methanol: acetic acid, 3: 1) and spread on glass slides by the air-drying method. Specimens were stained with a 3% Giemsa solution in 0.07 M phosphate buffer (pH 6.8) for 7 min. For determination of both chromosome aberrations (gaps, breaks, exchanges, dicentric chromosomes, ring chromosomes and fragmentations) and chromosome number, 100 metaphases per experimental group were scored. Achromatic lesions greater than the width of the chromatid were scored as gaps unless there was displacement of the broken piece of chromatid. If there was displacement, these were recorded as breaks.

Results

No growth stimulating activities were observed in SHE cells treated at 0.3 to 10 μg/ml with these Es tested. Each E inhibited SHE cell growth in a dose-dependent manner. The growth-inhibitory effect of each E was ranked as follows: 2-OHE$_1$ ≈ 4-OHE$_1$ ≈ 2-OHE$_2$ > 4-OHE$_2$ > 2-MeOE$_1$ ≥ E$_2$ >. E$_1$ ≈ 16α-OH E$_1$ ≈ E$_3$.

Dose-dependent increases in the frequencies of morphological transformation in SHE cells were induced by treatment of cells at 0.3 to 10 μg/ml for 48 hr with each E other than E$_3$. The transforming activity of E$_1$ was similar to E$_2$. Although 2-OHE$_2$ exhibited the transforming activity similar or greater than E$_1$ or E$_2$, other three catechol Es, 2-OHE$_1$, 4-OHE$_1$ and 4-OHE$_2$, showed the activities higher than E$_1$ or E$_2$. The transforming activities of 2-MeOE$_1$ and 16α-OHE$_1$ were lower than that of E$_2$.

Treatment of SHE cells with 4-OHE$_1$, 2-MeOE$_1$ or 4-OHE$_2$ at 0.3 to 10 μg/ml for 48 hr induced somatic mutations at the Na$^+$/K$^+$ATPase and/or *hprt* loci in SHE cells. The mutation frequencies at the Na$^+$/K$^+$ATPase locus were within 2.8 x 10^{-6}-2.1 x 10^{-5}, and those at the *hprt* locus were within 1.2 x 10^{-5}-2.5 x 10^{-5}. In untreated cells, the frequencies at the Na$^+$/K$^+$ATPase locus and the *hprt* locus were 3.3 x 10^{-7} and 1.2 x 10^{-6}, respectively. No significant increases in the mutation frequencies were observed in cells treated with any of other Es examined.

Significant levels of chromosome aberrations in SHE cells were elicited by exposure for 24 hr to E$_1$, 2-OHE$_1$, 4-OHE$_1$, 2-OHE$_2$ or 4-OHE$_2$ at the highest concentrations examined (3 or 10 μg/ml).

The effect of the Es on the induction of aneuploidy was measured by determining the chromosome number in metaphase cells, 48 or 72 hr after the start of treatment. Statistically significant increases in the percentage of aneuploid cells in the near diploid range were induced by treatment at 1 to 30 µg/ml with each E, except for 4-OHE$_1$ and E$_3$. The level of aneuploidy induction was varied with each E examined. The high inducibility was observed in cells treated with E$_2$ or 2-MeOE$_1$, and the intermediate or low inducibility was exhibited in cells treated with 2-OHE$_2$, or in cells treated with E$_1$, 2-OHE$_1$, 16α-OHE$_1$ or 4-OHE$_2$, respectively.

Discussion

We examined the abilities of E$_2$ and its eight metabolites to induce cellular transformation and genetic effects using the SHE cell model to investigate a direct involvement of genotoxic effects of the Es in the initiation of hormonal carcinogenesis. Morphological transformation was induced in a dose-dependent manner in cells treated with all Es examined, except for E$_3$. The morphological transformation induced by these Es was stable because the cells were treated and the chemicals removed for a week before the transformed colonies were scored. This finding indicates that the chemicals have the ability to exert directly a heritable change in the cellular phenotype that initiates the cells to lead to neoplastic transformation. Catechol Es other than 2-OHE$_2$ exhibited transforming activities higher than E$_2$ or other E$_2$ metabolites. Because the transforming activities correspond to the abilities of these catechol Es to induce chromosome aberrations and gene mutations in SHE cells, it is suggested that chromosome mutation and/or gene mutation act as one of causal mechanisms of catechol E-induced cellular transformation in SHE cells. However, it is not yet clear whether the high transforming activity of the catechol Es is attributed to the intrinsic feature or the metabolic fate of the chemicals. In the hamster kidney tumor model, 4-hydroxy catechol Es are carcinogenic whereas 2-hydroxy catechol Es are not (16, 17). However, our results that a direct treatment of SHE cells with 2-hydroxy catechol Es (2-OHE$_1$ and 2-OHE$_2$) induced morphological transformation in the cells suggest the intrinsic carcinogenic activity of 2-hydroxy catechol Es. 2- or 4-Hydroxy catechol Es could undergo metabolic conversion in SHE cells to reactive intermediates such as quinone Es (CE-2,3-Q and CE-3,4-Q) that can form DNA adducts (18, 19), because SHE cells have endogenous metabolizing enzymes that exhibit oxidative and peroxidative activities (13, 14). This possibility is supported by our previous findings that when detected by the ^{32}P-postlabeling assay, treatment of SHE cells with E2 and 2- or 4-OHE2 induced covalent DNA adduct formation in the cells, corresponding to the induction of cellular transformation (11).

E$_2$ induced morphological transformation and aneuploidy in SHE cells, but failed to induce any detectable gene mutations and chromosome aberrations over the doses which induced cellular transformation, as described previously (10). Because aneuploidy and cellular transformation in SHE cells are mechanistically related (6, 7, 10, 20), the ability of E_2 to induce aneuploidy could participate in SHE cell transformation by E_2.

E_1 induced cellular transformation, chromosome aberrations and aneuploidy in SHE cells. However, somatic mutations at the Na^+/K^+ATPase and *hprt* loci were not elicited in SHE cells by E_1. No effects at two genetic endpoints including chromosome aberrations and gene mutations are also demonstrated in CHO cells and V79 cells (21, 22). Clastogenic and/or aneugenic activities could play a role in the induction of SHE cell transformation by E_1.

The transforming activity of 16α-OHE$_1$ was lower than E_2, which is consistent with observation that 16α-OHE$_1$ has low carcinogenic activity in hamster kidney relative to E_2 or 4-OHE$_2$ (17, 23). 16α-OHE$_1$ induced aneuploidy in SHE cells. Microtubule disruption is induced in V79 cells by 16α-OHE$_1$(24). As the interaction between Es and microtubules may mediate the induction of aneuploidy in mammalian cells (21, 25), and aneuploidy is mechanistically related to SHE cell transformation, aneuploidy induction might be involved in SHE cell transformation by 16α-OHE$_1$.

Table 1. Effects of 17β-estradiol and its eight metabolites on four genetic endpoints in SHE cells.

Genetic endpoint	E$_2$ and its metabolites								
	E$_2$	E$_1$	2-OH E$_1$	4-OH E$_1$	2-Me OE$_1$	16 α-OH E$_1$	2-OH E$_2$	4-OH E$_2$	E$_3$
Morphological transformation	+	+	+	+	+	+	+	+	−
Chromosome aberration	−	+	+	+	−	−	+	+	−
Aneuploidy*	+	+	+	−	+	+	+	+	−
Gene mutation	−	−	−	+	+	−	±	+	−

*Numerical abnormality of chromosomes in the near diploid range.

Treatment of SHE cells with 2-MeOE$_1$ resulted in cellular transformation, somatic mutations at the Na^+/K^+ATPase locus, and aneuploidy in SHE cells. The results suggest that 2-MeOE$_1$ is genotoxic and potentially carcinogenic. E_3 exhibited no effects at four genetic endpoints including cellular transformation, chromosome aberrations, aneuploidy, and gene mutations in

SHE cells. Very few reports are available to evaluate the genotoxic effects of E_1.

In summary, the transforming activities of all Es tested corresponded to at least one of genetic effects by each E, i.e., chromosome aberrations, aneuploidy or gene mutations (Table 1), suggesting the involvement of the genetic effects in the initiation of E-induced carcinogenesis.

References

1. IARC, IARC (1979) Monographs on the Evaluation of the Carcinogenic Risk of Chemicals to Humans, Sex Hormones (II). Lyon: International Agency for Research on Cancer Vol 21: 139-362.
2. Yager JD Jr, Yager R (1980) Oral contraceptive steroids as promoters of hepatocarcinogenesis in female Sprague-Dawley rats. Cancer Res 40:3680-3685.
3. Barrett JC, Huff J (1991) Cellular and molecular mechanisms of chemically induced carcinogenesis. Renal Failure 13:211-225.
4. Tsutsui T, Barrett JC (1997) Neoplastic transformation of cultured mammalian cells by estrogens and estrogenlike chemicals. Environ Health Perspect 105:619-624.
5. Barrett JC, Wong A, McLachlan JA (1981) Diethylstilbestrol induces neoplastic transformation without measurable gene mutation at two loci. Science 212:1402-1404.
6. Tsutsui T, Maizumi H, McLachlan JA et al (1983) Aneuploidy induction and cell transformation by diethylstilbestrol: a possible chromosomal mechanism in carcinogenesis. Cancer Res 43:3814-3821.
7. Tsutsui T, Maizumi H, Barrett JC (1984) Colcemid-induced neoplastic transformation and aneuploidy in Syrian hamster embryo cells. Carcinogenesis 5:89-93.
8. Tsutsui T, Suzuki N, Maizumi H et al (1986) Alteration in diethylstilbestrol-induced mutagenicity and cell transformation by exogenous metabolic activation. Carcinogenesis 7:1415-1418.
9. Tsutsui T, Degen GH, Schiffmann D et al (1987) Dependence on exogenous metabolic activation for induction of unscheduled DNA synthesis in Syrian hamster embryo cells by diethylstilbestrol and related compounds. Cancer Res 44:184-189.
10. Tsutsui T, Suzuki N, Fukuda S et al (1987) 17β-Estradiol-induced cell transformation and aneuploidy of Syrian hamster embryo cells in culture. Carcinogenesis 8:1715-1719.
11. Hayashi N, Hasegawa K, Barrett JC et al (1996) Estrogen-induced cell transformation and DNA adduct formation in cultured Syrian hamster embryo cells. Mol Carcinog 16:149-156.
12. Korach KS, McLachlan JA (1985) The role of the estrogen receptor in diethylstilbestrol toxicity. Arch Toxicol 58(Suppl 8):33-42.

13. Pienta RJ (1980) Transformation of Syrian hamster embryo cells by diverse chemicals and correlation with their reported carcinogenic and mutagenic activities. In: de Serres FJ and Hollaender A (eds) Chemical Mutagens, Principles and Methods for their Detection. Plenum Press, New York, Vol 6:175-202.

14. Degen GH, Wong A, Eling TE et al (1983) Involvement of prostaglandin synthetase in the peroxidative metabolism of fibroblast cell cultures. Cancer Res 43:992-996.

15. Barrett JC, Bias NE, Ts'o POP (1987) A mammalian cellular system for the concomitant study of neoplastic transformation and somatic mutation. Mutat Res 50:121-136.

16. Liehr JG, Fang WF, Sirbasku DA et al (1986) Carcinogenicity of catechol estrogens in Syrian hamsters. J Steroid Biochem 24:353-356.

17. Li JJ, Li SA (1987) Estrogen carcinogenesis in Syrian hamster tissues: role of metabolism. Fed Proc 46:1858-1863.

18. Liehr JG, Roy D, Ulubelen AA et al (1990) Effect of chronic treatment of Syrian hamsters on microsomal enzymes mediating formation of catechol estrogens and their redox cycling: implications for carcinogenesis. J Steroid Biochem 35:555-560.

19. Cavalieri EL, Stack DE, Devanesan PD et al (1997) Molecular origin of cancer: Catechol estrogen-3,4-quinones as endogenous tumor initiators. Proc Natl Acad Sci USA 94:10937-10947.

20. Tucker RW, Barrett JC (1986) Decreased numbers of spindle and cytoplasmic microtubules in hamster embryo cells treated with a carcinogen, diethylstilbestrol. Cancer Res 46:2088-2095.

21. Drevon C, Piccoli C, Montesano R (1981) Mutagenicity assays of estrogenic hormones in mammalian cells. Mutat Res 89:83-90.

22. Kochhar TS (1985) Inducibility of chromosome aberrations by steroid hormones in cultured Chinese hamster ovary cells. Toxicol Lett 29:201-206.

23. Li JJ, Li SA, Oberley TD et al (1995) Carcinogenic activities of various steroidal and nonsteroidal estrogens in the hamster kidney: relation to hormonal activity and cell proliferation. Cancer Res 55:4347-4351.

24. Aizu-Yokota E, Susaki A, Sato Y (1995) Natural estrogens induce modulation of microtubules in Chinese hamster V79 cells in culture. Cancer Res 55:1863-1868.

25. Wheeler WJ, Cherry LM, Downs T et al (1986) Mitotic inhibition and aneuploidy induction by naturally occurring and synthetic estrogens in Chinese hamster cells in vitro. Mutat Res 171:31-41.

Evidence for an Initiation Mechanism of 17β-Estradiol Carcinogenesis

Fu-Li Yu, Mian-Ying Wang, and Wanda Bender

Summary

17β-estradiol (E_2), the endogenous female hormone, is carcinogenic causing uterine and breast cancers. The mechanism is unknown. We found that E_2 could be activated by the epoxide-forming oxidant dimethyldioxirane (DMDO) and proposed that E_2 epoxidation is the mechanism of E_2 carcinogenesis. One of the critical tests of our hypothesis is to determine whether E_2-DNA adducts are formed *in vivo*. When female ACI rats were given intramammillary injections of E_2 and DMDO-activated E_2, identical DNA adducts were formed. However, the activated E_2 was at least 25,000-fold more active than E_2 forming DNA adducts *in vivo*.

Introduction

Breast cancer leads all cancer incidence among American women accounting for 30% of the 1998 estimated new cases in the USA and is the second leading cause of cancer deaths estimated at 44,000 per year (1). Estrogens (Es), natural or synthetic, used widely in a variety of clinical conditions, from hormone replacement therapy to cancer treatment, are themselves carcinogenic, causing uterine (2) and breast cancer (3). The mechanism of their carcinogenic action is still not well understood. Because Es are required for the growth and development of their target tissues, it has long been believed that Es are cancer promoters. Recently, we found that estrone (E_1), 17β-estradiol (E_2), diethylstilbestrol (DES), and the anti-E tamoxifen (TAM) could be activated by the epoxide-forming oxidant dimethyldioxirane (DMDO) resulting in the inhibition of rat liver nuclear and nucleolar RNA synthesis in a dose-dependent manner *in vitro* (4). Since epoxidation is often required for the activation of carcinogens (5), we proposed that E epoxidation is the underlying mechanism for the initiation of E carcinogenesis (4). It is well established that chemical carcinogenesis is a multistage process involving initiation, promotion, and progression (6). Initiation, the most critical first step in carcinogenesis, requires

444

the binding of a chemical carcinogen to DNA forming DNA adducts. For this reason, one of the critical tests of our hypothesis was to determine whether Es, after activation, are able to bind DNA. In support of our hypothesis, we found that [^{3}H[-E$_1$ and -E$_2$ were able to bind DNA only after DMDO activation (7- 8). Furthermore, E$_1$ - and E$_2$ -DNA adducts were detected by [^{32}P]-post labeling analysis (7-8). However, since these are *in-vitro* experiments, these results can only suggest that the formation of E$_1$- and E$_2$-DNA adducts is possible. For the hypothesis to be biologically relevant, it is critical that E-DNA adducts are detected *in vivo*. The female ACI rat is an ideal animal model to study E carcinogenesis. A recent report has shown that female ACI rats continuous treated with E$_2$, delivered through silastic tubing implants, developed 100% mammary tumors (9). Herein, we report that when female ACI rats were treated by intramammallary injection of E$_2$ or DMDO-activated E$_2$, identical DNA adducts were formed *in vivo*, and that the DMDO-activated E$_2$ was at least 25,000-fold more active than E$_2$ in forming of DNA adducts in the ACI mammary gland. The data presented, represent the first *in-vivo* findings providing evidence in support of our proposed E epoxidation hypothesis, in the potential initiation role of E$_2$ carcinogenesis.

Materials and Methods

For the detection of E$_2$-DNA adducts in the mammary glands *in vivo* (Figure 1), female ACI rats, five-weeks old (100-110 g body weight), were used. The animals were divided into three groups (3 rats/group). A. Control group, rats were given a single intramammallary injection of the solvent, 20% DMSO in corn oil, and sacrificed 24 h later. B. E$_2$ group, rats treated with a single E$_2$ injection of 250 µg/mammary gland/day/3 consecutive days before the animals were killed (only 5 of the right mammary glands of each rat were used). C. DMDO-activated E$_2$ group, rats were treated as those in the E$_2$ group, except a single injection of 1µg /mammary gland of the DMDO-activated E$_2$ was given, and the rats were killed 24 h later. Mammary DNA was extracted and purified. DNA aliquots (10 µg) from each group were used for [^{32}P[-postlabeling analysis to detect DNA adducts (7-8). Autoradiograms were obtained using Cronex^r 10T Medical X-ray films with Dupont Lighting Plus intensifying screens, after the samples were exposed for 24 h at -80^{0}C.

To determine whether the major DNA adducts, namely spots # 1, 2, and 3 (Figure 1) , from both the E$_2$ and the DMDO-activated E$_2$ groups were identical, these [^{32}P]-postlabeling DNA adducts were excised, eluted, and concentrated. Then, they were then re-spotted on polyethyleneimine-cellulose thin-layer chromatography plates and run under four different solvent systems as indicated (Figure 2). Solvent B: 0.4 M Tris-HCl, 0.4 M H$_3$BO$_3$, 8 mM EDTA, 1.04 M NaCl, and 6.4 M urea (pH 8). Solvent I: isopropanol, 4 N NH$_4$OH (1:1, v/v).

Solvent L: 0.56 M LiCl, 0.24 M NaH_2PO_4, 0.4 M Tris-base, and 6.8 M urea (pH 4.5). Solvent P: 0.64 M NaH_2PO_4, 0.4 M Tris-HCl, and 6.8 M urea (pH 8.0). a. Spots 1, 2, and 3 were the corresponding three major DNA adducts from E_2 group as shown in Figure 1. b. Spots 1, 2, and 3 were the corresponding three major DNA adducts from the DMDO-activated E_2 group. Autoradiograms were obtained using Cronex[r] 10T Medical X-ray films with intensifying screens after exposing the samples for 3 days at -80^0C .

For the dose-response $[^{32}P]$-postlabeling E_2-DNA adduct studies (Figure 3), groups of female ACI rats were treated with intramammallary injections as described in Figure 1. Except for this study, different doses of DMDO-activated E_2 were injected per mammary gland. B, 100 µg; C, 10 µg; D, 1 µg; E, 0.1 µg; F, 0.01 µg. A, the control received only the solvent. All the animals were killed 24 h later. Autoradiograms were obtained using Cronex[r] 10T Medical X-ray films with intensifying screens after exposing the samples for 16 h at -80^0 C.

To obtain the E_2-DNA adduct dose-response curve of the female ACI rats after given intramammallary injections of the DMDO-activated E_2 (Figure 4), the major spots of the DNA adducts, namely 1, 2 and 3 (Figure 3) were excised. The radioactivity of each spot was determined by Cerenkov counting. The relative adduct level (RAL) for each injected dose was calculated and expressed as E_2-DNA adducts/10^{10} nucleotides.

Results

The results shown in Figure 1 clearly indicate that there were three major DNA adducts, labeled 1, 2 and 3, produced after female ACI rats were treated with intramammallary injection of either E_2 or DMDO-activated E_2. No detectable DNA adducts from the control group, except an unknown spot marked "b" that appeared in all groups, and the internal standard DNA adduct marker labeled as "is" that was included in each sample to monitor the efficiency of the $[^{32}P]$-postlabeling procedure and to reflect the relative amount of DNA adducts from each sample when compared.

Although the migration positions of the three DNA adduct spots on the two-dimensional $[^{32}P]$-postlabeling maps from both the E_2 and the DMDO- activated E_2 groups were similar, it was important to determine whether they are identical DNA adducts. For this reason, the three DNA adduct spots from each group were cut and eluted. After concentration, these DNA adducts from both groups were re-spotted in parallel on the polyethyleneimine-cellulose thin-layer chromatography plates and separated under four different solvents. Results from this study (Figure 2) indicate that the three DNA adducts formed in the mammary glands from both the E_2 and the DMDO-activated E_2 injected groups were identical.

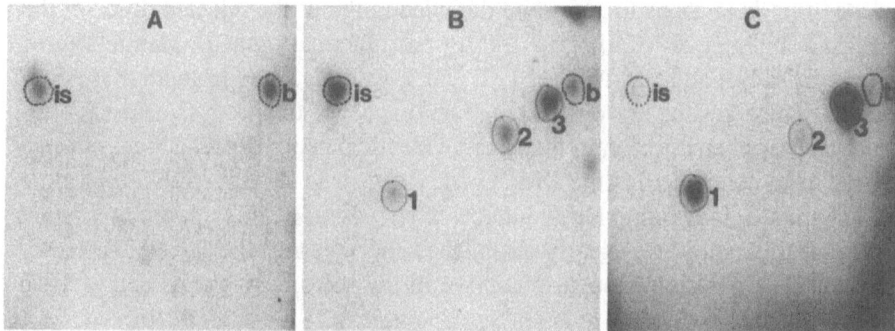

Figure 1. Detection of E_2-DNA adducts in ACI female rats treated by intramammallary injection of either E_2 or DMDO-activated E_2 *in vivo*. A, control group; B, E_2 group; rats treated with a single E_2 injection of 250 μg/ mammary gland/day for 3 days; and C, DMDO-activated E_2 group. Rats were treated with a single injection of 1μg/mammary gland of DMDO-activated E_2.

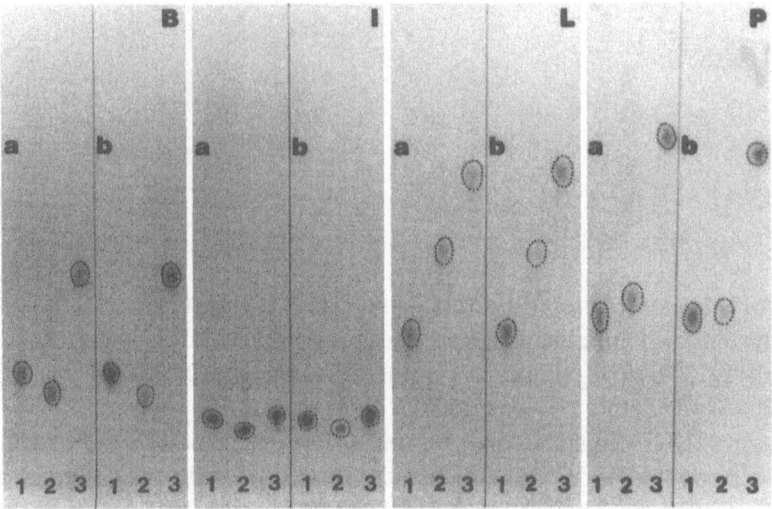

Figure 2. Evidence for the formation of identical *in vivo* E_2 DNA adducts in the ACI female mammary glands treated by intramammallary injection of either E_2 or DMDO-activated E_2. See Materials and Methods for details.

Figure 3 shows dose-response [^{32}P]-postlabeling E_2-DNA adduct maps of female
ACI rats treated with intramammallary injections of DMDO-activated E_2. It is
clear from these maps that, despite the wide range of the injected doses of the
DMDO-activated E_2 (0.01µg to 100 µg per mammary gland), identical three
major E_2-DNA adducts, marked 1, 2, and 3, were detected from all these dose
points. These results not only strengthen our belief that both E_2 and DMDO-
activated E_2 when injected produced three identical major DNA adducts, but also
allow us to conclude that the DMDO-activated E_2 is at least 25,000-fold more
active than E_2 in forming DNA adducts *in vivo*. Finally, it is important to point
out that this study has clearly established the fact that the injected DMDO-
activated E_2 is stable enough to survive in the mammary glands and to form
DNA adducts.

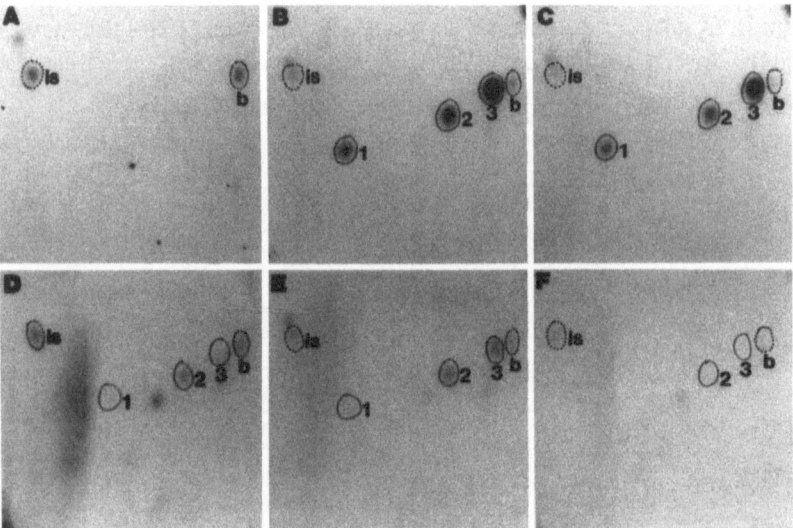

Figure 3. Dose-response [^{32}P]-postlabeling E_2-DNA adduct maps of female ACI
rats treated with intramammallary injections of DMDO-activated E_2 .   A,
Control; B, 100 µg; C, 10 µg; D, 1 µg; E, 0.1 µg; and F, 0.01 µg.

To obtain the E_2-DNA adduct dose-response curve, the three major DNA adducts
(Figure 3) were excised. The radioactivity from each spot was determined by
Cerenkov counting. The relative adduct level (RAL) for each injected dose was
calculated and expressed as E_2-DNA adducts per 10^{10} nucleotides. The results
from this analysis are shown in Figure 4.
    It is interesting to note that the formation of the E_2-DNA adducts is linearly
correlated with the log dose of the injected DMDO-activated E_2. Thus, when

0.01, 0.1, 1.0, 10, and 100 µg DMDO-activated E_2/mammary gland were injected, there were 38, 63, 86, 107, and 136 E_2-DNA adducts per 10^{10} nucleotides formed, respectively, 24 h after the initial injection.

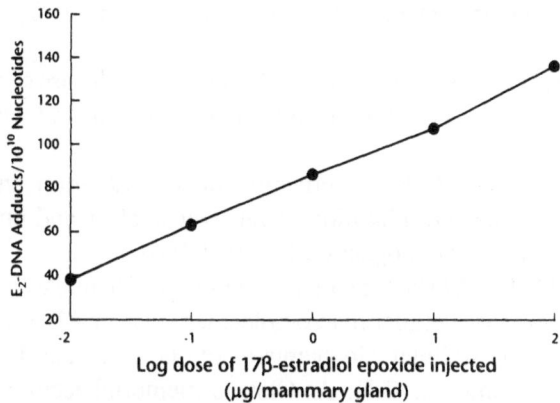

Figure 4. An E_2-DNA adduct dose-response curve of female ACI rats treated with an intramammallary injection of DMDO-activated E_2.

Conclusions

1. We detected by [^{32}P]-postlabeling three major DNA adducts formed in vivo after female ACI rats were given intramammallary injection of either E_2 or the DMDO activated E_2.
2. Evidence is presented to show that the three DNA adducts formed in the mammary glands after E_2 injection were identical to the three DNA adducts formed after the injection of the DMDO activated E_2.
3. Since it required 250 µg E_2/ mammary gland for the injection per day for three consecutive days to detect the DNA adducts in the mammary glands, and it required only 0.01µg DMDO activated E_2/mammary gland for a single injection and sacrifice 24 hrs later to detect the DNA adducts, it is concluded that the DMDO activated E_2 is at least 25,000-fold more active than E_2 in forming DNA adducts in vivo.
4. These experimental results, which are all first time findings, have provided the critical in vivo evidence needed to support our proposed E epoxidation hypothesis, and the potential initiation role of E_2 carcinogenesis.

Acknowledgment

This work was supported by PHS grant # CA-70466 awarded by National Cancer Institute, DHHS.

References

1. Landis SH, Murray T, Bolden S et al (1998) Cancer Statistics 1997. CA Cancer J Clin 48: 6-29.
2. Grady D, Gebretsakid T, Kerlikowske K et al (1995) Hormone replacement therapy and endometrial cancer: A meta-analysis. Obstet Gynecol 85: 304-313.
3. Colditz GA, Hankinson SE, Hunter DJ et al (1995) The use of estrogens and progestins and the risk of breast cancer in postmenopausal women. N Engl J Med 332: 1589-1593.
4. Yu FL, Bender W (1996) Activation of 17β-estradiol and estrone by dimethyldioxirane and inhibition of rat liver nuclear and nucleolar RNA synthesis in vitro. Carcinogenesis 17: 1957-1961.
5. Miller EC, Miller JA (1981) Searches for ultimate chemical carcinogens and their reactions with cellular macromolecules. Cancer 47: 2327-2345.
6. Farber E (1984) Cellular biochemistry of the stepwise development of cancer with chemicals: G.H. A. Clowes memorial lecture. Cancer Res 44:5463-5474.
7. Yu FL, Wang MY, Li DH et al (1998) Evidence for the DNA binding and adduct formation of estrone and 17β-estradiol after dimethyldioxirane activation. Chemico-Biological Interactions 110: 173-187.
8. Yu FL, Bender W, Zheng WY et al (1998) The transcriptional effects and DNA- binding specificities of 17β-estradiol after dimethyldioxirane activation. Carcinogenesis 19:1127-1131.
9. Shull JD, Spady TJ, Snyder MC et al (1997) Ovary-intact, but not ovariectomized female ACI rats treated with 17β-estradiol rapidly develop mammary carcinoma. Carcinogenesis 18:1595-1601.

Estradiol Metabolism by Rat Liver Microsomes from Strains Differing in Susceptibility to Mammary Carcinogenesis

Gregory A. Reed, Angela M. Wilson, and Janette K. Padgitt

Summary

Rat strains are known to differ markedly in their susceptibility to estrogen (E)-induced mammary tumors. Specifically, the ACI strain is extremely sensitive to Es, whereas the Sprague-Dawley (SD) strain is relatively resistant. We have compared the metabolism of estradiol (E_2) by liver microsomes from these two rat strains. Both strains exhibit hydroxysteroid dehydrogenase activity, with estrone (E_1) being the major product at E_2 concentrations above 1 μM. Some A-ring hydroxylation also is seen. As the E_2 concentration is decreased, however, hydroxylation becomes a more dominant pathway for both strains. In the SD preparations this still yields E_1 as the major product. ACI liver, however, produces primarily hydroxylated-E_2 at these concentrations. This difference is most apparent at E_2 concentrations below 100 nM. This difference in the disposition of E_2 and its being most pronounced at E_2 concentrations nearing the physiological range, suggest that this difference may contribute to the relative sensitivity of these strains to E_2 carcinogenicity.

Introduction

The identification of carcinogenic risks may be derived from two complementary approaches: the first is epidemiological analysis of human populations, while the second is by extrapolation from controlled exposure studies with experimental animals. The association between Es and breast cancer has been supported by ample data from both approaches. Despite the clear association between Es and breast cancer, the mechanisms involved in this effect are not clear. A pronounced strain difference in sensitivity to mammary carcinogenesis by Es provides an opportunity to identify key mechanistic features of the process. The

ACI rat is sensitive to Es as mammary carcinogens (1-4). Sprague-Dawley rats, in contrast, are relatively resistant to E carcinogenicity (2,5). By comparing E metabolism and resultant effects in the two strains it not only is possible to look for differences in metabolism and responses, but also to try and correlate these responses with susceptibility to carcinogenesis. The examination of estradiol (E_2) metabolism by liver microsomal preparations from these two strains represents the first step in these comparative studies.

Materials and Methods

Female Sprague-Dawley and ACI rats, 6 to 7 weeks old, were purchased from Harlan Laboratories. The livers were homogenized and microsomes prepared by differential centrifugation. Microsomal pellets were resuspended in phosphate-$MgCl_2$ buffer, pH 7.4, and stored at -80° C.

[^{3}H]-E_2 was incubated with RLM (1 mg protein/ml) in 50mM Tris-HCl buffer, pH 7.4, containing 5 mM MgCl2, 5 mM glucose-6-phosphate, and 1 mM ascorbate at 37° C. The NADPH generating system, where noted, included 1 U/ml glucose-6-phosphate dehydrogenase and was initiated by the addition of 1 mM NADP. Reactions with NADP or NAD as cofactors were initiated by the addition of these compounds, again to a final concentration of 1 mM. Incubations were continued for 10 to 60 min, as indicated, depending on substrate concentration. The reaction was stopped by the rapid extraction with 2 x 3 vol of ethyl acetate. The combined extracts were evaporated under vacuum, and the residue dissolved in the initial acetonitrile-methanol-water-acetic acid mix of the HPLC elution.

Separation of metabolites was performed on a Supelcosil C18 column (5 μ, 4.6 mm x 25 cm) at 30° C using a gradient of acetonitrile, methanol, water, and 0.1% acetic acid (6). Unlabeled metabolite standards were detected by monitoring absorbance at 280 nm, whereas labeled metabolites were detected by a Packard Flo-One Beta detector with Ultima Flo M liquid scintillant.

Results

Liver microsomal preparations from female ACI and SD rats both catalyze extensive NADPH-dependent metabolism of E_2. Oxidation of E_2 to E_1 and aromatic hydroxylation of E_2 were the only products observed with these preparations. Maximal rates of E1 formation exceed 300 pmol mg^{-1} min^{-1} in both strains, whereas maximal rates of aromatic hydroxylation are greater than 6 pmol mg^{-1} min^{-1} in SD microsomes and 30 pmol mg^{-1} min^{-1} in ACI liver microsomes. Extensive metabolism was observed not only at the commonly used micromolar concentrations of E_2 (7-10), but at substrate concentrations as low as 3 nM.

Although the metabolite profiles derived from the two strains are nearly identical at high substrate concentrations, a pronounced divergence emerges as the E_2 concentration drops below 1 µM (Figure 1). For both strains, aromatic hydroxylation becomes more pronounced as the E_2 concentration is decreased, but this shift is far more extensive in the ACI rat. As shown, at 100 nM E_2 aromatic hydroxylation to yield catechol Es becomes the dominant pathway for E_2 oxidation, comprising 73% of total metabolism. In the SD rat preparation, however, the fraction of metabolism resulting from aromatic hydroxylation only reaches 36% of the total. An additional 16% of the metabolites produced by the SD rat are catechol E_1 derivatives, which have undergone both 17β-dehydrogenation but also aromatic hydroxylation. Even combining the E_1 and E_2 catechol metabolites still only comprises 52% of total metabolism, as compared to the 73% catechols formed by the ACI liver microsomes under these same conditions.

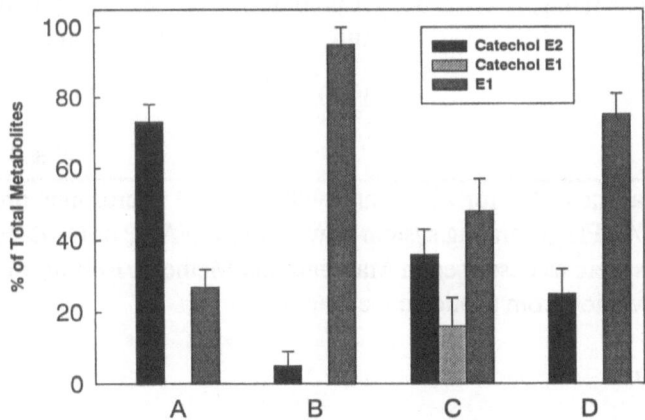

Figure 1. Product Distribution from E2 Oxidation by ACI and SD Rat Liver Microsomes: Effect of Substrate Concentration. Indicated concentrations of [^{3}H]-E_2 were incubated with 1 mg/ml microsomal protein with an NADPH generating system for 20 minutes. Extraction and analysis were as described. All data represent mean ± standard deviation from triplicate incubations. A, ACI rat, 100 nM E_2; B, ACI rat, 30 µM E_2; C, SD rat, 100 nM E_2; D, SD rat, 30 µM E_2.

The formation of hydroxylated products is assumed to be a cytochrome P450-dependent reaction, and thus NADPH-dependent, whereas the conversion to E_1 is a dehydrogenation which may utilize either NAD or NADP as a cofactor. This is borne out by the cofactor specificity demonstrated in Table 1. With the active glucose-6-phosphate dehydrogenase generating system maintaining most NADPH in the reduced form, fully 75% of E_2 metabolism is by hydroxylation, rather than dehydrogenation. The use of NADP, without the generating system for reduction of the cofactor, results in a 3.5-fold increase in the rate of dehydrogenation to E_1, and a 70% decrease in aromatic hydroxylation. The residual hydroxylation presumably results from reduction of NADP via the 17β-hydroxysteroid dehydrogenase reaction. Finally, when NAD is added as the cofactor, which is fully active as a 17β-hydroxysteroid dehydrogenase cofactor but inactive as a cytochrome P450 cofactor in either its oxidized or reduced form, no hydroxylation is observed and 100% of the E_2 is converted to E_1. These cofactor studies clearly support the assignment of E_1 formation to 17β-hydroxysteroid dehydrogenase and the aromatic hydroxylation as a cytochrome P450-dependent reaction.

Table 1. Cofactor effect on E_2 oxidation by ACI rat liver microsomes.

Cofactor	Aromatic Hydroxylation	Dehydrogenation
NADPH generating system	25.8 ± 1.1 pmol mg^{-1} min^{-1}	8.7 ± 2.2 pmol mg^{-1} min^{-1}
NADP	6.3 ± 0.8	20.5 ± 0.5
NAD	0	50 ± 0

1 μM E_2 was incubated for 20 minutes with 1 mg/ml microsomal protein and either the NADPH generating system or with 1 mM NADP or NAD. Extraction and analysis were as described in Materials and Methods. Results are means ± standard deviation from triplicate incubations.

Conclusions

1. Rat liver microsomes efficiently oxidize E_2 at concentrations as low as 3 nM.
2. 17β-Hydroxysteroid dehydrogenase is a relatively low affinity but high capacity system for E_2 oxidation in RLM. Cytochrome P450-dependent aromatic hydroxylation of E_2 is a relatively high affinity but low capacity system for E_2 oxidation in RLM.
3. RLM from the female ACI rat differ from those from other rat strains in that aromatic hydroxylation of E_2 is more dominant than it is in the SD rat.

Acknowledgment

This work was supported by DAMD17-97-1-7155 and ES-07079.

References

1. Dunning WF, Curtis MR (1952) The incidence of diethylstilbestrol-induced cancer in reciprocal F1 hybrids obtained from crosses between rats of inbred lines that are susceptible and resistant to the induction of mammary cancer by this agent. Cancer Res 12: 702-706.
2. Stone JP, Holtzman S, Shellabarger CJ (1979) Neoplastic responses and correlated plasma prolactin levels in diethylstilbestrol-treated ACI and Sprague-Dawley rats. Cancer Res 39: 773-778.
3. Shellabarger CJ, McKnight B, Stone JP et al (1980) Interaction of dimethylbenzanthracene and diethylstilbestrol on mammary adenocarcinoma formation in female ACI rats. Cancer Res 40: 1808-1811.
4. Shull JD, Spady TJ, Snyder MC et al (1997) Ovary-intact, but not ovariectomized female ACI rats treated with 17β-estradiol rapidly develop mammary carcinoma. Carcinogenesis 18: 1595-1601.
5. Sydnor KI, Butenandt O, Brillantes FP et al (1962) Race-strain factor related to hydrocarbon-induced mammary cancer in rats. J Natl Cancer Inst 29: 805-814.
6. Brueggemeier, RW, personal communication.
7. Dannan GA, Porubek DJ, Nelson SD et al (1986) 17β-Estradiol 2- and 4-hydroxylation catalyzed by rat hepatic cytochrome P-450: Roles of individual forms, inductive effects, developmental patterns, and alterations by gonadectomy and hormone replacement. Endocrinology 118: 1952-1960.
8. Watanabe K, Takanishi K, Imaoka S et al (1991) Comparison of cytochrome P-450 species which catalyze the hydroxylations of the aromatic ring of estradiol and estradiol 17-sulfate. J Steroid Biochem Molec Biol 38: 737-743.
9. Kerlan V, Dreano Y, Bercovici JP et al (1992) Nature of the cytochromes P450 involved in the 2-/4-hydroxylations of estradiol in human liver microsomes. Biochem Pharmacol 44: 1745-1756.
10. Suchar LA, Chang RL, Thomas PE et al (1996) Effects of phenobarbital, dexamethasone, and 3-methycholanthrylene administrqation on the metabolism of 17β-estradiol by liver microsomes from female rats. Endocrinology 137: 663-676.

Induction of Breast Cancer in Noble Rats Treated with a Combination of Estrogen and Testosterone

Y.C. Wong, B. Xie, and S.W. Tsao

Summary

Despite extensive research, the precise mechanisms of breast carcinogenesis remain unclear. We have developed an animal model of breast carcinogenesis using a combination of estradiol and testosterone. We found that chronic treatment with a combination of these hormones induces a much higher incidence of breast cancer in Noble rats, than either hormones alone. Although the dosage of testosterone does not influence the cumulative tumor incidence, it does affect the tumor latency period. This suggests that testosterone may act as a promoter in breast tumorigenesis. This study provides in vivo evidence that both estrogens and androgens are important factors for mammary tumorigenesis and that androgens may work synergistically as a promoter to shorten the latency period.

Introduction

Breast cancer is the most common cancer and the second most frequent cause of cancer death in women (1). From among the various recognized risk factors, age of menarche, age of first pregnancy, and age of menopause, suggest that endogenous sex hormones may play the predominant role at all stages in the development of breast cancer (2). Estrogens (Es), especially estrone and estradiol, have long been linked to the risk of breast cancer (3). Furthermore, animal studies have shown repeatedly that Es are able to induce and promote mammary tumors whereas the removal of ovaries, or administration of antiestrogenic drugs, achieves the opposite effect (4).

Considerable efforts have been made in the past attempting to show that women with a high risk of breast cancer and/or those who subsequently develop the disease, have abnormal endocrine profiles. The evidence for elevated urinary and plasma steroids is stronger for androgens than for Es in predicting breast cancer. Based on these observations, androgens have also been proposed as a possible carcinogenic factor in breast cancer (5). This proposal is mainly supported by the fact that the incidence of breast cancer is high in post-menopausal women when androgenic levels are high. More recently, a number of researchers have demonstrated that, among all plasma steroids, the evidence for association of testosterone levels with breast cancer is strongest, although they could not determine whether this association is a cause or an effect of malignancy (6).

Materials and Methods

Animals. The animals were housed under standard conditions (22±2 C, 40-70% relative humidity, 12 hours light/12 hours dark) and fed with rat chow with tap water ad libitum. All surgical operation were done under Pentobarbitone anesthesia. Animals were killed at the end of experiments by cervical dislocation.

Hormonal treatment. At 3 mo. of age sexually mature female Noble rats, weighing 180-210 gm, were randomly divided into six groups. Groups I rats were surgically implanted s.c. in the inguinal regions, with four 2.0 cm Silastic tubings (i.d.1.6mm, o.d.3.2mm) tightly packed with testosterone propionate (T) and one 1.0 cm Silastic tubing containing 17β-estradiol benzoate (E_2). Groups II and III rats were implanted s.c. with one 1.0 cm E_2 and four 2.0 cm T, tubings respectively. Group IV received one 1.0 cm E_2 and two 2.0 cm T tubings. Group V rats received empty Silastic tubings. All tubings were replaced at 3 mo. intervals. The rats were palpaped regularly for mammary tumors starting from 2 mo. after treatment.

Histopathological examination. Breast tumors of various size were removed and paraffin sections (4 μm in thickness) were prepared and stained with hematoxylin and eosin (H&E) for histopathological examination, using the criteria and classification of mammary tumors as outlined by Young and Hallowes (7). The Iball's index is defined as the ratio of incidence (%) to the average latency period in days multiplied by 100 (8). Statistical analyses were carried out using Fisher's exact probability test for incidence, and Student's t-test to determine the level of significance between two mean values.

Results

Incidence of breast carcinogenesis . The results of hormone-induced breast carcinogenesis are summarized in Table 1 and   Figure 1. Spontaneous development of mammary tumor was not observed (Group V) during the experimental period of 12 mo. Compared with other Groups, the rats in Group I showed a significantly increased incidence of breast cancer (52.78%), with a latency period of 5.82±1.77 mo. with an average of just over one tumor per tumor-bearing rat (1.16±0.37). Although multiple tumors had been observed in animals, most rats had only one tumor at the time of sacrifice. Furthermore, the majority of induced tumors were detected in thoracic mammary gland. Only very rarely were tumors observed in cervical, abdominal or inguinal mammary glands (rat has four pairs of mammary glands). The tumor incidence was 22.22% in Group II (E_2 alone) and 16.67% in Group III (T alone), which was not statistically different.   The highest Iball's index score for the overall development of mammary tumor was observed in Group I, which was 3-fold higher than that in Group II and 4-fold higher than that of Group III. The Iball's index of Group I was also significantly higher than that in Group IV which received one E_2 and two T capsules. As shown in Figure 1, the first tumors were observed about 1-2 mo. earlier in the Group I than in Groups II, III, and IV. Significant differences in the cumulative incidence of tumors were initially observed at 6.8 mo. between Group I (44.44%) and Group II (11.11%). On the other hand, the difference in latency period between Group I and Group IV was statistically significant although there was no difference in the cumulative incidence among them (52.78% and 53.33%, respectively). (As shown in Figure 1 and Table 1.)

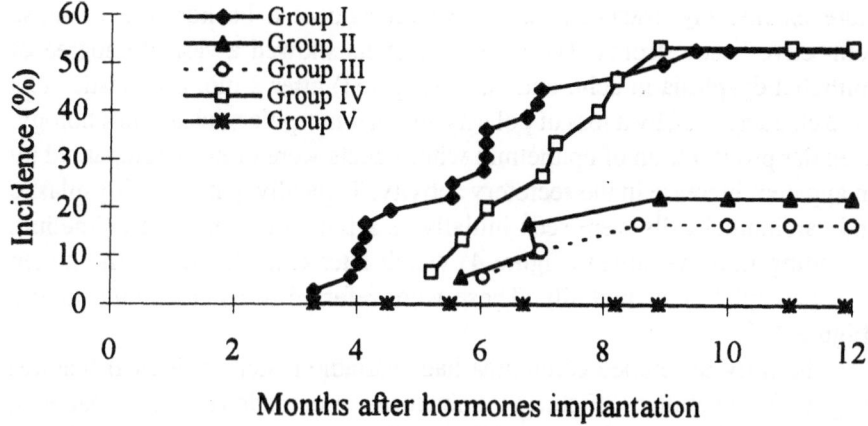

Figure 1. Cumulative incidence of breast tumors in hormone treated Noble rats. The tumor incidence in Group 1 rats is significantly higher (P<0.05) than Groups II and III after 6 mo. The difference between the tumor incidence of Group II and III and between Group I and Group IV is not significant (P>0.05).

Table 1. Induction of breast tumors in hormone treated Noble rats.

Group	Treatment	No. of rats	Rats with tumor No.	Rats with tumor %[a]	No. of tumors Total	No. of tumors Tumors/rat[b]	Latency period (months)[b, c]	Iball's index
I	1E+4T	36	19	52.78	23	1.16±0.37	5.82±1.77	30.23
II	1E	18	4	22.22	4	1.00±0.00	7.07±1.35	10.48
III	4T	18	3	16.67	3	1.00±0.00	7.19±1.28	7.72
IV	1E+2T	15	8	53.33	9	1.13±0.35	7.03±1.29	25.31
V	Control	30	0	0	0	0	0	0

[a]Differences: I versus II and III, P<0.05; I versus IV, P>0.05.

[b]Mean ± SE.

[c]Differences: I versus II, III, IV, P<0.05.

Histopathology. Mammary glands from age-matched control animals were characterized by sparse clusters of epithelial tubules, embedded in small amounts of connective tissue and surrounded by large fat pad. The epithelial ducts had small lumen and darkly stained cuboidal epithelial cells (Figure 2). Mammary glands of all rats implanted with a combination of T and E_2 had a more extensively branched ductal system against a background of loose connective tissue stroma. The alveoli or ducts showed a variable degree of epithelial dysplasia in acini and ducts (Figure3) after 2 mo. Dysplastic cells were characterized by a loss of polarity and pleomorphic nuclear morphology. Irregular proliferation of epithelium within ducts were often accompanied by an apparent increase in the secretory activity. Typically, patches of dysplastic and carcinomal cells were seen initially as a focal thickening of epithelium extending into the lumen (Figure 4) which later extended to fill the lumen either completely or partially. These were referred to as carcinoma in situ (Figure 4, 5).

The fully developed carcinoma had variable histopathological features ranging from papillary (Figure 5), cribriform, or comedo (Figure 6) patterns, either alone or in combination. The papillary pattern consists of bulbous, seemingly fragile, neoplastic epithelial projections protruding into the lumen of the duct (Figure 5) which were often seen in early development. These projections were composed of relatively uniform cells with small nuclei, arranged haphazardly or at right angles to the long axis of the papillae. The cribriform pattern was characterized by neoplastic cells which extended into the ductal lumen to form bridges of anastomosing arcades with many vacuole-like structure. Very often, tumors appeared as multilayered cells surrounding a central necrotic debris, characterized as a comedo pattern (Figure 6). Central necrosis with dystrophic calcification was particularly common in this pattern. As the tumors enlarged further, they invaded the stroma, forming the typical infiltrating ductal or lobular carcinoma (Figure 7). Infiltrating ductal carcinoma also could develop into papillary, cribriform, or comedo patterns.

The well-differentiated type of infiltrating ductal carcinoma retained a tendency to form tubules and alveoli (Figure 7), while the moderately differentiated type was characterized by some features of glandular formation within the tumor masses. The poorly differentiated carcinoma was characterized by solid masses of poorly organized tumors virtually devoid of glandular formation (Figure 8). Very often, isolated islets or single tumor cell were seen infiltrating the connective tissue stroma (Figure 8). Although the breast tumors induced by testosterone and estradiol were of all ranges, the predominant type was solid carcinomas with moderate stroma with obvious evidence of local invasiveness. One metastatic tumor was observed in the uterus, while another one was believed to have invaded the underlying thoracic muscular layer. The histopathology of tumors induced by E_2 or testosterone alone were similar to those induced by a combination of T and E_2.

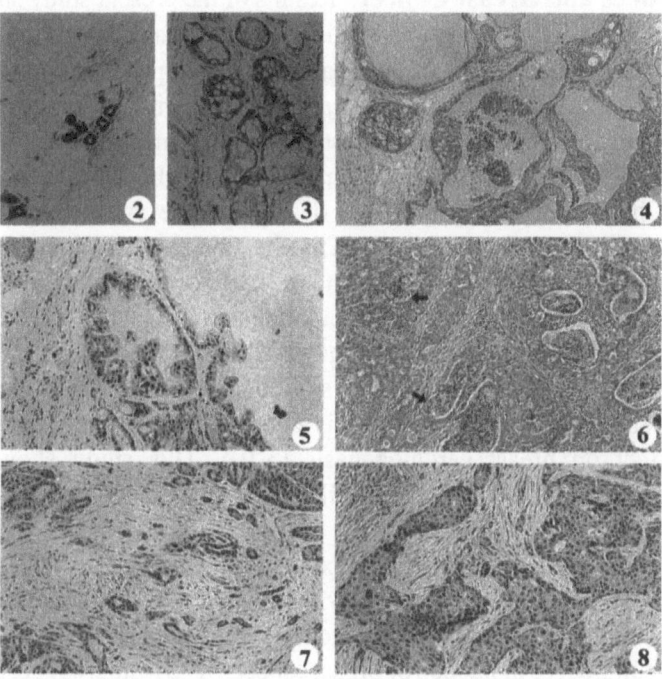

Figure 2. Mammary gland from age-matched control animal. Sparse clusters of epithelial tubules, embedded in small amount of connective tissue and surrounded by a large fat pad. The epithelial ducts had small lumen and darkly stained cuboidal epithelial cells. H&E, 60x; **Figure 3.** Epithelial dysplasia of ducts originating from mammary gland of Nb rat in Group I. Focal areas of dysplastic cells (arrows) are seen in these mildly dilated breast ductal tubules. H&E, 150x; **Figure 4.** Focal ductal carcinoma originating from the mammary gland of Nb rat from Group I. Focal carcinoma in situ are seen extending into the lumen, which is dilated with secretion. H&E, 60x; **Figure 5.** Ductal carcinoma in situ, papillary type. Note the typical papillary projection of epithelial ridges into the lumen. H&E, 150x; **Figure 6.** Ductal carcinoma in situ, comedo type. It is characterized by large cords of closely packed malignant cells often with central necrosis (arrows). Tumor cells are large with pleomorphic morphology. H&E, 60x; **Figure 7.** Infiltrating ductal carcinoma. This picture shows a mixture of well-formed glandular structures and more solid tumor cell nests, suggesting a moderately differentiated carcinoma. H&E, 60x; **Figure 8.** Infiltrating ductal carcinoma. Note the small clumps or single carcinoma cells among stromal connective tissue. H&E, 150x.

Discussion

Sex Hormones and Breast Cancer. Results of the present study show that in the rat, mammary tumors can be readily induced by a combination of 17β-estradiol and testosterone. Over 50% of animals developed breast cancer after sex hormones implantation, with an overall latency period of about 6 mo. We believe this is a better model for studying the mechanisms of breast carcinogenesis, as it closely mimics the natural human breast cancer. Further, the tumors induced by a combination of testosterone and estradiol bear a striking resemblance, not only in growth patterns but also in histopathology, to the human   (9). Thus, this model can be used to elucidate the role and mechanism of sex hormones in breast carcinogenesis.

Epidemiological evidence shows that androgens are strongly associated with breast cancer risk. It is still unclear whether androgens are a cause or an effect of breast carcinogenesis and whether they have a direct or an indirect effect on breast carcinogenesis (5,10). This study showed that testosterone implanted alone had the ability to induce breast tumors in female Noble rats.

The incidence and Iball's index in the rats treated with T and E_2 is significantly higher than those treated with either T or E_2 alone. Reduction in T dosage, while keeping the E_2 level unchanged, increases the latency period but not the cumulative incidence of breast cancers. The results suggest that the two hormones act synergistically on mammary gland, and in breast carcinogenesis, with T playing a crucial role in the process.

Androgens and Breast Cancer. Although the amount of T implanted which was aromatized to estradiol is not known, the coexistence of Es (natural and converted) and T can be established. We believe a synergistic effect of E and T continues to exist in this situation. Compared to estradiol-treated rats, treatment with a combination of T and E_2 shortens the latency period. When the dosage of T was reduced to half (E_2+2T) of those used in Group I (E_2+4T), although no significant difference in cumulative incidence was observed but the latency period was significantly longer than in Group I. On the other hand, treatment of intact male rats with T alone does not induce breast tumor, while a combination of T and E_2 does (data not shown). Taken together, these observations lead us to speculate that T may act as an endogenous promoter in breast carcinogenesis and this role may be through stimulation of secretion of growth factors and oncogenes in mammary glands rather than stimulation of breast cell proliferation.

Conclusion

The present study demonstrates that long-term treatment with a combination of E_2 and T induces a higher incidence of breast cancer in Noble rats, regardless of the dosage of T used. The histopathological patterns of the induced tumors and the number of tumors per tumor-bearing animal bear close resemblance to human mammary tumors. Furthermore, the dosage of T though does not influence the tumor incidence, but does effect the tumor latency period. This suggests that T may act as a promoter in the mammary tumorigenesis. Additionally, we offer a useful animal model for exploring the role of androgens in mammary tumorigenesis.

References
1. Parker SL, Tong T, Bolden S et al (1997) Cancer statistics 1997. CA Cancer J Clin 47:5-27.
2. Boyle P (1988) Epidemiology of breast cancer. Baillieres Clin Oncol 2:1.
3. King RJB (1991) A discussion of the roles of oestrogen and progestin in human mammary carcinogenesis. J Steroid Biochem Mol Bio 39(5B):811.
4. Dao TL (1981) The role of ovarian steroid hormones in mammary carcinogenesis. In: Pike M.C., Siiteri, P.K., Welsch C.W. (eds) Hormones and Breast Cancer, Banbury Report No 8. Cold Spring Harbor Laboratory Press, New York, pp. 281-295.
5. Bernstein L, Ross RK (1993) Endogenous hormones and breast cancer risk. Epidemiol Rev 15:48-65.
6. Dorgan JF, Longcope C, Stephenson HE et al (1997) Serum sex hormone levels are related to breast cancer risk in postmenopausal women. Environ Health Perspectives, 105(Suppl.):583-585.
7. Young S, Hallowes RC (1973) Tumors of the mammary gland. In Turusov, VS (ed) Pathology of Tumors in Laborotory Animals, vol. 1. IARC Scientific Publications, Lyon, France, pp. 31-74.
8. Iball J (1939) The relative potency of carcinogenic compounds. Am J Cancer 35:188-190.
9. Veronesi U, Goldhirsch A, Yarnold J (1995) Breast cancer. In: Peckham, M, Pinedo, H, and Veronesi, U (eds) Oxford textbook of oncology.. Oxford University Press, Oxford, England, pp. 1243-1289.
10. Berrino F, Muti P, Micheli A et al (1996) Serum sex hormone levels after menopause and subsequent breast cancer. J Natl Cancer Inst 88:291-296.

Isolation and Purification of Breast Carcinoma Cell Lines From a Noble Rat

B. Xie, Y.C. Wong, and S.W. Tsao

Summary

We report here the establishment of a culture of breast epithelial cells derived from breast carcinoma of a male rat induced by implantation of a combination of 17β-estradiol and testosterone propionate. This serially cultivated cell line has been demonstrated, by a variety of criteria, to be a neoplastic rat mammary epithelial cell line. The criteria used include morphological and growth characteristics, presence of specific antigens, steroid hormone receptors, hormone responsiveness, and karyotype analysis. These cell lines may be useful for a number of *in-vitro* studies to explore the mechanism(s) of hormonal carcinogenesis. Inasmuch as the cell line expresses androgen receptor, it may serve as a valuable in vitro model in which to assess the effects of endogenous and exogenous androgens known to play an important role in breast carcinogenesis.

Introduction

Breast cancer is the most common malignancy and the leading cause of cancer death in women in the Western world (1). From among the various recognized risk factors, estrogens, especially estrone and estradiol, have long been linked to the risk of breast cancer (2). More recently, a number of researchers have demonstrated that, among all plasma steroids, the evidence for association of testosterone levels with breast cancer is strongest, although they could not determine whether this association is a cause or an effect of malignancy (3).

Recently, we have developed an animal model for breast cancer using testosterone and estradiol as a carcinogen to carry out detailed investigations. Furthermore, we also have established a serially cultivated cell line from this animal model. The environment of cultured cells can be controlled to a far greater extent than that of an *in-situ* solid tumor and *in-vitro* experiments can be performed without interference from host related factors such as stroma-epithelial interaction which is very important and complicated factor in hormonal carcinogenesis. Establishment of neoplastic mammary epithelial cells, therefore, can provide a valuable model with which to investigate the direct cellular effects on breast carcinogenesis.

Materials and Methods

Breast cancers were induced in male Noble rats by a modification of the procedure of Noble et al. (4). Cell isolation and routine subculture methods were essentially as described in (5). Growth curve and hormone responsiveness were determined by MTT labeling method (6). Chromosome analysis was by a modification of standard cell culture procedures (7). The markers used for determining epithelial origin of the cells were anti-cytokeratin 18, anti-myosin, and anti-vimentin. The expression of these markers, as well as estrogen receptor, androgen receptor, and some growth factors as listed in Table 2, was detected by routine immunocytochemistry method.

Results

The histopathological examination confirmed that rats treated with testosterone and estradiol showed a typical ductal carcinoma of breast in a high percentage of animals. This cell line was derived from a ductal carcinoma cell culture. A summary of characterizing features of the cell line is listed in Table 1. The typical growth curve in terms of absorbances of ELISA reader can be seen in Figure 1. The tumor cells *in vitro* readily attached to the surface of plastic flasks. Following initial removal of larger pieces of tumor tissue and other cell debris, the cells were subcultured every two days, with a plating efficiency of approximately 93% in plastic flasks. Saturation density was 210,000 cells/cm2 surface area. Population doubling time during logarithmic growth was 20.54 hours. The cells grew mainly in monolayer cultures, although some clustering with occasional heaps could be seen. Morphologically, the cells were epithelial-like with nuclear polymorphism. The major part of the cells had abundant cytoplasm, but cells with scanty cytoplasm were also found. The pleomorphic nuclei usually contained abundant nucleolar material, indicating a high degree of metabolic activity. Figure 2 (A) is a photomicrograph showing tumor cells from passage 70 as seen by phase contrast microscopy. From then on, more than 50 sequential passages have been performed and microscopic observations of the culture carried out routinely every two days. No changes in cellular morphology and growth characteristics have been observed.

Table 1. Summary of characterization of the cell line.

Subculture	More than 240 passages
Population Doubling Level	3.5 population doublings
Population Doubling Time	20.54 hours per doubling
Saturation Density	21.08 H10⁴ cells/cm²
Plating Efficiency	93%
Morphology	Epithelial-like cell (polygonal)
Dome formation	Yes
Chromosome analysis	Aneuploid (Normal: 2N=42)
Loss of contact inhibition	Yes
Growth in soft agar	Positive
Growth in nude mice	Negative

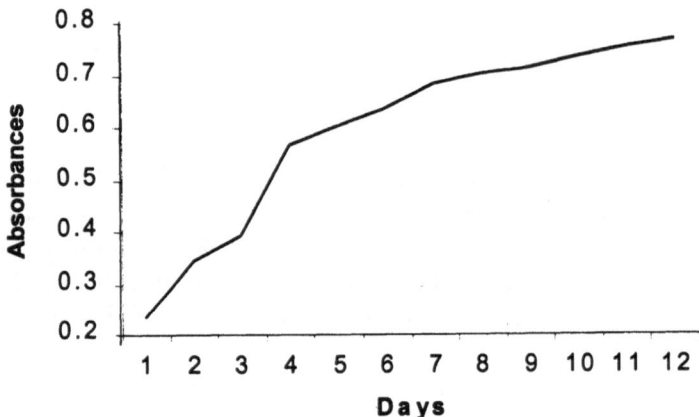

Figure 1. Growth curve of the cell line. Cells (Passage 107) were plated at 5000/well in RPMI-1640 supplemented with 10% FBS. The medium was changed every 3 days.

Table 2. Summary of immunocytochemical staining patterns of the cell line.

Cytokeratin 8	+	Estrogen receptor	+	EGF receptor	+
Cytokeratin 18	+	Progesterone receptor	+ /-	VEGF	+
Cyto keratin 19	+	Androgen receptor	+	Flk-1	+
Myosin	-	TGF-α	+	Flt-1	+ /-
Vimentin	-	Neu	+		

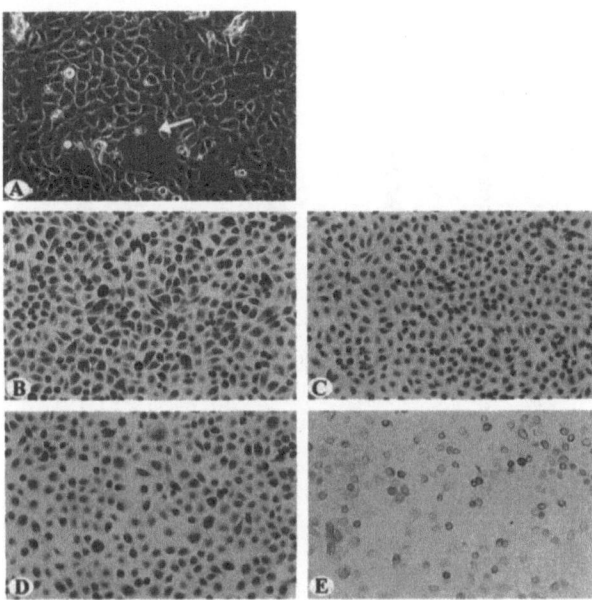

Figure 2. Morphological and immunocytochemical study on the cell line. (A) Phase contrast photomicrograph. Note Acobblestone@ growth pattern. Arrow denote a multinuclear giant cell. 200x. (B) Expression of cytokeratin 18 in the cells. 100x. (C) Absence of myosin in the cells. 100x. (D) Expression of VEGF in the cells. 100x. (E) Expression of Flk-1 in the cells. 100x.

The growth effect of hormones on the cells is shown in Figure 3. The difference between normal medium and control medium is that the former was supplemented with 5% FBS, whereas the later contained only 1% FBS. Compared to control group, when the cells treated with estradiol, hydrocortisone, and insulin the proliferation of the cells increased significantly. In contrast, dihydrotestosterone (DHT) appeared to inhibit the proliferation of the cells. Further, combination of hydrocortisone, EGF, and insulin could stimulate growth to near maximal levels (compared to normal medium).

Karyotype analyses revealed a widely distributed number of chromosomes per metaphase at passage 102. In some metaphase spreads as many as 168 chromosome were counted. In addition, a small percentage of haploid, diploid or triploid metaphases were observed. The majority of the cells had 80 to 90 chromosomes. The typical chromosome spread can be seen in Figure 4 and the distribution of chromosome per metaphase can be seen in Figure 5.

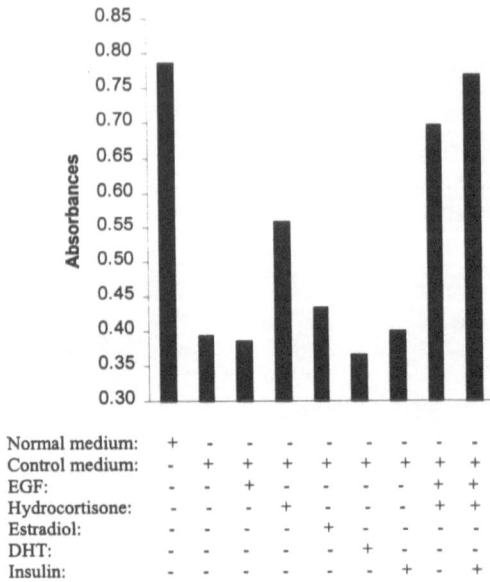

Normal medium:	+	-	-	-	-	-	-	-	-
Control medium:	-	+	+	+	+	+	+	+	+
EGF:	-	-	+	-	-	-	-	+	+
Hydrocortisone:	-	-	-	+	-	-	-	+	+
Estradiol:	-	-	-	-	+	-	-	-	-
DHT:	-	-	-	-	-	+	-	-	-
Insulin:	-	-	-	-	-	-	+	-	+

Figure 3. Effect of various hormones and growth factors on the growth of the cell line.

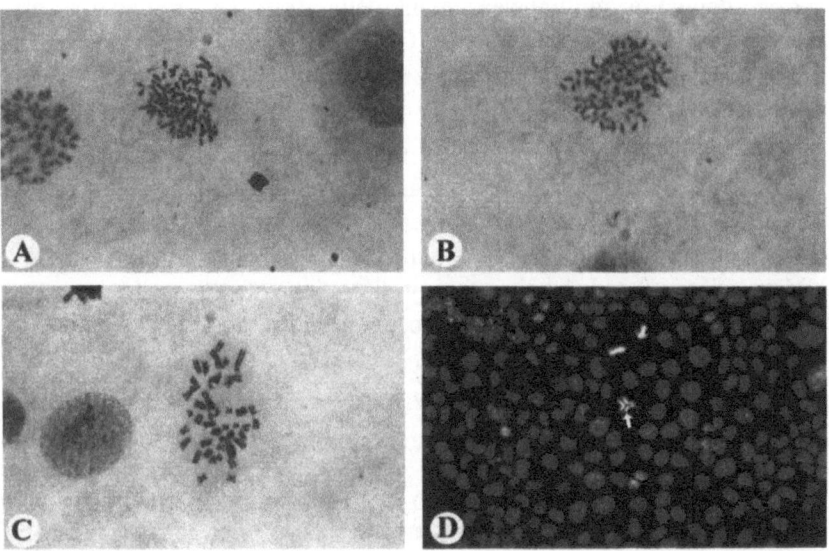

Figure 4. Chromosome analysis of cells at passage 102. Most of the cells have 70 to 90 chromosomes (A, B), with a small percentage of diploid (C) and triploid (D, arrow) cells. 1000x.

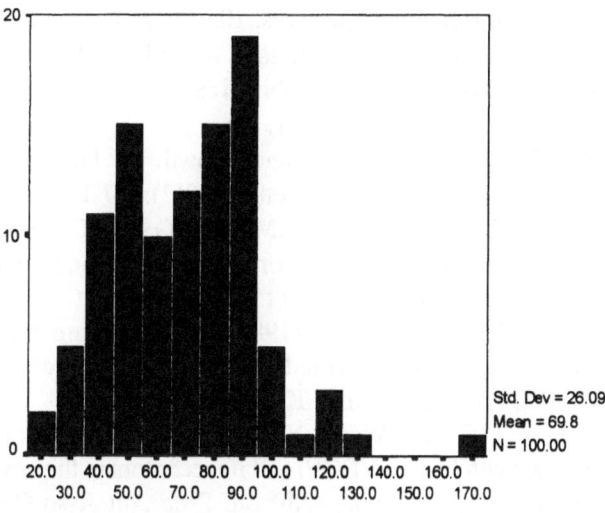

Number of chromosome per cell

Figure 5. The chromosomal distribution of cells at Passage 102.

Discussion

The results presented here indicate that the cell line developed in our laboratory is a neoplastic rat mammary epithelial cell line. The polygonal morphology and the Acobblestone@ growth pattern suggested their epithelial origin. This suggestion is supported by the presence of cytokeratin 18, 19, and 8 and absence of myosin and vimentin, and responsiveness to hydrocortisone combined with EGF and insulin. Furthermore, proliferation of the cells can be stimulated by estradiol and inhibited by DHT revealed that the cells derived from mammary gland epithelium.

In our study, the ability of the cells to growth in nude mice was not observed. However, the neoplastic nature of the cell line could be inferred from its immortal growth behavior, its ability to growth in multilayered patterns, and its high modal chromosome number. More important, the neoplastic nature of the cells also supported by its ability to growth in soft agar which correlated well with in vivo tumorgenicity (9) .

References
1. Parker SL, Tong T, Bolden S et al (1997) Cancer statistics 1997. CA Cancer J Clin. 47:5-27.
2. King RJB (1991) A discussion of the roles of oestrogen and progestin in human mammary carcinogenesis. J Steroid Biochem Mol Biol. 39(5B):811.

3. Dorgan JF, Longcope C, Stephenson HE et al. (1997) Serum sex hormone levels are related to breast cancer risk in postmenopausal women. Environ Health Perspectives. 105(Suppl.):583-585.
4. Noble RL (1976) A new characteristic transplantable type of breast carcinoma in Nb rats following combined estrogen-androgen treatment. Proc Am Assoc Cancer Res. 17:221.
5. Stampfer MR (1985) Isolation and growth of human mammary epithelial cells. J Tissue Culture Methods. 9(2):107-115.
6. Park JC, Kramer BS, Steinberg SM et al (1987) Chemosensitivity testing of human colorectal carcinoma cell lines using a tetrazolium colorimetric assay. Cancer Res. 47(15):5875-5879.
7. Rooney DE, Czepilkowski BH (1986) Tissue culture methods. In: Rooney DE, Czepulkowski BH (eds) Human cytogenetics. A practical approach. IRL Press Ltd, United Kingdom, pp20-22.
8. Xie, B, Tsao GT, and Wong YC (1998) Expression of vascular endothelial growth factor (VEGF) and its receptors in the development of breast cancer in the Noble (Nb) rat. Proc Am Asso Cancer Res. 39:375.
9. Cohen LA (1982) Isolation and characterization of a serially cultivated, neoplastic, epithelial cell line from the N-nitrosomethylurea induced rat mammary adenocarcinoma. In Vitro. 18(6):565-575.

The ACI Rat as a Genetically Defined Animal Model for the Study of Estrogen Induced Mammary Cancers

Martin Tochacek, Eric A. VanderWoude, Thomas J. Spady, Djuana M. E. Harvell, Mary C. Snyder, Karen L. Pennington, Tanya M. Reindl, and James D. Shull

Summary

We have demonstrated that physiologic levels of 17β-estradiol (E_2) rapidly induce mammary cancer development in ovary intact, but not ovariectomized, female ACI rats. Susceptibility to E_2 induced mammary cancers in F1, F2 and backcross (BC) progeny from a genetic cross between the highly susceptible ACI strain and the highly resistant Copenhagen (COP) rat strain, has now been examined. Susceptibility in progeny from a cross between the ACI strain and a second highly resistant rat strain, Brown Norway (BN), is currently being evaluated. Data from these genetic studies strongly suggest that the unique susceptibility of the ACI rat strain to development of E_2 induced mammary cancers is conferred by a limited number of genes, making mapping and eventual cloning of these genes experimentally tractable. The phenotypically defined F2 and BC progeny are being used in linkage studies to identify the genetic loci that confer and/or modulate susceptibility to E_2 induced mammary cancers. Data accumulated to date indicate that: 1) the genetic etiology of estrogen induced mammary cancers in the ACI rat is distinct from that of dimethylbenz-*a*-anthracene induced mammary cancers; and 2) the rat homologs of the known human breast cancer susceptibility genes *BRCA1* and *BRCA2* do not confer susceptibility to estrogen induced mammary cancer in the ACI rat strain.

Introduction

Although numerous epidemiological studies indicate the importance of estrogens in the etiology of breast cancer(BC), the molecular mechanisms through which estrogens contribute to development of BCs in humans are not presently defined. We have recently demonstrated that the ACI rat strain exhibits a unique susceptibility to development of mammary cancers when treated with physiologic levels of E_2 (1). We hypothesize that the homologs of the genes that confer and/or modulate the susceptibility of the ACI rat strain to development of E_2 induced mammary cancers may modulate susceptibility to BCs in humans. To test this hypothesis we are pursuing genetics and genomics based experimental approaches toward identification of the genes that confer and/or modulate susceptibility to development of estrogen induced mammary cancers in this rat strain.

Materials and Methods

ACI and Brown Norway (BN) rats were obtained from Harlan Sprague-Dawley (Indianapolis, IN). Copenhagen (COP) rats were obtained from the National Cancer Institute Animal Breeding Program (Bethesda, MD). All experimental procedures with animals were approved by the Institutional Animal Care and Use Committee of the University of Nebraska Medical Center. Silastic tubing implants containing 27.5 mg of E_2 were prepared and surgically inserted over the scapulae when the animals were 63 ± 2 days of age, as described previously (1). Each animal was examined twice weekly for appearance of palpable mammary tumors. When a tumor reached 1-2 cm in diameter, the animal was sacrificed by decapitation and subjected to necropsy. Data on latency to appearance of each palpable mammary tumor, tumor growth rate, and tumor location were collected. Trunk blood serum was collected for assay of circulating hormone levels. Mammary tissues, both grossly normal and tumors, were collected for histologic evaluation as described previously (1-2). The spleen was removed and stored at -80 C.

DNA from spleen was isolated using Qiagen (Valencia, CA) spin columns. Each F2 and backcross (BC) animal was genotyped, using a polymerase chain reaction (PCR) based assay (3), at a panel of previously mapped loci distributed across the rat genome (4). PCR primers were obtained from Research Genetics (Huntsville, AL). The PCR products were analyzed on 8% denaturing polyacrylamide gels and visualized using a Phosphorimager. The association between phenotype (i.e., latency or tumor number) and genotype was evaluated by Chi square analysis. LOD scores across genomic intervals were calculated using MAPMAKER/QTL (5).

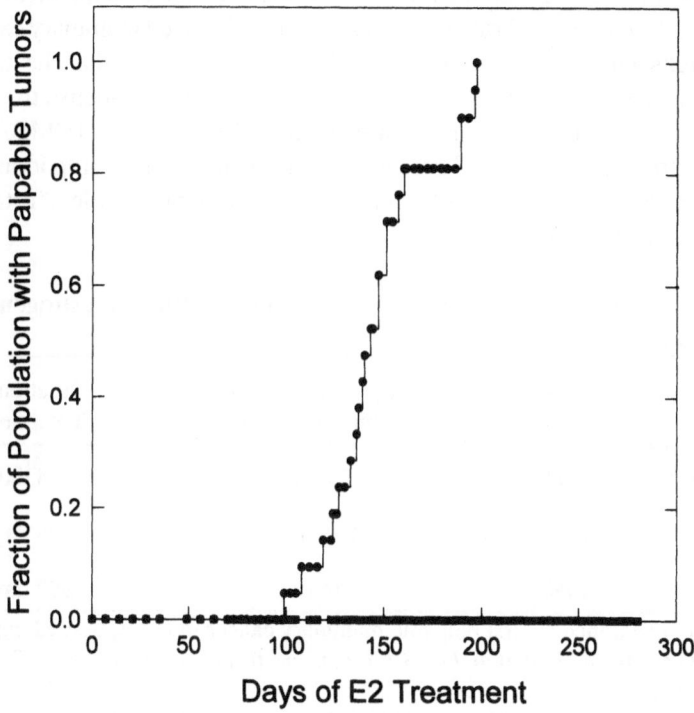

Figure 1. E_2 Rapidly Induces Mammary Cancers in Female ACI Rats. Each data point represents the time after initiation of E_2 treatment at which an animal exhibited its initial palpable mammary tumor. Symbols: filled circle, E_2 treated animals; filled square, untreated control animals. From: Shull, *et al.* (1).

Results

Our laboratory has provided data that chronic treatment with near physiologic levels of E_2 induces rapid development of mammary carcinomas in the female ACI rat (1). Palpable mammary cancers have been observed as early as 70 days following initiation of E_2 treatment (unpublished data); however median latency in several independent experiments approximated 140 days (Figure 1 and unpublished data). In these experiments, virtually 100% of the E_2 treated ACI females developed mammary carcinomas, and most exhibited multiple cancers (1 and unpublished data). In contrast, untreated, but ovary intact, ACI rats did not develop mammary cancers. Rapid development of mammary cancers in response to administered E_2 required the presence of a functional ovary, suggesting that an unidentified ovarian factor contributed to the genesis of these cancers (1). Hyperprolactinemia resulting from the presence of estrogen induced pituitary tumors was demonstrated to be insufficient to explain the unique susceptibility of the ACI rat to development of E_2 induced mammary cancers (1, 2, unpublished data). Studies reviewed by us (1) indicate that the ACI rat is highly resistant to development of mammary cancers in response to treatment with chemical carcinogens such as dimethylbenz[a]anthracene (DMBA) and N-methlynitrosourea (MNU). These data illustrate the potential importance of the ACI rat as a physiologically relevant model for studying the role of estrogens in the etiology of BC in humans.

Table 1. The ACI rat displays a unique susceptibility to estrogen-induced mammary cancers.

Strain	Incidence	Appearance of First Mammary Tumor[1]	Duration of Treatment[2]
ACI	100%	99 days	238 days
COP	20%	223 days	378 days
BN	27%	314 days	392 days

[1]Data of appearance of first palpable mammary cancer in the E_2 treated populations. ACI data are from Shull et al. (1). COP data are from Spady, *et al.* (2). BN data are unpublished.
[2]Experiments in which ACI and COP rats were examined were terminated following indicated periods of E_2 treatment. BN experiment remains in progress.

We are utilizing a genetics based approach to elucidate the molecular mechanisms through which E_2 induces mammary cancer development in the ACI rat. A requisite step in this approach was to identify rat strains that are highly resistant to development of E_2 induced mammary cancers. The COP strain was initially examined for this purpose, because this rat strain has been demonstrated to be highly resistant to mammary cancer development, both spontaneously arising and DMBA or MNU induced (2 and references cited within). Female COP rats displayed a high degree of resistance to development of E_2 induced mammary cancers; in a population of five E_2 treated COP females, a single carcinoma was detected 223 days following initiation of hormone treatment (2). More recently, we have determined that the BN strain is also highly resistant to development of E_2 induced mammary cancers (unpublished data). The relative susceptibilities of the ACI, COP and BN strains to E_2 induced mammary cancers are illustrated in Table 1.

In our genetic studies, we mated female ACI rats to males of either the COP and BN strains and evaluated the relative susceptibilities of the derived F1, F2

(F1 male x F1 female) and BC (F1 male x ACI female) progeny to development of E_2 induced mammary cancers. Populations of F1 ACI/COP and ACI/BN progeny displayed susceptibility to development of E_2 induced mammary cancers, although susceptibility in these F1 populations appeared to be somewhat reduced relative to that observed in the parental ACI strain; although the incidence of E_2 induced mammary cancers in the F1 progeny approached 100%, latency was prolonged. Susceptibility in populations of ACI/COP and ACI/BN BC progeny more closely resembled that of the ACI strain. As expected, populations of ACI/COP and ACI/BN F2 progeny exhibited phenotypes ranging over the extremes defined by the highly susceptible ACI strain and the resistant COP and BN strains. The data from these unpublished studies strongly suggest that susceptibility to E_2 induced mammary cancer development in the ACI/COP and ACI/BN intercross progeny was inherited as a complex genetic trait conferred and/or modulated by two to four genes. The genetic model most consistent with the data from the ACI/COP intercross suggests that the ACI allele of a single gene acts in a dominant manner to confer susceptibility, whereas the actions of this susceptibility gene are modified by dominantly acting COP alleles of one or more additional genes (6). Analysis of linkage to markers on rat chromosome 10, on which the homolog of the human BC susceptibility gene *BRCA1* resides, and rat chromosome 12, on which the homolog of *BRCA2* resides, strongly suggested that these genes do not confer or modulate susceptibility to development of E_2 induced mammary cancers in the ACI/COP intercross (unpublished data). Similarly, analysis of association between susceptibility to development of E_2 induced mammary cancers and inheritance of ACI and COP markers at four loci determined by Gould, *et al.* (7-8) to modulate susceptibility to development of DMBA induced mammary cancers, strongly suggested that the molecular mechanisms through which estrogen induced mammary cancers develop are distinct from those that give rise to development of DMBA induced mammary cancers (unpublished data).

Conclusions

1. The ACI rat exhibits a unique susceptibility to development of E_2 induced mammary cancers, while at the same time displaying resistance to spontaneous development of mammary cancers and development of mammary carcinomas induced by the chemical carcinogens DMBA and MNU.
2. Mammary cancers develop rapidly in female ACI rats in which circulating E2 is chronically maintained near the upper boundary of the physiologic range.
3. Rapid development of E2 induced mammary cancers requires the presence of a functional ovary.

4. Hyperprolactinemia resulting from development of estrogen induced pituitary tumors is insufficient to account for the unique susceptibility of the ACI rat strain to development of estrogen induced mammary cancers.

5. The COP and BN rat strains are resistant to development of E2 induced mammary cancers.

6. Susceptibility to development of E2 induced mammary cancers is inherited in progeny of an ACI/COP intercross as a complex genetic trait.

7. The rat homologs of BRCA1 and BRCA2 do not appear to modulate development of E2 induced mammary cancers in the ACI rat.

8. The genetic etiology of E2 induced mammary cancers appears to be distinct from that underlying development of DMBA induced mammary cancers.

References

1. Shull JD, Spady TJ, Snyder MC et al (1997) Ovary intact, but not ovariectomized female ACI rats treated with 17β-estradiol rapidly develop mammary carcinoma. Carcinogenesis 18:1595-1601.

2. Spady TJ, Harvell DME, Snyder MC et al (1998) Estrogen-induced tumorigenesis in the Copenhagen rat: disparate susceptibilities to development of prolactin-producing pituitary tumors and mammary carcinomas. Cancer Lett 124:95-103.

3. Remmers EF, Du Y, Zha H et al (1995) Ten polymorphic DNA loci, including five in the rat MYC (RT1) region, form a single linkage group on rat chromosome 20. Immunogenetics 41:316-319.

4. Jacob HJ, Brown DM, Bunker RK et al (1995) A genetic linkage map of the laboratory rat, Rattus norvegicus. Nature Genetics 9:63-69.

5. Lander ES, Botstein D (1989) Mapping Mendelian factors underlying quantitative traits using RFLP linkage maps. Genetics 121:185-199.

6. Shull JD, Snyder MC, Spady TJ et al (1997) A single, dominantly acting, gene confers susceptibility to estrogen induced mammary carcinoma in a genetic cross between ACI and Copenhagen rats. Breast Cancer Research and Treatment 46:111.

7. Hsu L-C, Kennan WS, Shepel LA et al (1994) Genetic identification of Mcs-1, a rat mammary carcinoma suppressor gene. Cancer Research 54:2765-2770.

8. Shepel LA, Lan H, Haag JD et al (1998) Genetic identification of multiple loci that control breast cancer susceptibility in the rat. Genetics 149:289-299.

Characteristics of Dehydroepiandrosterone-induced Hepatocarcinogenesis in the Rat

Doris Mayer, Christel Metzger, Dirk Nehrbass, and Peter Bannasch

Summary

Dehydroepiandrosterone (DHEA) induces and enhances hepatocarcinogenesis in the rat, the tumor incidence being higher in females than in males. Preneoplastic and neoplastic lesions induced by DHEA belong to the amphophilic cell lineage of hepatocarcinogenesis. Moreover, DHEA modulates preneoplastic liver foci of the glycogenotic/basophilic cell lineage induced by the hepatocarcinogen N-nitrosomorpholine (NNM) to amphophilic cell foci (APF). This process is associated with profound changes in the expression of key enzymes of energy metabolism and a down-regulation of the expression of insulin receptor substrate-1, a signaling molecule activated by tyrosine kinase receptors, which is over-expressed in glycogenotic lesions. This suggests a cross-talk of the steroid-mediated signaling pathway with tyrosine kinase receptor-activated signal transduction pathways during enhancement of hepatocarcinogenesis by DHEA.

Introduction

DHEA is the main adrenal steroid in primates including humans and a precursor in the biosynthesis of estrogens and androgens. In the rat, DHEA acts as a peroxisome proliferator and liver carcinogen when given at high doses (1, 2). The hepatocarcinogenic effect of DHEA has been attributed to its properties as a peroxisome proliferator (1). However, peroxisome proliferation occurs mainly in the perivenular hepatocytes, whereas hepatocellular neoplasms develop in the periportal areas of the liver lobules, distant from the zone of peroxisome proliferation. Furthermore, hepatocellular carcinomas (HCC) were also induced by DHEA in rainbow trout, a species which is insensitive to peroxisome proliferation (3). These findings permitted the conclusion that peroxisome proliferation is not the major cause for DHEA-induced hepatocarcinogenesis (2).

Two main hepatocellular lineages have been distinguished during hepatocarcinogenesis in the rat, the glycogenotic/basophilic and the amphophilic cell lineage (4). These lineages show characteristic sequential changes in the morphological and biochemical phenotype of the hepatocytes, indicating fundamental aberrations in gene expression and cellular metabolism during neoplastic cell conversion (5, 6). The glycogenotic/basophilic cell lineage starts with small focal preneoplastic lesions storing excessive amounts of glycogen, which develop via mixed cell foci into basophilic neoplasms. Typically, this lineage occurs in livers of rats treated with various oncogenic agents including nitrosamines (4, 5). In the amphophilic lineage hepatocellular neoplasms develop from small glycogen-poor preneoplastic lesions designated as APF (2). APF are induced by peroxisome proliferators including DHEA. More recently, we observed that DHEA modulates hepatocarcinogenesis induced by NNM from the glycogenotic/basophilic to the amphophilic lineage (5, 7). This process is associated with a profound change in the expression of key enzymes of energy metabolism (6) and of insulin receptor substrate-1 (IRS-1) (8, 9), a central protein in the tyrosine receptor kinase signaling pathway. We present recent results on neoplastic development and changes in gene expression induced by DHEA.

Materials and Methods

Preneoplastic and neoplastic liver lesions were induced in male and female Sprague-Dawley strain rats with DHEA (0.6% in the diet) given for up to 84 weeks, or with NNM (120 mg/liter drinking water, 7 weeks) given either alone or followed by DHEA (6, 7). Liver slices were fixed in Carnoy's fixative and embedded in Paraplast, or snap-frozen at −150°C in isopentane pre-cooled with liquid nitrogen. Liver sections stained with H&E or treated with the periodic acid Schiff-reaction were used for identification of the preneoplastic liver foci [glycogen storage foci, GSF; mixed cell foci, MCF; amphophilic cell foci, APF; basophilic cell foci, BCF; (Bannasch, 1996)] and the neoplasms (hepatocellular adenomas, HCA; hepatocellular carcinomas, HCC). The methods for histochemical demonstration and evaluation of enzyme activities and for immunohistochemistry of IRS-1 have been described in detail recently (6, 9).

Results

Incidence of Liver Neoplasms Induced by DHEA- and NNM/DHEA-treatment in Male and Female Rats

The incidence of liver neoplasms in male and female rats treated with DHEA and/or NNM is summarized in Table 1. While the tumor incidence was similar in both sexes treated with NNM alone, it was significantly higher in females than in males when DHEA was given either alone or in combination with NNM. In both males and females, NNM/DHEA-treatment resulted in a higher tumor incidence as compared to NNM-treatment alone, which clearly points to a tumor enhancing effect of DHEA. The higher incidence of neoplasms observed in females was mainly due to an increase in HCC. These findings indicate a higher sensitivity of female rats as compared to males towards the hepatocarcinogenic and tumor enhancing effect of DHEA.

Table 1. Incidence of hepatic adenomas and carcinomas in male and female rats treated with DHEA, NNM, or NNM/DHEA. Percentage of tumor-bearing rats is given in brackets.

Treatment [a]	Female rats		Male rats	
	HCA	HCC	HCA	HCC
DHEA [b]	3/9 (33%) [c]	4/9 (44%) [c]	0/9 (0%)	1/9 (11%)
NNM	10/30 (33%)	8/30 (27%)	10/30 (33%)	9/30 (30%)
NNM/ DHEA	12/30 (40%)	14/30 (47%) [c, d]	13/30 (43%) [d]	11/30 (37%)

[a] Rats were treated with NNM followed either by standard diet or by diet containing DHEA. Groups of rats were killed immediately after stoppage of NNM-treatment and at 4, 20, 32, 70 and 84 weeks of DHEA-treatment. In DHEA-treated rats tumors occurred only after 70-84 weeks, in NNM and NNM/DHEA-treated rats tumors were observed between 4 and 32 weeks after stop of NNM-treatment. [b] Only rats killed after 70-84 weeks of DHEA-treatment are included in this line. [c] Significantly different from males, [d] and from NMM, $P \leq 0.05$.

Modulation of Enzyme Expression in Preneoplastic and Neoplastic Liver Lesions by DHEA

Morphometric measurements showed that DHEA-treatment not only results in the induction of APF and amphophilic neoplasms, but also modulates GSF and MCF induced by NNM into APF (7). This modulation is accompanied by a significant decrease in the glycogen content and by changes in the activity and expression of key enzymes of energy metabolism. These changes are summarized in Table 2. The activity of mitochondrial enzymes (COX, G3PDH, SDH) is increased in APF reflecting the strong proliferation of these organelles (2). Similarly, increased peroxisomal hydratase and AOX activities are in accordance with the increase in the number of peroxisomes observed in these by electron microscopy (2). G6Pase activity which is reduced in GSF, is increased in APF, whereas G6PDH and ME which are very high in GSF, are down-regulated in APF. The pattern of enzyme activities observed in HCA and HCC developing in NNM/DHEA-treated liver is similar to that in APF. The enzyme patterns in GSF and APF are in many respects opposite. They reflect different metabolic states which have been described as energy-preserving or insulinomimetic in the case of GSF, and as energy-wasting or thyromimetic in the case of APF (5, 6). Figure 1 shows the biplot (10) of the enzyme pattern of GSF and APF. It is evident that GSF and APF represent two populations with different enzyme patterns.

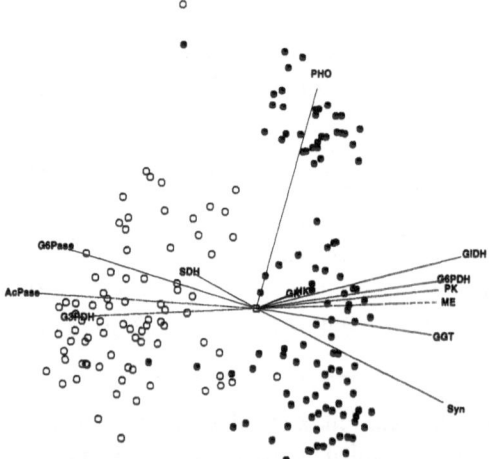

Figure 1. Biplot analysis of enzyme alterations in GSF (●) and APF (○). Each symbol represents an individual focus. The lines from the origin show the positive direction of the changes of enzyme activities, and their length explains the importance of the enzymes for the distinction of the two types of lesions (from 6).

Modulation of IRS-1 Expression in Preneoplastic Liver Foci by DHEA

IRS-1, a central docking protein in the tyrosine kinase receptor signaling pathway, is over-expressed in GSF (Figure 2), which agrees with the insulinomimetic metabolic state in these lesions (9). IRS-1 is also increased in GSF within MCF and HCA, indicating a correlation of IRS-1 over-expression with this specific metabolic state. IRS-1 is not detectable in APF (8). Since DHEA-treatment modulates GSF into APF it can be concluded that IRS-1 expression is down-regulated by DHEA. APF clearly represent a more advanced stage in hepatocarcinogenesis than GSF. Since IRS-1 is also down-regulated within the glycogenotic/basophilic cell lineage in BCF representing late stages of hepatocarcinogenesis and in basophilic tumors, it is assumed that down-regulation of IRS-1 is related to tumor progression.

Table 2. Enzyme alterations of GSF, APF, BCF and HCA and HCC compared to normal liver tissue* (from 6).

Parameter	Type of lesion									
	GSF		APF		BCF		HCA+MC, amphophilic		HCC	
	n=155	%	n=84	%	n=24	%	n=42	%	n=8	%
Glycogen	●●●	100	OOO	100	OOO	100	OOO	93	OOO	88
Basophilia	O	60	●●●	100	●●●	100	●●●	100	●●●	100
SYN	(●)	49	OO	75	OOO	100	OO	72	OOO	100
PHO	O	58	OO	78	OOO	100	OOO	85	OO	80
HK	n.c.	76	n.c.	90	n.c.	100	n.c.	70	●	57
PK	(●)	43	OO	74	●●	78	OO	64	OO	75
G6PDH	●●●	96	n.c.	64	●●●	86	●	66	●●●	100
ME	●●●	94	n.c.	64	●	50	●	53	●●●	88
G6Pase	OO	76	●	60	OOO	89	●	55	●	63
COX	n.c.	77	●●	75	●	58	●●	78	●●●	86
G3PDH	n.c.	64	●●	79	(●)	44	●●●	98	●●	71
SDH	n.c.	65	(●)	43	O	57	●	65	●	63
GlDH	●●	70	O	64	(●)	43	OO	77	O	50
AcPase	O	67	●●	76	●	63	OO	77	●	63
GGT	●●●	90	n.c.	91	●●●	80	n.c.	100	n.c.	57
PH	OOO	90	●●	75	n.d.		O	50	O/●	50/50
Catalase	OOO	100	n.c.	50	n.d.		n.c.	83	n.c.	100
AOX	OOO	90	●	70	n.d.		O	50	●●	75

* The table shows the prevailing groups of the respective lesions which have either increased, decreased or unchanged activity, and the percentage of lesions which show the respective activity changes. ●●●, increase in >80%; ●●, increase in 70-80%; ●, increase in 50-70%; (●), increase in <50% of the lesions. OOO, decrease in >80%; OO, decrease in 70-80%; O, decrease in 50-70% of the lesions; n.c., no change; n.d., not determined.

Abbreviations: MC, microcarcinomas; SYN, glycogen synthase; PHO, glycogen phosphorylase; G6Pase, glucose-6-phosphatase; HK, hexokinase; GK, glucokinase; PK, pyruvate kinase; G6PDH, glucose-6-phosphate dehydrogenase; COX, cytochrome c oxidase; G3PDH, glycerol-3-phosphate dehydrogenase; SDH, succinate dehydrogenase; ME, malic enzyme; GlDH, glutamate dehydrogenase; AcPase, acid phosphatase; GGT, γ-glutamyltranspeptidase; PH, peroxisomal hydratase, AOX, acyl-CoA oxidase.

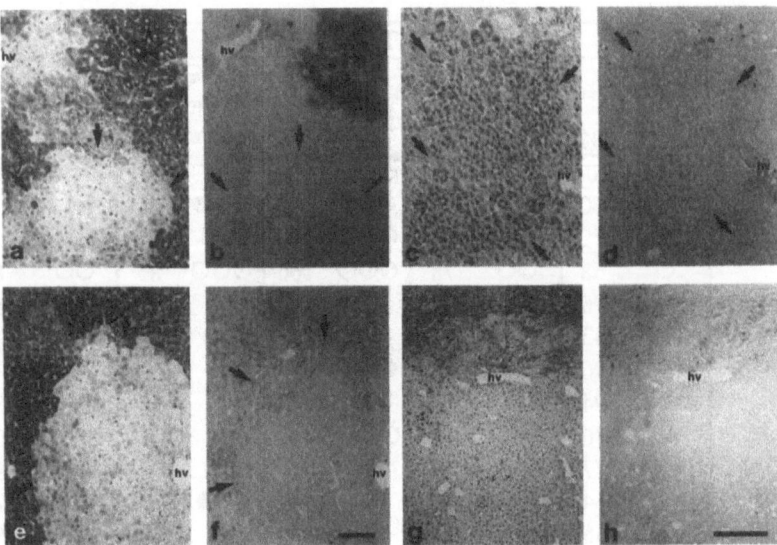

Figure 2. Correlation of glycogen content (PAS-reaction) (a, c, e, g) with the expression of IRS-1 demonstrated by immunostaining (b, d, f, h) in preneoplastic lesions and a HCC induced in rat liver with NNM followed by DHEA. a and b, c and d, e and f, g and h are serial sections, respectively.

Preneoplastic GSF (asterisks in a and b) showing a strong overexpression of IRS-1 in contrast to the negative reaction in the surrounding tissue; APF (a, b, e, f, demarcated by arrows), and IRS-1-negative intermediate cell foci (c, d) composed of cells showing both a slightly increased glycogen content and an increased basophilia as compared to the surrounding parenchyma. An amphophilic HCC containing single glycogenotic cells (g, h) also shows a negative or only very weak IRS-1 immunoreaction. Bar in f, 100 µm (same magnification in a - f); bar in h, 1 mm; hv, hepatic venule.

Conclusions

DHEA induces and enhances hepatocarcinogenesis in the rat. DHEA-treatment results in a modulation of NNM-induced hepatocarcinogenesis from the glycogenotic/basophilic to the amphophilic phenotype. This switch is accompanied by profound alterations in the expression of key enzymes of energy metabolism and a down-regulation of IRS-1 in preneoplastic and neoplastic lesions. This points to a cross-talk between steroid receptor-mediated signaling pathways and tyrosine kinase receptor-mediated signaling pathways which seems to result in enhanced tumor progression.

References

1. Rao MS, Subbarao V, Yeldandi AV et al (1992) Hepatocarcinogenicity of dehydroepiandrosterone in the rat. Cancer Res 52:2977-2979.
2. Metzger C, Mayer D, Hoffmann H et al (1995) Sequential appearance and ultrastructure of amphophilic cell foci, adenomas, and carcinomas in the liver of male and female rats treated with dehydroepiandrosterone. Toxicol Pathol 23:591-605.
3. Orner GA, Mathews C, Hendricks JD et al (1995) Dehydroepiandrosterone is a complete hepatocarcinogen and potent tumor promoter in the absence of peroxisome proliferation in rainbow trout. Carcinogenesis 16:2893-2898.
4. Bannasch P (1996) Pathogenesis of hepatocellular carcinoma: Sequential cellular, molecular, and metabolic changes. Prog Liver Dis 14:161-197.
5. Bannasch P, Klimek F, Mayer D (1997) Early bioenergetic changes in hepatocarcinogenesis: preneoplastic phenotypes mimic responses to insulin and thyroid hormone. J Bioenerg Biomembr 29:303-313.
6. Mayer D, Metzger C, Leonetti P et al (1998) Differential expression of key enzymes of energy metabolism in preneoplastic and neoplastic rat liver lesions induced by N-nitrosomorpholine and dehydroepiandrosterone. Int J Cancer (Pred Oncol) 79:232-240.
7. Metzger C, Bannasch P, Mayer D (1997) Enhancement and phenotypic modulation of N-nitrosomorpholine-induced hepatocarcinogenesis by dehydroepiandrosterone. Cancer Lett 121:125-131.
8. Nehrbaß D, Klimek F, Mayer D et al (1998) Differential expression of insulin receptor substrate-1 in various types of preneoplastic hepatic foci. Proc Amer Assoc Cancer Res 39:485.
9. Nehrbaß D, Klimek F, Bannasch P (1998) Overexpression of insulin receptor substrate-1 emerges early in hepatocarcinogenesis and elicits preneoplastic hepatic glycogenosis. Am J Pathol 152:341-345.
10. Gabriel KR, Odoroff CL (1990) Biplots in biomedical research. Statistics in Medicine 9:469-485.

Hepatic Toxicity of Estrogen in Armenian and Chinese Hamsters

John E. Coe, Kamal G. Ishak, and M.J. Ross

Summary

High serum levels of estrogen result in clinically detectable hyperbilirubinemia in two closely related Cricetulus hamsters, the Armenian hamster (*Cricetulus migratorius*) and the Chinese hamster (*Cricetulus griseus*). In previous studies, hepatic tumors developed in most Armenian hamsters after chronic estrogen treatment, but in the present study, we found that the livers of Chinese hamsters were remarkably free of neoplastic change under similar conditions. Also, when compared with the responses in the Armenian hamsters, signs of hepatic destruction and regeneration were less prevalent in estrogen-treated Chinese hamsters and the bilirubin levels were lower and of shorter duration. In contrast to the findings in Armenian hamsters, bile canaliculi were severely affected in livers of estrogen-treated Chinese hamsters, and hepatic microvesicular steatosis, indicative of an unusual lipodystrophy caused by estrogen, was prominent. An additional lesion peculiar to the Chinese hamster was a striking sinusoidal dilatation. Although these two hamster species are genetically similar, the genes activated by estrogen receptor show remarkable heterogeneity when their respective livers are examined. Comparisons within these species may provide information about specific gene activation responsible for particular pathologic events.

Introduction

Estrogens (Es) are remarkably toxic to the liver of the Armenian hamster (*Cricetulus migratorius*). A few days after estrogen administration, they become profoundly icteric, and their livers show histologic evidence of degenerative and regenerative change (1). With chronic E treatment, neoplastic changes occur so that adenomas and hepatocellular carcinomas are detected in livers of virtually all treated animals (2, 3). A wide variety of Es, natural (17β-estradiol, Zeranol) and synthetic (ethinyl estradiol, diethylstilbestrol), are effective, and the acute and chronic effects can be inhibited by the concomitant administration of Tamoxifen (TAM) (3,4), suggesting that the hepatic effects are mediated by estrogen receptor (ER).

The mechanism by which E produces these unusual effects in the liver of the Armenian hamster is unclear. In this report we studied the effect of E when administered to another *Cricetulus* hamster, the Chinese hamster (*Cricetulus griseus*), a very close relative of the Armenian hamster.

Materials and Methods

Hamsters were injected with various Es, such as diethylstilbestrol (DES) and Resorcylic acid lactone (RAL), and the acute and chronic effects on liver were monitored by measuring changes in serum constituents and by observing changes in hepatic structure as seen grossly and by light and electron microscopy (5).

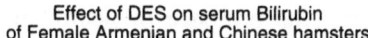

Effect of DES on serum Bilirubin
of Female Armenian and Chinese hamsters

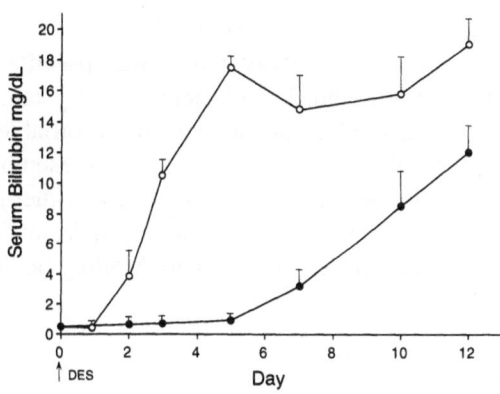

Figure 1. Effect of 15 mg DES pellet (implanted day 0) on serum bilirubin in female Armenian (n=5) (--O--) and Chinese (n=5) (--●--) hamsters.

Results

The kinetics of E-induced hyperbilirubinemia is different in the Armenian and the Chinese hamster (Figure 1). All Armenian hamsters became icteric within 48 hrs of treatment, whereas 7 days were required before the onset of icterus in the Chinese hamsters, even when a massive dose of E was given. Also, the serum levels of bilirubin were greater and tended to last longer in the Armenian hamster than in the Chinese hamster. Chinese hamsters were also given RAL (pellets with 36 mg of Zeranol), an E dose that produces consistent hyperbilirubinemia in Armenian hamsters (3), and only about 25% of Chinese hamsters developed detectable serum icterus (serum bilirubin greater than 2 mg%).

Effects of Long-term Estrogen Treatment

Chronic exposure to exogenous Es is associated with the occurrence of hepatic tumors in virtually all Armenian hamsters (3). This hepatic carcinogenesis did not occur in Chinese hamsters. Over 50 Chinese hamsters treated from 4 to 12 mo. with DES or RAL were examined and only one hepatic tumor was found.

When the livers of Chinese hamsters treated with DES for 12 mo. were examined microscopically, we found three E-induced pathologic changes that were not common to the Armenian hamster.

All livers showed patchy (non-zonal) enlargement of liver cells with microvesicular steatosis; the presence of neutral lipid in the vacuoles was confirmed in frozen sections stained with oil red-O. Moderate to marked sinusoidal dilatation was observed in all the livers with the formation of pelioid cavities and subendothelial prolapse of liver cells.

In all livers, canaliculi were variably dilated with pseudogland formation and many canaliculi were surrounded by clusters of foamy xanthomatous cells. When examined ultrastructurally, canaliculi showed variable dilatation and swelling and shedding of microvilli. No dense pigment resembling human bile was seen in canaliculi or in the cytoplasm of liver cells. Other general changes affecting liver cells included moderate to marked anisonucleosis, scattered apoptotic bodies, occasional clusters of cells with Mallory bodies and scattered mitotic figures.

Conclusions

The Armenian hamster and the Chinese hamster share not only the same chromosome number (2n=22), but also a variety of anatomical features and their serum proteins show many common antigens (unpublished). We are not aware of a successful hybrid derived from these two Cricetulus species.

E is known to alter hepatocyte physiology and impair hepatobiliary function although an E-induced dysfunction severe enough to cause hyperbilirubinemia is unusual, except in these two genetically susceptible hamsters and in certain genetically susceptible women (6, 7) who develop cholestatic jaundice of pregnancy or have an idiosyncratic reaction to estrogenic compounds. The pathophysiology responsible for the jaundice may be different in the human and the hamster. For that matter, there are marked differences in pathophysiology between the two hamster species (Table I), suggesting different mechanisms responsible for the jaundice induced by E. In both, the ER is the presumed mediator because a variety of Es with different structures can be used and their effect is blocked by concomitant injections of TAM. The Chinese hamster is definitely more resistant because even with massive doses of a potent E, like DES, clinical icterus requires weeks to appear in the Chinese hamster versus days in the Armenian hamster. Even so, the complete absence of any evidence of tumor formation in the Chinese hamster after one year of treatment with DES was unexpected, because neoplastic change was detected in the Armenian hamster after only 60 days of exposure to E (2). Also, Zeranol, a weak E, was a very effective carcinogen in the Armenian hamster liver (3). It is of interest that Mallory bodies appeared early and were abundant in livers of E treated Armenian hamsters (1, 3), whereas they were rare in similarly treated Chinese hamsters. Hepatic destruction with attendant regeneration (mitotic figures) appears more prevalent in E-treated Armenian hamsters than in similarly treated Chinese hamsters and this hepatic regeneration may be a critical feature necessary for hepatic transformation in the Armenian hamster.

In contrast to the Armenian hamster, the major hepatic pathology in the Chinese hamster was centered on canalicular damage, an alteration of fat metabolism, and striking sinusoidal dilatation. Other than the absence of bile accumulation, canalicular changes are not unlike those seen in human cholestasis of intra- or extrahepatic causation. E has a dramatic effect on fat metabolism in the Chinese hamster (hyperlipidemia) (unpublished) and we believe this effect readily explains the hepatic steatosis and accumulation of cholesterol noted in these animals microscopically. The dramatic sinusoidal dilatation in the Chinese hamster lacks the zonality but otherwise is similar to the sinusoidal dilatation reported in women on long-term oral contraceptives (8, 9).

The ER has been highly conserved during evolution and functions at the molecular level as a regulator of gene transcription. After E activation, conformational changes in its structure permit it to bind to E response elements and modulate expression of E responsive genes. The effect of ER on transcription is quite different in liver of these two closely related hamsters. They demonstrate an array of E-induced pathophysiologic changes, including a common hepatobiliary dysfunction, a remarkable hepatocarcinogenesis specific for the Armenian hamster, and extensive lipodystrophy-canalicular aberration and sinusoidal lesions peculiar to the Chinese hamster. Comparative studies in these two species of hamster may reveal the gene activation responsible for these particular events.

Table 1. Effect of E on the livers of two species of hamster.

	Armenian	Chinese
All estrogens, DES, EE, Zeranol	+++	+
Inhibition by Tamoxifen	+++	+++
Susceptibility	+++	+
Rapidity	+++	+
Hepatocyte Transformation	+++	0
Lipid Changes	+	+++
Histologic Changes:		
Mitotic Figures	+++	+
Mallory Bodies	+++	+
Canalicular Changes	+	+++
Sinusoidal Dilatation	+	+++
Microvesicular Steatosis	0	+++
Neoplastic Change	+++	0

Abbreviations: 0=absent; += mild or minimal; ++= Moderate; +++= Marked

References

1. Coe JE, Ishak KG, Ross MJ (1983) Diethylstilbestrol-induced jaundice in the Chinese and Armenian hamster. Hepatology 3:489-496.
2. Coe JE, Ishak KG, Ross MJ (1990) Estrogen induction of hepatocellular carcinomas in Armenian hamsters. Hepatology 11:570-577.
3. Coe JE, Ishak KG, Ward JM et al (1992) Tamoxifen prevents induction of hepatic neoplasia by Zeranol, an estrogenic food contaminant. Proc Natl Acad Sci USA 89:1085-1089.
4. Coe JE, Ross MJ (1988) Tamoxifen inhibits estrogen-induced hepatic injury in hamsters. Endocrinology 122:137-144.
5. Coe JE, Ishak KG, Ross MJ (1998) Estrogen-induced hepatic toxicity and hepatic cancer: Differences between two closely related hamster species. Liver 18:343-351.
6. Dalen E, Westerholm B (1974) Occurrence of hepatic impairment in women jaundiced by oral contraceptives and in their mothers and sisters. Acta Med Scand 195:459-463.
7. Sherlock S (1966) Biliary secretory failure in man: the problem of cholestasis. Ann Intern Med 65:397-408.
8. Winkler K, Poulsen H (1975) Liver disease with periportal sinusoidal dilatation. A possible complication to contraceptive steroids. Scand J Gastroenterol 10:699-704.
9. Heresbach D, Deugnier Y, Brissot P et al (1988) Dilatations sinusoidales et prise de contraceptifs oraux. A propos d'un cas avec revue de la litterature. Ann Gastroenterol Hepatol 24:189-191.

Suppression of Liver Tumor Formation by the Liver Microenvironment of Female, but Not Male, Syngeneic Hosts

Gary J. Smith, Sharon C. Presnell, William B. Coleman, and Joe W. Grisham

Summary

Chemical-induced liver cancer in animal models, and primary human liver cancers are mainly male diseases. Sex-related differences in metabolism/detoxification of carcinogenic agents and cultural practices may contribute to the striking sensitivity of males to hepatocellular carcinoma development. No physiological mechanisms have been identified to explain the relative insensitivity of females to liver carcinogenesis. We compared the capacity of the male versus female liver tissue microenvironment to support/suppress tumorigenicity of orthotopically transplanted tumor liver cells. GN6TF rat liver epithelial cells, that are 100% tumorigenic at ectopic sites, were transplanted into the liver microenvironment of male and female syngeneic hosts that were fed ad libitum or were maintained on a caloric restricted diet. The liver microenvironment of young adult (3-9 mo.) ad lib-fed male rats suppressed tumor formation completely. Transplanted cells migrated into liver plates where they underwent hepatocytic differentiation. Transplantation of GN6TF cells into the livers of old male hosts (18-24 mo.) resulted in the formation of tumors within 90 days (66-100% of hosts, respectively). Transplantation of GN6TF cells into the livers of old male, caloric restricted animals were followed by rapid formation of tumors (latency = 40 days). In contrast, transplantation of GN6TF cells into female rats resulted in suppression of the tumorigenic phenotype in 85% of old and 100% of young female rats. These data suggest that hormonal-directed epigenetic suppression of tumorigenicity contributes to the sex-specific sensitivity to liver carcinogenesis.

Introduction

The liver is a target tissue for sex hormones; normal hepatocytes express appreciable levels of androgen receptor (AR) and estrogen receptor (ER). Hepatic AR levels decrease significantly after partial hepatectomy or after chronic exposure to ethanol, and increased expression of AR has been associated with several liver diseases, including aplastic anemia and hepatocellular carcinoma (HCC). Epidemiological data demonstrate that HCC is predominantly a disease of males, with an incidence in females only a fraction (as small as 11%) of the incidence in males (1). Chronic dietary exposure of rats to N-2-fluorenyldiacetamide (2-FdiAA) leads to the development of cirrhosis, hyperplasia, and HCC in males, while the response in females was limited to the development of hyperplastic nodules that did not progress to tumors (2). Suppression of 2-FdiAA-induced tumor genesis was observed when males were castrated and/or treated with diethylstilbestrol (DES), and female rats developed tumors upon removal of the ovaries. Moreover, transplantation of hyperplastic nodules from 2-FdiAA-treated females into syngeneic males resulted in growth and progression of the nodule into HCC, which suggested that lower tumor incidence in females was due to suppressive effects of the female microenvironment and/or permissive effects of the male microenvironment. Another chemical hepatocarcinogenesis model demonstrated that all intact males and no intact females developed HCC after a single dose of diethylnitrosamine (DEN), a potent hepatocarcinogen (3). Gonadectomized mice after DEN treatment caused the incidence of HCC to fall in males (100% to 18%) and rise in females (0% to 40%). Similar patterns of sexual dimorphism were observed for the sensitivity to spontaneous HCC in mice. These data support the hypothesis that the observed difference in incidence of HCC among males and females is due both to the growth-promoting effects of an androgen environment and the growth-suppressive effects of an estrogen environment. However, the target cell for the effect of androgen is not clear. Studies of DEN-induced hepatocarcinogenesis in female livers mosaic for *Tfm* (testicular feminization) demonstrated that while functional AR must be present in the liver to observe the development of HCC, the target cell for transformation does not require expression of AR (4). Furthermore, the lower incidence of HCC in females may be due in part to suppressive effects of the female microenvironment on initiated cells, rather than a decrease in the actual number of initiated cells in females vs. males. This hypothesis is supported by the observation that while AR usually is expressed in HCC at levels greatly elevated relative to the surrounding normal liver, the expression of ER frequently is lost (5, 6). Consequently, the role of the tissue microenvironment surrounding a cell with a potentially tumorigenic genotype may be able to determine epigenetically the ultimate expression of the tumorigenic phenotype.

In the present study, we sought to determine whether the liver microenvironment of young and/or old females was capable of suppressing the tumorigenic phenotype of a liver tumor cell line. BAG2-GN6TF cells are aggressively tumorigenic when transplanted ectopically, are equally tumorigenic in prepubertal males and females, and are suppressed for tumorigenicity in the liver of young adult males, but form hepatic tumors in 100% of aged animals (7, 8). In addition, we evaluated intrahepatic tumorigenic potential of BAG2-GN6TF in aged calorie-restricted male and female hosts. Calorie-restriction is a unique model that has been shown to extend life span as well as to prolong the androgen responsiveness of the liver of males.

Methods

Animals. Age-controlled male and female Fischer-344 rats were obtained from the Aged Rat Colony of the National Institute of Aging (Harlan Sprague-Dawley, Indianapolis IN) and aged caloric restricted Fischeer 344 rats were obtained from the National Center for Toxicologic Research (Jefferson, Arkansas). Rats were fed either ad libitum or with a 40% calorie-reduced diet (NIH 31 Chow, vitamin supplemented) from 16 weeks of age. Average consumption of chow among ad-lib rats at the time of experimentation (18 mo.-old rats) was 19 g/day for males and 15 g/day for females. Age-matched caloric restricted rats received 11.5g/day (males) and 9 g/day (females).

Cell Line and Transplantation. The GN6TF cell line was established from a tumor that arose following subcutaneous transplantation of a chemically transformed cell line (GN6) derived from WB-F344 rat liver epithelial stem-like cells. For the purpose of identification of transplanted cells, the GN6TF cells were infected with a replication-defective retrovirus carrying a β-galactosidase reporter gene (LacZ) and the neomycin resistance gene, and the resulting cell line was designated BAG2-GN6TF (7, 8). Cells were prepared for transplantation by brief trypsinization, followed by enumeration with a hemacytometer. Aliquots of 5×10^6 cells were pelleted at 1000 RPM and washed twice in Thilly's buffer, followed by resuspension in 250µl of Thilly's buffer. Rats were placed under light ether anesthesia, a midline incision was made, and cells were injected into the left liver lobe via syringe fitted with a 27G needle. Rats were monitored daily for signs of tumor formation. Rats that developed tumors were euthanized, and liver tissue removed and processed for histological evaluation.

β-Galactosidase Histochemistry. At necropsy, liver tissue was examined for the presence of tumor nodules. Liver tissue from each rat was used for preparation of frozen sections (7μ). Liver cryosections were fixed in an ice-cold solution of 1.0% glutaraldehyde containing 100 mM $NaPO_4$ (pH 7.0) and 1.0 mM $MgCl_2$ for 15 minutes and rinsed in a buffer containing 100 mM $NaPO_4$ (pH 7.0), 100 mM NaCl, and 5.0 mM $MgCl_2$. Fixed sections were incubated at 37°C in a buffer composed of 0.2 mg/ml 5-bromo-4-chloro-3-indoyl-β-D-galactopyranoside (X-gal substrate), 100 mM $NaPO_4$ (pH 7.0), 150 mM NaCl, 1.0 mM $MgCl_2$, 3.3 mM $K_4Fe(CN)_6 \cdot 3H_2O$, and 3.3 mM $K_3Fe(CN)_6$. Sections were counterstained with Mayer's hematoxylin.

Results

Part 1:

Intrahepatic Tumorigenicity, Male vs. Female. BAG2-GN6TF cells were aggressively tumorigenic when introduced into the livers of old (18-24 mo.) syngeneic male hosts, forming tumors in 13/16 rats within 3 mo. (Table 1). In contrast, the tumorigenic phenotype was suppressed in the livers of all (16/16) young male rats examined, indicating that the hepatic microenvironment of young rats is able to inhibit tumor formation. In contrast, young adult female rats that received hepatic injections of BAG2-GN6TF cells did not develop liver tumors (0/5). Intrahepatic transplantation of BAG2-GN6TF cells into old female rats also failed to produce liver tumors (0/5), suggesting that the female liver is able to suppress, or at least delay, expression of the tumorigenic phenotype.

Table 1. Intrahepatic tumorigenicity: Male vs. female, young vs. old

	Male	Female
Young (3-9 mo.)	0/16	0/5
Old (18-24 mo.)	13/16	0/5

5×10^6 BAG2-GN6TF cells injected directly into the liver.
Duration of experiment = 3 mo.

Part 2:

Intrahepatic Tumorigenicity and Caloric Restriction. BAG2-GN6TF cells were injected intrahepatically into male and female aged rats (18-mo.) that were maintained on a 40%-reduced calorie diet. Age-matched animals fed ad-libitum were included as controls. The aged male rats developed liver tumors in 13/14 cases, regardless of their diet (Table 2). Calorie-restricted male rats displayed a significantly shorter average latency (40 days) than age-matched ad-lib male rats (58 days). During 3 mo. after transplantation, a time interval during which 93% of the male animals had developed liver tumors, only 2/10 ad-lib fed females and 3/14 calorie-restricted females developed detectable liver tumors. Microscopic examination of tumor cryosections revealed widely distributed β-galactosidase (+) BAG2-GN6TF hepatocyte-like cells and small foci of phenotypically aberrant β-galactosidase (+) BAG2-GN6TF cells were present in the female livers. These foci disrupted the architecture of the liver but had not progressed into macroscopic tumors within the 3-mo. incubation period.

Table 2. Intrahepatic tumorigenicity: Male vs. female & ad-lib vs. calorie-restricted

Treatment Group	Tumor Incidence	Average Latency (days)
Male (Ad Lib)	13/14	58
Male (Calorie-Restricted)	13/14	40
Female (Ad Lib)	2/10	40
Female (Calorie-Restricted)	3/14	19

18 mo.-old rats, injected with 5 x 10^6 BAG2-GN6TF cells, directly into the liver.

Discussion

The mechanism(s) responsible for the male predominance for development of HCC are unresolved. Androgen, through the androgen receptor (AR), has been demonstrated to have strong promotional effects for HCC in both males and females (1,9). Consistent with this role for androgens, hormonal ablation in males with HCC slows tumor growth in a subset of patients (5, 10, 11). In contrast, estrogens acting alone or through the ER appear to have an anti-carcinogenic effect in the liver (12-14). Consistent with the hypothesis that androgens and estrogens have opposing effects in the liver is the observation that AR is often over expressed and expression of ER is often lost in HCC (5, 6). However, the target of the steroid hormone is not clear. Kemp, *et al.* (4) demonstrated in the *Tfm* mouse that presence of AR in the tissue microenvironment, but not the target cell, is sufficient to allow development of chemically induced HCC. This observation suggested that the role of androgen is promotional and is mediated through the liver micro-environment. BAG2-GN6TF cells were introduced into the liver microenvironment of young and old male and female syngeneic rats. Despite aggressive tumor formation at extrahepatic sites in all test groups, the tumorigenic potential of BAG2-GN6TF cells in the liver was suppressed in young rats of both sexes and in old (> 18 mo.) female rats, while tumors formed readily in aged male hosts. Development of microscopic tumor foci in aged females supports the hypothesis that the rate of tumor progression, rather than the frequency of transformation, is influenced by the female microenvironment. Therefore, our experimental data support the hypothesis that differences in HCC incidence in males and females are not due to variations in the number of initiated cells, but are due rather to the slower rate of progression of initiated cells into tumors in the female liver microenvironment.

Caloric restriction has been demonstrated to increase life expectancy and reduce tumor incidence in both normal and genetically compromised animals. However, in this study caloric restricted aged male rats developed tumors at the same frequency, but with a shorter latency, than their ad-lib fed counterparts. The lack of suppression of growth of the orthotopically transplanted cells in caloric restricted males suggests the reduced tumor formation reported in other studies may be due to decreased levels of initiation in caloric restricted animals and not epigenetic effects mediated through the tissue microenvironment. The mechanisms contributing to rapid tumor growth of transplanted GN6TF cells in caloric restricted males are unclear. However, the differential growth potential of the same tumor cell line in male versus female hosts demonstrates the importance of the tissue microenvironment in tumor progression.

References

1. Erdstein J, Wisebord S, Mishkin SY et al (1989) The effect of several se steroid hormones on the growth rate of three Morris hepatoma tumor lines. Hepatology 9: 621-624.
2. Reuber MD, Firminger HI (1962) Effect of progesterone and diethylstilbesterol on hepatic carcinogenesis and cirrhosis in A X C rats fed N-2-fluorenyldiacetamide. J Nat Cancer Inst 29: 933-946.
3. Vesselinovitch SD (1987) Certain aspects of hepatocarcinogenesis in the infant mouse model. Toxicological Pathol 15: 221-228.
4. Kemp CJ, Leary CN, Drinkwater NR (1989) Promotion of murine hepatocarcinogenesis by testosterone is androgen receptor-dependent but not cell autonomous. Proc Nat Acad Sci (USA) 86: 7505-7509.
5. Nagasue N, Kohno H, Chang Y et al (1990) Specificity of androgen receptors of hepatocellular carcinoma and liver in humans. Hepato-gastroenterol 37: 474-479.
6. Ohnishi S, Murakami T, Moriyama T et al (1986) Androgen and estrogen receptors in hepatocellular carcinoma and in the surrounding noncancerous liver tissue. Hepatology 6: 440-443.

7. McCullough KD, Coleman WB, Smith GJ et al (1994) Age-dependent regulation of the tumorigenic potential of neoplastically transformed Rat liver epithelial cells by the liver microenvironment. Cancer Res 54: 3668-3671.

8. McCullough KD, Coleman WB, Smith GJ et al (1997) Age-dependent induction of hepatic tumor regression by the tissue microenvironment following transplantation of neoplastically transformed rat liver epithelial cells into the liver. Cancer Res 57: 1807-1813.

9. Yu M-W, Chen C-J (1993) Elevated serum testosterone levels and risk of hepatocellular carcinoma. Cancer Res 53: 790-794.

10. Forbes A, Wilkinson ML, Iqbal MJ et al (1987) Response to cyproterone acetate treatment in primary hepatocellular carcinoma is related to fall in free 5a-dihydrotestosterone. Eur J Cancer Clin Oncol 23: 1659-1664.

11. Yu L, Nagasue N, Makino Y et al (1995) Effect of androgens and their manipulation on cell growth and androgen receptor (AR) level in AR-positive and –negative human hepatocellular carinomas. J Hepatol 22: 295-302.

12. Mancici MA, Song CS, Rao TR et al (1992) Spatio-temporal Expression of estrogen sulfotransferase within the hepatic lobule of male rats: implication of in situ estrogen inactivation of androgen action. Endocrinol 131: 1541-1546.

13. Francavilla A, Polimno L, DiLeo A et al (1989) The Effect of estrogen and tamoxifen on hepatocyte proliferation in vivo and in vitro. Hepatology 9:614-620.

14. Roy AK, McMinn DM, Biswas NM (1975) Estrogenic inhibition of the hepatic synthesis of a2υ-globulin in the rat. Endocrinology 97:1501-1508.

Dietary Energy Restriction Inhibits Estrogen Induced Pituitary Tumorigenesis in a Rat Strain Specific Manner

Djuana M. E. Harvell, Thomas J. Spady, Tracy E. Strecker, Athena M. Lemus-Wilson, Karen L. Pennington, Fangchen Shen, Diane F. Birt, Rodney D. McComb, and James D. Shull

Summary

We are investigating modulation by dietary energy consumption of estrogen action in the regulation of cell proliferation and survival and induction of prolactin (PRL)-producing pituitary tumors in different inbred rat strains. Summarized herein are data which indicate that a 40% restriction of energy consumption virtually abolishes development of estrogen induced pituitary tumors in the inbred Fischer 344 (F344) rat strain and that this inhibition occurs through modulation of estrogen regulation of pituitary cell survival, not inhibition of estrogen stimulated cell proliferation. Data are also presented which indicate that the inhibitory effect of energy restriction on estrogen induced pituitary tumorigenesis is rat strain specific. Whereas energy restriction markedly inhibited development of pituitary tumors in the F344 and Copenhagen (COP) rat strains, no inhibitory effect was observed in the ACI strain. Genetic studies have been initiated to elucidate the molecular bases of the strain specific inhibitory actions of dietary energy restriction on development of estrogen induced pituitary tumors in the genetically related COP and ACI rat strains.

Introduction

Estrogens (Es) are important regulators of growth and development and are implicated in the etiology of a variety of human cancers. Dietary energy consumption is also considered to be an important modulator of carcinogenesis.

The ability of dietary energy restriction, defined herein as a 40% reduction in energy consumption relative to that consumed by animals allowed to feed ad libitum, to modulate E action in the rat pituitary gland was investigated. This gland serves as a well defined experimental model for studying E regulation of cell number homeostasis and E induced tumorigenesis. Data summarized herein represent the first indication that energy consumption modulates the manner in which a defined target cell population responds to E and provide unique insight into interactions between endocrine, environmental and genetic factors in the regulation of cell proliferation and survival.

Materials and Methods

The sources of experimental animals, reagents and supplies as well as the methods relating to care, feeding and hormonal treatment of animals have been described previously (1-4). Pituitary lactotroph proliferation was assayed as described previously (4). Expression of *TRPM2* mRNA was assayed as a surrogate marker of apoptosis (4). Statistical significance was assessed by ANOVA or two tailed t test. Values of $p \leq 0.05$ were considered statistically significant.

Results

Dietary Energy Restriction Inhibits Estrogen Induced Pituitary Tumorigenesis in a Rat Strain Specific Manner

It is well established that administered Es induce development of PRL-producing pituitary tumors in specific inbred rat strains, including F344 (3-5), COP (2), and ACI (1, 6). We have recently reported that a 40% restriction of energy consumption virtually abolishes development of E induced pituitary tumors in the F344 rat (3, 4). We have now extended these studies to the COP and ACI rat strains, two genetically related strains that develop PRL-producing pituitary tumors when treated with Es (1-2, 6). Dietary energy restriction markedly inhibited development of pituitary tumors in female COP rats treated with E_2 for 12 weeks, as evidenced by measurements of pituitary weight (Figure 1A), which is proportional to pituitary cell number and gland DNA content (1-5), pituitary weight to body weight ratio (Figure 1B) and circulating PRL (Figure 1C). Data from an experiment in which F344 rats were treated with E_2 for 10 weeks (4) is illustrated for comparison. In contrast, no inhibition of E_2 induced pituitary tumor development was apparent in female ACI rats treated with E_2 for 12 (Figure 1) or 20 (data not shown) weeks.

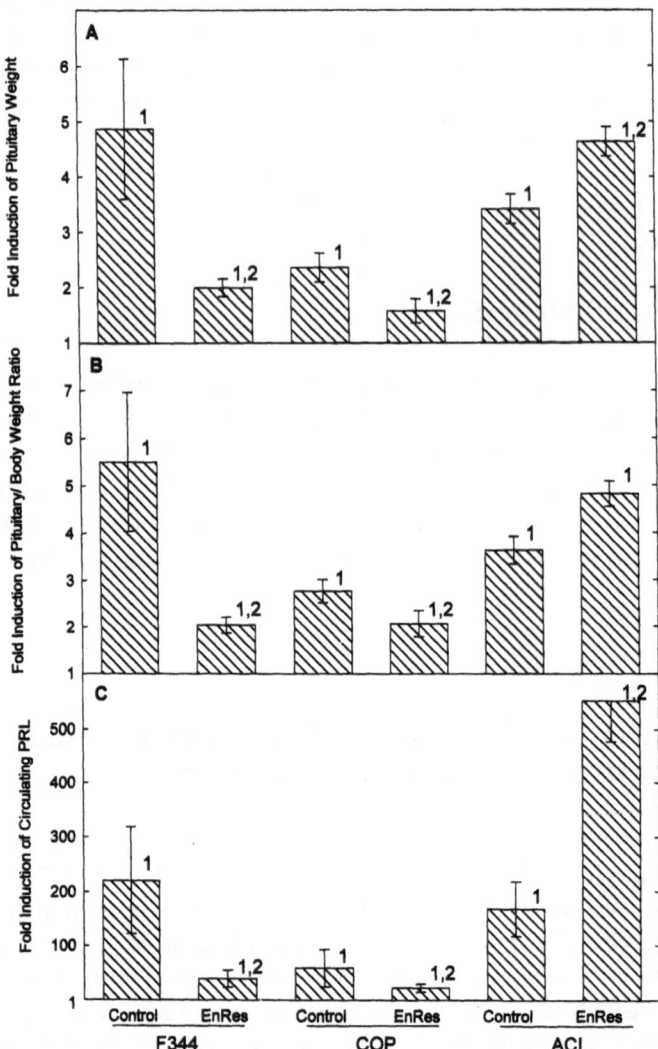

Figure 1. Dietary energy restriction inhibits development of estrogen induced pituitary tumors in a rat strain specific manner. Experimental details are summarized in the text and detailed in cited literature. Each data bar represents the mean fold induction of the indicated parameter in E_2 treated rats relative to untreated control rats fed the same experimental diet. A. Pituitary wet weight in milligrams was measured. B. The ratio of pituitary weight to body weight was calculated. C. Prolactin in the systemic circulation was measured by radioimmunoassay.

Dietary Energy Restriction Modulates Estrogen Regulation of Pituitary Cell Homeostasis

We have evaluated the effects of E_2 and dietary energy restriction on proliferation within the PRL-producing lactotroph population, employing a double immunohistochemical protocol that detects PRL and 5-bromo-2'-deoxyuridine (BrdU) that was incorporated into the DNA of replicating cells during the 4 hour period preceding sacrifice. Administered E_2 significantly stimulated lactotroph proliferation in ovariectomized female F344 rats and a 40% restriction of energy consumption did not inhibit this induction of lactotroph proliferation (4). These data indicate that the antitumorigenic actions of energy restriction in the F344 pituitary gland were not mediated at the level of lactotroph proliferation. E_2 similarly induced lactotroph proliferation in ovariectomized ACI rats treated with E_2 for 20 weeks, and again energy restriction did not inhibit this induction (data not shown).

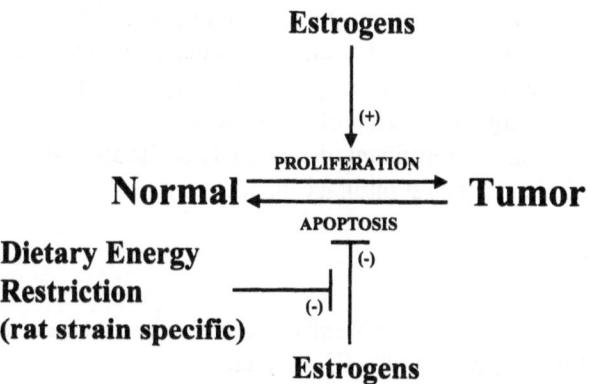

Figure 2. Dietary energy restriction appears to exert its rat strain specific inhibitory actions on development of E induced pituitary tumors by modulating regulation by E of pituitary cell survival.

Messenger RNA for *TRPM2* (7) was quantified as an indicator of apoptotic activity in the anterior pituitary gland. In ovariectomized female F344 rats allowed to feed *ad libitum*, the level of *TRPM2* mRNA was decreased by approximately 80% following 10 weeks of E_2 treatment (4). *TRPM2* mRNA was similarly decreased following 20 weeks of E_2 treatment in ovariectomized female ACI rats allowed to feed *ad libitum*. These data suggest that administered E_2 exerts an antiapoptotic action in the pituitary gland of the F344 and ACI rat strains and that this contributes to the development of PRL-producing pituitary tumors in these strains. Interestingly, no reduction in the level of *TRPM2* mRNA was observed in response to E_2 in the pituitary glands of energy restricted F344 rats (4). In contrast, E_2 reduced *TRPM2* mRNA in energy restricted ACI rats in a manner similar to that observed in animals allowed to feed *ad libitum* (data not shown). These data suggest that dietary energy restriction modulates the ability of E_2 to exert its antiapoptotic action in the pituitary gland of the F344, but not ACI, rat strain, and provide a potential mechanism for the rat strain specific inhibitory effects of energy restriction on development of E induced pituitary tumors (Figure 2).

Genetic Bases of Estrogen Induced Pituitary Tumor Development

The observation that the COP and ACI rat strains differ in sensitivity to the inhibitory action of dietary energy restriction on E induced pituitary tumor development is particularly noteworthy because these rat strains are closely related genetically. We have initiated efforts to define the genetic bases of E induced pituitary tumor development in the ACI and COP strains. Data from these studies indicate that the pituitary gland of the ACI rat displays approximately twice the growth response to administered E, relative to that of the COP anterior pituitary, and that this additional growth response appears to be conferred by the ACI allele of a single gene acting in a dominant manner. We are presently mapping the location of this gene within the rat genome in order to evaluate its role as a determinant of sensitivity to the antitumorigenic actions of energy restriction in the rat pituitary gland.

Conclusions

1. Dietary energy restriction virtually abolishes development of E induced pituitary tumorigenesis in the F344 rat strain.
2. Inhibition of E induced pituitary tumorigenesis in the F344 rat occurs through modulation of E regulation of pituitary cell survival, not inhibition of E stimulated cell proliferation.
3. The inhibitory effects of energy restriction on E induced pituitary tumorigenesis are rat strain specific. Whereas energy restriction markedly inhibits development of E induced pituitary tumors in the F344 and COP rat strains, no inhibition is observed in the ACI rat strain.
4. The COP and ACI rat strains display a quantitative difference in their pituitary growth response to administered E. In progeny of a genetic cross between the ACI and COP strains, the ACI phenotype is inherited as a dominant genetic trait that appears to be conferred through the actions of a single gene.

References

1. Shull JD, Spady TJ, Snyder MC et al (1997) Ovary intact, but not ovariectomized female ACI rats treated with 17β-estradiol rapidly develop mammary carcinoma. Carcinogenesis 18:1595-1601.
2. Spady TJ, Harvell DME, Snyder MC et al (1998) Estrogen-induced tumorigenesis in the Copenhagen rat: disparate susceptibilities to development of prolactin-producing pituitary tumors and mammary carcinomas. Cancer Lett 124:95-103.
3. Shull JD, Birt DF, McComb RD et al (1998) Estrogen induction of prolactin-producing pituitary tumors in the Fischer 344 rat: modulation by dietary energy, but not protein consumption. Mol Carcinogenesis 23:96-105.
4. Spady TJ, Lemus-Wilson AM, Pennington KL et al (1998) Dietary energy restriction abolishes development of prolactin-producing pituitary tumors in Fischer 344 rats treated with 17β-estradiol. Mol Carcinogenesis 23:86-95.
5. Wiklund J, Wertz N, Gorski J (1981) A comparison of estrogen effects on uterine and pituitary growth and prolactin synthesis in F344 and Holtzman rats. Endocrinology 109:1700-1707.
6. Holtzman S, Stone JP, Shellabarger CJ (1979) Influence of diethylstilbestrol treatment on prolactin cells of female ACI and Sprague-Dawley rats. Cancer Res 39:779-784.
7. Buttyan R, Olsson CA, Pintar J et al (1989) Induction of the *TRPM-2* gene in cells undergoing programmed death. Mol Cell Biol 9:3473-3481.

Estrogen-induced Prolactinoma Development: A Role for Cell-Cell Communication

Shane T. Hentges and Dipak K. Sarkar

Introduction

Estrogen (E) has been linked to tumorogenesis in various endocrine tissues including the pituitary. There are subsets of the population that display hypersensitivity to the mitotic effect of E on the pituitary in both humans and animals. The Fischer-344 strain of rats is one such example among animals. 17β-estradiol (E_2) treatment rapidly results in the formation of prolactin-secreting adenomas (prolactinomas) in the pituitaries of Fischer-344 rats. This animal model has been useful in elucidating some of the roles of E in tumor formation; however, the mechanisms of E action are not well understood (1).

The mitotic action of E on lactotropes involves the regulation of the production of growth factors from the lactotropes themselves. Utilizing *in vivo* and *in vitro* animal models, we have previously shown that lactotropes produce and secrete transforming growth factor (TGF)-β1 and TGF-β3. The transforming growth factor-βs belong to a family of multifunctional polypeptide growth factors with varied actions, including regulation of differentiation, proliferation, and cell adhesion. The actions of TGF-β1 on lactotropes have been described by us previously (2, 3). TGF-β1 inhibits lactotropic cell proliferation. E_2 has an inhibitory effect on TGF-β1 production from anterior pituitary tissue. However, preliminary data indicate that E_2 increases the production of TGF-β3 from the anterior pituitary. The altered expression of TGF-β3 induced by E_2 led us to examine the action of this growth factor on lactotropic cell proliferation. We show that TGF-β3 stimulates lactotropic cell proliferation and that this action of TGF-β3 is mediated by a paracrine mechanism involving the agranular folliculo-stellate (FS) cells.

Materials and Methods

Primary Cultures of Pituitary Cells . Adult female Fischer-344 rats were ovariectomized and implanted sc with a 1-cm silastic capsule filled with 17β-estradiol (E_2) . The capsules maintain plasma E_2 levels at 215±20 pg/ml.

Seven to ten days post ovariectomy, pituitaries were collected from sacrificed Fischer-344 rats and enzymatically dissociated. Cells were pelleted and resuspended in Dulbecco's Modified Eagle's (DME) medium:F-12 (1:1; Sigma, St. Louis, MO) with 100 units/ml penicillin, 100 μg/ml streptomycin and 10% fetal calf serum. Lactotropes were enriched using percoll separation. Dissociated anterior pituitary cells were suspended in 1x Earl's balanced salts solution and layered on top of the discontinuous percoll gradient (4). The cells from the 35/50% interface were collected as enriched lactotropes. The cells were grown on poly-L-lysine-coated coverslips in 24-well plates. After 24 h, the media was changed to DME:F12 containing 2.5% fetal calf serum and 10% horse serum. On day 4 of culture the media was changed to DME:F-12 containing serum supplement (100 μM human transferrin, 5 μM insulin, and 1 μM putrescine) and the treatment. Control wells received serum supplement and 10 nM 17β-estradiol (Sigma). The treatment groups were treated like the controls, but also received recombinant human TGF-β3 (R&D, Minneapolis, MN) added at .001, .01 ng/ml, .1 ng/ml, 1 ng/ml or 10 ng/ml. The media with treatments were changed at 48 hours, and at 92 hours 5-bromo-2'-deoxyuridine (BrdUrd, Sigma; 0.1 mM) was added for 4 hours before termination of the experiment at 96 hours. Primary cultures from E_2-treated rats contained 40-60% lactotropes. Percoll separation enriched the lactotropic population to approximately 75-80%. FS cells were not detectable in the enriched lactotropic populations as determined by staining for S-100.

Folliculo-stellate Cell Line. We established a folliculo-stellate (FS) cell line from a primary culture of anterior pituitary cells from Fischer-344 rats. The dissociated cells were subjected to percoll separation as above with the exception that the cells from the 50/60% interface were plated on a 100-mm culture dish. The culture was maintained in 10% FCS until confluent then the cells were split to multiple plates. After 10 passes, immunohistochemical procedures for S-100 detection revealed that the culture contained only folliculo-stellate cells. S-100 detection was carried out using S-100 antibody (Zymed, San Francisco, CA) and stained with NBT-BCIP (Zymed). The FS cell line was maintained in DME:F-12 (1:1; Sigma) supplemented with 10% FCS (Hyclone, Logan, UT). The FS cells used in these experiments were between generation 20 and 30.

Lactotropic Cell Proliferation. Lactotropic cell proliferation was determined by double staining for BrdU and prolactin (PRL) immunoreactivities as previously described by us (5). Cells displaying immunoreactivites for both PRL and BrdU (a marker of S phase) were considered dividing lactotropes. Five areas from each coverslip were counted (approximately 500 cells/area).

Results

TGF-β3 Stimulates Lactotropic Cell Proliferation in Primary Cultures of Anterior Pituitary Cells in the Presence of Estradiol.

Lactotropes displayed an increase in proliferation in primary cultures treated with TGF-β3 and E_2 as compared to cultures treated with E_2 alone. The lowest dose of TGF-β3 tested (.001 ng/ml) elicited only a marginal increase in lactotropic proliferation while all other doses significantly increased lactotropic proliferation in primary cultures of anterior pituitary cells. The 1 ng/ml dose of TGF-β3 resulted in more than a two-fold increase in lactotropic proliferation compared to the E_2 -only control and was the dose used in the subsequent studies.

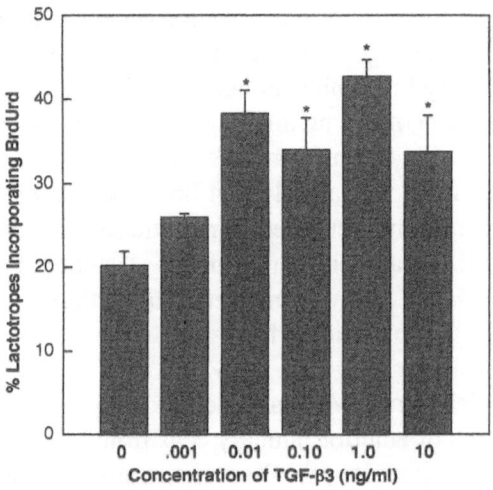

Figure 1. Primary cultures of anterior pituitary cells were treated with various doses of TGF-β3 (0-10 ng/ml) with 10 nM E_2 then stained for BrdU and PRL immunoreactivities. The number of dividing lactotropes is expressed as the percentage of total lactotropes in the culture. *, $p<0.05$ compared to the control group receiving E_2 alone. N=4-8.

TGF-β3 Has No Proliferative Effect on Lactotropes in the Rc/4-bc Cell Line Unless Co-cultured with Fs Cells .

The proliferative effect of TGF-β3 on lactotropes was determined in the RC/4-BC cell line. This cell line was utilized as it contains all of the secreting cell types of the anterior pituitary, but is devoid of FS cells. Interestingly, we found that unlike the lactotropes in primary cultures, the lactotropes in the RC/4-BC cell line do not proliferate in response to TGF-β3 treatment. However, when RC/4-BC cells were co-cultured with FS cells, the lactotropes did proliferate following TGF-β3 treatment, implying a potential mediating role for FS cells.

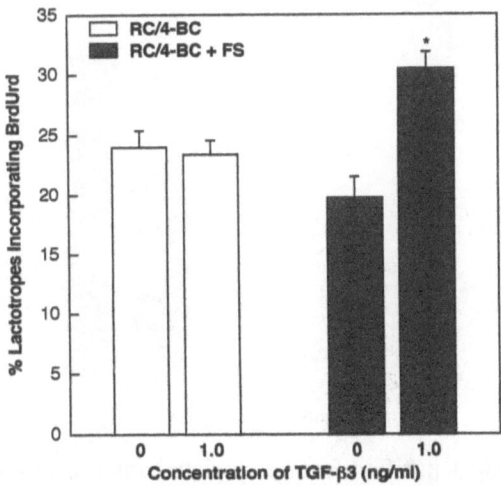

Figure 2. RC/4-BC cells were plated alone (RC/4-BC) or co-cultured with FS cells (RC/4-BC + FS; 200,000 RC/4-BC cells and 50,000 FS cells). The cultures were treated with 1 ng/ml of TGF-β3 in the presence or absence of E_2 ("0" dose). The percentage of lactotropes undergoing cell division in each treatment group was determined. There was no significant effect of TGF-β3 on lactotropic cell proliferation in RC/4-BC cells alone (p>0.1). In co-cultures, TGF-β3 stimulated lactotropic cell proliferation. *, p<0.05 as compared to the group treated with E_2 alone. N=8.

TGF-β3 Stimulates Lactotropic Cell Proliferation   Only in the Presence of Fs Cells. To determine if the modulatory effect of FS cells on TGF-β3-stimulated lactotropic cell proliferation was specific to lactotropes in the RC/4-BC cell line or was also true for lactotropes in primary culture, we utilized cultures of enriched lactotropes. Dissociated anterior pituitary cells were separated by density gradient and cells from the layer containing mostly lactotropes and no detectable FS cells were plated and treated with TGF-β3 and E_2 . Purified lactotropes did not proliferate in response to TGF-β3, but rather, the growth response of these cells was moderately inhibited by this growth factor. This is in contrast to the effect observed in primary cultures of mixed anterior pituitary cell types (Figure 1). Similar to the lactotropes of the RC/4-BC cell line, lactotropes purified from primary cultures displayed increased proliferation in response to TGF-β3 when co-cultured with FS cells.

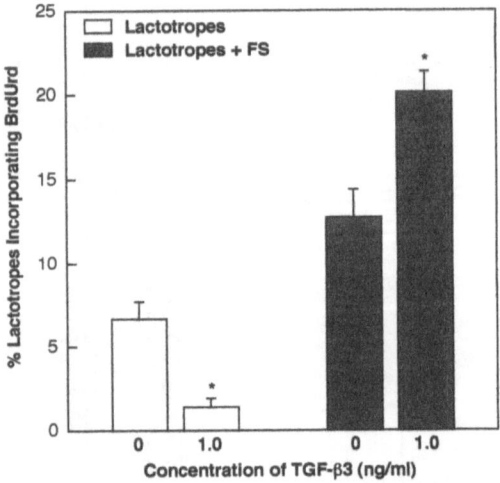

Figure 3. Lactotropes purified from dissociated anterior pituitary cells were plated alone (Lactotropes) or with FS cells (Lactotropes + FS;   200,000 lactotropes and 50,000 FS cells) and treated with TGF-β3 in the presence or absence of 10-nM E_2 ("0" dose). The percentage of lactotropes undergoing cell division in each treatment group was determined. *, $p<0.05$ compared to the "0"-dose group. N=8.

Discussion

The E-hypersensitive Fischer-344 rat strain has proven to be a useful model to study the process of E-induced tumorogenesis. From this strain of rat we utilized cells that were not transformed, but were undergoing rapid cell division, we were able to identify a growth-promoting action of TGF-β3 in the lactotropes of the anterior pituitary in the presence of E_2 .

The TGF-β family of peptide growth factors has been widely studied in relation to cell proliferation and differentiation. The various isoforms of TGF-β are highly conserved among species and each isoform shares high amino acid sequence homology with the others. However, despite the similarity in structure of these peptides, they have distinct promoters and differential expression (6), which indicates that isoform-specific functions may exist for the TGF-βs.

The data presented here indicate that a growth-stimulatory role may exist for TGF-β3 during E-induced tumorogenesis. In most epithelial cells, TGF-β1 is considered an inhibitor of cell proliferation. Here we have presented evidence that, while TGF-β3 inhibits lactotropic proliferation in enriched cultures, TGF-β3 stimulates lactotropic cell proliferation in cultures of mixed anterior pituitary cells containing other endocrine and FS cells (Figure 1). These data suggest that the *in vivo* actions of E_2 and TGF-β3 are complex and involve cell-to-cell interactions. The studies determining the actions of TGF-β3 on lactotropes in the RC/4-BC cell line identified a mediating role of FS cells in TGF-β3 action on lactotropes. This is verified by the data showing that TGF-β3 stimulation of lactotropes requires the presence of FS cells both in primary pituitary culture and in the RC/4-BC cell line models. Hence it can be hypothesized that *in vivo* FS cells regulate the growth-promoting action of E_2 on lactotropes.

In several tissues, it appears that the growth of cells depends not only on the mitogenic stimulus, but also on cell-to-cell interactions. For example, in uterine, ovarian, and mammary tissues, the communication with mesenchymal cells facilitates the growth of epithelial cells (7-9). In some cell types (e.g., mesenchymal cells) where various TGF-β isoforms stimulate cell proliferation, the actions of these peptides on the cells appear to be indirect via increasing the production of other growth factors (10). Our present data indicate that, like some other E-responsive tissues, the pituitary may be another site where TGF-β action is mediated by cell-to-cell interactions. Whether or not communication between FS cells and lactotropes requires cell-cell contact or paracrine mediation involving growth factors is unknown.

FS cells produce several growth factors including bFGF, TGF-α, and IGF-1 (11-13). The expression and actions of these growth factors are affected by E. In addition, bFGF, TGF-α, and IGF-1 are secreted by FS cells and have proliferative effects on lactotropes. FS cells may mediate lactotropic cell proliferation in response to E_2 by increasing production and/or secretion of one or more of these or other growth factors. Elucidating the cell-cell communication between FS cells and lactotropes will lend further insight into the mechanisms involved in E-induced cell proliferation and transformation in the anterior pituitary.

References

1. Sarkar DK, Hentges ST, De A et al (1998) Hormonal control of pituitary prolactin-secreting tumors. Front Biosci 3:d934-d943.
2. Sarkar DK, Kim KH, Minami S (1992) Transforming growth factor-β1 mRNA and protein expression in the pituitary gland and its action on PRL secretion and lactotropic growth. Mol Endocrinol 6:1825-1833.
3. Pastorcic M, De A, Boyadjieva N et al (1995) Reduction in the expression and action of transforming growth factor β1 on lactotropes during estrogen-induced tumorigenesis inthe anterior pituitary. Cancer Res 55:4892-4898.
4. Burris TP, Freeman ME (1993) Low concentrations of dopamine increase cytosolic calcium in lactotrophs. Endocrinology 133:63-68.
5. De A, Boyadjieve N, Pastorcic M et al (1995) Potentiation of estrogen's mitogenic effect on the pituitary gland by alcohol consumption. Int J Onco 7:643-48.

6. Roberts AB, Kim S, Noma T (1991) Multiple forms of TGF-β: distinct promoters and differential expression. In: Bock GR, Marsh J (eds). Clinical applications of TGF-β. John Wiley & Sons, Chichester, pp. 7-15.
7. Parrot JA, Vigne JL, Chu BZ et al (1994) Mesenchymal-epithelial interactions in the ovaries follicle involve keratinocyte and hepatocyte growth factor production by theca cells and their action on granular cells. Endocrinology 135:569-575.
8. Bigsby RM, Li A, Everett L (1993) Stromal-epithelial interactions regulating cell proliferation in the uterus. In: Magness RR, Naftolin F (eds) Local systems in reproduction. Raven Press, New York, pp. 171-188.
9. Venkateswaren V, Oliver SA, Ram TG et al (1993) Salivary mesenchyme cells that induce mammary epithlial hyperplasia up-regulate EGF receptors in primary cultures of mammary epithelium within collagen gels. Growth Regul 3:138-45.
10. Moses HL, Yang EY, Pietenpol JA (1990) TGF-β stimulation and inhibition of cell proliferation: new mechanistic insights. Cell 63:254-257.
11. Ferrara N, Schweigerer L, Neufeld G et al (1987) Pituitary follicular cells produce basic fibroblast growth factor. Proc Natl Acad Sci USA 84:5773-5777.
12. Korbin MS, Asa SL, Samsoondar J et al (1987) α-Transforming growth factor in the bovine anterior pituitary gland: secretion by dispersed cells and immunohistochemical localization. Endocrinology 121:1412-1415.
13. Bach MA, Bondy CA (1992) Anatomy of the pituitary insulin-like growth factor system. Endocrinology 131:2588-2594.

Combined Administration of Transplacental Ethylnitrosourea and Postnatal Diethylstilbestrol Induces Neural Differentiation in Interstitial Cells of the Golden Hamster Kidney

Amando Peydro-Olaya, Carmen Carda, and Antonio Llombart-Bosch

Summary

Diethylstilbestrol produces kidney tumors with nephroblastoma-like structure in the Syrian golden hamster. Their controversial histogenesis is commonly related to the kidney interstitial cells, in which are probably undifferentiated nephrogenic or blastemal cells with epithelial, mesenchymal, and neuroectodermal potentialities. On the other hand, transplacental administration of ethylnitrosourea induces neural tumors in animals, and in the golden hamster it also causes nephroblastomas. The present study seeks the addition of the neurogenic and nephrogenic effects in the kidney hamster following ethylnitrosourea and diethylstilbestrol treatment. Our ultrastructural study demonstrates in this dual intoxicated kidney model, axons are in direct relationship with interstitial cells (hyperplastic or not) and also in association with tumoral cells. These findings suggest the existence of neural crest cell derivatives in the interstitial renal spaces which may represent the predecessors of kidney nephroblastoma.

Introduction

Experimental transplacental administration of ethylnitrosourea (ENU) induces in animals neural tumors, and in Syrian golden hamster (GH) also ENU+DES-hamster kidney tumor causes nephroblastomas (1). Diethylstilbestrol (DES) produces kidney tumors in GH, in both intact and castrated animals. These tumors display nephroblastoma-like structures (2). Their origin remains controversial, but from morphological and immunohistochemical data, we have postulated an interstitial neuroectodermal-cell origin (3). Interstitial cell hyperplasia and tubular dysplasia have been considered as preneoplastic lesions, and in the most early DES-kidney tumoral stages, prior to the infiltrating macroscopic tumors, are typified as microtumors or tumorlets (3-6). The present study seeks the addition of the nephrogenic and neurogenic effects in the hamster kidney by DES and ENU, particularly in order to obtain ultrastructural evidence of the presence of neural structures in the interstitial intoxicated kidney, and in the kidney tumorlets and tumors.

Materials and Methods

Three series of 25 GH were used. Series I received 25 mg of DES implanted subcutaneously after castration at 3 mo. of age. Series II were intoxicated by transplacental means, with 100 mg/kg of weight of ENU (day 15 of pregnancy), in a single intraperitoneal injection. Series III combined the administration of ENU with 25 mg of DES at 3 mo. of age after castration. Animal kidneys were processed for histology and electron microscopy at 5, 7 and 9 mo. following the initiation of the study (2, 4 and 6 mo. of the DES administration).

Results

The DES-kidney induced lesions of Series I were similar to those previously described (2,3), mainly with epithelial-like configuration. All the kidneys of the animals of Series I possessed some preneoplastic lesions. In four cases, one at 4.0 mo. and three at 6.0 mo. of the DES administration, the preneoplastic lesions appeared mixed and with a concomitant macroscopic infiltrating tumor. No tumors or pretumoral kidney changes were found in ENU, the group of Series II.

In Series III the incidence of interstitial cell hyperplasia and tubular dysplasia of the kidney was lower than observed in the animals of Series I, and only ten cases with kidney preneoplasic changes, six of them with small tumoral foci, could be detected, and two with nodular infiltrating tumors. On histologic and ultrastructural examination, the DES+ENU kidney tumors exhibited an architectural pattern similar to that described in the DES tumors (2). All were solid, ciliated and sourrounded by a continuous basal membrane. But the DES+ENU tumors showed a predominant neuroepithelial-like character. This neural character was confirmed by electron microscopy with evidence of neural-like characteristics (neurofilaments, neurotubules, neurosecretory granules) in the A. Peydro-Olaya, *et al.*tumor cells, and for the presence of numerous peripheral axons. In the apparently normal interstitial kidney (Figs. 1a,1b) and interstitial hyperplasia, the axons appeared grouped conforming to typical peripheral non-myelinated nerve fibers. In the tumors, the axons made direct contact with tumoral cells, with non-myelinated and aberrant myelinated organizations (Figures 2, 3).

Conclusions

The ultrastructural evidence of axons in the DES+ENU hamster treated kidney in direct relationship with interstitial cells (hyperplastic or not) and mainly, the presence of numerous intra-tumoral axons, in direct contact with the tumor cells, without any intervening basement membrane, both in early tumoral focus and in infiltrating tumor, contributed to reinforcing our hypothesis of the existence of neural crest cell derivatives in the interstitial renal spaces which may represent predecessors of the DES-hamster nephroblastoma.

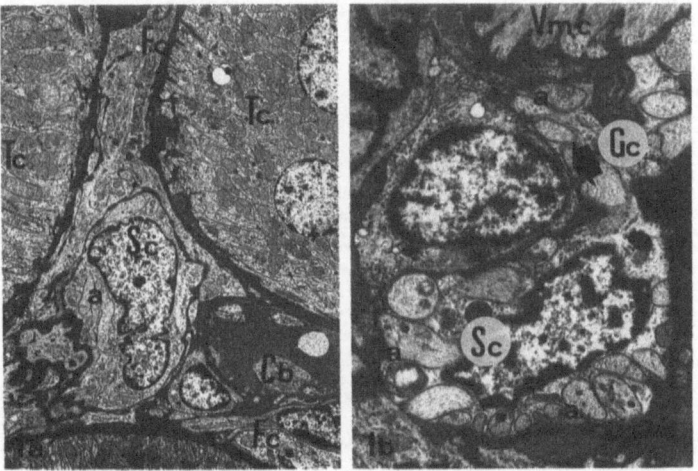

Figure 1. DES+ENU hamster kidney. a. Interstitial intertubular kidney. **b.** Interstitial perivascular kidney. Abbreviations: Fibroblastic-like cell (Fc), Schwann cell (Sc), Axon (a), Ganglionar cell (Gc), Tubular cell (Tc), Capillary blood (Cb), Vascular smoth muscle cell (Vmc).

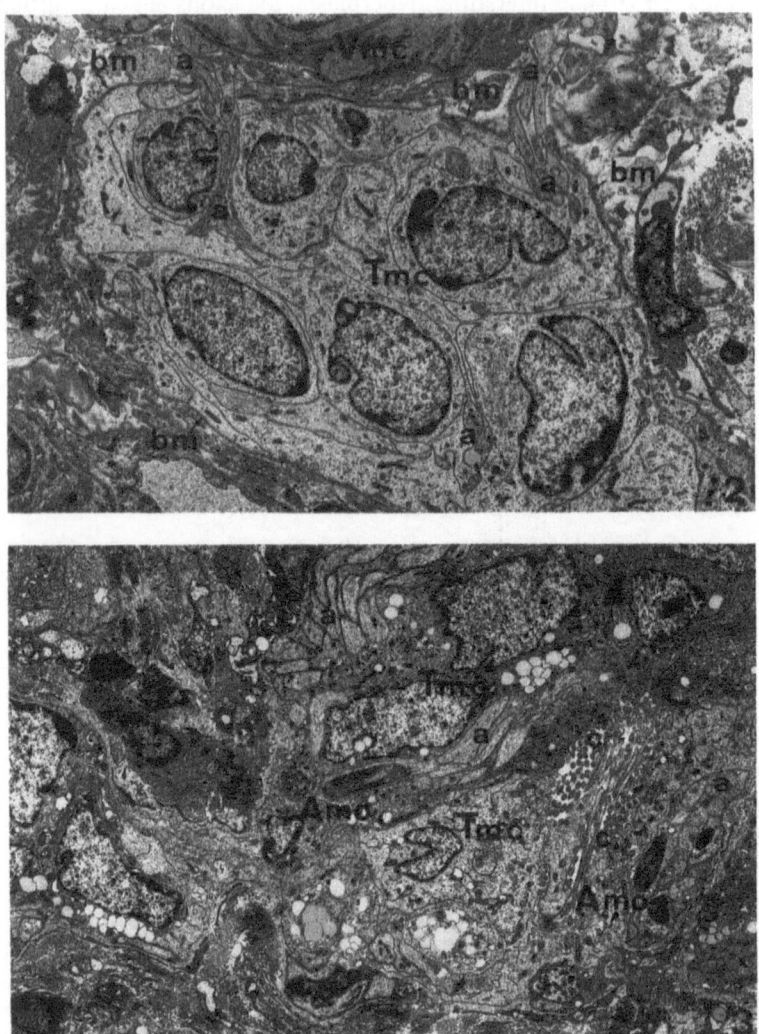

Figure 2. Microtumor. **Figure 3.** Infiltrating tumor. **DES+ENU-treated hamster kidney.** Abbreviations: Tumor cell (Tmc), Cilia (c), Axon (a), basal membrane (bm), Aberrant myelinated organization (Amo), Vascular smoth muscle cell (Vmc).

References

1. Mennel HD, ZŸlch KJ (1972) Zur Morphologie transplacentar erzeugter neurogener Tumoren beim Goldhamster. Acta Neuropathol (Berlin) 21: 194-203.
2. Llombart-Bosch A, Peydro-Olaya A (1998) Estrogen-induced malignant tumour, kidney, Syrian golden hamster. In: Jones TC, Hard GC, Mohr U (eds) Urinary System, Monographs on Pathology of Laboratory Animals, 2nd ed, ILSI. Springer-Verlag, Berlin, pp. 179-198.
3. Cortés-Vizcáno V, Peydro-Olaya A, Llombart-Bosch A (1994) Morphological and immunohistochemical support for the interstitial cell origin of oestrogen-induced kidney tumours in the Syrian golden hamster. Carcinogenesis 15: 2155-2162.
4. Gonzalez A, Oberley TD, Li JJ (1989) Morphological and immunohistochemical studies of the estrogen-induced Syrian hamster renal tumor: probable cell of origin. Cancer Res 49:1020-1028.
5. Goldfarb S, Pugh T (1990) Morphology and anatomic localization of renal microneoplasms and proximal tubule dysplasias induced by four different estrogens in the hamster. Cancer Res 50:113-119.
6. Oberley TD, Gonzalez A, Lauchner LJ et al (1991) Characterization of early kidney lesions in estrogen-induced tumors in the Syrian hamster. Cancer Res 51:1922-1929.

Aromatase Overexpression: Is Aromatase an Oncogene

Rajeshwar Rao Tekmal, Kiran Gill, and Nameer Kirma

Summary

To directly test the role of aromatase overexpression in tumorigenesis, we have developed a transgenic mouse model and demonstrated for the first time that increased tissue estrogens due to the overexpression of aromatase in mammary glands leads to the induction of various preneoplastic and neoplastic changes that are similar to early breast cancer. Increased estrogenic activity in breast tissue alters the regulation of genes involved in apoptosis, cell cycle and cell proliferation, as well as the levels of various growth factors. Tissue aromatase overexpression is sufficient to induce and maintain early preneoplastic and neoplastic changes in female mice without circulating ovarian estrogen. Overexpression of aromatase in male mammary glands leads to different histopathological changes that are similar to gynecomastia. Increased estrogenic activity in male mice changes the hormonal milieu of testis and results in the induction of Leydig cell tumors. These studies indicate a direct role of aromatase in preneoplastic and neoplastic changes seen in both mammary glands and testis.

Introduction

Breast cancer is one of the most prevalent types of cancer observed in women. The mitogenic and proliferative effects of estrogens (Es) have long been recognized and are known to correlate with E and progesterone receptors in breast tumor tissue. Interestingly, the proportion of patients with hormone sensitive tumors is higher among postmenopausal patients than premenopausal patients (1, 2). In addition, the source of sex steroids differ between pre- and postmenopausal women. The biosynthesis of Es is catalyzed by an enzyme called aromatase, a cytochrome P450 enzyme localized in the endoplasmic reticulum (3). Breast tumors from postmenopausal women maintain a high E content, even though the plasma levels of E_2 fall to low levels following menopause. In postmenopausal women, adipose tissue is the main source of circulating Es, since Es are no longer synthesized by the ovaries. As a result of the functional cessation of the ovaries, plasma E levels decrease dramatically in postmenopausal women and remain unchanged or increase slightly by the time of breast carcinoma development. In contrast, concentrations of 17β-estradiol (E_2) in breast tumors from post menopausal patients remain as high as in premenopausal patients plasma (4-6). In addition, E concentrations are higher in breast tumor tissue than those in normal breast tissue. Maintenance of high tumor E_2 concentrations reflects the *in-situ* E_2 production from plasma E precursors. One pathway for *in-situ* synthesis involves the conversion of androstenedione to estrone/E_2 catalyzed by aromatase (6). Since aromatase was first detected in breast tumors, the problem of assessing its functional significance has attracted considerable attention and controversy. A number of recent studies provide evidence to support a biological role for tumor aromatase.

An intriguing hypothesis is that local E is directly involved in the initiation of either preneoplastic or neoplastic (or both) changes in mammary epithelium. To address this question directly, we have generated an aromatase transgenic mice model and showed for the first time that the transgenic virgin and postlactational females that overexpress aromatase develop various preneoplastic histopathological changes (7).

Materials and Methods

The generation of aromatase transgenic mice (*MMTV-int-5 aromatase*) and their characterization has been described previously (7). Briefly, aromatase was expressed under the control of mouse mammary tumor virus promoter (MMTV). MMTV promoter which is active in both mammary glands and male reproductive organs. Aromatase transgenic mice overexpressing aromatase were maintained in a centralized, fully accredited animal facility. Histological examination of mammary glands and expression of various biochemical markers both at messenger RNA and protein level has been carried out as described previously (7, 8).

Results and Discussion

Mammary glands from nontransgenic virgin females of 7-8 weeks old consisted of extensive ducts, with a few alveoli growing from terminal branches at the end buds of the ducts. In transgenic virgin females we observed both the increased and enlarged ductal growth, compared to nontransgenic litter mates. Of these ducts several had hyperplastic and dysplastic lesions and fibroadenomas (7). This suggests that early estrogenic activity as a result of aromatase overexpression is sufficient for hyperplastic changes to occur in mammary epithelial cells of transgenic mice.

Mammary glands from postlactational nontransgenic females consisted of extensive ducts with the presence of minimal lobular alveolar growth. In contrast, mammary glands of transgenic females showed significant alveolar hyperplasia throughout the mammary glands. In the transgenic mice there were abundant alveolar glands and numerous terminal ducts as compared to nontransgenic animals, which had retained only simple ductal development after involution.

Histological examination of mammary glands of transgenic female mice that had gone through one pregnancy, and 3 weeks of postlactational involution showed a range of histologic abnormalities including formation of HAN, atypical ductal and glandular hyperplasia, ductal and lobular dysplasia, and hyperplastic lesions with excessive fibrous tissue around them, similar to fibroadenomas. In addition, mammary glands in transgenic mice exhibited an increased occurrence of multinucleated cells and some nuclei were enlarged (karyomegaly), with a hyperchromatic appearance. In general, the involuted mammary glands of transgenic mice contain a pattern of post-pregnancy involution different than the control. There is a significant increase in periductal, peri and intralobular fibrosis. Interestingly these changes are similar to what is observed in the breast tissue from women with a history of breast cancer (7).

Persistence of ductal hyperplasia and dysplasia was evident even after several months of involution in mammary glands from transgenic females. In many postlactational females, the progression of hyperplastic and dysplastic changes to more prominent preneoplastic/neoplastic changes was very significant with age. Ductal enlargement, extensive hyperplasia and other histopathological changes consistent with preneoplastic/neoplastic abnormalities similar to early breast cancer progressed significantly with age. Other secondary events are probably necessary for the advanced disease to manifest, as suggested by the lack of any frankly invasive tumors in these animals. Our data also show that preneoplastic and neoplastic changes persist even in the absence of ovarian E in ovariectomized virgin and postlactational females (Figure 1). These results clearly demonstrate that increased mammary E alone without the influence of circulating ovarian E is sufficient to maintain various preneoplastic/neoplastic changes.

Development of preneoplastic/neoplastic lesions to complete, invasive tumors is rare in this model. Nonetheless the data indicate that continued mammary estrogenic activity is involved in the progression of preneoplastic changes to neoplastic changes and provide evidence that mammary E is involved in the initiation and progression of breast cancer.

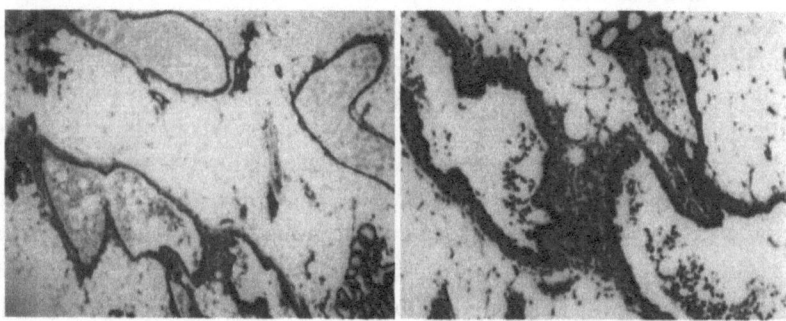

Figure 1. Continued hyperplastic and dysplastic mammary growth in ovariectomized aromatase transgenic mice.

To test whether the increased mammary E as a result of aromatase overexpression is responsible for various epigenetic changes in this tissue, we examined the expression of various growth factors that are known to be involved in breast cancer. Figure 2 clearly shows the overexpression of a number of growth factors in aromatase transgenic mammary glands as compared to nontransgenic mammary glands. These observations suggests that increased estrogenic activity up regulates various growth factors that may be responsible for increased mammary growth and hyperplasia associated with this growth. We have also observed the up regulation of a number of genes involved in cell cycle and anti-apoptotic process that is consistent with increased mammary proliferation (8).

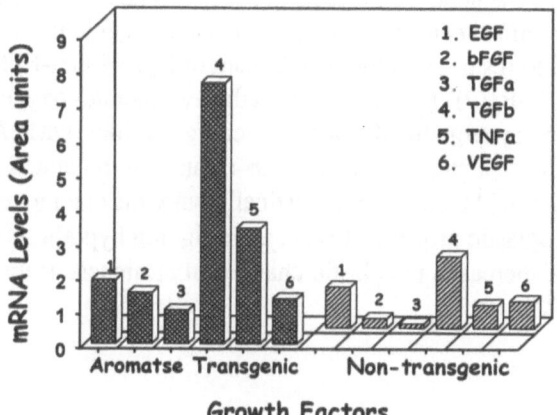

Figure 2. Effect of aromatase overexpression on growth factor induction in transgenic female mammary glands.

Our studies also show that overexpression of aromatase in male transgenic mice results in the increased epithelial glandular growth as early as 10 weeks of age. Histological examination of these glands show a clear evidence of hyperplastic and dysplastic changes that are similar to gynecomastia (a benign condition). These results clearly demonstrate that increased mammary E, without the influence of circulating ovarian E, is sufficient to induce various proliferative changes and which support the prior hypothesis that increased aromatase may contribute to gynecomastia. Transgenic males not only overexpress aromatase in reproductive tissues but also contributes to increased circulating Es. Compared to nontransgenic males, circulating E_2 levels in transgenic males is increased by 3-4 fold. Change in hormonal milieu resulted in male infertility and about 40% of the males develop testicular Leydig cell tumors. These studies clearly indicate increased estrogenic activity as a result of overexpression of aromatase is sufficient to induce gynecomastia and testicular cancer in males (Figure 3). Consistent with increased estrogenic activity in mammary glands and reproductive organs due to overexpression of aromatase, we have also observed changes in the regulation of genes involved in cell cycle and cell proliferation. Representative data with gene involved in cell cycle is shown in Figure 4. Other genes involved in cell cycle and cell proliferation that are influenced by E follow the same pattern. Increased estrogenic activity also alters the levels of various growth factors. These observations clearly indicate the direct effect of E on the regulation of various genes involved in mammary tumorigenesis, and are in complete agreement with previous observations with breast tumor tissue samples and breast cancer cell lines.

Steroidal Es are thought to act as carcinogens by alternate metabolic transformations. The genotoxic effects of specific metabolites of E can be at the origin of many human cancers. For example, carcinogenic mechanism that has been suggested to result from the metabolism of E_2 to 4-OH-E_2 to 3,4 quinone and back to 4-OH-E_2 (9). This metabolic pathway generates oxygen free radicals which may act synergistically with carcinogens like DMBA to produce neoplasms. Increased production of E in tissues, as mediated by aromatase overexpression would then act synergistically with this carcinogen to induce or enhance the neoplastic process. This is an intriguing hypothesis to explain our observations of increased neoplastic changes in aromatase transgenic animals receiving DMBA (10).

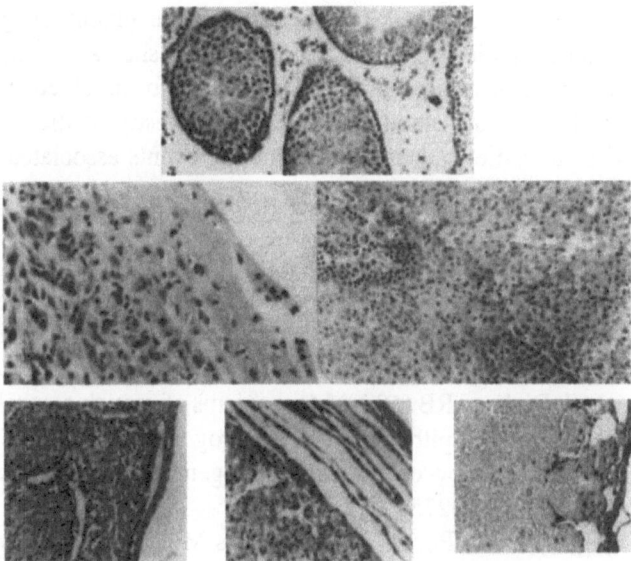

Figure 3. Overexpression of aromatase in transgenic male mice leads to the induction of testicular tumors. Note: Normal nontransgenic testis (top panel) and different stages of testicular tumors in transgenic mice.

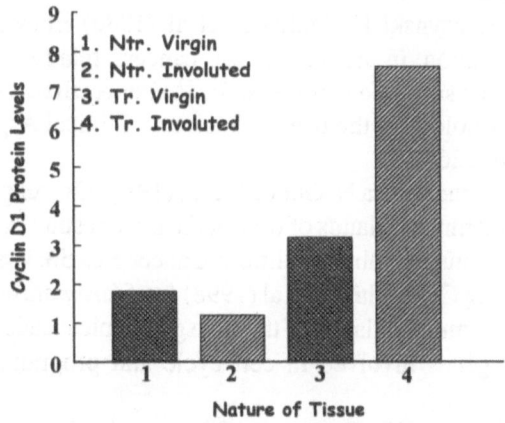

Figure 4. Cyclin D1 expression in mammary tissues.

Conclusions

Our study clearly indicates that overexpression of aromatase leads to increased estrogenic activity in both male and female mammary glands, and in male reproductive tissues, which results in the initiation of various preneoplastic/neoplastic changes in female and male mammary glands and Leydig cell tumor formation in males. Our data clearly shows overexpression of aromatase leads to various epigenetic changes that may be involved in E-induced tumorigenesis. This model should be useful to investigate the mechanisms involved in E mediated epigenetic and genotoxic events associated with both mammary and testicular tumorigenesis.

References

1. McGuire WL (1980) An update on estrogen and progesterone receptors in prognosis for primary and advanced breast cancer. In: Iacobelli S, et al., (eds) Hormones and Cancer. Raven Press, New York, pp. 337-344.
2. Lippman ME, Dickson RB (1989) Mechanisms of growth control in normal and malignant breast epithelium. Recent Prog Hormone Res 45:383-440.
3. Siiteri PK (1982) Review of studies on estrogen biosynthesis in the human. Cancer Res 42:3269s-3275s.
4. van Landeghem AAJ, Poortman J, Nabuurs M et al (1985) Endogenous concentration and subcellular distribution of estrogens in normal and malignant human breast tissue. Cancer Res 45:2900-2906.
5. Toniolo PG, Levitz M, Zeleniuch-Jacquotte A et al (1995) A prospective study of endogenous estrogens and breast cancer in postmenopausal women. J Natl Cancer Inst 87:190-197.
6. Santen RJ, Leszczynski D, Mallet N et al (1986) Enzymatic control of estrogen production in human breast cancer: relative significance of aromatase versus sulfatase pathways. In: Angel A, Bradlow HL, Dogliotti L (eds) Endocrinology of the Breast: Basic and Clinical Aspects. Acad Sci, New York, pp. 126-137.
7. Tekmal RR, Ramachandra N, Gubba S et al (1996) Overexpression of int-5/ aromatase in mammary glands of transgenic mice results in the induction of hyperplasia and nuclear abnormalities. Cancer Res 56:3180-3185.
8. Keshava N, Fang G, Bhalla KN et al (1998) Int-5/aromatase overexpression in involuting mammary glands of the transgenic mice leads to change in the regulation of genes involved in cell cycle and programmed cell death. Oncogene (in press).
9. Cavalieri EL, Stack DE, Devanesan PD et al (1997) Molecular origin of cancer: catechol estrogen-3,4-quinones as endogenous tumor initiators. Proc Natl Acad Sci USA 94:10937-42.
10. Keshava N, Kirma N, Tekmal RR (1998) Acceleration of mammary neoplasia in int-5/aromatase transgenic mice by 7,12-dimethylbenzanthracene. Environ Mol Mutagenesis (in press).

Genetic Toxicity In Vitro of Bisphenol A-Diglycidylether (BADGE) and its Hydrolysis Products

Erika Pfeiffer and Manfred Metzler

Summary

The detection of bisphenol A-diglycidylether (BADGE) in food from cans with interior lacquer-coatings has raised questions concerning the genotoxicity of BADGE and its putative metabolites. In this study, we report that BADGE is very stable in the absence of metabolizing enzymes (S9-mix) but is rapidly hydrolyzed to a diglycol (BADGE*2H$_2$O) by S9-mix. BADGE, but not BADGE*2H$_2$O, induced micronuclei and gene mutations at the HPRT locus in cultured Chinese hamster V79 cells. The induced micronuclei consisted of acentric chromosomal fragments and did not contain whole chromosomes/chromatids, as was shown by staining with CREST antikinetochore antibodies. This is in contrast to bisphenol-A, which induced exclusively micronuclei with whole chromosomes/chromatids in V79 cells. We conclude that BADGE exhibits clastogenic and mutagenic potential, which is lost after hydrolysis of the epoxide rings and converted to aneuploidogenic potential after cleavage to bisphenol-A.

Introduction

Bisphenol A-diglycidylether (BADGE, Figure 1) is released from epoxy resins and organosoles, which are used for the interior lacquer-coating of food cans (1). Metabolic transformations of BADGE may comprise (i) hydrolysis of the epoxide rings leading to a diglycol (BADGE*2H$_2$O, Figure 1) and (ii) cleavage of the ether bonds leading to bisphenol A (BP-A, Figure 1) (2). We have recently reported that BP-A induces metaphase arrest and micronuclei with whole chromosomes in cultured Chinese hamster V79 cells, indicative of an aneuploidogenic potential (3). The health implications of BADGE and its putative hydrolysis products are yet unclear. We have therefore studied the induction of micronuclei and gene mutations in V79 cells by BADGE with and without metabolizing system (S9 mix).

$H_2C-HC-H_2C-O-O-\langle\rangle-C(CH_3)(CH_3)-\langle\rangle-O-CH_2-CH-CH_2$

BADGE

$H_2C-HC-H_2C-O-O-\langle\rangle-C(CH_3)(CH_3)-\langle\rangle-O-CH_2-CH-CH_2$ (OH OH ... OH OH)

BADGE*2H₂O

$HO-\langle\rangle-C(CH_3)(CH_3)-\langle\rangle-OH$

BP-A

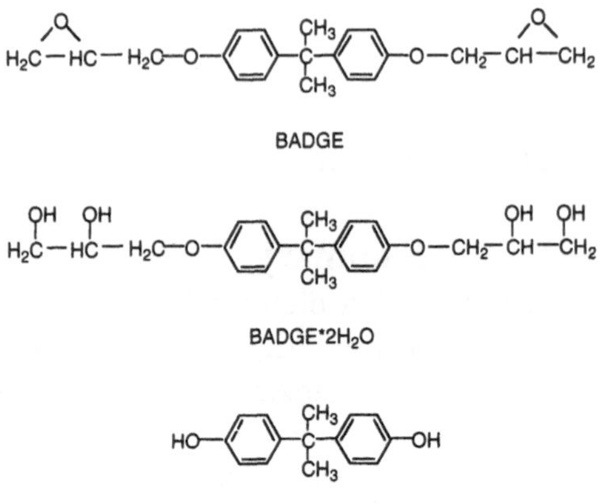

Figure 1. Chemical structures of BADGE, BADGE*2H$_2$O, and BP-A.

Materials and Methods

Chemicals. BADGE (purity > 98% according to HPLC and GC/MS) was purchased from Sigma Chemical Co. (DER resin 332). BADGE*2 H$_2$O (purity >98% according to HPLC and GC/MS) was synthesized by refluxing BADGE for 3 h with 10% aqueous acetic acid containing 15% dioxane, followed by extraction with ethylacetate and recrystallization from ethylacetate/heptane.

Preparation of Metabolizing System. The 9,000 g supernatant (S9 fraction) was prepared from liver homogenates of aroclor-treated male rats and stored in 150 mM aqueous KCl solution (25% w/v) at -80¡C. The metabolizing system (S9 mix) prepared in 100 mM phosphate buffer pH 7.4 or culture medium contained 5 mM glucose-6-phosphate, 4 mM NADP$^+$ and 0.1 ml S9 fraction/ml and was stored on ice until used.

Micronucleus Assay with CREST Staining. V79 cells were plated onto sterile glass slides in small Petri dishes. Each dish received about 8 x 10^5 cells in 5 ml Dulbecco's modified Eagle's medium (DMEM) supplemented with 10% fetal calf serum (FCS). 24 h after seeding, the medium was replaced and various concentrations of the test compounds were added in DMSO (final concentration 1% v/v). 0.1 ml of S9 mix were added per ml medium in those assays performed in the presence of metabolizing system. 3 or 6 h later, the cells were rinsed with phosphate-buffered saline (PBS) and kept in fresh medium for 0, 3, 6, 12, 18 and 24 h prior to fixation in methanol at -20°C for at least 1 h. Slides were then immersed for 10 min in acetone at-20°C, soaked in PBS, covered with CREST serum for 1 h at 37°C, rinsed with PBS, incubated with FITC-labelled anti-human IgG for 45 min at 37°C, rinsed again with PBS and stored at 4°C for 24 h in Soerensen buffer pH 8.0. Slides were randomly coded and scored after treatment with antifade solution containing DAPI and propidium iodide.

HPRT Mutation Assay. 10^6 V79 cells in log phase were seeded in 75-cm^2 dishes, grown for 24 h, and then incubated with the test compounds for 3 h in FCS-free DMEM in the presence and absence of S9 mix. After treatment, cells were washed and trypsinized. Cytotoxicity was determined as the decrease in plating efficiency by plating 500 cells in 10-cm dishes with 10 ml DMEM (5% FCS). 7 days later the colonies were fixed, stained and counted. Plating efficiency was calculated as the ratio of colonies over the number of seeded cells per 10-cm dish.. For phenotypic expression, the remaining cells were reseeded into new flasks at about 1 x 10^6 cells per 250-ml flask in DMEM (5% FCS). After an expression period of 6 days with two subcultures, cells were replated at a density of 10^6 in 10-cm Petri dishes in medium containing 7 µg/ml 6-thioguanine for the selection of mutants (3 replicate plates). The plates were fixed and stained, and the colonies were counted after 10 days.

Results and Discussion

BADGE was very stable in cell culture medium at pH 7.5 and 37°C, after 24 h, only unchanged BADGE was present in an ethylacetate extract analyzed by HPLC. However, a few min after adding S9 mix, BADGE had disappeared and the only product found in the extract was BADGE*2H$_2$O. When FCS was present in the culture medium in the absence of S9 mix, 80% of BADGE was covalently bound to serum proteins after 3 h incubation; in contrast, more than 90% of BADGE was extractable as BADGE*2H$_2$O when S9 mix was present.

BADGE induced micronuclei (MN) in V79 cells: after treatment with 50 µM BADGE for 6 h, the cells were kept in fresh medium for 3, 6, 12, 18, and 24 h. The number of BADGE-induced MN was 18 per 2000 cells at 3 and 6 h post-treatment and thereafter increased steadily to a maximum of 140 MN per 2000 cells at 24 h; about the same time course and yield of MN was obtained with 0.5 µM 4-nitroquinoline-N-oxide (NQO), an established clastogen used as a reference compound in our study.

In order to elucidate the effect of the metabolizing system on the activity of BADGE to induce MN, V79 cells were treated with various concentrations of BADGE in the presence and absence of S9 mix for 6 h, followed by a post-treatment period, in fresh medium, of 24 h which is the maximum of MN induction. The MN were characterized with CREST antikinetochore antibodies to distinguish MN containing acentric chromosomal fragments (generated by clastogenic agents) from MN containing whole chromosomes/chromatids (generated by aneuploidogenic agents). BADGE without S9 mix gave rise to a significant induction of CREST negative, but not CREST positive, MN in a concentration-dependent manner, whereas BADGE in the presence of S9 mix did not induce any MN (Figure 2).

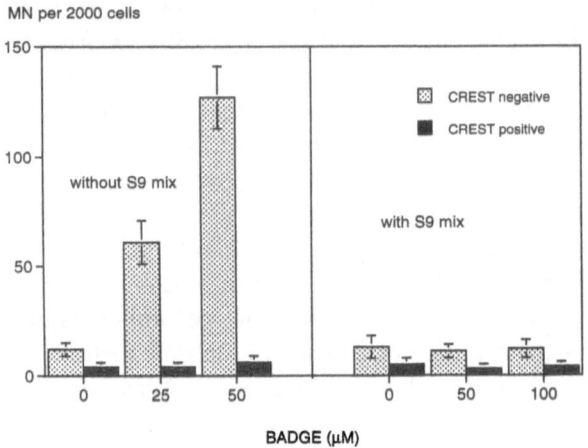

Figure 2. Induction of MN by BADGE with and without S9 mix, and characterization of the MN with CREST antikinetochore antibodies. Treatment time was 6 h, followed by a post-treatment period of 24 h in fresh medium.

Because BADGE was found to covalently bind to serum proteins (see above), the effect of fetal calf serum (FCS) on the induction of MN was studied. The cell culture medium used for 6 h incubations is supplemented with 10% FCS to ensure the viability of the V79 cells. In the absence of FCS, only incubation periods of 3 h are tolerated by the cells. We have therefore compared the activity of BADGE to induce MN in V79 cells after 3 h incubation in the presence and absence of FCS. No difference in the yield of MN was found between 3 and 6 h of treatment in the presence of FCS in the culture medium. In the absence of FCS, BADGE induced the same rate of MN at a tenfold lower concentration and became cytotoxic at 10 μM. This finding is in agreement with the assumption that most of the BADGE is trapped by FCS.

In order to rule out the formation of CREST positive MN by the hydrolysis product of BADGE, a post-treatment time of 3 to 6 h is required where the induction of CREST positive MN is at its maximum. But after exposure in the presence of S9 mix, cells displayed changes in cell morphology and growth inhibition for up to 10 h after treatment. Therefore, we have synthesized BADGE*2H$_2$O and tested it at high concentrations and under the same conditions as BP-A. BP-A induced CREST positive MN, whereas no induction of MN was observed with synthetic BADGE*2H$_2$O even at 200 μM (Figure 3). Synthetic BADGE*2H$_2$O was also tested at 200 μM concentration for CREST negative MN with a post-incubation time of 24 h and found to be inactive.

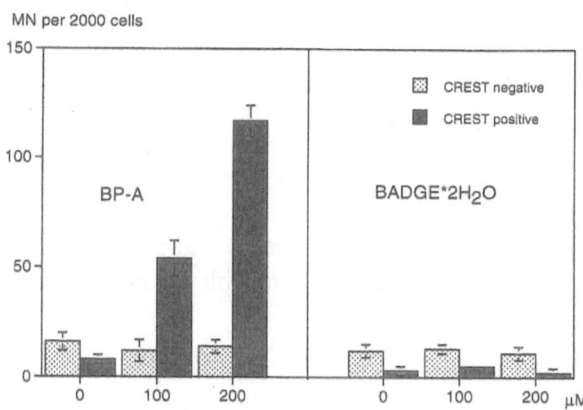

Figure 3. Induction of MN in V79 cells by BP-A and BADGE*2H$_2$O, and characterization with CREST antikinetochore antibodies. Treatment time was 3 h and post-incubation time 3 h.

Finally, the ability of BADGE and its hydrolysis product to induce gene mutations at the hypoxanthine guanine phosphoribosyltransferase (HPRT) gene locus was assayed. The data obtained for the plating efficiencies and mutation frequencies with various concentrations of BADGE (with and without S9 mix) in FCS-free medium for 3 h are depicted in Figure 4. In the absence of S9 mix, the plating efficiency was still high with 10 μM BADGE but decreased in a concentration-dependent manner to 4 - 36% with 20 μM BADGE. The number of thioguanine-resistant mutants was elevated over controls with 10 and 15 μM BADGE, although with a large variation; a significant increase of mutants was only obtained at the cytotoxic concentration of 20 μM BADGE. In the presence of S9 mix, 100 μM BADGE was neither cytotoxic nor mutagenic.

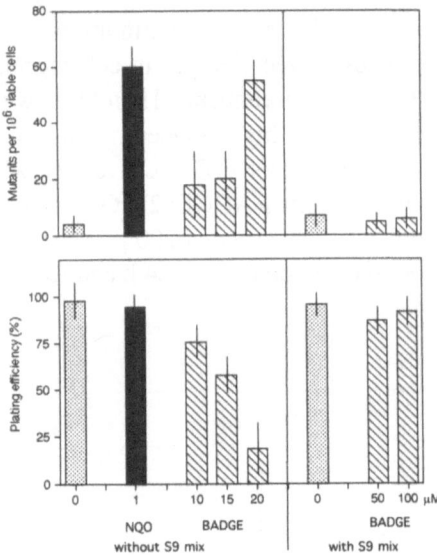

Figure 4. Effect of BADGE in the absence and presence of S9 mix on the mutation frequencies at the HPRT locus and plating efficiencies of V79 cells.

Conclusions

The present study provides evidence that BADGE acts as a clastogen and gene mutagen in cultured V79 cells and is very resistant to chemical hydrolysis, but is rapidly inactivated by enzymatic epoxide hydrolysis to a non-genotoxic metabolite.

Acknowledgment

This study was supported by the Deutsche Forschungsgemeinschaft (Grant 574/9-2).

References

1. Biedermann M, Bronz M, Grob K et al (1997) BADGE and its accompanying compounds in canned oily foods: Further results. Mitt Gebiete Lebensm Hyg 88:277-292.
2. Steiner S, Honger G, Sagelsdorff P (1992) Molecular dosimetry of DNA adducts in CH3 mice treated with bisphenol A diglycidylether. Carcinogenesis 13:969-972.
3. Pfeiffer E, Rosenberg B, Deuschel S et al (1997) Interference with microtubules and induction of micronuclei in vitro by various bisphenols. Mutat Res 390:21-31.

Lack of Genotoxicity of Major Mammalian and Plant Lignans at Various Endpoints In Vitro

Sabine E. Kulling, Eric Jacobs, and Manfred Metzler

Summary

We have investigated the genotoxic potential of the four lignans enterolactone, enterodiol, matairesinol and secoisolariciresinol by measuring their effects on cell-free microtubule assembly and at the following endpoints in cultured male Chinese hamster V79 cells: disruption of the cytoplasmic microtubule complex, induction of mitotic arrest and micronuclei, and mutations at the HPRT gene locus. The aneuploidogen diethylstilbestrol and the clastogen 4-nitroquinoline-N-oxide were used as positive reference compounds. None of the four lignans was active at any of the endpoints studied, implying that they are devoid of genetic toxicity.

Introduction

The mammalian lignans enterolactone (ENL, Figure 1) and enterodiol (END) are formed by intestinal bacteria from the plant lignans matairesinol (MAT) and secoisolariciresinol (SEC), respectively, which are ingested with cereals, vegetables, fruits and other types of plant-derived food (1, 2).

ENL and END are weak estrogens. According to epidemiological and biological studies, lignans may act as anticarcinogens (1, 3), but little is known about their genotoxic potential. We have therefore investigated the effects of ENL, END, MAT and SEC on cell-free microtubule assembly and at the following endpoints in cultured male Chinese hamster V79 cells: disruption of the cytoplasmic microtubule complex, induction of mitotic arrest, induction of micronuclei and their characterization by staining with CREST antikinetochore antibodies, and mutations at the HPRT gene locus.

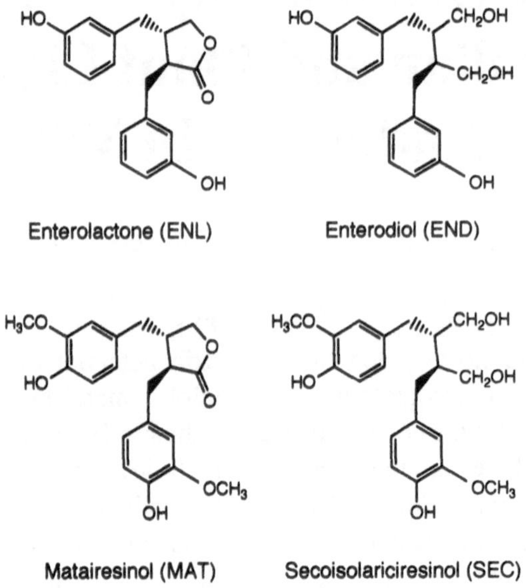

Figure 1. Chemical structures of ENL, END, MAT and SEC.

Materials and Methods

(±)-ENL and (±)-END were synthesized in our laboratory according to the method of Pelter *et al.* (4). (-)-MAT and (±)-SEC were kindly provided by Dr. Kaspar (University of Berlin) and Dr. Schšttner (University of Bayreuth), respectively. The purity of all compounds was >99% according to GC/MS analysis of the trimethylsilylated derivatives. All other chemicals were obtained from Sigma, Fluka or Serva and were of the highest purity available.

Microtubule (MT) proteins were prepared and the MT polymerization assay performed as recently reported (5). Male Chinese hamster V79 cells were cultured as described (5, 6). The sulforhodamine B (SRB) assay, the trypan blue assay, the staining of tubulin in the cytoplasmic microtubule complex (CMTC) and mitotic spindle, the micronucleus assay and CREST staining, and the HPRT mutation assay wera also carried out as reported earlier (5, 6).

Results

The four lignans ENL, END, MAT and SEC were tested at concentrations of 200 μM in the cell-free system and 100 μM in cultured V79 cells, which represents the limit of solubility in each assay. The established aneuploidogen diethylstilbestrol (DES) and the clastogen 4-nitroquinoline-N-oxide (NQO) were used as positive reference compounds.

When the effect on cell-free microtubule (MT) assembly was studied, none of the four lignans affected MT formation, in contrast to DES, which caused a 50% inhibition at 40 µM concentration (data not shown). Likewise, the lignans did not affect the cytoplasmic microtubule complex (CMTC) or mitotic spindles in cultured V79 cells, whereas 20 µM DES led to an almost complete loss of the CMTC and seriously damaged spindles (data not shown).

Studies were then conducted on the growth inhibitory and cytotoxic effects of the ligans on V79 cells in order to find suitable concentrations for the genotoxicity tests. The sulforhodamine B (SRB) test and the trypan blue assay were used to assay growth inhibition and cytotoxicity. ENL, END and SEC at 100 µM concentration for 48 h exhibited a 40%, 18% and 52% inhibition of cell growth, respectively, in the SRB assay without causing an increase in dead cells over that in untreated controls (<1%) in the trypan blue test. 100 µM MAT also was not cytotoxic at all but inhibited cell growth by 80%. In contrast, 20 µM DES caused a 80% reduction in cell growth accompanied by a marked elevation of dead cells (>20%). Likewise, 1 µM NQO gave rise to an almost complete inhibition of cell growth and 36% dead cells.

As 100 µM concentrations of the lignans were tolerated by the V79 cells for 48 h without any signs of cytotoxicity, this concentration was used in the assays for mitotic arrest, induction of MN and induction of HPRT mutations. When the number of metaphase and anaphase cells per 1000 cells was determined after 6 h exposure to the four lignans at 50 and 100 µM, no increase over that in untreated control cells was observed (data not shown). In contrast, 10 µM DES caused a 10-fold elevation of metaphase cell number.

For assaying the induction of micronuclei, V79 were incubated with the test compounds for 6 h and then kept in fresh medium for various lenghts of time ranging from 3 to 24 h. Subsequently, cells were stained with DAPI and propidium iodide to detect micronuclei (MN), and with CREST antikinetochore antibodies to distinguish between MN containing whole chromosomes/chromatids (CREST-positive) and chromosomal fragments (CREST-negative). As shown in Figure 2, none of the four lignans at 100 µM was able to induce MN of either type, whereas 20 µM DES clearly induced CREST-positive MN (with a maximum at 6 h post-treatment time) and 0.5 µM NQO led to an marked in crease of CREST-negative MN (with a maximum at 24 h).

MN per 2000 cells

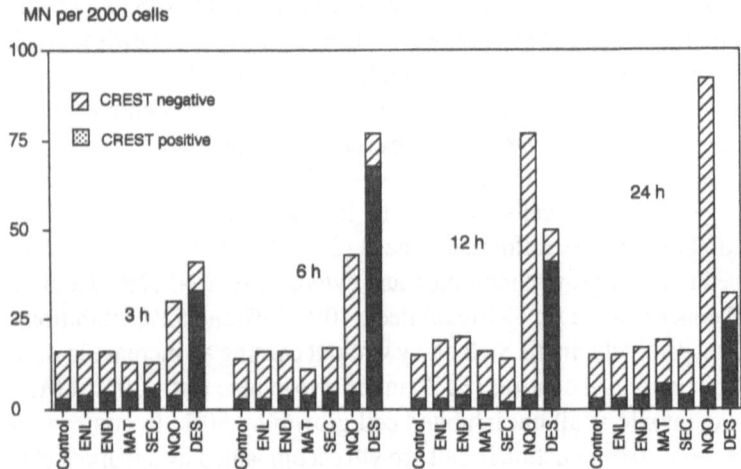

Figure 2. Induction of micronuclei (MN) in V79 cells by the four lignans (at 100 µM), NQO (at 0.5 µM) and DES (20 µM). Mean of two independent experiments.

The four lignans were also negative when assayed for the induction of HPRT mutations, as measured by the number of mutants resistant against 6-thioguanine (6-TG, Figure 3). As expected, the reference mutagen NQO caused a significant increase of 6-TG-resistant cells even at 1 µM concentration.

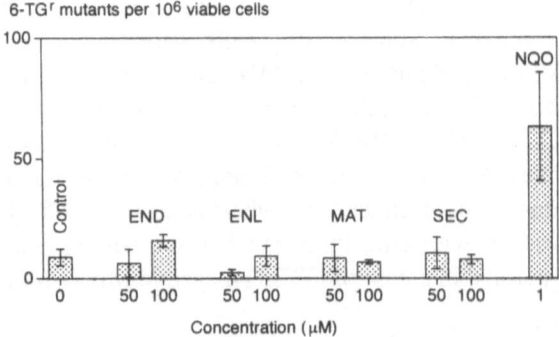

Figure 3. Mutation frequencies at the HPRT locus of V79 cells after treatment with various lignans and with NQO. Data are the mean ± S.D. of three independent experiments. Exposure time was 6 h and plating efficiencies of the treated cells were >80% for all compounds.

Conclusion

The results, summarized in Table 1, indicate that the mammalian lignans ENL and END and their metabolic precursors MAT and SEC are devoid of genotoxicity at the *in vitro* endpoints and under the experimental conditions used in this study. In this respect, lignans differ from two other important classes of phytoestrogens, i.e. isoflavones and coumestans, because genistein and coumestrol have recently been shown to act as clastogens and to induce DNA strands breaks, micronuclei with acentric fragments and HPRT mutations in cultured V79 cells (6).

Table 1. Comparison of the effects of the mammalian lignans ENL and END, the plant lignans MAT and SEC, and the reference compounds DES and NQO at various endpoints for genotoxicity.

Compound	ENL	END	MAT	SEC	DES	NQO
Inhibition of MT Assembly	-	-	-	-	+	n.t.[a]
Induction of Mitotic Arrest	-	-	-	-	+	n.t.
Disruption of CMTC	-	-	-	-	+	n.t.
Induction of Micronuclei						
CREST-Positive	-	-	-	-	+	-
CREST-Negative	-	-	-	-	-	+
Induction of HPRT Mutations	-	-	-	-	-	+

[a]n.t, not tested

The lack of genotoxic potential of lignans is comforting in view of the widespread exposure to these important food constituents. However, we have recently observed that both ENL and END are oxidatively metabolized to several products carrying an additional hydroxy group in the para- and ortho-positions of the existing phenolic groups (7). Such metabolites were found in human hepatic microsomes incubated with ENL or END *in vitro*, and also in the urine of female and male adults ingesting flaxseed as a source of plant lignans. These metabolites are presently studied for genotoxic potential in our laboratory.

Acknowledgments

We are grateful to Mrs. Sybille Mayer and Cornelia Hodapp for their help with parts of this work, and to the Deutsche Forschungsgemeinschaft for financial support (Grant Me 574/9-2).

References

1. Setchell KDR (1988) Mammalian lignans and phyto-oestrogens - recent studies on their formation, metabolism and biological role in health and disease. In: Rowland IR (ed) Role of the Gut Flora in Toxicity and Cancer. Academic Press, London, pp. 315-345.
2. Thompson LU, Robb P, Serraino M et al (1991) Mammalian lignan production from various foods. Nutr Cancer 16:43-52.
3. Adlercreutz (1995) Phytoestrogens: epidemiology and a possible role in cancer protection. Environ Health Perspect 103:103-112.
4. Pelter A, Ward RS, Satyanarayana P (1983) Synthesis of lignan lactones by conjugate addition of thioacetal carbanions to butenolide. J Chem Soc Perkin Trans I 643-647.
5. Pfeiffer E, Rosenberg B, Deuschel S et al (1997) Interference with microtubules and induction of micronuclei in vitro by various bisphenols. Mutat Res 390:21-31.
6. Kulling SE, Metzler M (1997) Induction of micronuclei, DNA strand breaks and HPRT mutations in cultured chinese hamster V79 cells by the phytoestrogen coumoestrol. Food Chem Toxicol 35:605-613.
7. Jacobs E, Metzler M (1998) In vitro- and in vivo-metabolism of the mammalian lignans enterolactone and enterodiol. Naunyn-Schmiedeberg's Arch Pharmacol 357 Suppl: R138.

Index

A

Acetylation, and chromosome structure, 9-10

Acetylcholine, effects on vasodilatation, 378

α-Actin, expression in normal prostate and tumors, 325

Actinomycin D (ACT D), blocking of vascular endothelial growth factor formation by, 241

Adenocarcinomas
  human mammary, centrosome aberrations in, 194
  human prostatic, stroma of, 324-325

Adenomatous polyposis coli gene (APC), as gatekeeper for colon cancer, 320-321

Adenylate cyclase, stimulation by estrogen in breast cancer cells, 271

Adhesion system
  effect of ovarian hormones on, 204
  expression of adhesion molecules by injured endothelial cells, 378

Adipocyte differentiation, of 2T3 osteoblasts, induction by PPARγ ligand, 353

Adipose tissue, as a postmenopausal source of estrogens, 514-515

Adrenal androgens, activation of androgen receptors of prostate tumors by, 336

African-Americans, study of breast cancer in, 47

Age

and hepatocellular carcinoma development, 491

and intrahepatic tumorigenicity, 492

and ovarian cancer, 311-313

and plasma concentration of IL-6, 278-279

and prostate cancer, 88

Alzheimer's disease, effect of estrogens on development of, 144

Amphiregulin, effect of P_4 on mRNA for, in the uterine epithelium, 202

Amphophilic cell foci (APF), induction by dehydroepiandrosterone, 479

Amphophilic cell lineages, in hepatocarcinogenesis in the rat, 478

Amplification
  chromosomal, in prostate cancer, 104
  gene, survey in prostate cancer progression, 108-110

Androgen-dependent cells, progression to androgen-independent cells, 301-306

Androgen-independent cell line, androgen receptor expression in, 333-334

Androgen insensitivity (AIS), inherited form of, mutations in, 339

Androgen receptor (AR)
  binding of dihydrotestosterone to, 88
  gene for
    amplification in prostate cancer, 104
    and androgen-independent prostate cancer, 301-306
  of hepatocytes, 490
  role in suppression of prostate tumors, 304